Pediatrics Morning Report: Beyond the Pearls

Series Editors

RAJ DASGUPTA, MD, FACP, FCCP, FAASM

Assistant Professor of Clinical Medicine
Division of Pulmonary/Critical Care/Sleep Medicine
Associate Program Director of the Sleep Medicine Fellowship
Assistant Program Director of the Internal Medicine Residency
Keck School of Medicine of the University of Southern California
Los Angeles, California

R. MICHELLE KOOLAEE, DO

Rheumatologist, Healthcare Partners Medical Group
Assistant Professor of Medicine
Division of Rheumatology
University of Southern California
Los Angeles, California

Volume Editors

ADLER SALAZAR, MD

Assistant Professor of Clinical Pediatrics
Director of Pediatric Residency Program
Pediatric Critical Care Medicine
Los Angeles County and the University of Southern California
Keck School of Medicine of the University of Southern California
Los Angeles, California

RANDALL Y. CHAN, MD

Medical Director, Pediatric Hematology-Oncology
Los Angeles County and the University of Southern California Medical Center;
Assistant Professor of Clinical Pediatrics
Keck School of Medicine of the University of Southern California
Los Angeles, California

MICHELLE PIETZAK, MD

Assistant Professor of Clinical Pediatrics
Department of Pediatric Gastroenterology
Keck School of Medicine of the University of Southern California;
Attending
Department of Pediatric Gastroenterology
Children's Hospital of Los Angeles and the Los Angeles County Hospital
Los Angeles, California

ELSEVIER

ELSEVIER

1600 John F. Kennedy Blvd.
Ste 1800
Philadelphia, PA 19103-2899

Executive Content Strategist: James Merritt
Senior Content Development Manager: Katie DeFrancesco
Content Development Specialist: Meghan Andress
Publishing Services Manager: Julie Eddy
Book Production Specialist: Carol O'Connell
Design Direction: Bridget Hoette

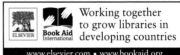

Pediatrics Morning Report:
Beyond the Pearls

We would like to dedicate this book to our two beautiful children, Mina and Aiden Dasgupta. They are very precious to us and we love them dearly. They continue to impress us every day and bring so much joy and happiness to our lives. – RD and RMK

I dedicate this book to Michelle, Anthony, and Aidan. My heartfelt gratitude goes out to my colleagues, residents, and faculty alike, who contributed to this book. –AS

To my amazing wife, Jenny, for her endless patience, wisdom, insight, and support without which my contribution would not have been possible. –RYC

To my loving, dedicated husband, and bright, beautiful daughter, who support me in all things; and to all of my teachers from college, medical school, residency, and USC who stimulate the search for knowledge and inspire to serve the underserved. – MP

Ananta Addala, DO, MPH
Fellow Physician, Pediatric Endocrinology,
Stanford University Medical Center,
Stanford, California

Audrey Ahn, DO
Attending Physician, Pediatrics, Los Angeles
County and University of Southern
California Medical Center, Los Angeles,
California

Monika Alas-Segura, MD
Associate Program Director, Pediatrics
Residency, Los Angeles County and the
University of Southern California Medical
Center; Assistant Professor of Clinical
Pediatrics, Keck School of Medicine of
the University of Southern California,
Los Angeles, California

Sunniya Basravi, DO
Chief Resident Physician, Department of
Pediatrics, Los Angeles County and the
University of Southern California Medical
Center, Los Angeles, California

Solomon Behar, MD
Attending Physician, Pediatric Emergency
Department, Long Beach Memorial/
Miler Children's Hospital and Children's
Hospital Los Angeles, Los Angeles,
California; Voluntary Faculty, Department
of Pediatrics, University of California
Irvine, Irvine, California

Vrinda Bhardwaj, MD
Assistant Professor of Pediatrics, Division
of Gastroenterology, Keck School of
Medicine of the University of Southern
California; Hepatology and Nutrition,
Children's Hospital Los Angeles, Los
Angeles, California

Russell K. Brynes, MD
Professor of Clinical Pathology, Department
of Pathology, Section of Hematopathology,
Keck School of Medicine of the University of
Southern California, Los Angeles, California

Rowena G. Cayabyab, MD, MPH
Assistant Professor of Clinical Pediatrics,
Keck School of Medicine of the University
of Southern California, Los Angeles,
California

Randall Y. Chan, MD
Medical Director, Pediatric Hematology-
Oncology, Los Angeles County and the
University of Southern California Medical
Center; Assistant Professor of Clinical
Pediatrics, Keck School of Medicine of
the University of Southern California,
Los Angeles, California

June Chapin, DO
Chief Resident Physician, Pediatrics, Los
Angeles County and the University of
Southern California Medical Center,
Los Angeles, California

Purva Chhibar, MD
Rheumatology Fellow, University of Southern
California, Los Angeles, California

Stratos Christianakis, MD
Assistant Professor of Medicine, Division of
Rheumatology, Keck School of Medicine
of the University of Southern California,
Los Angeles, California; Program Director,
Internal Medicine Residency, Huntington
Memorial Hospital, Pasadena, California

Mikhaela Cielo, MD
Assistant Professor of Clinical Pediatrics,
Keck School of Medicine of the University
of Southern California, Los Angeles,
California

Raj Dasgupta, MD, FACP, FCCP, FAASM
Assistant Professor of Clinical Medicine,
Division of Pulmonary/Critical Care/Sleep
Medicine, Associate Program Director of
the Sleep Medicine Fellowship, Assistant
Program Director of the Internal Medicine
Residency, Keck School of Medicine of
the University of Southern California,
Los Angeles, California

Catherine DeRidder, MD
Associate Program Director, Violence
 Intervention Program, Los Angeles County
 and the University of Southern California
 Medical Center, Los Angeles, California

Aileen Dickinson, DO, MPH
Resident Physician, Pediatrics, Los Angeles
 County and the University of Southern
 California Medical Center, Los Angeles,
 California

Vidhi Doshi, MD
Chief Resident Physician, Combined Internal
 Medicine-Pediatrics, Los Angeles County
 and the University of Southern California
 Medical Center, Los Angeles, California

Kelly Fan, MD
Fellow, Pulmonary and Critical Care
 Medicine, Los Angeles County and the
 University of Southern California Medical
 Center, Los Angeles, California

Franklyn Fenton, MD
Resident, Department of Internal Medicine
 and Medicine Pediatrics, Los Angeles
 County and the University of Southern
 California Medical Center, Los Angeles,
 California

Richard Fine, MD
Professor of Pediatrics, Stony Brook University
 School of Medicine, Stony Brook, New
 York; Professor of Pediatrics, Keck School
 of Medicine of the University of Southern
 California, Los Angeles, California

Rebecca Graves, DO
Resident Physician, Department of Pediatrics,
 University of Southern California, Los
 Angeles, California

Justin Greenberg, DO
Chief Resident Physician, Department of
 Pediatrics, Los Angeles County and the
 University of Southern California Medical
 Center, Los Angeles, California

Melissa Harada, MD
Fellow, Developmental and Behavioral
 Pediatrics, Mattel Children's Hospital of
 the University of California at Los Angeles,
 Los Angeles, California

John Harlow, MD
Resident Physician, Pediatrics, Los Angeles
 County and the University of Southern
 California Medical Center, Los Angeles,
 California

Asma Hasan, MD
Fellow, Endocrinology, Los Angeles County
 and University of Southern California
 Medical Center, Los Angeles, California

Cynthia Hayek, MD
Neonatology, Los Angeles County and
 University of Southern California Medical
 Center, Los Angeles, California

Alauna K. Hersch, DO
Fellow, Division of Gastroenterology,
 Hepatology, and Nutrition, Children's
 Hospital Los Angeles, Los Angeles,
 California

Cynthia H. Ho, MD
Hospitalist, Department of Internal Medicine,
 Southern California Permanente Medical
 Group, Kaiser Permanente Los Angeles
 Medical Center, Los Angeles, California

Thomas C. Hofstra, MD
Assistant Professor of Clinical Pediatrics,
 Keck School of Medicine of the University
 of Southern California, Los Angeles,
 California

James Homans, MD, MPH
Associate Professor of Clinical Pediatrics,
 Division of Infectious Disease, Department
 of Pediatrics, Los Angeles County and
 the University of Southern of California
 Medical Center, Keck School of Medicine
 of the University of Southern California,
 Los Angeles, California

Alyssa Huang, MD
Pediatric Endocrinology Fellow, Division of
 Endocrinology, University of California,
 San Francisco, San Francisco, California

Mohammad Jami, MD
Pediatric Gastroenterologist, Lucille Packard
 Children's Hospital Stanford, Los Gatos,
 California

Jeffrey Johnson, MD
Associate Chief of Pediatrics, Los Angeles
    County and the University of Southern
    California Medical Center; Clinical
    Assistant Professor of Pediatrics, Keck
    School of Medicine of the University
    of Southern California, Los Angeles,
    California

Mayra Jones-Betancourt, MD
Resident Physician, Pediatrics, Los Angeles
    County and the University of Southern
    California Medical Center, Los Angeles,
    California

Christine Kassissa-Mourad, DO
Chief Resident, Department of Pediatrics,
    Los Angeles County and the University of
    Southern California Medical Center, Los
    Angeles, California

David T. Kent, MD
Assistant Professor, Otolaryngology,
    Vanderbilt University Medical Center,
    Nashville, Tennessee

Aslam Khan, DO
Resident Physician, Pediatrics, Los Angeles
    County and the University of Southern
    California Medical Center, Los Angeles,
    California

R. Michelle Koolaee, DO
Rheumatologist, Healthcare Partners Medical
    Group, Assistant Professor of Medicine,
    Division of Rheumatology, University
    of Southern California, Los Angeles,
    California

Robyn Kuroki, MD
Pediatric Hospitalist, Complex Care Team,
    Department of Hospital Medicine,
    Children's Hospital of Los Angeles,
    Assistant Professor of Clinical Medicine,
    Department of Pediatrics, University
    of Southern California, Los Angeles,
    California

Arathi Lakhole, MD, MPH
Associate Pediatric Gastroenterologist,
    Department of Pediatric Gastroenterology,
    Hepatology, and Nutrition, UCSF Benioff
    Children's Hospital at Oakland, Oakland,
    California

Keith Lewis, MD
Assistant Professor of Pediatrics, Department
    of Pediatrics, Los Angeles County and the
    University of Southern California Medical
    Center, Keck School of Medicine of the
    University of Southern California, Los
    Angeles, California

Spencer Liebman, MD
Resident Physician, Combined Internal
    Medicine-Pediatrics, Los Angeles County
    and the University of Southern California
    Medical Center, Los Angeles, California

Quin Y. Liu, MD
Assistant Professor of Clinical Medicine
    and Pediatrics, David Geffen School of
    Medicine at UCLA, Digestive Disease
    Center, Cedars-Sinai Medical Center, Los
    Angeles, California

Patricia Lorenzo, MD
Division of Endocrinology, Diabetes, and
    Metabolism, University of Southern
    California, Los Angeles, California

Neha Mahajan, MD
Doctor, Department of Internal Medicine and
    Pediatrics, Los Angeles County and the
    University of Southern California Medical
    Center, Los Angeles, California

Julio Martinez, MD
Resident Physician, Department of Pediatrics,
    Los Angeles County and University of
    Southern California Medical Center, Los
    Angeles, California

Joseph Meouchy, MD
Nephrology and Hypertension, Keck School
    of Medicine of the University of Southern
    California, Los Angeles, California

Rebecca Meyer, MD, MEd
Fellow, Department of Pediatrics, Division of
    Neonatology, Los Angeles County and the
    University of Southern California Medical
    Center, Keck School of Medicine of the
    University of Southern California, Los
    Angeles, California

Brittany Middleton, MD
Clinical Instructor, Department of Pediatrics–
  Pediatric Hospital Medicine Division,
  University of California at Los Angeles
  Mattel Children's Hospital, Los Angeles,
  California

Lindsey Miller, MD
Clinical Assistant Professor of Pediatrics, Keck
  School of Medicine of the University of
  Southern California, Los Angeles, California

Aaron Mochizuki, DO
Fellow Physician, Pediatrics, University of
  California, Los Angeles, Los Angeles,
  California

Steven M. Naids, MD
Ophthalmology, Icahn School of Medicine at
  Mount Sinai, New York, New York

Amrita Narang, MD
Fellow, Division of Gastroenterology,
  Hepatology, and Nutrition, Children's
  Hospital Los Angeles, Los Angeles,
  California

Caroline T. Nguyen, MD
Assistant Professor of Clinical Medicine,
  Division of Endocrinology, Diabetes,
  and Metabolism, University of Southern
  California, Los Angeles, California

Lawrence Opas, MD
Chief, Department of Pediatrics, Los Angeles
  County and the University of Southern
  California Medical Center; Professor
  of Clinical Pediatrics, Department of
  Pediatrics, Keck School of Medicine of
  the University of Southern California, Los
  Angeles, California

Pranay Parikh, MD
Nocturnist, Internal Medicine, Good Samaritan
  Hospital, Los Angeles, California

Arthur Partikian, MD
Director, Division of Child Neurology, Los
  Angeles County and the University of
  Southern California Medical Center;
  Clinical Associate Professor of Neurology
  and Pediatrics (Clinician Educator), Keck
  School of Medicine of the University
  of Southern California, Los Angeles,
  California

Iris A. Perez, MD
Associate Professor of Clinical Pediatrics,
  Keck School of Medicine of the University
  of Southern California; Children's Hospital
  Los Angeles, Los Angeles, California

Michelle Pietzak, MD
Assistant Professor of Clinical Pediatrics,
  Department of Pediatrics, Keck School of
  Medicine of the University of Southern
  California; Chief, Division of Pediatric
  Gastroenterology, Los Angeles County
  Hospital; Attending Gastroenterologist,
  Division of Gastroenterology, Hepatology,
  and Nutrition, Children's Hospital Los
  Angeles, Los Angeles, California

Suraiya Rahman, MD, MACM
Pediatric Hospitalist, Los Angeles County
  and the University of Southern California
  Medical Center; Assistant Professor
  of Clinical Pediatrics, Keck School of
  Medicine of the University of Southern
  California, Los Angeles, California

Swetha Ramachandran, MD
Resident Physician, Internal Medicine,
  Boston University Medical Center, Boston,
  Massachusetts

Michael Regalado, MD
Associate Professor of Clinical Pediatrics,
  Department of Pediatrics, Keck School of
  Medicine of the University of Southern
  California, Los Angeles, California

Reza Ronaghi, MD
Chief Fellow, Pulmonary and Critical Care
  Medicine, Los Angeles County and the
  University of Southern California Medical
  Center, Los Angeles, California

Ann Sahakian, MD
Pediatrician, Descanso Pediatrics, Huntington
  Health Physicians, La Cañada Flintridge,
  California

Adler Salazar, MD
Assistant Professor of Clinical Pediatrics,
  Director of Pediatric Residency Program,
  Pediatric Critical Care Medicine, Los
  Angeles County and the University of
  Southern California, Keck School of
  Medicine of the University of Southern
  California, Los Angeles, California

Nicole Samii, MD
Resident Physician, Los Angeles County
and the University of Southern California
Medical Center, Los Angeles, California

Tracey Samko, MD
Associate Program Director, Combined
Internal Medicine-Pediatrics Residency,
Attending Physician, Internal Medicine
and Pediatrics, Los Angeles County and
the University of Southern California
Medical Center, Los Angeles, California

Smeeta Sardesai, MD, MS Ed, FAAP
Associate Professor of Pediatrics, Associate
Program Director for Neonatal Perinatal
Medicine, Keck School of Medicine of
the University of Southern California, Los
Angeles, California

Paola Sequeira, MD MPH
Attending Physician, Pediatric Endocrinology,
Los Angeles County and the University of
Southern California Medical Center, Los
Angeles, California

Hui Yi Shan, MD
Assistant Professor of Clinical Medicine,
Associate Program Director of Nephrology
Fellowship, Medicine, Keck School of
Medicine of the University of Southern
California, Los Angeles, California

Priya Shastry, DO
Neonatology Fellow, Department of
Pediatrics, Los Angeles County and the
University of Southern California Medical
Center, Los Angeles, California

Jennifer Shepherd, MD
Assistant Professor of Clinical Pediatrics,
Fetal and Neonatal Institute, Division of
Neonatology, Children's Hospital Los
Angeles, Department of Pediatrics, Keck
School of Medicine of the University
of Southern California, Los Angeles,
California

Erica Z. Shoemaker, MD, MPH
Assistant Professor of Clinical Psychiatry,
Department of Psychiatry, University
of Southern California, Los Angeles,
California

Mark Sims, MD
Resident, Medicine-Pediatrics, Los Angeles
County and University of Southern
California Medical Center, Los Angeles,
California

Cynthia Stotts, DO, MS
Assistant Professor of Clinical Pediatrics,
Associate Service Chief of Pediatrics,
Department of Pediatrics, Los Angeles
County and the University of Southern
California Medical Center, Keck School
of Medicine of the University of Southern
California, Los Angeles, California

Jocelyn Supan, DO, MPH
Resident Physician, Pediatrics, Los Angeles
County and the University of Southern
California Medical Center, Los Angeles,
California

Huynh Tran, MD, DPD
Postdoctoral Clinical Fellow, Rheumatology/
Internal Medicine, University of Southern
California, Los Angles, California

Rashmi Tunuguntla, DO
Department of Pediatrics, Los Angeles
County and the University of Southern
California Medical Center, Los Angeles,
California

Merujan Uzunyan, MD
Director of Pediatric Cardiology, Department
of Pediatrics, Los Angeles County and the
University of Southern California Medical
Center, Keck School of Medicine of the
University of Southern California, Los
Angeles, California

Colette Vassilian, DO
Pediatric Resident Physician, Department of
Pediatrics, Los Angeles County and the
University of Southern California Medical
Center, Los Angeles, California

Maria Vergara-Lluri, MD
Assistant Professor of Clinical Pathology,
Department of Pathology, Section of
Hematopathology, Keck School of
Medicine of the University of Southern
California, Los Angeles, California

Patricia F. Villegas, DO
Resident Physician, Pediatrics, Los Angeles
County and the University of Southern
California Medical Center, Los Angeles,
California

Laura Wachsman, MD, MSEd
Adjunct Clinical Professor of Pediatrics, Keck
School of Medicine of the University of
Southern California, Los Angeles County
and the University of Southern California
Medical Center, Los Angeles, California

Cecilia Weaver, MD
Pediatrics Department, Los Angeles County
and the University of Southern California
Medical Center, Los Angeles, California

Marc J. Weigensberg, MD
Associate Professor of Clinical Pediatrics,
Keck School of Medicine of the University
of Southern California, Los Angeles,
California

Jenny L. Wong, DMD, MD
Adjunct Assistant Professor of Clinical
Dentistry, Division of Dental Public
Health and Pediatric Dentistry, Herman
Ostrow School of Dentistry; Adjunct
Clinical Instructor, Department of Medical
Education, Keck School of Medicine of
the University of Southern California, Los
Angeles, California

Loren Fox Yaeger, DO
Neonatology Fellow, Department of
Pediatrics, Los Angeles County and the
University of Southern California Medical
Center, Los Angeles, California

Shoji Yano, MD, PhD
Director, Genetics Division, Department of
Pediatrics, Los Angeles County and the
University of Southern California Medical
Center; Associate Professor of Clinical
Pediatrics, Keck School of Medicine of
the University of Southern California, Los
Angeles, California

Mariya Zakiuddin, MD
Pediatric Resident, Department of Pediatrics,
Los Angeles County and the University of
Southern California Medical Center, Los
Angeles, California

Anne Zepeda-Tiscareno, MD
Neonatology Fellow Physician, Department
of Pediatrics, Department of Newborn
Medicine, Los Angeles County and the
University of Southern California Medical
Center, Los Angeles, California

Stephanie K. Zia, MD, MACM, FAAP, FACP
Assistant Dean for Career Advising, Clinical
Assistant Professor of Internal Medicine
& Pediatrics, Keck School of Medicine of
the University of Southern California, Los
Angeles, California

PREFACE

It is with great pleasure once again that we present to you our third book, *Pediatric Morning Report: Beyond the Pearls,* First Edition. Writing the "perfect" review text has been a dream of mine ever since I was a first-year medical student. Dr. Koolaee and I envisioned a text that incorporates U.S. Medical Licensing Examination (USMLE) Steps 1, 2, and 3 along with up-to-date evidence-based clinical medicine. We wanted the platform of the text to be drawn from a traditional theme, such as the "morning report" format that many of us are familiar with from residency. This book is geared toward a wide audience, from medical students to attending physicians practicing general pediatrics. Each case has been carefully chosen and covers scenarios and questions frequently encountered on the pediatric boards, shelf exams, and wards integrating both basic science and clinical pearls.

We would like to sincerely thank all the many contributors who have helped to create this text. Your insightful work will be a valuable tool for medical students and physicians in order to gain an in-depth understanding of pediatrics. It should be noted that while a variety of clinical cases in pediatrics were selected for this book, it is not meant to substitute a comprehensive pediatric reference.

Dr. Koolaee and I would like to thank our volume editors, Dr. Salazar, Dr. Pietzak, and Dr. Chan, for all their hard work and dedication to this book. It was truly a pleasure to work with all of you, and we look forward to our next project together.

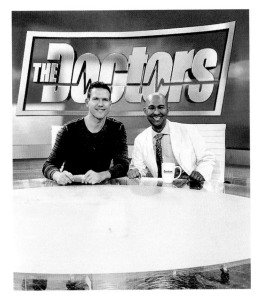

Drs. Dasgupta and Koolaee are to be congratulated for developing the new and much needed series of case-based books for in-training and practicing medical professionals, *Morning Report: Beyond the Pearls*. With pediatric volume editors, Drs. Adler Salazar, Michelle Pietzak, and Randall Chan, the team has succeeded in delivering what every Pediatrician can use: in-depth, user-friendly clinical cases with practical take-home facts. Whether for the medical student, the resident, or the clinician in practice, *Pediatrics: Morning Report* will keep us fresh, current, and sharp. After knowing "Dr. Raj" for 6 seasons on *The Doctors* television show, I am not surprised that this book is as passionate, energetic, and informative as his segments on the show. "Dr. Raj" is a pleasure to work with and embodies the core attributes of a great physician: the love for teaching, practicing, and constant learning.

Travis Stork, MD
Emmy®-nominated host of award-winning talk show *The Doctors*
#1 New York Times Bestselling author
Board-certified Emergency Medicine physician

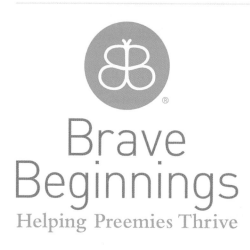

Brave
Beginnings

Helping Preemies Thrive

The Brave Beginnings program received a great deal of credibility and notoriety when Dr. Raj hosted one of our symposiums. Dr. Raj understands the challenges that NICU healthcare professionals face daily, due to the high level of premature births in the United States. We can't thank him enough for lending his support to our mission to provide NICUs with the equipment they need so every preemie has a chance to thrive.

CONTENTS

20-Month-Old With a Limp

Aaron Mochizuki ■ Maria Vergara-Lluri ■ Randall Y. Chan

A 20-month-old child presents with 8 weeks of right leg pain and limping. She otherwise has had no fever, bleeding, or other joint pain.

What is the differential diagnosis for a toddler with a limp?

A painful limp may have a number of causes. The most common are likely to be trauma-related, ranging in severity from overuse injuries to severe fractures with neurovascular compromise. Generally, trauma-related injuries will be readily diagnosed after elicitation in the history of an associated traumatic event. It is not uncommon for a toddler to present with a spiral fracture of the tibia after a minor fall or twisting of the leg, often without family members remembering any specific traumatic event. This fracture after minor injury is known as a *toddler's fracture*.

CLINICAL PEARL	STEP 2/3

A fracture presenting with compartment syndrome or neurovascular compromise is a medical emergency.

In a child with acute pain and a limp in the absence of trauma, septic arthritis and transient synovitis should be considered. Both would present with arthritis (i.e., a hot, swollen joint). The former is a medical emergency requiring antibiotics and drainage, whereas the latter is managed expectantly. The former is more likely to present with fever, leukocytosis, an elevated erythrocyte sedimentation rate, and an inability to bear weight (the Kocher criteria). More chronic pain and a limp suggest osteomyelitis. Finally, malignancy should be considered.

Case Point 1.1

Physical examination is remarkable for mild conjunctival and sublingual pallor, as well as anterior cervical and submandibular lymphadenopathy. Her right leg is not tender to palpation or passive range of motion testing, and there is no swelling or erythema.

A complete blood count is drawn due to pallor, which demonstrates a white blood cell count of 2.4×10^9/L (12% neutrophils, 84% lymphocytes, 4% monocytes), hemoglobin of 7.5 g/dL, hematocrit of 21.5%, and platelet count of 82×10^9/L.

What are causes of pancytopenia?

Pancytopenia is the combined failure of the erythroid, myeloid, and megakaryocytic cell lines. This may be due to marrow aplasia or malignant infiltration. Congenital causes of marrow aplasia include inherited bone marrow failure syndromes such as Fanconi anemia and dyskeratosis congenita. Secondary causes of marrow aplasia include viral infection (e.g., parvovirus B19, human immunodeficiency virus [HIV]); drugs (e.g., chloramphenicol, busulfan, gold, chlorpropamide); malnutrition (e.g., copper deficiency, anorexia nervosa, marasmus, kwashiorkor, even pregnancy); end-stage neoplastic myelofibrosis, in which the bone marrow becomes fibrotic and hypocellular due to mutations in *JAK2* or *MPL*, causing cytokine-independent proliferation (e.g., primary myelofibrosis, postpolycythemic myelofibrosis); paroxysmal nocturnal hemoglobinuria, caused by the clonal expansion of one or more hematopoietic stem cell lines; and aplastic anemia of an unknown cause.

In our case, however, the patient's pancytopenia, lymphadenopathy, and bone pain are concerning for malignant infiltration—in particular, acute leukemia.

BASIC SCIENCE/CLINICAL PEARL   **STEP 1/2/3**

Pancytopenia in the setting of acute leukemia occurs when leukemic blasts have infiltrated the bone marrow extensively enough to suppress normal myelopoiesis. Therefore, pancytopenia should increase the concern for malignancy. On the other hand, the absence of pancytopenia does not rule it out.

What is the next indicated procedure in this patient and why?
Given the depression in multiple hematopoietic lineages without an obvious cause, examination of the bone marrow is indicated. Acute leukemia is diagnosed when the bone marrow contains more than 20% abnormal blasts. Marrow hypocellularity would suggest aplastic anemia. Abnormal fibrosis could indicate neoplastic or nonneoplastic myelofibrosis. Granulomas may suggest an infectious cause.

BASIC SCIENCE/CLINICAL PEARL   **STEP 1/2/3**

If abnormal lymphoblasts or myeloblasts are found circulating in the peripheral blood in high enough numbers, an accurate diagnosis of acute leukemia can be made prior to marrow examination (or without marrow examination).

Case Point 1.2

A bone marrow aspiration and trephine biopsy is performed on the patient. Her bone marrow is markedly hypercellular, with sheets of small to medium-sized lymphoblasts replacing normal cells (**Fig. 1.1**).

What is the next step?
The specific type of leukemia has to be determined (e.g., acute vs. chronic, mature vs. immature precursor, B-cell vs. T-cell, lymphoid vs. myeloid, disease-defining genetic vs. molecular abnormalities). This is achieved by a multimodal diagnostic approach with integration of the results of the morphologic examination, cytochemical staining, immunophenotypic analysis of blasts by immunohistochemistry and/or flow cytometry, cytogenetic aberrations and, occasionally, molecular testing. Each specific type is treated differently (Table 1.1).

BASIC SCIENCE   **STEP 1**

The vast majority of ALL cases arise from either B- or T-cell precursors. Although morphologically identical and treated similarly, the two lineages are driven by different genetic mutations and are clinically different diseases. Precursor B-cell ALL is more common in children and also carries a more favorable prognosis.

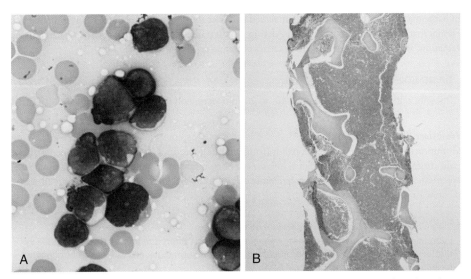

Fig. 1.1 (A) Bone marrow aspirate shows variably sized lymphoblasts. The lymphoblasts have irregular to delicately lobulated nuclear contours, finely dispersed chromatin, small nucleoli, and very scant cytoplasm without granules (Wright-Giemsa stain, 1000× magnification). (B) Bone marrow trephine biopsy demonstrates a markedly hypercellular bone marrow, with near-complete replacement of the medullary cavity by lymphoblasts. Normal hematopoietic elements are sparse to absent (H&E stain, 20× magnification).

TABLE 1.1 ■ **Treatment of Leukemia: Varies by Type**

Leukemia Type	Basic Treatment Principles
Acute lymphoblastic leukemia	Intensive therapy × 6–8 months; maintenance for 2–3 years
Mature B cell leukemia, lymphoma (i.e., Burkitt leukemia, lymphoma)	Lymphoma-style therapy (2 months induction, 2–4 months maintenance)
Acute myeloid leukemia	2–4 months of intensive chemotherapy ± bone marrow transplantation, no maintenance
Chronic myeloid leukemia	Lifelong therapy with tyrosine kinase inhibitor, transplantation only for treatment failure
Juvenile myelomonocytic leukemia	Immediate bone marrow transplantation

Case Point 1.3

Analysis of the leukemic blasts in our patient shows positivity of cell surface markers specific to abnormal precursor B cells on flow cytometric analysis.

Diagnosis: precursor B cell acute lymphoblastic leukemia.

What are the known causes of childhood acute lymphoblastic leukemia (ALL)? What is the risk to siblings?

The cause of ALL is unknown. Several genetic factors are associated with an increased risk of ALL, though inherited factors are recognized in a minority of patients. Of note, the identical twin of a child who develops leukemia in the first 5 years of life has a 20% risk of developing leukemia; siblings of leukemia patients have a four-fold increased risk over the general population. Environmental risk factors that have been associated with ALL in children include traffic pollution, benzene, ionizing radiation, and alkylating agents. These causes account for a minority of cases.

BASIC SCIENCE/CLINICAL PEARL   **STEP 1/2/3**

Patients with Down syndrome have 10- to 20-fold increased risk of leukemia.

How does ALL commonly present?

Common symptoms include fever, pallor (from anemia), bleeding (from thrombocytopenia), bone pain (from bone marrow or periosteal invasion or bone infarction), lymphadenopathy, and hepatosplenomegaly (from extramedullary leukemic cell infiltration). Each patient may exhibit all, some, or none of these symptoms.

CLINICAL PEARL   **STEP 2/3**

Lymphadenopathy seen in a primary care setting is most often due to infection, but nodes that are very large (>2.5 cm), fixed on palpation, or in a supraclavicular site are all concerning for malignancy.

CLINICAL PEARL   **STEP 2/3**

Bone pain in leukemia mimics a very common diagnosis in primary care—growing pains. Growing pains generally occur only at night with resolution by morning and in the setting of a normal physical examination. A child who is refusing to bear weight or who is limping at presentation should trigger a more thorough search for an underlying cause.

Central nervous system (CNS) involvement occurs in less than 5% of children with ALL at initial diagnosis, but they may present with headache, morning vomiting, papilledema, and/or sixth cranial nerve palsy. Testicular involvement usually manifests as painless enlargement of the testis in 10% to 20% of boys, usually in the setting of relapsed disease. The kidneys, gastrointestinal tract, skin, and lungs may also be involved.

What presenting signs and symptoms suggest a medical emergency?

Medical emergencies include leukostasis, superior mediastinal syndrome, tumor lysis syndrome, and overwhelming infection.

Leukostasis can result in a myriad of CNS, pulmonary, genitourinary, and vascular symptoms. CNS symptoms include blurred vision, confusion, stupor, coma, and/or papilledema. Pulmonary symptoms can present as tachypnea, dyspnea, and/or hypoxia. Genitourinary symptoms can include priapism, oliguria, and/or anuria. Finally, vascular symptoms may present in the form of diffuse intravascular coagulation (DIC), retinal hemorrhage, myocardial infarction, and/or renal vein thrombosis. Hyperleukocytosis is the major risk factor for leukostasis.

Superior mediastinal syndrome (SMS), a syndrome characterized by compression of the trachea and superior vena cava via a large anterior mediastinal mass (usually seen in T-cell ALL) is also a medical emergency, with a high mortality rate. Cough, hoarseness, orthopnea, stridor, dysphagia, and chest pain (symptoms that worsen when the patient is in a supine position) should raise suspicion for SMS.

Tumor lysis syndrome (TLS) is a condition in which the rapid release of intracellular metabolites (e.g., phosphorus, potassium, uric acid) may lead not only to urate nephropathy, but also to cardiac arrhythmias, renal failure, seizures, coma, DIC, and death. Although often a consequence of initiating chemotherapy, it can be seen prior to introduction of chemotherapy in patients with a high tumor burden.

Our patient had an absolute neutrophil count of 300×10^6/L. Patients with an absolute neutrophil count <500×10^6/L (or <1000×10^6/L and decreasing) are considered neutropenic. The most important factor in a patient's susceptibility to bacterial and fungal infections is the number of circulating neutrophils. Additional factors that make patients with ALL susceptible to rapid progression of infections include foreign bodies (e.g., central venous catheters), chemotherapy, and impaired humoral and cell-mediated immunity. Febrile patients should be rapidly treated with empiric antibiotics.

CLINICAL PEARL	STEP 2/3

A patient with a mediastinal mass may appear well but can develop obstructive respiratory failure when sedated (e.g., during sedation for a bone marrow aspiration and biopsy). Endotracheal intubation would not likely rescue the patient due to the distal nature of the obstruction. Always get a chest x-ray in any patient suspected of having leukemia!

Case Point 1.4

A radiograph of the left leg was taken at the time of initial presentation (**Fig. 1.2**).

What is the significance of radiolucent lines in the metaphyses of long bones? What other radiographic findings can be seen in acute lymphoblastic leukemia?
Metaphyseal bands are seen in 9.8% of patients with ALL; these are transverse lines of increased density indicative of growth arrest secondary to a nutritional dysfunction that interferes with osteogenesis at the growth plate. Other radiographic changes seen in ALL include osteolytic lesions involving the medullary cavity and cortex, osteopenia, subperiosteal new bone formation, osteosclerosis, permeative patterns, and pathologic fractures. About 40% of ALL patients will have a radiographic abnormality at presentation, although no finding is specific for leukemia. Late radiologic changes in acute leukemia include vertebral collapse and aseptic necrosis.

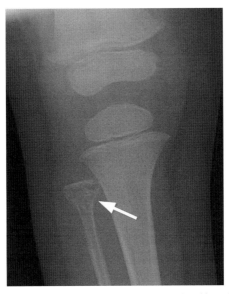

Fig. 2.2 Permeative irregularity and expansion of the proximal right fibula, with cortical erosions and periosteal reaction *(arrow)*, as well as diffuse metaphyseal lucencies.

Case Point 1.5

> Therapy was started in our patient with a three-drug regimen based on a modified Berlin-Frankfurt-Münster regimen using vincristine, peg-asparaginase, and dexamethasone, along with intrathecal chemotherapy. She went into complete remission, with no detectable minimal residual disease after 1 month of induction chemotherapy. She will have to complete 2 years of chemotherapy and then 5 to 10 years of surveillance after therapy to be considered cured.

What are the principles of therapy for ALL?

The various treatment regimens for childhood ALL are similar and include several phases. Induction therapy lasts 4 to 6 weeks and includes a glucocorticoid, vincristine, asparaginase, an optional anthracycline, and intrathecal chemotherapy. Almost all patients achieve remission. However, relapse occurs in all patients without additional chemotherapy, which includes the following phases:

- 6–8 weeks of intensive combination chemotherapy to prevent remission and the development of CNS leukemia (consolidation)
- interim maintenance phase
- 8-week delayed intensification phase
- low-intensity, antimetabolite-based therapy for 18 to 30 months (maintenance)

Therapy is risk-adapted; patients are stratified based on a uniform approach initially adopted in 1993, with more recent incorporation of cytogenetic abnormalities and minimal residual disease (MRD) assessment after therapy. Overall survival rates are now up to 90%.

BASIC SCIENCE/CLINICAL PEARL   **STEP 1/2/3**

Prior to CNS prophylaxis in the 1970s, remissions were achievable, but relapses into the CNS were almost guaranteed. Cranial irradiation improved outcomes, but it was intrathecal chemotherapy that dramatically enhanced survival to rates comparable to those that are currently seen.

BASIC SCIENCE/CLINICAL PEARL   **STEP 1/2/3**

Response to induction chemotherapy is a critical predictor of final outcome, and therapy is adapted to this. The recent use of flow cytometric analysis, polymerase chain reaction testing, and next-generation sequencing to detect minimal residual disease (MRD) has improved our ability to detect the subset of patients at the highest risk for relapse.

Case Summary

See Box 1.1.

Complaint/History: A 20-month-old child presents with 8 weeks of right leg pain and limping.

Findings: Mild conjunctival and sublingual pallor, as well as anterior cervical and submandibular lymphadenopathy.

Labs/Tests: White blood cell count of $2.4 \times 10^9/L$ (12% neutrophils, 84% lymphocytes, 4% monocytes), hemoglobin, 7.5 g/dL, hematocrit, 21.5%, and platelet count, $82 \times 10^9/L$. Her bone marrow demonstrated hypercellularity, with sheets of small to medium-sized lymphoblasts replacing normal cells.

Diagnosis: Acute lymphoblastic leukemia.

Treatment: Chemotherapy.

BEYOND THE PEARLS

- Of ALL cases, 85% arise from B cell precursors, and 15% from T cell precursors. T cell precursors have different driver mutations and overall have a worse outcome.
- Acute lymphoblastic leukemia (ALL) can mimic juvenile idiopathic arthritis. In one study, low white blood cell count, low-normal platelet count, and nighttime pain were the strongest predictors of ALL. Rash and a positive antinuclear antibody (ANA) test result were not helpful in ruling out ALL. An accurate diagnosis is critical because pretreating ALL patients with glucocorticoids worsens prognosis.
- A small subset of ALL patients harbor a t(5;14) translocation, fusing the IgH-promoter gene with the interleukin (IL)-3 gene. The resulting IL-3 overproduction can result in a very impressive eosinophil count, with blood eosinophils reaching 100,000/mm^3 (100 × 10^9/L). The eosinophils are not malignant, however, and simply reflect the elevated IL-3 levels.
- A t(9;22) chromosomal translocation (the Philadelphia [Ph] chromosome), creating the *BCR-ABL1* fusion gene, is present in 3% to 5% of childhood ALL cases (Ph+ ALL). This mutation traditionally has resulted in the worst outcomes of any subset of ALL patients, with event-free survivals of less than 30%. This poor outcome has been mitigated by the addition of tyrosine kinase inhibitors (TKIs), which can block the BCR-ABL1 fusion protein; TKI therapy combined with chemotherapy has more than doubled the survival rate for patients with Ph+ ALL.
- Other important cytogenetic abnormalities portending a poor prognosis include *KMT2A* gene rearrangement (often seen in infant ALL cases), hypodiploidy, and intrachromosomal amplification of chromosome 21 (iAMP21). Additionally, there has been a recently described subset of ALL patients known as *Ph-like ALL*; although they do not have the *BCR-ABL1* fusion, they display a gene expression profile similar to that of Ph+ ALL. Several aberrations in genes that lead to a kinase-driven phenotype, including *CRLF2* and *JAK1/JAK2*, have been implicated. Clinical trials using TKIs designed to block the pathways stemming from these kinase alterations are underway.
- The use of high-dose glucocorticoid therapy—in particular, dexamethasone, which is 6.5 times more potent than prednisone—has increased the rates of symptomatic osteonecrosis of weight-bearing joints. The incidence has risen above 20% in some therapeutic trials for high-risk ALL. Although symptomatic management (including operative joint replacement) has been used to intervene, the focus of the pediatric oncology community has been to reduce the overall incidence through therapeutic protocol modifications.

Bibliography

Gutierrez A, Silverman LB. Acute lymphoblastic leukemia. In: Orkin SH, Fisher DE, Ginsburg D, Look AT, Lux SE, Nathan DG, eds. *Nathan and Oski's Hematology of Infancy and Childhood.* Saunders; 2015:1527–1554.

Herman MJ, Martinek M. The limping child. *Pediatr Rev.* 2015;36.5:184–195.

Hunger SP, Mulligan CG. Acute lymphoblastic leukemia in children. *New Engl J Med.* 2015;373(16):1541–1552.

Jones Olcay Y, et al. A multicenter case-control study on predictive factors distinguishing childhood leukemia from juvenile rheumatoid arthritis. *Pediatrics.* 2006;117.5:e840–e844.

Sinigiglia, et al. Musculoskeletal manifestations in pediatric acute leukemia. *J Pediatr Orthoped.* 2008;20:20–28.

9-Year-Old Male With Jaw Pain

Aileen Dickinson ■ Jenny L. Wong ■ Maria Vergara-Lluri ■
Randall Y. Chan

A 9-year-old male presents complaining of progressive left jaw pain and swelling. He has been having intermittent epistaxis for 2 weeks, and 1 week ago he noticed left-sided jaw swelling. At that time, he was prescribed amoxicillin for a presumed infectious cause. He did not respond to the antibiotics, however, and developed increasing pain in his left jaw, accompanied by trismus and a 3-kg weight loss.

What are common causes of jaw swelling with pain in a child?
Orofacial infection, facial trauma, and pathologic processes together account for the bulk of clinical presentations of jaw pain with swelling.

Orofacial infection may be odontogenic or nonodontogenic in origin. Odontogenic infections arise from the teeth (e.g., dental caries) and periodontal tissues (e.g., gingivitis, periodontitis, periodontal abscess, pericoronitis.)

Dental caries are the most likely cause of odontogenic infections in children. They are asymptomatic in the early stages but progress to cause sensitivity and eventual pain as the caries advance into the pulp and periapical tissues. Resulting periapical abscesses can track within bone, leading to either self-drainage or continued spread, with resulting infection of bone (osteomyelitis) and neighboring soft tissues (fascial space infections). Significant soft tissue swelling and pain can accompany either osteomyelitis or fascial space infections.

CLINICAL PEARL STEP 2/3

Deep fascial space infections require emergent intervention to prevent or mitigate life-threatening complications, such as airway obstruction, sepsis, or spread to vital structures such as the cavernous sinus or mediastinum.

Pain with swelling in the mandibular region caused by nonodontogenic infections is also common. Salivary gland swelling can arise from infections (e.g., mumps) or sialolithiasis (salivary stones). Tuberculosis, infective mononucleosis, and cat scratch disease can also cause lymphadenopathy in the vicinity of the mandible and upper neck.

Traumatic causes of jaw pain and swelling include trauma to the dentoalveolar structures (teeth, periodontal tissues, alveolar bone, and soft tissues of the oral region) and injury to facial structures, such as the mandible and temporomandibular joint. In children younger than 5 years, the most common cause of dentoalveolar trauma is falls. Motor vehicle accidents and play accidents are mostly responsible for dentoalveolar injuries in children 5 to 15 years of age.

CLINICAL PEARL STEP 2/3

Regardless of patient age, facial trauma may be an indicator of child abuse.

Finally, pediatric mandibular swelling with pain can indicate the presence of a neoplasm (benign or malignant). Benign masses may be inherently painful (e.g., osteoblastoma, osteoid osteoma). Other masses become painful after the development of a secondary infection (e.g., soft tissue cysts, osseous cysts, osseous masses). Malignancies that can present in the pediatric mandible include osteosarcoma, Ewing sarcoma, Langerhans cell histiocytosis, and lymphomas, including Burkitt lymphoma and Hodgkin lymphoma.

BASIC SCIENCE/CLINICAL PEARL   **STEP 1/2/3**

New-onset paresthesia and tooth mobility in conjunction with pain and swelling suggest a malignant process.

Case Point 2.1

The physical examination reveals a cachectic-appearing boy in mild distress secondary to jaw pain. A soft, fixed, 6- × 6-cm tender nonerythematous mass in the left jaw region is palpable. The oral examination reveals only multiple dental caries. A firm, fixed, tender 6-cm mass is palpable in the right lower quadrant of his abdomen. The remainder of his examination is normal.

What is your differential diagnosis for a right lower quadrant abdominal mass in this child?
A palpable right lower quadrant mass in a child should elicit a high suspicion for malignancy, particularly in a male. The most common causes of primary abdominal malignancies in school-age children include lymphomas and soft tissue sarcomas, including rhabdomyosarcoma. Ovarian masses (including benign cysts) are also possible in females.

Non-Hodgkin lymphomas (NHLs) account for 10% of all childhood cancers and include primarily Burkitt lymphoma (BL), diffuse large B-cell lymphoma (DLBCL), anaplastic large cell lymphoma (ALCL), and lymphoblastic lymphoma (LBL). The sporadic form of BL commonly presents with an abdominal mass, whereas the endemic type generally presents with bony facial masses (see earlier). DLBCL often presents with abdominal or mediastinal masses, and ALCL with lymphadenopathy and extranodal disease, whereas LBL can have a varied presentation.

Rhabdomyosarcoma is the most common pediatric soft tissue sarcoma, usually involving the head and neck (25%) and genitourinary tract (24%) and, less commonly, the orbit and extremities. In children younger than 2 years, neuroblastoma, hepatoblastoma, and Wilms tumors are most commonly seen.

In a female, ovarian germ cell tumors, including dysgerminomas and the more aggressive malignant teratomas and endodermal sinus tumors, should be considered. Although rare, gonadoblastoma should be considered in males. Benign masses that may mimic a malignancy include mature cystic teratomas and cystadenomas.

BASIC SCIENCE/CLINICAL PEARL   **STEP 1/2/3**

Consider non-Hodgkin lymphoma in a child or adolescent with rapidly growing peripheral lymph nodes and/or a mediastinal or abdominal mass, particularly if the patient presents with weight loss, fevers, hepatomegaly, or splenomegaly.

Case Point 2.2

A computed tomography (CT) scan of the patient's face reveals a 5.3- × 4.2- × 5.8-cm mass centered in the left masticator space, with obliteration of the intramuscular fat planes (Fig. 2.1). A CT scan of the patient's abdomen reveals a second mass (Fig. 2.2).

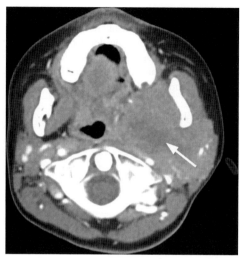

Fig. 2.1 This computed tomography scan reveals a large mass in the left masticator space *(arrow)*.

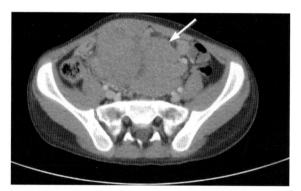

Fig. 2.2 This computed tomography scan reveals a large mass in the lower abdomen extensively involving the duodenum, jejunum, and ileum *(arrow)*.

What is the next step?

Evaluating tissue morphology and cellular expression via biopsy is critical to determine a diagnosis and provide the patient with a prognosis and treatment plan. Tissue from the primary mass should be removed via excisional or incisional biopsy whenever possible or by needle core biopsy in select cases. The initial morphologic evaluation of the tissue will guide the pathologist in determining which studies are required to make a definitive diagnosis. These studies include histopathologic assessment, tissue immunohistochemistry, immunophenotyping by flow cytometry, and genetic or molecular evaluation.

Case Point 2.3

A core needle biopsy is performed (Fig. 2.3).

Diagnosis: Burkitt lymphoma.

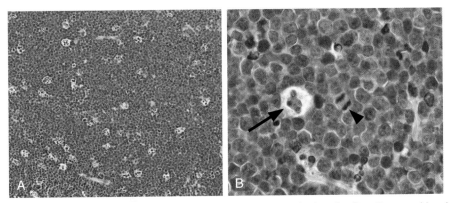

Fig. 2.3 (A) Low-power magnification of Burkitt lymphoma. The neoplastic cells efface the normal lymph node architecture and are monotonous cells. Note the tingible body macrophages embedded singly and dispersed within the tumor, imparting the so-called starry sky appearance (H&E stain, 200× magnification). (B) High-power magnification. The neoplasm is composed of monotonous medium-sized cells with finely speckled chromatin, small nucleoli, and scant to moderate amounts of cytoplasm. This is a highly proliferative neoplasm. Note the mitotic figure *(arrowhead)* at the center. A tingible body macrophage *(arrow)* can be seen to the left of the mitotic figure (H&E stain, 1000× magnification).

What is Burkitt lymphoma?

BL is a highly aggressive B cell NHL arising from germinal center B cells due to a translocation between the long arm of chromosome 8 and one of three immunoglobulin genes—t(8;14), t(2;8), or t(8;22)—leading to fusion of *c-MYC* with *IgH*, *Igκ*, or *Igλ*, respectively. The resulting fusion gene gives rise to increased expression of the MYC transcription factor, in turn leading to cellular immortality and ultimately tumorigenesis.

The three types of BL differ by epidemiology, clinical manifestations, and genetic features, although they share an identical histology. These include the endemic, sporadic, and immunodeficiency-associated types. Endemic BL is seen primarily in equatorial zones, primarily in Africa, Papua New Guinea, and Brazil. It is highly associated with Epstein Barr virus (EBV) infection (95% of cases) as well as malaria. It presents with bony face or jaw involvement, with a peak incidence at 6 years old.

The sporadic type is seen in the United States and Europe; it commonly presents with an abdominal mass and is driven by EBV infection in only 10% to 15% of cases. The median age of presentation is 6 to 8 years old. Associated complications of abdominal involvement, particularly in the ileocecal region, include intussusception, obstruction, and ascites. In addition to abdominal presentations, sporadic BL may also present with the involvement of lymph nodes throughout the body and spleen. Metastatic disease may include bone marrow, central nervous system, and solid organs, including the ovaries, testes, kidneys, omentum, and breast.

Immunodeficiency-associated BL is associated with acquired immunodeficiency syndrome (AIDS) caused by the human immunodeficiency virus (HIV), as by well as post–organ transplantation states.

BASIC SCIENCE/CLINICAL PEARL　　　　　　　　　　　　　　　　　　**STEP 1**

Burkitt lymphoma is thought to arise from germinal center B lymphocytes. Morphologically, it appears as a sheet of densely packed tumor cells with occasional interspersed tingible body macrophages (i.e., the characteristic "starry sky" appearance).

CLINICAL PEARL   **STEP 2/3**

Although rare, Burkitt lymphoma should be considered in any patient with intussusception outside of the typical age range for idiopathic ileocolic intussusception.

BASIC SCIENCE/CLINICAL PEARL   **STEP 1/2/3**

Immunodeficiency syndromes often predispose patients to lymphoma.

What presentations of Burkitt lymphoma are acutely an emergency?

Large mediastinal masses can cause dyspnea, orthopnea, cough, chest pain, facial swelling, and/or plethora due to airway obstruction and venous congestion (superior mediastinal syndrome). Large, fast-growing neck masses can cause upper airway compromise. Suspected airway obstruction in the setting of a suspected lymphoma is best evaluated with CT scanning, given its increased sensitivity to airway impingement; it is critical to perform this prior to further workup, which may require sedatives.

Patients with abdominal pain and/or a peritonitic abdominal examination—rigid abdomen, no bowel sounds, rebound tenderness—should be immediately evaluated for perforation, obstruction, or intussusception secondary to an abdominal mass. An urgent surgical consultation may be warranted.

Tumor lysis syndrome (TLS) may occur as a result of a high tumor cell turnover rate, resulting in hyperuricemia, hyperkalemia, hyperphosphatemia, and hypocalcemia. The resulting renal failure, cardiac arrhythmias, and seizures are life-threatening.

BASIC SCIENCE/CLINICAL PEARL   **STEP 1**

Burkitt lymphoma has the shortest doubling time of any known tumor.

What is the next step?

Once oncologic emergencies have been ruled out or mitigated, and a pathologic diagnosis has been made, the next step in managing this patient would be to evaluate all locations in the body affected by the lymphoma by radiographic and imaging studies. This process, known as staging, is important because the information collected will ultimately guide the length and intensity of therapy, as well as the therapeutic modalities used. In children, the most commonly used staging system for non-Hodgkin lymphoma is the St. Jude (Murphy) staging system.

Tumors are staged from I to IV. Stage I signifies a single lymph node involved (not abdominal or mediastinal), stage II signifies two or more involved areas on the same side of the diaphragm (or single abdominal tumor), stage III signifies nodal involvement on both sides of the diaphragm (or a mediastinal tumor), and stage IV signifies metastatic disease.

Case Point 2.4

Positron emission tomography–computed tomography (PET-CT) reveals extensive tumor involvement of the head and neck region, thyroid, stomach, small intestine, and adrenal glands (Fig. 2.4). An evaluation of his cerebrospinal fluid and examination of his bone marrow is negative for extranodal metastatic disease.

How is Burkitt lymphoma treated?

Intensive risk-adapted chemotherapy protocols have resulted in survival rates greater than 90% to 95%. Important chemotherapy drugs used include vincristine, cyclophosphamide, doxorubicin, prednisone, and methotrexate. Rituximab is a monoclonal antibody to CD20 that has rapidly

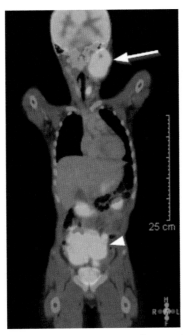

Fig. 2.4 This positron emission tomography–computed tomography scan shows tumor involvement of cervical *(arrow)* and abdominal *(arrowhead)* nodes.

become an important component of therapy for aggressive non-Hodgkin lymphoma in children (and adults). Surgery is generally reserved for emergent situations given the high response rate to chemotherapy, although certain nonemergent scenarios do warrant resection.

CLINICAL PEARL　　　　　　　　　　　　　　　　　　　　　　　**STEP 2/3**

Burkitt lymphoma and diffuse large B-cell lymphoma are treated identically in children.

The patient underwent four cycles of intensive chemotherapy with vincristine, cyclophosphamide, doxorubicin, prednisone, methotrexate, and rituximab and went into complete remission. He continues to be followed in the oncology clinic for disease surveillance and survivorship care.

BEYOND THE PEARLS

- Burkitt lymphoma makes up nearly 50% of all non-Hodgkin lymphomas in children younger than 15. In children older than 15, it only makes up about 25% of all non-Hodgkin lymphomas.
- Burkitt lymphoma frequently involves a group of specific lymphoid tissues in the head and neck collectively known as Waldeyer's ring. Waldeyer's ring includes the pharyngeal tonsil, Eustachian tonsils, palatine tonsils, and lingual tonsils.
- The site of abdominal disease often differs according to the type of BL. Sporadic BL often involves the ileum and cecum. Endemic BL often involves the mesentery and omentum.
- Ileocecal lymphoma is invariably Burkitt lymphoma.
- Disease restricted to the bone marrow with circulating peripheral blasts can occur. This is known as Burkitt leukemia and was previously considered a subtype of acute lymphoblastic leukemia. It is treated in an identical fashion to Burkitt lymphoma.

Case Summary

  Complaint/History: A 9-year-old male presents complaining of progressive left jaw pain and swelling.

  Findings: A soft, fixed, 6- × 6-cm tender nonerythematous mass in the left jaw region is palpable.

  Labs/Tests: A CT scan of the patient's face reveals a 5.3- × 4.2- × 5.8-cm mass centered in the left masticator space with obliteration of the intramuscular fat planes. A second mass is seen in the abdomen as well.

  Diagnosis: Burkitt lymphoma.

  Treatment: Chemotherapy.

Bibliography

Cameron A, Widmer R. *Handbook of Pediatric Dentistry*. 4th ed. Mosby Elsevier; 2013.

Neville BW, Damm DD, Allen CM, Chi AC. *Hematologic Disorders. Oral and Maxillofacial Pathology*. 4th ed. St. Louis, MO: Elsevier; 2016:533–571.

Gross TG, Perkins SL. Malignant non-Hodgkin lymphomas in children. In: Pizzo PA, Poplack DG, eds. *Principles and Practice of Pediatric Oncology*. 6th ed. Philadelphia, PA: Lippincott Williams and Wilkins; 2011.

Prusakowski Melanie K, Cannone Daniel. Pediatric oncologic emergencies. *Emerg Med Clin North Am*. 2014;32(3):527–548. Web.

Shukla N, Trippett T. Non-Hodgkin's lymphoma in children and adolescents. *Curr Oncol Rep*. 2006;8:387–394.

15-Year-Old Female With Pain and Neck Stiffness

Alyssa Huang ■ Maria Vergara-Lluri ■ Russell K. Brynes ■ Randall Y. Chan

A 15-year-old female presents with pain, trismus, and neck stiffness for approximately 5 days. She is able to eat but has pain with chewing and swallowing. She also has right ear pain and a diffuse headache. She has otherwise not had any sore throat, cough, or hoarseness.

On physical examination, she experiences pain during palpation of the right lateral neck. She has decreased range of motion of the neck laterally and on flexion and extension. Her oral pharynx appears unremarkable.

A radiograph of her neck reveals a retropharyngeal abscess. A CT scan of her neck confirms a rim-enhancing retropharyngeal fluid collection (Fig. 3.1).

BASIC SCIENCE PEARL	STEP 1

A retropharyngeal abscess is an infection arising from draining lymph nodes between the posterior pharyngeal wall and prevertebral fascia. It is most common in prepubertal children because the lymph nodes atrophy during puberty. It can be an immediately life-threatening infection due to airway impingement or direct extension into the mediastinum.

CLINICAL PEARL	STEP 2/3

Retropharyngeal abscesses can be visualized on plain radiography but overreliance on the modality can lead to overdiagnosis. Computed tomography is ideal for making a definitive diagnosis and for surgical planning (60% of patients will not need surgery).

Case Point 3.1

A complete blood count reveals a white blood count of 25.4×10^9/L, hemoglobin of 11.4 g/dL, hematocrit of 34.7%, and platelet count of 2808×10^9/L (Fig. 3.2).

BASIC SCIENCE/CLINICAL PEARL	STEP 1/2/3

A normal platelet count is 150 to 400×10^9/L. This is true essentially from birth to death, unless a patient is born extremely prematurely. A fetus has a slightly higher normal range, which reaches adult values at about 30 weeks of gestation.

What is the most common cause of thrombocytosis in a hospitalized patient?

The most common cause of a high platelet count is reactive thrombocytosis (RT) in both children and adults, even in cases of extreme thrombocytosis (platelet counts greater than 1000×10^9/L). RT

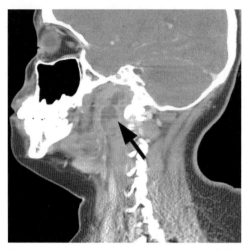

Fig. 3.1   A 3.8-cm abscess is seen in the retropharyngeal soft tissues *(arrow).*

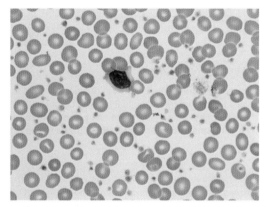

Fig. 3.2   Peripheral smear shows a reactive lymphocyte, normal red blood cell morphology, and numerous platelets.

refers to thrombocytosis in patients who have a medical or surgical condition likely to be associated with an increased platelet count and in whom the platelet count normalizes after the resolution of the condition (Box 3.1). Thrombopoietic growth factors and cytokines (e.g., thrombopoietin or interleukin-6 [IL-6], respectively) have been implicated as resulting in RT of various causes.

Case Point 3.2

> The retropharyngeal abscess is successfully treated with surgical drainage and IV clindamycin. The patient is followed for 12 months. The inflammation completely resolves but the platelet count remains high, with values ranging from 1600 to 3200 × 10^9/L.

What is the differential diagnosis for the persistent thrombocytosis in this patient?

An elevated platelet count may be the result of a cytokine-driven mechanism (reactive or secondary thrombocytosis; see Box 3.1) or the result of overproduction of platelets by neoplastic

---

BOX 3.1 ■ Major Causes of Reactive Thrombocytosis.

Nonmalignant Hematologic Conditions

- Acute blood loss
- Acute hemolytic anemia
- Iron deficiency
- Treatment of vitamin B_{12} deficiency
- Rebound effect after treatment of immune thrombocytopenia (ITP)
- Rebound effect after ethanol-induced thrombocytopenia

Malignant Conditions

- Metastatic tumors
- Lymphoma
- Rebound effect following use of myelosuppressive agents

Acute and Chronic Inflammatory Conditions

- Rheumatologic disorders, vasculitides
- Inflammatory bowel disease
- Celiac disease
- Kawasaki disease
- Nephrotic syndrome

Tissue Damage

- Thermal burns
- Myocardial infarction
- Severe trauma
- Acute pancreatitis
- Postsurgical period, especially postsplenectomy

Infections

- Chronic infections
- Tuberculosis
- Acute bacterial and viral infections

Reactions to Medications

- Vincristine
- Epinephrine, glucocorticoids
- Interleukin-1B
- All-trans retinoic acid
- Thrombopoietin
- Low-molecular-weight heparins

Others

- Exercise
- Allergic reactions
- Functional and surgical asplenia

Adapted from Dame C, Sutor AH. Primary and secondary thrombocytosis in childhood. *Br J Haematol.* 2005;129(2):165–177; and Schafer A. Thrombocytosis. *N Engl J Med.* 2004;350(12):1211–1219.

---

megakaryocytes (clonal or primary thrombocytosis). Although RT remains in the differential diagnosis, it is less likely given the lack of resolution over time as the inflammation abates. Causes of clonal thrombocytosis—including myeloproliferative neoplasms, especially essential thrombocythemia (ET)—must be considered.

| BASIC SCIENCE/CLINICAL PEARL | STEP 1/2/3 |

Reactive thrombocytosis is far more common than clonal thrombocytosis from a myeloproliferative neoplasm.

What is the next step to make a diagnosis?

The 2016 World Health Organization (WHO) diagnosis of ET requires the following:

- Sustained platelet count greater than or equal to 450×10^9/L
- Bone marrow biopsy showing mainly megakaryocyte lineage proliferation
- Not meeting WHO criteria for other myeloid neoplasms (e.g., *BCR-ABL1*+ chronic myelogenous leukemia, polycythemia vera, primary myelofibrosis, myelodysplastic syndrome)

Plus:

- Presence of a clonal genetic marker (e.g., *JAK2*, *CALR*, *MPL*) *or* exclusion of other causes (e.g., RT)

Thus the patient should undergo molecular testing on peripheral blood with single-gene panels or next-generation sequencing panels that will identify *JAK2*, *CALR*, and *MPL* mutations (Table 3.1). If testing is negative and clinical suspicion is still high for ET, then the patient should have a bone marrow examination. Molecular testing alone cannot distinguish ET from other myeloproliferative neoplasms.

| BASIC SCIENCE PEARL | STEP 1 |

Whereas 45% of ET in adults is clonal, only 20% of cases of ET in children is clonal. Most are due to *JAK2* V617F mutations. Because *JAK2* V617F mutations can be seen in other MPNs, the morphologic findings on a bone marrow biopsy must be integrated with the results of molecular testing to arrive at a definitive diagnosis.

| BASIC SCIENCE/CLINICAL PEARL | STEP 1/2/3 |

ET is 60 times more common in adults than in children. There is a childhood incidence of 1/1 million children.

TABLE 3.1 ■ **Mutations Seen in Essential Thrombocythemia**

Mutation	Function	No. of Patients (%)
Janus kinase 2 (*JAK2* V617F)	Turns on thrombopoietin receptor permanently	50–60 (seen in 90% of patients with PV and PMF)
Myeloproliferative leukemia virus oncogene (*MPL*)	Codes for thrombopoietin receptor protein → promotes growth and proliferation of megakaryocytes	3–5
Calreticulin (*CALR*)	Encodes for calreticulin protein found in ER; role in gene activity, cell growth and proliferation, migration, adhesion, and apoptosis.	25
Thrombopoietin (*THPO*)	Encodes for TPO → proliferation of megakaryocytes	Rare cases

ER, Endoplasmic reticulum; *PMF*, primary myelofibrosis; *PV*, polycythemia vera; *TPO*, thrombopoietin.

Case Point 3.3

Genetic testing is negative for *JAK2*, *CALR*, and *MPL* mutations. Bone marrow biopsy reveals a normocellular bone marrow with normal numbers of granulocytic and erythroid elements, but with a striking megakaryocytic hyperplasia (Fig. 3.3).

Diagnosis: Essential Thrombocythemia (ET).

BASIC SCIENCE/CLINICAL PEARL	STEP 1/2/3

Of note, all other myeloid neoplasms must be excluded prior to making the diagnosis of ET. These include chronic myelogenous leukemia, polycythemia vera, primary myelofibrosis, and myelodysplastic syndromes (MDSs; e.g., 5q– syndrome, MDS with ring sideroblasts and thrombocytosis [MDS-RS-T, an MDS-MPN overlap syndrome]).

How does essential thrombocythemia present?
Symptoms vary from vasomotor, thrombotic, and/or hemorrhagic symptoms (Table 3.2). Up to half of patients with ET may be asymptomatic at presentation.

Children with ET tend to have more of a benign course compared to adults, but about one-third will experience thrombotic or mild bleeding complications. Other possible findings include fatigue, weight loss, night sweats, and splenomegaly on examination.

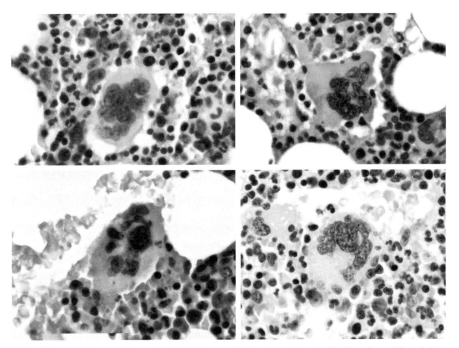

Fig. 3.3 Characteristic megakaryocytopoiesis in essential thrombocythemia with giant, hyperlobated, "stag-horn-like" megakaryocytes.

TABLE 3.2 ■ **Symptoms Associated with Essential Thrombocythemia**

Type of Symptom	Features
Vasomotor	Headaches; lightheadedness; syncope; chest pain; acral paresthesia; erythromelalgia (characterized by intense burning pain, severe redness and increase temperature of affected extremities); transient visual disturbances— amaurosis fugax, scintillating scotoma, ophthalmic migraines
Thrombotic	Qualitative and quantitative platelet alterations; stroke, transient ischemia attacks, retinal artery and venous occlusion coronary artery ischemia; pulmonary embolism; hepatic or portal vein thrombosis; deep vein thrombosis; digital ischemia
Hemorrhagic	Bleeding (infrequent)

What complications occur in essential thrombocythemia?
There is an increased risk of thrombotic events, which is thought to be due to more than simply platelet count elevation. Risk factors include age older than 60 years, previous history of thrombosis, presence of cardiovascular risk factors, leukocytosis greater than $11 \times 10^9/L$, and the presence of a *JAK2* V617F mutation. Cardiovascular risk factors also associated with thrombosis in patients with ET include the use of tobacco, hypertension, and diabetes mellitus.

ET is also associated with hemorrhagic complications, including epistaxis, gingival bleeding, and easy bruising. Gastrointestinal (GI) hemorrhage is usually rare but can be seen in patients with exceptionally high platelet counts. Of note, when platelet counts exceed $1000 \times 10^9/L$, there is a loss of intermediate and large von Willebrand factor (vWF) multimers, which leads to acquired von Willebrand disease (vWD) and a higher risk of bleeding. Reduction of platelet counts to less than $1000 \times 10^9/L$ can restore intermediate and large vWF multimers and resolve the acquired vWD.

BASIC SCIENCE/CLINICAL PEARL   **STEP 1/2/3**

Reactive thrombocytosis rarely presents with complications (bleeding or thrombosis), and thus the high platelet count alone is not the cause of the complications. The presence of clotting or bleeding should increase the suspicion for ET over RT.

CLINICAL PEARL   **STEP 2/3**

ET patients do not have a clotting tendency or bleeding tendency. The same patient can simultaneously have both clotting and bleeding.

How is essential thrombocythemia treated?
Treatment can vary from observation alone to aggressive cytoreductive therapy; the therapy is individualized with goals of care to minimize thrombotic and hemorrhagic complications. Treatments have not been shown to prevent disease transformation or prolong survival, but are key in controlling symptoms and minimizing complications. Individualization of treatment is based specifically on the risk for thrombosis (summarized in Fig. 3.4).

For those who are asymptomatic, observation and interval monitoring of counts are sufficient. When patients develop low-intensity symptoms and have low risk for thrombosis, therapy is initiated with antiplatelet therapy, typically low-dose aspirin in the pediatric population.

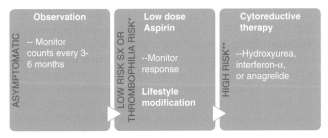

Fig. 3.4 Treatment is based on risk factors. *Low-risk symptoms: hepatosplenomegaly, headaches, erythromelalgia, cardiac risk factors, additional thrombophilia or bleeding risk factors. **High- risk symptoms: failed low-risk therapy, or history of thrombosis, severe bleeding, or persistent extreme thrombocytosis.

For those with high-risk symptoms and/or features, cytoreductive therapy is generally recommended. In the pediatric population, cytoreductive therapy is not usually offered without a history of thrombosis, severe bleeding, or extremely severe thrombocytosis. Options include the following:

- Hydroxyurea, an antimetabolite and the preferred cytoreductive agent for most patients. This is because it is effective at reducing platelet counts and decreasing thrombotic risk. Doses are adjusted to achieve platelet counts in the range of 100 to 400×10^9/L. It is generally well tolerated, with minimal side effects (e.g., oral ulcers, hyperpigmentation, rash). It is, however, a teratogen and may cause myelosuppression.
- Anagrelide, which suppresses megakaryocyte differentiation. Side effects include palpitations, cardiac arrhythmias, and edema.
- Pegylated interferon-α, which controls thrombocytosis, with once weekly dosing. It is generally well tolerated. Side effects include fatigue, flulike symptoms, myelosuppression, depression, and autoimmune disease. This agent is not well tolerated in those with mental health disorders. It is the first-line agent for those who are pregnant.

CLINICAL PEARL   **STEP 2/3**

Acetylsalicylic acid (ASA [aspirin]) therapy is generally considered to be contraindicated in patients with ET with acquired vWD because this will worsen bleeding risk. Patients with platelet counts higher than 1500×10^9/L should be checked for vWD prior to any empiric ASA therapy.

Case Point 3.4

The patient was not started on cytoreductive therapy but instead was monitored frequently with a plan to start cytoreductive therapy only if she develops a thrombotic or hemorrhagic complication. She has continued to do well.

CLINICAL PEARL   **STEP 2/3**

In young and otherwise healthy patients, complications are unusual, even if the platelet count exceeds 2000×10^9/L.

What is the prognosis for a patient with essential thrombocythemia?
Life expectancy is near normal in adults with ET. Of all the myeloproliferative neoplasms, ET has the lowest mortality rate. There is a risk of transformation to myelofibrosis, termed *post–essential*

thrombocythemia myelofibrosis; however, it is low at 3% in the first 5 years and then 4% to 15% by 15 years. Additionally, there is a risk to progression of acute myeloid leukemia (AML), with rates of 1% to 3% in 10 years and 8% by 20 years. Once transformation to AML has occurred, the long-term prognosis is considered to be very poor, with median survival from 2 to 7 months.

The prognosis for children with ET is less clear but thought to be better than that for adults with ET. Children should be at lower risk for vascular complications and thrombosis due to having minimal risk factors (e.g., low rates of diabetes and atherosclerosis) and overall healthier vasculature. However, early diagnosis in childhood means that they will be thrombocythemic for several more decades and have prolonged exposure to endothelial damage and platelet derangement, which could potentially increase a later risk of long-term complications.

BASIC SCIENCE/CLINICAL PEARL   **STEP 1/2/3**

Tobacco use has been shown to be an independent predictor of poor survival in those with ET.

CLINICAL PEARL   **STEP 2/3**

Although the prognosis in children is overall very good, the cumulative annual risk over a long remaining life span translates to significant risk for complications over a lifetime.

BEYOND THE PEARLS

- Patients with ET can present with high serum potassium levels due to pseudohyperkalemia. The patient actually has a normal serum potassium level, but intracellular potassium is released as platelets degranulate in vitro.
- Unlike erythropoietin levels, which can distinguish between primary and secondary causes of erythrocytosis, thrombopoietin levels are not helpful in distinguishing ET from RT. However, C-reactive protein may be a helpful marker because it tracks well with IL-6 levels, a mediator of liver synthesis of thrombopoietin in RT.
- Even asymptomatic patients who normally do not need cytoreductive therapy may benefit from therapy prior to surgery because surgery has been shown to increase the risk of thrombosis. In addition, the use of nonsteroidal antiinflammatory drugs (NSAIDs) after surgery can increase the risk of bleeding.
- The platelets in ET are qualitatively abnormal. In a patient presenting with significant hemorrhage, a transfusion of normal platelets may be necessary to control bleeding regardless of high platelet count in the patient. Transfusion of von Willebrand protein or plateletpheresis to lower the platelet count may also be necessary.
- In those with ET, pregnancy is complicated by spontaneous abortions, placental infarction, placental abruption, intrauterine growth retardation, and other major thrombotic events. The patient's platelet count in the setting of ET is not predictive when assessing pregnancy risk.

Case Summary

Complaint/History: A 15-year-old female diagnosed with retropharyngeal abscess is found to have thrombocytosis that does not resolve with resolution of the abscess.

Findings: No abnormal findings on the physical examination; platelet count, 2808×10^9/L.

Labs/Tests: Bone marrow biopsy reveals a normocellular bone marrow with normal numbers of granulocytic and erythroid elements, but with a striking megakaryocytic hyperplasia.

Diagnosis: Essential thrombocythemia.

Treatment: Observation.

Bibliography

Carobbio A, et al. Risk factors for arterial and venous thrombosis in WHO-defined essential thrombocythemia: an international study of 891 patients. *Blood*. 2011;117(22):5857–5859.

Chiarello P, et al. Thrombocytosis in children. *Minerva Pediatr*. 2011;63(6):507–513.

Kucine N, et al. Primary thrombocytosis in children. *Haematologica*. 2014;99(4):620–628.

Michiels JJ. Acquired von Willebrand disease due to increasing platelet count can readily explain the paradox of thrombosis and bleeding in thrombocythemia. *Clin Appl Thromb Hemost*. 1999;5(3):147–151.

Scherer S, Ferrari R, Rister M. Treatment of essential thrombocythemia in childhood. *Pediat Hematol Oncol*. 2003;20(5):361–365.

11-Year-Old Male With New-Onset Chest Pain and Palpitations

Ananta Addala ▦ Lindsey Miller ▦ Jeffrey Johnson ▦ Merujan Uzunyan

---

An 11-year-old male presents to the emergency room with chest pain, palpitations, diaphoresis and dizziness while playing soccer earlier in the day. He describes the chest pain as occurring in the center of his chest and squeezing in nature. He notes that the palpitations occurred suddenly and clearly preceded the chest pain. On the onset of symptoms, he had immediately stopped playing. The symptoms resolved after 5 minutes and he attempted returning to play, but the symptoms recurred and have since persisted over the last 3 hours.

What is the differential diagnosis of chest pain in a child or adolescent?

Chest pain is a common complaint both at the pediatrician's office and in the emergency department. Despite frequent patient and parental concern for cardiac disease, a cardiac cause accounts for only 0.5% to 1% of pediatric patients with chest pain.

Overuse, trauma, costochondritis, Tietze syndrome, idiopathic chest wall pain, and slipping rib syndrome are common musculoskeletal considerations. Pediatric patients with concomitant chronic diseases may have musculoskeletal complications that manifest as chest pain, such as patients with sickle cell disease who develop acute chest syndrome or vasoocclusive crisis.

Due to the innervation pattern of the lungs and pleura, intrinsic lung pathology such as pleural effusion, pneumothorax, pneumonia, or asthma may present as chest pain. Additionally, significant and prolonged increased work of breathing in patients with asthma or other compensated pulmonary conditions may result in muscular strain due to excessive muscle use.

Gastrointestinal disease such as reflux, peptic ulcer disease, esophagitis, and cholecystitis may also present with chest pain. Neurologic conditions such as hyperesthesia due to herpes zoster or anxiety are also in the differential for pediatric chest pain. Chest or mediastinal neoplasms such as lymphoma may also precipitate a chief complaint of chest pain.

BASIC SCIENCE/CLINICAL PEARL	STEP 1/2/3

Chest pain is rarely cardiac in origin in a pediatric patient.

What symptoms, examination findings and/or findings in family history suggest a cardiac cause of chest pain, in contrast to noncardiac chest pain?

Symptoms such as syncope, exertional chest pain or syncope, exercise intolerance, symptoms of heart failure, or palpitations increase suspicion for a cardiac cause. Chest pain or syncope with activity is a red flag symptom that is consistent across different cardiac abnormalities. Exercise intolerance (dyspnea on exertion), orthopnea, dependent edema, and—in an infant—tachypnea, poor feeding and excessive sweating all may suggest congestive heart failure. Palpitations may suggest an arrhythmia.

CLINICAL PEARL   **STEP 2/3**

Sudden-onset tachycardia and palpitations with abrupt cessation is consistent with arrhythmia, whereas sinus tachycardia (and some arrhythmias) have a more gradual onset and return to baseline.

Eliciting a social history may reveal potential intoxication with illicit substances such as cocaine or a methamphetamine. Family history is a very important piece in the evaluation of a chest pain. A history of early death in the family due to any cause may be an indication of an undiagnosed hereditary arrhythmia syndrome (e.g., long QT syndrome, catecholaminergic polymorphic ventricular tachycardia, arrhythmogenic right ventricular dysplasia, Brugada syndrome) or familial cardiomyopathy syndromes such as hypertrophic, dilated, or restrictive cardiomyopathy.

On the physical examination, pathologic murmurs, rubs, clicks, gallops or irregular rhythm noted on auscultation are more suggestive of a cardiac cause. Extracardiac findings such as pectus excavatum or carinatum, joint hyperflexibility, or dysmorphism may also suggest a connective tissue disease (e.g., Marfan syndrome) that may have an associated cardiac disease.

CLINICAL PEARL   **STEP 2/3**

Chest pain or syncope during exercise should raise concern for cardiac pathology.

Case Point 4.1

There is no past medical history or family history for cardiac disease or sudden death.

Vitals on evaluation are notable for a temperature of 98.6°F, pulse rate of 224/min, blood pressure of 142/92 mm Hg, respiratory rate of 20/min, and oxygen saturation of 100% on room air. Examination findings are notable for diaphoresis and an extremely fast heartbeat.

What is the most likely diagnosis, given the magnitude of the tachycardia?
Heart rates exceeding 200 beats/min are concerning for supraventricular tachycardia (SVT), the most common arrhythmia identified in children. The average heart rate in a pediatric patient with SVT is 235 beats/min. This is dependent on age; infants in the first 9 months of life present with an average heart rate of 270 beats/min, whereas older children present with an average heart rate of 210 beats/min.

CLINICAL PEARL   **STEP 2/3**

Heart rate more than 220 beats/min in infants and more than 180 beats/min for children should trigger an evaluation for SVT.

Children with very high heart rates may still be in sinus tachycardia, however. This can be difficult to determine at high heart rates because P waves may be difficult (or impossible) to appreciate. Furthermore, the presence of P waves does not rule out SVT due to an ectopic atrial pacemaker. A 12-lead electrocardiogram (ECG) can help identify the source of a P wave. The character of the heart rate may also assist in identifying a sinus rhythm; in SVT, the heart rate is fixed and nonvariable, whereas in sinus tachycardia, beat to beat variations with activity and vagal tone can be appreciated.

BASIC SCIENCE/CLINICAL PEARL   **STEP 1/2/3**

SVT does not show variability in rhythm and rate. The timing and polarity of P waves in relationship to R waves help elicit the mechanism of SVT (e.g., a retrograde P wave with negative polarity in inferior leads [II, III, aVF] would indicate an orthodromic accessory pathway).

Case Point 4.2

The electrocardiogram shows a narrow complex, fixed-rate tachycardia (Fig. 4.1).

What is the differential diagnosis of supraventricular tachycardia?
The two major subcategories of SVT in the pediatric population are reentrant (reciprocal) atrioventricular (AV) tachyarrhythmias (RAVTs) and ectopic or automatic tachyarrhythmias.

RAVTs occur when electrical conductance occurs in a rapid loop from the atria to the ventricles and back, passing through the AV node in at least one direction; an accessory pathway may be involved in the opposite direction (Fig. 4.2). RAVTs may occur due to a preexcitatory accessory pathway (e.g., Wolff-Parkinson-White [WPW] pattern) in association with congenital heart malformations (e.g., Ebstein's anomaly) or after cardiac surgery. Up to 50% of pediatric patients with RAVTs, particularly infants, do not have any underlying heart disease.

Ectopic and automatic tachyarrhythmias include an ectopic pacemaker, multifocal atrial tachycardia, atrial flutter, atrial fibrillation, and junctional (nodal) ectopic tachycardia. RAVTs are far more common in children than ectopic or automatic tachyarrhythmias.

What are the immediate next steps to assess and/or stabilize this child?
Determining hemodynamic stability dictates the next steps. Hypotension, signs of heart failure, and/or altered levels of consciousness indicate hemodynamic instability and mandates emergency treatment. In an infant, an altered level of consciousness can vary from irritability to poor feeding to lethargy. If a patient is hemodynamically unstable, a rapid trial of adenosine to terminate the aberrant rhythm is indicated if intravenous/intraosseous (IV/IO) access is already available. In patients without IV/IO access, or those who do not respond to adenosine, the immediate next step would be synchronized cardioversion at 0.5 to 1 J/kg.

CLINICAL PEARL   **STEP 2/3**

Whenever termination of SVT is attempted—whether via chemical or electrical means—emergency resuscitation equipment (e.g., a crash cart) and appropriate personnel should be on hand to treat a potential cardiac arrest.

CLINICAL PEARL   **STEP 2/3**

If a patient is in cardiac arrest, cardiopulmonary resuscitation (CPR) should be initiated, regardless of the underlying electrical rhythm.

For hemodynamically stable SVT, vagal maneuvers such as an ice bag over the face for 15 to 30 seconds or a Valsalva maneuver may be sufficient to terminate SVT. The use of carotid massage and/or orbital pressure to elicit vagal tone is no longer recommended.

If the patient does not respond to vagal maneuvers, adenosine may be given at an initial dose of 0.1 mg/kg rapid bolus IV-IO to a maximum dose of 6 mg. A second dose at double the amount may be given immediately after this if there is no response to the first dose. Continuous electrocardiographic

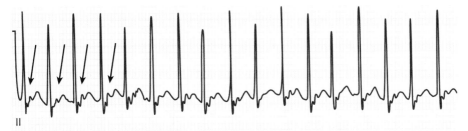

Fig. 4.1 The electrocardiogram shows a narrow complex tachycardia. P waves are retrograde in character *(arrows)*, and beat to beat rate variability is not appreciated. (From Samson RA, Atkins DL. Tachyarrhythmias and defibrillation. *Pediatr Clin North Am.* 2008;55[4]:887–907.)

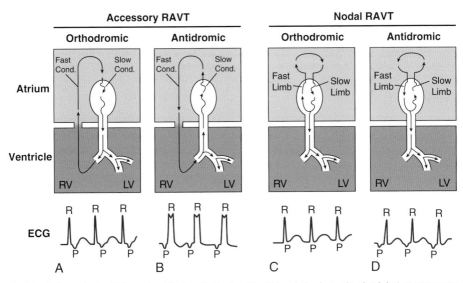

Fig. 4.2 Atrioventricular (AV) reentrant tachyarrhythmias. The AV node is always involved, but an accessory pathway may also be involved in either antegrade (A) or retrograde (B) conduction. Alternately, the AV node may provide the pathway for both antegrade and retrograde conduction (C, D). *Cond.,* Conduction; *LV,* left ventricle; *RAVT,* reentrant (reciprocating) atrioventricular tachycardia; *RV,* right ventricle. (From Park MK, Guntheroth WG. *How to Read Pediatric ECGs,* ed. 4. Philadelphia: Mosby; 2006.)

recording should be performed during adenosine administration because the electrocardiographic response could be diagnostic (e.g., atrial flutter may be more clearly seen). SVT that is refractory to vagal maneuvers and adenosine may require IV antiarrhythmic therapy or transesophageal pacing.

CLINICAL PEARL	**STEP 2/3**

Because the half-life of IV adenosine is so short, it must be pushed as fast as possible and as close to the central circulation as possible to be effective.

CLINICAL PEARL	**STEP 2/3**

Vagal maneuvers may be attempted in a hemodynamically unstable patient if it can be done without leading to a delay in definitive therapy with adenosine and/or synchronized cardioversion.

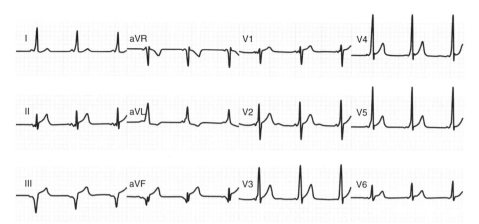

Fig. 4.3 This 12-lead electrocardiogram obtained from the patient shows a normal sinus rhythm with the presence of a δ wave in V2 to V5, with a shortened PR interval. (From Tsao S, Deal BJ. Management of symptomatic Wolff-Parkinson-White syndrome in childhood. *Prog Pediatr Cardiol.* 2012;35[1]:7–15.)

Case Point 4.3

Given that he is hemodynamically stable, the decision is made to give adenosine, 6 mg, in an attempt to terminate his arrhythmia. He does not respond to the first dose of adenosine, but a second dose of 12 mg results in a brief asystole followed by sinus rhythm at a rate of 110/min.

What tachyarrhythmias terminate with adenosine?

Adenosine causes a temporary block in the conduction of the AV node and interrupts reentry circuits that involve the AV node, thereby blocking the propagation of supraventricular arrhythmias that require the AV node as part of the circuit. The temporary AV node block is enough to terminate most RAVTs and therefore can differentiate them from ectopic or automatic tachyarrhythmias because the latter do not respond to adenosine.

The use of adenosine is not indicated in wide-complex tachycardia because it may worsen the overall clinical picture. Notable side effects of adenosine include chest pain, flushing, dyspnea, bronchospasm, and cardiac arrhythmias. A brief period of asystole is usually noted with successful termination of the SVT, but the asystole can rarely be prolonged; asystolic arrest has been reported.

Case Point 4.4

A 12-lead ECG was performed after termination of the arrhythmia (Fig. 4.3), confirming the presence of an RAVT as the source of SVT. A delta wave is seen on the ECG.

Diagnosis: Wolff-Parkinson-White syndrome.

What is WPW syndrome?

Patients may present with either an asymptomatic WPW pattern or a symptomatic WPW syndrome. Patients with a WPW pattern on an ECG manifest ventricular preexcitation in the form of a shortened PR interval, with slurred upstroke of the Q wave (i.e., a delta [δ] wave) and a resulting widened QRS complex. The δ wave indicates early, aberrant, antegrade AV conduction through an accessory pathway along the annulus of atrioventricular valves. These findings may or may not occur in association with ST or T wave changes. The findings are most sensitive in leads V2 to V4 but may be found in all the leads. Additional electrocardiographic abnormalities may include left axis deviation, absence of Q waves in V6, or widened Q waves.

WPW syndrome is the combination of a WPW pattern on the ECG and paroxysmal symptomatic RAVT. Whereas accessory conduction is antegrade during sinus rhythm, resulting in a δ wave, conduction becomes retrograde during episodes of orthodromic RAVT. This results in the disappearance of the δ wave (and retrograde P waves). An RAVT episode is usually triggered by an atrial premature complex occurring at a moment in time when the AV node is receptive, and the accessory pathway is refractory. As the refractory pathway in turn becomes receptive, retrograde conduction then occurs, starting the conductance loop that rapidly overtakes sinus pacing.

Thus, in general, the essential requirement for WPW syndrome is the capacity of the accessory pathway to conduct in both directions. However, in 5% to 7% of patients with WPW syndrome, the retrograde conduction occurs in the AV node. The resulting RAVT is known as *antidromic circus movement tachycardia* (i.e., SVT with aberrancy). Such a rhythm is a diagnostic dilemma because it mimics the appearance of ventricular tachycardia (VT).

CLINICAL PEARL	STEP 2/3

Although antidromic circus movement tachycardia mimics the appearance of VT, the treatment of the two phenomena are very different.

In addition to orthodromic and antidromic RAVTs, patients with WPW syndrome may also present with atrial fibrillation, with rapid conduction to the ventricle. Atrial fibrillation in WPW syndrome presents with a characteristic, irregular, wide complex tachycardia. Rapid conduction through an accessory pathway results in disorganized ventricular depolarization, manifested on the ECG as wide QRS complexes, and therefore have the potential for more serious arrhythmias, such as ventricular fibrillation.

BASIC SCIENCE/CLINICAL PEARL	STEP 1/2/3

Atrial fibrillation associated with WPW syndrome is notoriously wide, complex, very fast, and very irregular.

What is the overall prognosis in WPW syndrome?

The overall prognosis of WPW syndrome is in part dependent on the presence of comorbid or associated conditions. Patients with WPW syndrome without comorbid conditions are still at risk for heart failure and hemodynamic instability, but such complications are rare. Ventricular arrhythmias in particular are a significant risk factor for mortality, which would be sudden in presentation.

Risk factors associated with cardiac arrest and sudden death include rapid antegrade conduction through an accessory pathway, tachyarrhythmia, and/or multiple accessory pathways capable of potentiating life-threatening arrhythmias. Risk stratification may be performed via an exercise treadmill test—the loss of preexcitation in a single beat suggests low risk. In a patient with comorbid atrial fibrillation, a short preexcited RR interval (<220 ms) also indicates a higher risk for cardiac arrest.

CLINICAL PEARL	STEP 2/3

Although rare, WPW syndrome may present with cardiac arrest and sudden death due to ventricular fibrillation.

How is WPW treated?

Long-term management for WPW syndrome in almost all patients will be ablation of the accessory pathway. Most pathways can be ablated by catheter; thus, surgery is rarely indicated. A select few patients can be managed with observation and/or antiarrhythmic medications (e.g., beta blockers) to prevent the episodic tachyarrhythmias, but some controversy exists as to whether the risks of ablation outweigh the true risk of sudden death. The management of patients with an asymptomatic WPW pattern is also controversial.

Case Point 4.5

No further episodes of tachyarrhythmias occur during a 24-hour monitoring period in the pediatric intensive care unit. Echocardiography is performed but does not reveal an anatomic cause for an accessory pathway. The patient is started on atenolol and discharged home.

A follow-up electrophysiology (EP) study performed during a cardiac catheterization procedure reveals a right-sided accessory pathway. The pathway is successfully ablated via catheter, and no further episodes of tachyarrhythmias occur.

CLINICAL PEARL   **STEP 2/3**

An arrhythmia presenting with presyncope or syncope is life-threatening, even if it has reverted to sinus rhythm before a diagnosis is made. These patients should not be worked up on an outpatient basis.

BEYOND THE PEARLS

- The WPW pattern is present in 0.1% to 0.3% of the general population, but only about 2% of those with a preexcitation pattern on the electrocardiogram (ECG) will have WPW syndrome.
- Multiple algorithms have been developed to predict the location of the accessory pathway in patients with WPW using surface electrocardiographic findings.
- Children with WPW syndrome may have more than one accessory pathway. Multiple pathways put a child at higher risk for complications.
- AV reentry tachycardia is often inducible in patients with WPW syndrome electrocardiographic findings during invasive EP studies. This inducible arrhythmia does not necessarily predict eventual development of WPW syndrome.
- Left-sided accessory pathways are more readily ablated when compared with right-sided accessory pathways.
- Atrial fibrillation with rapid ventricular response can be fatal in WPW syndrome. Drugs generally used to treat unstable atrial fibrillation, however, often act on the AV node. In WPW syndrome, this may enhance conduction along the accessory pathway and hasten the onset of hypotension and/or cardiac arrest. Drugs that block accessory conduction are preferred instead (e.g., procainamide).
- Additionally, although adenosine is the drug of choice for terminating narrow complex SVTs, including those caused by WPW syndrome, its use is also typically contraindicated in preexcitation atrial fibrillation due to WPW syndrome. This is because AV nodal blockade may promote conduction through the accessory pathway.

Case Summary

    Complaint/History: An 11-year-old male presents to the emergency room with chest pain, palpitations, diaphoresis, and dizziness.

    Findings: An extremely fast heartbeat is noted on physical examination.

Labs/Tests: The ECG shows a narrow complex, fixed-rate tachycardia with retrograde P waves. The administration of adenosine restores sinus rhythm and reveals a preexcitation pattern.

Diagnosis: Wolff-Parkinson-White syndrome.

Treatment: Cardiac catheter–directed accessory pathway ablation.

Bibliography

Cannon BC, Snyder CS. Disorders of cardiac rhythm and conduction. *Moss & Adams' Heart Disease in Infants, Children, and Adolescents: Including the Fetus and Young Adult.* Philadelphia: Lippincott Williams & Wilkins; 2013:523–546.

Cohen MI, et al. PACES/HRS expert consensus statement on the management of the asymptomatic young patient with a Wolff-Parkinson-White (WPW, Ventricular Preexcitation) electrocardiographic pattern. *Heart Rhythm.* 2012;9(6):1006–1024.

Friedman KG, Alexander ME. Chest pain and syncope in children: a practical approach to the diagnosis of cardiac disease. *J Pediatr.* 2013;163(3):896–901.e1-3.

Kleinman ME, et al. Part 14: pediatric advanced life support. 2010 American Heart Association guidelines for cardiopulmonary resuscitation and emergency cardiovascular care. *Circulation.* 2010;122(suppl 3):S876–S908.

Link MS. Evaluation and initial treatment of supraventricular tachycardia. *N Engl J Med.* 2012;367: 1438–1448.

CASE 5

A Newborn Presenting With Profound Cyanosis

Aslam Khan ▪ Lindsey Miller ▪ Merujan Uzunyan

A girl is born at 35 weeks and 3 days gestation to a 26-year-old mother. Minimal prenatal care was given prior to delivery. She is born under considerable distress and is apneic on delivery. The child is noted to be cyanotic, with pulse oximetry measuring oxygen saturation of 50%. Initial resuscitation efforts are focused on ensuring adequate ventilation, but despite 100% inspired oxygen delivered via endotracheal tube, with evidence of gas exchange via carbon dioxide detector, the oxygen saturation remains at approximately 70%.

What are the causes of cyanosis in a neonate?

There are multiple causes of cyanosis (hypoxemia) in the neonate, commonly categorized by whether central or peripheral distribution of cyanosis is prominent. Central cyanosis can be visualized with a change of color on the lips and under the tongue. Central cyanosis can be caused by cardiac disease, pulmonary disease, or central nervous system (CNS) depression. Early central cyanosis is more likely secondary to cardiac causes, such as congenital heart disease with shunting of deoxygenated blood to the systemic circulation (i.e., right-to-left shunt); or it may have a pulmonary cause, such as parenchymal lung disease, pneumothorax, diaphragmatic hernia, or persistent pulmonary hypertension of the newborn. CNS causes are secondary to perinatal asphyxia, heavy maternal sedation, and intrauterine fetal distress.

Peripheral cyanosis can be caused by peripheral vasoconstriction in conditions such as hypothermia, shock, sepsis, or heart failure. It is more commonly seen in neonates as acrocyanosis, which is cyanosis restricted to the hands and feet and the perioral region. Acrocyanosis is a normal finding at birth that is thought to be due to vasomotor instability, and it can last hours to weeks.

BASIC SCIENCE PEARL	**STEP 1**

Cyanosis, or a bluish discoloration of the skin and other tissues, is due to capillary circulation of deoxygenated hemoglobin.

CLINICAL PEARL	**STEP 2/3**

Acrocyanosis, or cyanosis of only the hands and feet, is essentially universal at birth and resolves in 1 to 2 days.

Case Point 5.1

The physical examination reveals a dusky infant with a heart rate of 174 beats/min. A single S2 sound and harsh continuous murmur are appreciated. Although breath sounds are coarse, no focal lung findings are noted. No pallor is noted. Pulses are palpably strong in all extremities, and capillary refill is brisk.

A cardiac lesion is suspected.

What congenital cardiac malformations are suspected in the setting of cyanosis? What malformations are suspected in the setting of cardiogenic shock?

Cyanosis in heart disease occurs when obstruction to right ventricular outflow causes intracardiac right-to-left shunting or when there is a mixture of pulmonary and systemic venous return in the heart. Shunting in the above conditions may exist due to the persistence of fetal pathways such as a patent foramen ovale and ductus arteriosus, especially in the setting of pulmonary stenosis.

The five cyanotic congenital heart diseases usually referenced include *t*runcus arteriosus, *t*ransposition of the great arteries, *t*ricuspid atresia, *t*etralogy of Fallot, and *t*otal anomalous pulmonary venous return—the five Ts. Additional cardiac malformations include single-ventricle physiologies, a double-outlet right ventricle, pulmonary atresia, variations on the five Ts, such as partial anomalous pulmonary venous return, and other complex malformations. The latter is often associated with heterotaxy syndromes.

Any critical left-sided obstruction can present with symptoms of both cyanosis and heart failure leading to cardiogenic shock. Hypoplastic left heart syndrome (mitral or aortic valve atresia) is the classic example, although interrupted aortic arch and critical aortic stenosis are also possible causes.

BASIC SCIENCE   **STEP 1**

A commonly used mnemonic for cyanotic congenital heart disease is the five Ts—*t*runcus arteriosus, *t*ransposition of the great arteries, *t*ricuspid atresia, *t*etralogy of Fallot, and *t*otal anomalous pulmonary venous return. However, these five conditions do not encompass all the possible cardiac malformation syndromes presenting with cyanosis.

Case Point 5.2

A chest X-ray (CXR) and electrocardiogram (ECG) are obtained (Figs. 5.1 and 5.2).

What is the differential diagnosis given the above findings? What is the next step?

The physical examination and CXR suggest a cardiac cause of cyanosis because no pulmonary lesions are heard or seen. The continuous murmur suggests a patent ductus arteriosus (PDA)–dependent lesion. With decreased pulmonary vascularity, the differential includes disease processes with decreased pulmonary blood flow. Additionally, with relative left axis deviation on the ECG, it is reasonable to consider cardiac lesions resulting in pulmonary vasculature outflow obstruction (e.g., pulmonary stenosis or atresia or truncus arteriosus).

If not already performed (as in this case), a trial of 100% oxygen may help differentiate between central and peripheral causes of cyanosis, with the latter causes often responding to the increased inspired oxygen fraction. If possible, an echocardiogram should be obtained quickly to delineate

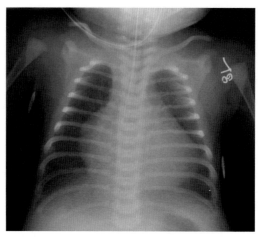

Fig. 5.1 This chest radiograph shows an enlarged cardiac silhouette and normal pulmonary vascularity. An endotracheal tube is also observed.

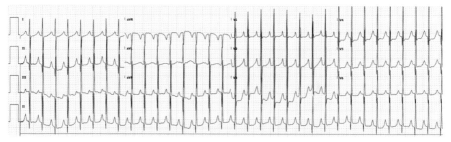

Fig. 5.2 Electrocardiogram shows relative left axis deviation. Neonates have rightward deviation compared to adults.

cardiac anatomy and obtain a diagnosis. Nevertheless, prostaglandin E1 (alprostadil) needs to be started to maintain a PDA. Finally, because sepsis has not yet been ruled out, empiric antibiotics should be given.

Case Point 5.3

A continuous infusion of alprostadil is started to maintain patency of the ductus arteriosus. Echocardiography reveals an atretic pulmonary valve with an intact ventricular septum and right ventricular hypoplasia (Fig. 5.3).

Diagnosis: Pulmonary atresia with intact ventricular septum (PA-IVS)

CLINICAL PEARL   **STEP 2/3**

With widespread use of fetal echocardiography, PA-IVS will often be diagnosed prior to birth. If the diagnosis is made prior to birth, delivery should be performed in a facility with a cardiac intensive care unit.

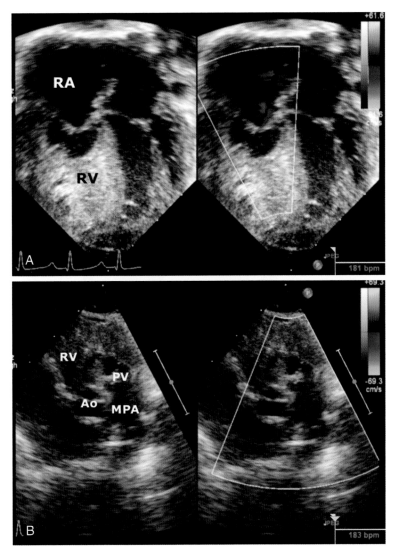

Fig. 5.3 Echocardiogram of the patient. (A) This four-chamber view shows a hypoplastic right ventricle. (B) The short-axis view shows an atretic pulmonary valve, with absence of flow into the main pulmonary artery. *Ao,* Aorta; *MPA,* main pulmonary artery; *PV,* pulmonary valve; *RA,* right atrium; *RV,* right ventricle.

What is the pathophysiology of pulmonary atresia with an intact ventricular septum?
In normal fetal circulation, oxygenated blood from the placenta shunts preferentially through the foramen ovale to the left atrium and then through the left ventricle and systemic circulation. Additionally, deoxygenated blood from the superior vena cava (SVC) passes through the right ventricle (RV) and the pulmonary artery (PA) through the PDA and aorta to reach the head and neck vessels. The remaining 10% of blood flow supply the lungs and shunts.

With PA-IVS, the blood supply traverses entirely from the right atrium (RA) through the foramen ovale to the left atrium and systemic circuit (Fig. 5.4). The blood supply to the lungs is

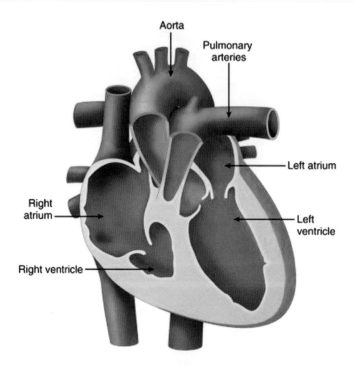

Fig. 5.4 Pathophysiology of pulmonary atresia with intact ventricular septum (PA-IVS). There is no blood flow from the right ventricle to the pulmonary arteries. All blood flow into the pulmonary arteries originates from the aorta via the ductus arteriosus. (From Szwast A. Pulmonary atresia with intact ventricular septum. *Fetal Cardiovasc Imaging.* 2012;25:275–286.)

entirely dependent on the ductus arteriosus, even after birth, and cyanosis (followed by death) will occur as the ductus arteriosus closes. The ductus itself will be small due to reduced blood flow during fetal life. Although a small amount of blood can pass from the RA to the RV, this blood will regurgitate back to the RA, given the intact ventricular septum and atretic pulmonary valve.

Given that there is no blood flow past the RV, it is hypoplastic, with a smaller cavity size. The musculature may be hypertrophied. Similarly, the proximal peripheral pulmonary arteries are not filling in typical fashion and are thus smaller. Additionally, coronary blood flow is compromised given the minimal flow through the aorta, which supplies coronary blood flow during diastole in normal anatomy.

BASIC SCIENCE PEARL	STEP 1

RV hypoplasia refers to the size of the RV cavity. The musculature is often hypertrophied, although it may be dilated.

BASIC SCIENCE PEARL	STEP 1

PA-IVS is the third most common of the cyanotic congenital heart diseases presenting in infancy, after transposition of the great arteries and tetralogy of Fallot.

How does the pathophysiology explain the physical examination, CXR, and ECG findings?
A patient with PA-IVS will present with cyanosis and a murmur. Tachypnea may be present due to hypoxia. As deoxygenated blood mixes with oxygenated blood at the level of the atrium, cyanosis will persist, even if the patient inspires pure oxygen.

Mild enlargement of the RA may be present due to regurgitant blood increasing the volume passing through the RA. This will manifest on the ECG as peaked P waves on leads I, II, and aVF and relative left axis deviation and will manifest on the CXR as normal or decreased pulmonary vascularity. Pulmonary blood flow is dependent on a PDA and collateral blood flow. There can be a systolic murmur due to tricuspid regurgitation, and a continuous, machine-like murmur can be heard from the PDA. The S2 heart sound is single and loud because the patient has a single semilunar valve.

BASIC SCIENCE PEARL   **STEP 1**

The ductal-dependent nature of blood flow in PA-IVS is due to the intact ventricular septum, leaving no outlet for the right ventricle. When PA is accompanied by a ventricular septal defect, the resulting defect—known as tetralogy of Fallot—causes intermittent right-to-left shunting and therefore only intermittent cyanosis.

BASIC SCIENCE/CLINICAL PEARL   **STEP 1/2/3**

Although the continuous murmur originating from the PDA would be expected to be the most prominent, an additional midsystolic murmur indicative of tricuspid regurgitation may also be appreciated.

CLINICAL PEARL   **STEP 2/3**

Cyanosis and PDA murmur may wax and wane with intermittent closure of the PDA. Eventually, the PDA will close permanently, which will be associated with deep cyanosis, disappearance of the murmur (and eventually death).

What other cardiac anomaly is associated with PA-IVS?
In addition to RA enlargement, RV hypertrophy, hypoplastic RV, or a dysplastic or stenotic tricuspid valve, there can be coronary abnormalities in up to 80% of patients, leading to significant morbidity. In normal physiology, the heart is perfused by diastolic flow from the aorta to the coronary arteries. In patients with PA-IVS, however, fistula formation with the coronaries and right ventricle, the absence of an aorta and coronary connection, and stenosis or connections between the left and right coronaries have all been described.

What is the next step?
Children with pulmonary atresia should be managed in a tertiary care center specializing in congenital cardiac care; transfer is therefore necessary after achieving hemodynamic stability by mimicking fetal circulation with prostaglandin E1 infusion if the patient is not already at a suitable care center.

The child may then undergo balloon atrial septostomy to improve right-to-left atrial shunting (modified atrial septal defect [ASD]), or insertion of a modified Blalock-Taussig shunt, which creates a connection with from the aorta to the pulmonary artery. The latter functions as a surgical PDA.

Once an initial surgery is performed, the child will need to be monitored closely while she or he grows large enough for further corrective surgery. The most common palliative procedures are insertion of a cavopulmonary shunt, followed by atriopulmonary anastomosis (Glenn and Fontan procedures, respectively); these result in a single-ventricle physiology. Biventricular repair is sometimes preferred, depending on the presence of coronary artery abnormalities, viability of the right ventricle, and level of atresia to the pulmonary valve.

Case Point 5.4

After diagnosis and stabilization, the child underwent balloon atrial septostomy and insertion of a modified Blalock-Taussig shunt. Plans were made for cavopulmonary anastomosis (Glenn procedure) to be performed at 6 months of age, followed by atriopulmonary anastomosis (Fontan procedure) at 3 years of age.

BEYOND THE PEARLS

- The ECG showing an adult pattern with the frontal plane axis more leftward than expected for a neonate suggests RV hypoplasia.
- Outcomes for those with pulmonary atresia with intact ventricular septum (PA-IVS) have been slowly improving, with recent overall survival at 5 years increasing to above 60%. Survival is higher for those who can undergo biventricular repair when compared with those for whom univentricular palliation is the only viable repair.
- Without any operative intervention, almost all children with PA-IVS will die in the first month of life. For the few who are able to survive into adulthood, the continuous right-to-left shunting will eventually result in Eisenmenger's physiology.
- In patients undergoing univentricular staged repair, cyanosis will persist throughout all stages prior to the Fontan procedure due to partial right-to-left shunting. Cyanosis after the Fontan procedure would not be expected, however, and, if present, would be an indication for further investigation.
- Post–univentricular palliation, patients remain at risk for a variety of complications throughout their lifetime, including heart failure, thrombosis, renal failure, liver disease, and protein-losing enteropathy.
- In patients with an adequately sized right ventricle, open surgery may be avoided entirely using percutaneous methods of pulmonary valve perforation to achieve biventricular repair. Wire, laser, and radiofrequency methods have all been described.

Case Summary

Complaint/History: A girl born at 35 weeks is apneic on delivery.

Findings: A single S2 sound and harsh continuous murmur.

Labs/Tests: Echocardiography reveals an atretic pulmonary valve, with an intact ventricular septum and right ventricular hypoplasia.

Diagnosis: Pulmonary atresia with intact ventricular septum.

Treatment: Balloon atrial septostomy and insertion of a modified Blalock-Taussig shunt, with planned multistage palliation surgery.

Bibliography

Ashburn DA, et al. Determinants of mortality and type of repair in neonates with pulmonary atresia and intact ventricular septum. *J Thorac Cardiovasc Surg.* 2004;127(4):1000–1007.

Daubeney PE, et al. Pulmonary atresia with intact ventricular septum: range of morphology in a population-based study. *J Am Coll Cardiol.* 2002;39(10):1670–1679.

Kliegman Robert. Pulmonary atresia with intact ventricular septum. In: *Nelson Textbook of Pediatrics.* 19th ed. Philadelphia: Elsevier/Saunders; 2011:1578–1579.

Lees Martin H, King Douglas H. Cyanosis in the newborn. *Pediatr Rev.* 1987;9(2):36–42.

Sasidharan Ponthenkandath P. An approach to diagnosis and management of cyanosis and tachypnea in term infants. *Pediatr Clin North Am.* 2004;51(4):999–1021.

4-Month-Old Male With Multiple Fractures

Jocelyn Supan ▦ Audrey Ahn ▦ Marc J. Weigensberg ▦
Paola Sequeira

A 4-month-old, ex–full-term African-American infant is brought in by ambulance to the emergency department (ED) after his mother witnessed him become unresponsive at home. The patient had just woken up from a nap and had one episode of nonprojectile, milk-colored emesis, immediately followed by stiffening of both arms, apnea, facial cyanosis, and both eyes rolling back into his head.

Upon arrival to the ED, his vital signs are significant for a temperature of 38.4°C and a pulse rate of 182/min. The physical examination reveals mild nasal congestion but is otherwise unremarkable. The workup to evaluate for the cause of the event is unrevealing and the cause is presumed to be due to a brief choking episode.

A serum chemistry panel is notable for an elevated alkaline phosphatase level of 987 U/L. The chest radiograph (CXR) reveals multiple healed posterior rib fractures (Fig. 6.1).

What is the differential diagnosis in an infant with multiple fractures?

There are many causes for multiple fractures, including genetic diseases such as osteogenesis imperfecta or neurofibromatosis type 1, but it is important to consider the possibility of nonaccidental trauma (a form of child abuse) in young children who present with multiple fractures or unexplained bruises, regardless of whether or not trauma was reported by the caregiver. There should also be a higher index of suspicion in infants who are nonambulatory.

The presence of metabolic bone disease must also be considered because this can also cause multiple fractures from increased bony turnover, as indicated by the markedly elevated alkaline phosphatase level.

BASIC SCIENCE/CLINICAL PEARL   **STEP 1**

Alkaline phosphatase levels vary with age and are higher in children when compared to adults due to increased osteoblast activity. The highest levels are typically seen in infants and adolescents, which coincide with periods of highest bone growth velocity.

Case Point 6.1

Due to concern for nonaccidental trauma, a further workup is performed. No evidence of abuse is found; however, skeletal survey radiographs show diffusely decreased bone mineral density, without associated metaphyseal fraying or physeal widening.

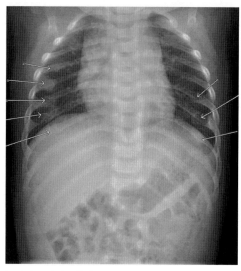

Fig. 6.1 Multiple healed posterior rib fractures are noted on the chest radiograph *(arrows).*

TABLE 6.1 ■ Simplified Differential Diagnosis of Decreased Bone Mineral Density with High Alkaline Phosphatase

	Level of:				
	Serum Calcium	Serum Phosphorus	Alkaline Phosphatase	Parathyroid Hormone	25(OH)-vitamin D
Vitamin D deficiency	N/↓	N/↓	↑	↑	↓
Nutritional (calcium, phosphorus) deficiency (e.g., rickets of prematurity)	N/↓	N/↓	↑	N/↑	N
Hypophosphatemic rickets	N	↓	↑	N	N

N, Normal.
Adapted from Chesney RW. Metabolic bone disease. *Pediatr Rev.* 1984;5:227–237.

What is the differential diagnosis in this patient with decreased bone mineralization?
The differential diagnosis for decreased bone mineralization includes disorders resulting in low total body calcium or phosphorus, summarized in Table 6.1.

The primary cause of low total body calcium in children is vitamin D deficiency. Nutritional vitamin D deficiency is most common, and secondary vitamin D deficiencies due to malabsorption, degradation, decreased hydroxylation, chronic kidney disease, and genetic mutations are also seen. Inadequate dietary calcium intake and malabsorption of calcium are also seen due to a low-calcium diet or milk allergy and malabsorptive disorders (e.g., celiac disease, cystic fibrosis, cholestatic liver disease, short bowel).

Low total body phosphorus is generally seen in cases of renal wasting, such as that due to Fanconi syndrome—global proximal tubule dysfunction—which is typically characterized by hypophosphatemia and phosphaturia. It can also be due to inadequate dietary phosphorus intake, malabsorptive disorders, and genetic disorders (e.g., X-linked, autosomal dominant, and autosomal recessive hypophosphatemic rickets; hereditary hypophosphatemic rickets with hypercalciuria).

BASIC SCIENCE/CLINICAL PEARL   **STEP 1/2/3**

Total body stores of calcium and phosphorus are not necessarily reflected by serum levels, except in severe deficiencies.

Case Point 6.2

Upon taking further history, the patient's mother states that he is exclusively breast-fed, without supplemental vitamin D. His family history is significant for vitamin D deficiency in several family members, including his mother.

The serum calcium level is 9.6 mg/dL (normal, 8.8–10.8 mg/dL). The phosphorus level is 4.3 mg/dL (normal, 3.8–6.8 mg/dL). The parathyroid hormone (PTH) level is 111 (normal, 10–60 pg/mL). The 25(OH)-vitamin D level is less than 12 ng/mL, which is the threshold of detection with this assay (normal > 20 ng/mL).

What is the significance of the vitamin D level?

Vitamin D is a fat-soluble vitamin that is derived from two natural sources, the skin and diet. There are two forms of vitamin D: vitamin D_2 (ergocalciferol, synthesized by plants) and vitamin D_3 (cholecalciferol, synthesized by mammals). The main source of vitamin D for humans is vitamin D_3, which is produced via exposure to ultraviolet B radiation in sunlight. This converts 7-dehydrocholesterol that is naturally present in skin to cholecalciferol, which subsequently binds to vitamin D–binding protein (DBP). This complex is transported to the liver, where 25-hydroxylase acts to convert it to 25-hydroxyvitamin D—25(OH)-D, known as *calcidiol*—which is then released back into the circulation and transported to the kidney bound to DBP. Once in the kidney, 25(OH)-D undergoes a second hydroxylation by 1-α-hydroxylase to become 1,25-dihydroxyvitamin D—1,25(OH)$_2$-D, known as *calcitriol*—the metabolically active form of vitamin D.

BASIC SCIENCE/CLINICAL PEARL   **STEP 1**

25-Hydroxylation of vitamin D occurs in the liver, and subsequent 1α-hydroxylation occurs in the kidney.

Vitamin D status is based on 25(OH)-D levels, as defined by the 2016 global consensus recommendations:
- Sufficiency: More than 20 ng/mL (>50 nmol/L)
- Insufficiency: 12 to 20 ng/mL (30–50 nmol/L)
- Deficiency: Less than 12 ng/mL (<30 nmol/L)

BASIC SCIENCE/CLINICAL PEARL   **STEP 1/2/3**

Direct measurement of vitamin D levels has no clinical utility due to the short half-life of vitamin D. Measurement of its direct metabolite, 25-hydroxyvitamin D—25(OH)-D—is used instead due to its long half-life and serum level stability.

Case Point 6.3

Diagnosis: Vitamin D deficiency and osteopenia.

What is the differential diagnosis for vitamin D deficiency?

Nutritional 25(OH)-D deficiency is the most common cause of rickets worldwide and often occurs in infants because of several risk factors that are specific to the perinatal period. Exclusively breast-fed infants are at increased risk for deficiency due to the low vitamin D content in breast milk, which is worsened if the mother is also deficient. Low vitamin D levels at birth may result from maternal vitamin D deficiency, as well as from premature birth, because the third trimester is a critical time for vitamin D and calcium transfer; this is when the fetal skeleton becomes calcified. Dark-skinned infants are also at higher risk for deficiency due to the increased amount of melanin, which, as a natural sunblock, reduces vitamin D synthesis.

There are also secondary causes of 25(OH)-D deficiency, such as inadequate intestinal absorption, decreased hydroxylation in the liver, and increased degradation. Patients with liver and gastrointestinal diseases (e.g., Crohn disease, cystic fibrosis, celiac disease, cholestatic liver disease, defects in bile acid metabolism) are particularly susceptible to vitamin D deficiency, both from fat malabsorption and a decrease in 25-hydroxylase activity. Medications including antiepileptics (e.g., phenobarbital, phenytoin, carbamazepine) and antituberculosis medications (e.g., isoniazid, rifampin) that induce the cytochrome P450 system also increase the risk of deficiency because they increase the degradation of vitamin D.

Vitamin D–dependent rickets, type 1, is an autosomal recessive disorder that results in a mutation causing decreased 1-α-hydroxylase activity. Unlike patients with classic vitamin D deficiency, they will have a normal 25(OH)-D level but a low 1,25(OH)$_2$-D level. Patients with hypoparathyroidism will also have low 1,25(OH)$_2$-D levels due to the decrease in parathyroid hormone (PTH) available to stimulate 1-α-hydroxylase activity in the kidney.

What are the recommendations for an adequate daily intake of calcium and vitamin D?

The recommendations for adequate daily intake of calcium and vitamin D, as outlined by the Food and Nutrition Board, National Research Council of the National Academy of Sciences, vary according to the age of the child.

Infants 0 to 12 months of age require 400 IU of vitamin D/day to prevent rickets and to maintain vitamin D concentrations at more than 20 ng/mL. All exclusively breast-fed infants will require supplementation to achieve adequate intake, beginning within a few days after birth and continuing until the infant is weaned. In 2010, the Institute of Medicine recommended daily allowance increases to 600 IU/day for healthy children 1 to 18 years of age. Natural dietary sources of vitamin D include fatty fish (e.g., salmon, mackerel, sardines), cod liver oil, and egg yolks. Fortified sources include infant formula, milk, some breakfast cereals, and breads.

CLINICAL PEARL   **STEP 2/3**

Few foods naturally contain vitamin D. Most children in industrialized countries receive vitamin D via fortified foods.

Infants 0 to 6 months of age require 200 mg of calcium/day, which increases to 260 mg at 6 to 12 months of age. At 1 year of age, the calcium requirement nearly triples to 700 mg. It increases to 1000 mg at 4 years of age and hits a peak of 1300 mg during the teenage years.

BASIC SCIENCE/CLINICAL PEARL   **STEP 1/2/3**

Calcium and vitamin D requirements during childhood are highest in the adolescent years to ensure maximal bone mineralization during this period of rapid growth.

BASIC SCIENCE/CLINICAL PEARL   **STEP 1/2/3**

Although adequate vitamin D levels can be obtained via sunlight exposure alone, the increased risk of sun damage and cancer generally outweigh the benefits of vitamin D photosynthesis when considering the ease of adequate dietary intake for most people.

BASIC SCIENCE/CLINICAL PEARL   **STEP 1/2/3**

Vitamin D supplementation can be taken to excess, a condition known as *hypervitaminosis D.* Hypercalcemia and hypercalciuria can be seen and—in severe cases—diffuse calcifications throughout the body.

What is the treatment for vitamin D deficiency?

High-dose replacement therapy should be initiated with either ergocalciferol or cholecalciferol at 2000 to 5000 IU/day for at least 8 to 12 weeks. Once treatment is complete, patients should be continued on supplemental vitamin D daily (400 IU/day for infants < 1 year or 600 IU/day for children ≥ 1 year). Infants should be monitored regularly on an outpatient basis.

Calcium supplementation should also be started if the patient has an elevated PTH level or evidence of rickets due to risk for so-called hungry bone syndrome, a phenomenon caused by the normalization of PTH levels, which leads to increased bone mineralization and precipitates hypocalcemia. The recommended dosage of oral elemental calcium is 30 to 75 mg/kg per day divided into three doses. In children who exhibit symptomatic hypocalcemia, intravenous calcium is required.

Case Point 6.4

The patient is started on 4000 IU/day of vitamin D, as well as calcium to prevent hungry bone syndrome. He is discharged home with close endocrinology follow-up given his risk for developing rickets.

What is the ultimate outcome of decreased bone mineralization if left untreated?

Prior to epiphyseal closure in late childhood, failure of mineralization while the growth plate cartilage and osteoid continue to expand causes growth plate thickening and circumferential increases of the growth plate and metaphysis, seen as widening of the wrists and ankles on radiography (Fig. 6.2). Softening of the bones is also seen, causing them to bend easily after being subjected to weight bearing or muscle pull. This results in a constellation of bone deformities known as *rickets.*

Deformities seen include delayed fontanelle closure, craniotabes (soft skull bones), frontal bossing, widening of the costochondral junctions (so-called rachitic rosary), and genu varum (bow legs) or valgum (knock knees; Fig. 6.3). Patients may also present with bone pain, irritability, motor delay, poor growth, delayed tooth eruption, and an increased susceptibility to infections—vitamin D modulates B and T lymphocyte function.

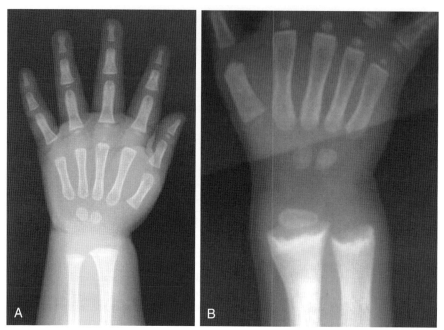

Fig. 6.2 (A) A normal wrist x-ray. (B) An abnormal wrist x-ray consistent with rickets. Note the widening, cupping, and fraying of the distal radius and ulna and the increased thickness of the growth plate. (From Greenbaum LA. Rickets and hypervitaminosis D. In: Kliegman R, Stanton B, St. Geme J, Schor N (eds): *Nelson Textbook of Pediatrics*. St. Louis: Elsevier; 2015:331–341.e1.)

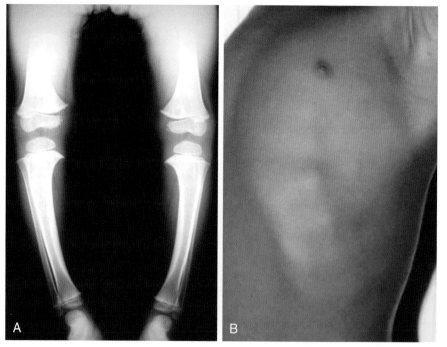

Fig. 6.3 (A) Bowing of the lower extremities (genu varum) in a child with rickets. (B) Rachitic rosary. (Courtesy T. Thacher, MD.)

BEYOND THE PEARLS

- Because humans (and most vertebrates) are able to synthesize sufficient vitamin D via photosynthesis in the skin, vitamin D is not a true vitamin.
- Commercially available supplemental vitamin D is produced via the irradiation of 7-dehyro-cholesterol (or ergosterol), a process that mimics ultraviolet (UV) photosynthesis in the skin.
- Unlike excessive dietary consumption of vitamin D, excessive sun exposure will almost never result in hypervitaminosis D because a negative feedback loop results in degradation of cutaneous vitamin D prior to entry into the circulation.
- The receptor for vitamin D resides in the cell nucleus and is a direct transcription factor.
- The optimal serum level of 25(OH)-D in relation to the risk of rickets is not known, but results of case series have associated rickets with 25(OH)-D levels below 10 mg/dL. Experts agree that 20 ng/mL is the minimum level for sufficient vitamin D.
- Persons with chronic renal failure develop a bone disease known as *renal osteodystrophy.* Because patients with renal osteodystrophy, by definition, do not have adequate renal function and thus do not have 1α-hydroxylation function, supplementation must be in the form of 1,25(OH)$_2$D or another biologically active analogue.

Case Summary

Complaint/History: A 4-month old is evaluated in the emergency department for brief unresponsiveness that is attributed to a brief choking episode.

Findings: Nasal congestion, otherwise unremarkable examination. The chest x-ray reveals multiple healed posterior rib fractures, and a serum chemistry panel is notable for an elevated alkaline phosphatase level of 987 U/L.

Labs/Tests: The parathyroid hormone level is elevated, and 25(OH)-vitamin D is undetectably low.

Diagnosis: Vitamin D deficiency and osteopenia.

Treatment: Vitamin D (high-dose) replacement therapy.

Bibliography

Gallo S, et al. Effect of different dosages of oral vitamin D supplementation on vitamin D status in healthy, breastfed infants: a randomized trial. *JAMA.* 2013;309.17:1785–1792.

Misra M, et al. Vitamin D deficiency in children and its management: review of current knowledge and recommendations. *Pediatrics.* 2008;122:398–417.

Munns Craig F, et al. Global consensus recommendations on prevention and management of nutritional rickets. *Hormone research in paediatrics.* 2016;85.2:83–106.

Ross AC, Taylo CL, Yaktine AL, Del Valle HB, eds. *Dietary Reference Intakes for Calcium and Vitamin D. Institute of Medicine of the National Academies.* Washington, DC: The National Academies Press; 2011. https://doi.org/10.17226/13050.2013.

Tieder JS, Bonkowsky JL, Etzel RA, et al. Clinical practice guideline: brief resolved unexplained events (Formerly apparent Life-Threatening Events) and evaluation of lower-risk infants. *Pediatrics.* 2016;137(5).

Wagner C, Greer F. Prevention of rickets and vitamin D deficiency in infants, children, and adolescents. *Pediatrics.* 2008;122(5):1142–1152.

13-Month-Old With Persistent Fever

John Harlow ▪ Swetha Ramachandran ▪ Randall Y. Chan ▪ James Homans ▪ Stephanie K. Zia

A 13-month-old male presents with 10 days of fever, fussiness, and cough. The patient was seen multiple times by his primary care physician, but thus far no source of fever has been found.

What is the differential diagnosis for a toddler with persistent fever lasting longer than 7 days?

Infections are the most common cause of persistent fever in children. Common viral infections implicated in persistent fever include adenovirus, enteroviruses, cytomegalovirus (CMV), Epstein-Barr virus (EBV), and hepatitis viruses. Bacterial infections causing persistent fever include *Mycobacterium tuberculosis*, *Bartonella henselae* (cat scratch disease), and *Salmonella*, *Brucella*, and *Rickettsia* spp. Invasive fungal infections (e.g., coccidiomycosis, blastomycosis, histoplasmosis), and parasitic infections (e.g., toxoplasmosis, malaria) are less common.

Localizing symptoms may point to infection of particular organ systems, including upper respiratory tract infections, urinary tract infections, infective endocarditis, osteomyelitis, and intraabdominal abscesses.

Rheumatologic causes of persistent fever include juvenile idiopathic arthritis (JIA), polyarteritis nodosa, and systemic lupus erythematosus. Malignancies such as leukemia and lymphoma should also be considered but are less common and frequently have manifestations other than fever. Other potential causes include drug fever, periodic fever, thyrotoxicosis, inflammatory bowel disease, hemophagocytic lymphohistiocytosis (HLH), and Kawasaki disease.

Despite an appropriate history, physical examination, and laboratory testing, many cases of persistent fever go undiagnosed.

BASIC SCIENCE/CLINICAL PEARL	STEP 1/2/3

Uncommon presentations of common illnesses are more common than common presentations of uncommon illnesses.

What questions are important to help narrow the differential diagnosis?

The fever pattern should be explored in detail. Questions regarding the duration, height, and pattern of the fever, how the fever was assessed, if the child appears ill or develops any other signs or symptoms during the febrile episode, whether the fever responds to antipyretic medication, and if the child returns to baseline between episodes are all helpful in pinpointing the cause of the fever.

Intermittent fevers with high spikes and rapid defervescence suggest pyogenic infection (but can also occur in patients with tuberculosis and JIA), whereas sustained fevers persisting with little or no fluctuation are suggestive of typhoid fever, typhus, or brucellosis. Relapsing fevers with 1 or more days between febrile episodes are characteristically seen with malaria. Fever is also a common reaction to drugs, and virtually any medication can cause a drug fever. When taking a medication history, it is important to include prescription, over-the-counter, and illicit drugs, as well as nutritional supplements and/or alternative therapies.

Information about sick contacts and specific exposures, including animals, recent travel, food consumption, behaviors, and medications may also be informative. For example, tuberculosis is more likely in patients living in endemic areas. Many fungal infections are endemic to specific regions of the world—for example, in the United States, *Coccidioides* sp. is found in the Southwest and the Central Valley of California, *Histoplasma capsulatum* is found in the central and southern United States and Mississippi and Ohio River Valleys, and *Blastomyces dermatitidis* is found in the upper Midwest and Great Lakes states. Tick bites can be suggestive of Lyme disease or Rocky Mountain spotted fever. Direct contact with cats (cat scratch disease, toxoplasmosis), rodents (tularemia), bird feces (psittacosis, cryptococcosis, histoplasmosis), opossums or rats (endemic typhus), and pet reptiles (salmonellosis), as well as consumption of raw meat or shellfish, can put children at risk for the respective listed infections. Additionally, recent international travel can put patients at risk for infections such as malaria, Zika virus, or dengue fever.

What physical examination findings are important to help narrow the differential diagnosis?

Localized signs and symptoms may be revealing. Bilateral nonexudative conjunctivitis with cracked red lips, a strawberry tongue, and edematous hands and feet in a child with an unexplained fever of more than 5 days is suggestive of Kawasaki disease. Limb or bone pain can be present in leukemia and osteomyelitis, but may be hard to determine in children who cannot vocalize their symptoms. Recurrent pharyngitis with ulcerations may suggest periodic fever with aphthous stomatitis, pharyngitis, and adenitis (PFAPA) syndrome.

A thorough skin examination may be revealing as well. Skin lesions and rashes are common in a number of conditions that can cause a prolonged fever and should be asked about because they can be transient. The macular salmon pink rash of JIA may be present only during fever and is characteristically evanescent. The rash of Rocky Mountain spotted fever typically begins distally on the palms and soles and spreads centrally to the trunk. Petechiae can be seen in infective endocarditis and bacteremia. Papular lesions in cat scratch disease, eschar in tularemia, and erythema migrans in tickborne diseases are all important skin findings that can help determine the cause of a prolonged fever.

Case Point 7.1

The mother states that the fever has been constant, although temporarily relieved by acetaminophen for 3 to 4 hours. The patient has taken no other drugs and has had no sick contacts or animal exposures. The patient's mother has not noted any conjunctivitis, rash, petechiae, ulcer, or other skin lesions. She denies any additional symptoms.

On examination, the patient was noted to have mild gingival bleeding, heart murmur, mild pallor, and moderate splenomegaly. He was noted to have fevers to 40°C. During febrile episodes, he displays marked tachycardia, diminished perfusion, and evidence of systemic toxicity.

What laboratory tests are warranted in this patient?

Although a completely nonfocal examination would point you to an infectious cause and a full workup for fever of unknown origin (FUO), the pallor and murmur suggest anemia, and the gum bleeding suggests thrombocytopenia. A complete blood count (CBC) with differential and visual examination of a peripheral blood smear would therefore be indicated to confirm depressions in these cell lineages.

In FUO, a full chemistry panel—including transaminases—is frequently helpful, because abnormalities may suggest certain processes. For example, elevated transaminase levels, although nonspecific, suggest a process that affects the liver. Urinalysis may reveal an infectious source as well. Multiple sets of blood cultures (at least three) should be sent when the patient is febrile, given the low sensitivity of a single culture.

Case Point 7.2

Laboratory tests are performed (Table 7.1).

What is the significance of the laboratory findings?

Our patient presents with fever, pancytopenia and splenomegaly, which expands the differential to hematologic malignancies such as leukemia and lymphoma. The remarkably elevated serum ferritin level (particularly >3000 ng/mL), however, should trigger consideration for HLH, a clinical syndrome resulting from dysregulated and self-damaging inflammation occurring in the setting of an underlying immune deficiency. The normal ability of T cells to induce apoptosis in activated immune cells leads to a self-amplifying cycle because the immune system essentially loses its ability to self-regulate. Excessive immune activation leads to dysfunction of macrophages and natural killer (NK) cells which produces a cytokine storm and eventual tissue destruction, with multiple organ involvement.

TABLE 7.1 ■ **Laboratory Values on Presentation**

Laboratory Test	Patient's Laboratory Values
White blood cell count	0.9×10^9/L
Hemoglobin	6.8 g/dL
Platelet count	71×10^9/L
Absolute neutrophil count	400×10^6/L
Absolute lymphocyte count	400×10^6/L
AST	364 U/L
ALT	179 U/L
Ferritin	5,333 ng/mL
Prothrombin time	15.4 sec
Activated partial thromboplastin time	35.8 sec
Fibrinogen	98 mg/dL
Triglycerides	846 mg/dL
Blood cultures	No growth
EBV IgM	Not detected
EBV IgG	Not detected
EBV PCR	92,150 copies/mL
Natural killer cell function	Decreased

ALT, Alanine aminotransferase; *AST,* aspartate aminotransferase; *EBV,* Epstein-Barr virus; *IgG,* immunoglobulin G; *IgM,* immunoglobulin M; *PCR,* polymerase chain reaction.

Using the diagnostic criteria from the international HLH-2004 trial, diagnosis of HLH can be made with definitive molecular array or with five or more of eight clinical criteria, as follows:

- Fever
- Splenomegaly
- Cytopenia affecting at least two of the three lineages in the peripheral blood (hemoglobin < 9 g/dL or hemoglobin < 10 g/dL in neonates, platelets < 100×10^9/L, neutrophils < 1000×10^6/L)
- Hypertriglyceridemia and/or hypofibrinogenemia (fasting triglyceride levels ≥ 265 mg/dL, fibrinogen < 1.5 g)
- Ferritin ≥ 500 ng/mL
- Hemophagocytosis in the bone marrow, spleen, or lymph nodes, with no sign of malignancy.
- Low or absent NK cell activity.
- Soluble CD25 > 2400 U/mL

CLINICAL PEARL   **STEP 2/3**

Ferritin is an acute-phase reactant, and thus mild to moderate elevation is nonspecific. Studies on HLH have shown that a ferritin level more than 10,000 ng/mL has a 90% sensitivity and 96% specificity for HLH in children; however, in adults, it is not nearly as useful.

Case Point 7.3

The diagnosis of HLH is considered based on the fever, splenomegaly, and pancytopenia in the setting of hyperferritinemia. A bone marrow examination is performed (Fig. 7.1).

Diagnosis: Hemophagocytic lymphohistiocytosis (HLH).

What is the cause of HLH? What infections are associated with HLH?

Whatever the underlying cause (genetic or acquired disease), the onset of clinical HLH is often triggered by any of a number of viral infections, including EBV, cytomegalovirus, parvovirus, herpes simplex virus, human immunodeficiency virus (HIV), varicella-zoster virus, measles virus, human herpes virus 8, and H1N1 influenza. In rare cases, HLH may also have an association with bacteria, fungi, or parasites.

Without treatment, median survival is approximately 2 months. The highest rate of incidence for HLH is in the pediatric population younger than 3 months, although it may present at any age. HLH occurring in infancy is almost always due to a genetic disorder, whereas HLH presenting later in life is often due to an underlying acquired disorder, such as a rheumatologic disorder.

CLINICAL PEARL   **STEP 2/3**

Despite the (unfortunate) name, hemophagocytosis as seen on bone marrow aspiration and biopsy is neither sensitive nor specific for HLH. Aspirate may fail to capture obvious evidence on hemophagocytosis, even in patients with active disease and, in rare cases, the process may be seen in patients without a clinical diagnosis.

BASIC SCIENCE/CLINICAL PEARL   **STEP 1/2/3**

Rapid diagnosis is critical because HLH is an almost uniformly fatal disease without therapy, and median survival is less than 2 months. In contrast, the 5-year survival rate of patients who were treated in the international HLH-94 trial was 54%.

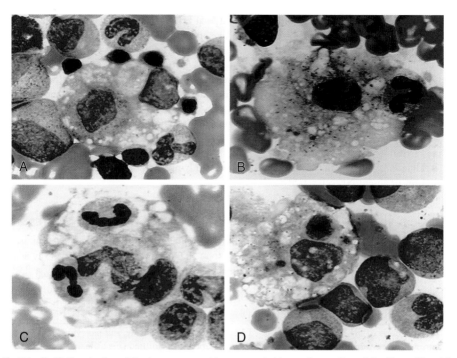

Fig. 7.1 (A–D) Examination of the bone marrow biopsy revealed hemophagocytic activity. (From Filipovich AH. Hemophagocytic lymphohistiocytosis and other hemophagocytic disorders. *Immunol Allergy Clin North Am.* 2008;28[2]:293–313.)

What is the difference between primary and secondary HLH?

Traditionally, patients with HLH have been divided into so-called primary or secondary groupings. Primary HLH is defined as occurrence of the disease with an established genetic link or within the context of a clear pattern of family inheritance. The typical patient is an infant, and the prognosis in primary HLH includes a high risk of recurrence. Because the immunologic defects in these patients are inherited, the immune dysregulation generally persists beyond a single disease flare, and excessive immune activation is likely to occur again and again without definitive treatment.

Conversely, patients who are said to suffer from secondary HLH present without any known family or genetic association. Instead, these patients typically have an infection, malignancy, or rheumatologic condition that is thought to serve as a trigger for the syndrome. Patients with secondary HLH are typically older and may have a complete resolution of disease after initial treatment. Typical triggering conditions include EBV infection, lymphomas or leukemias, and JIA. In the rheumatologic literature, secondary HLH is generally referred to as macrophage activation syndrome (MAS).

When categorizing a patient's disease as primary or secondary in nature, it is also important to note the subtlety of individual cases. Many primary HLH patients with a known genetic mutation will also have a triggering event such as EBV infection, whereas some patients with likely secondary HLH may later present with recurrent disease suggestive of an underlying genetic defect.

Case Point 7.4

As part of a FUO workup, a workup for EBV is sent. Antibodies are negative, but EBV viremia is detected via a polymerase chain reaction assay.

What organ systems are commonly involved in HLH, and how might they manifest symptoms?

Almost all patients with HLH will have liver involvement, and HLH hepatitis can lead to jaundice, elevated triglyceride levels, impaired hepatic synthesis, and/or disseminated intravascular coagulopathy. Approximately one-third of patients will have inflammation in the central nervous system, which may manifest as seizures, ataxic gait, encephalitis, headache, and/or alteration in consciousness. Additionally, patients may develop deteriorating respiratory function, renal disease, severe hypotension, or skin manifestations such as petechiae, purpura, rash, or erythroderma.

How is primary HLH treated? How is secondary HLH treated?

HLH is typically treated aggressively with multiple immunosuppressive agents (e.g., etoposide and dexamethasone). Patients with genetically proven familial HLH or recurrent disease require hematopoietic stem cell transplantation (HSCT). HLA typing and search for a suitable donor should be initiated as soon as possible to improve survival.

For patients with secondary HLH who are clinically stable, treating the triggering illness may be sufficient.

Case Point 7.5

The patient was initially treated with dexamethasone and etoposide. He responded initially but ultimately had multiple relapses and was unable to clear his EBV viremia. He eventually successfully underwent a hematopoietic stem cell transplantation from his brother.

BEYOND THE PEARLS

- Widely accepted and available HLH diagnostic criteria stem from the international HLH-2004 trial and are designed to differentiate HLH from other disorders. It does not include a full survey of commonly affected organ systems, such as the liver or central nervous system.
- Mutations in several genes have been implicated in HLH, but essentially all the genes play a role in the pathway that leads to perforin-mediated apoptosis of target cells by cytotoxic T lymphocytes or natural killer cells. The most commonly mutated gene in North America—and likely worldwide—is *PRF1* (also known as *FHL2*), which encodes for the perforin protein.
- Serum levels of many cytokines are elevated in HLH (e.g., IL-2, IL-6, tumor necrosis factor [TNF]) but measured cytokine levels are not available in the clinical setting. The soluble IL-2 receptor (sIL2R) level is a good marker of cytokine activity and tracks the course of the disease well. Repeating the sIL2R test during therapy can aid the clinician in assessing the degree of control of the pathologic inflammation.

BEYOND THE PEARLS—cont'd

- Hemophagocytosis is assessed in the marrow but can be seen anywhere in the reticu-loendothelial system, such as the spleen, liver, and lymph nodes (if these sites were to be biopsied). Because hemophagocytosis can be a late finding, it is often not evident on initial bone marrow aspiration or biopsy but may be present if the procedure were to be repeated.
- Pigmentary defects in newborns and young children should increase suspicion for a genetic HLH syndrome. Specifically, hypopigmented skin with silvery gray (metallic) hair in an infant should trigger suspicion for Griscelli syndrome (type 2 is caused by *RAB27A* mutations), or Chediak-Higashi syndrome (caused by the *LYST* gene). Both Griscelli type 2 and Chediak-Higashi syndromes predispose patients to HLH.

Case Summary

Complaint/History: A 13-month-old male presents with 10 days of fever, fussiness, and cough.

Findings: Intermittent fevers.

Labs/Tests: Hemoglobin, 6.8 g/dL; platelet count 71 × 10^9/L; neutrophils, 400 × 10^6/L; ferritin, 5333 ng/mL.

Diagnosis: Hemophagocytic lymphohistiocytosis.

Treatment: Chemotherapy followed by hematopoietic stem cell transplantation.

Bibliography

Gholam C, Grigoriadou, Gilmour KC, Gaspar HB. Familial haemophagocytic lymphohistiocytosis: advances in genetic basis, diagnosis, and management. *Clinical and Experimental Immunology*; 163: 271–283.

Henter JI, Samuelsson-Horne A, Arico M, et al. Treatment of hemophagocytic lymphohistiocytosis with HLH-94 immunochemotherapy and bone marrow transplantation. *Blood*. 2002;100:2367.

Jordan MB, Allen CE, Weitzman S, Filipovich AH, McClain KL. How I treat hemophagocytic lymphhistio-cytosis. *Blood*. 2011;118(15):4041–4052.

Mischler M, Flemng GM, Stanley TP, et al. Epstein-Barr virus–induced hemophagocytic lymphohistiocy-tosis and X-linked lymphoproliferative disease: a mimicker of sepsis in the pediatric intensive care unit. *Pediatrics*. 2007;119:e1212.

24-Month-Old Male With Loss of Speech

Julio Martinez ▪ Suraiya Rahman ▪ Erica Z. Shoemaker ▪ Michael Regalado

A 24-month-old male is seen for a routine well-child care visit. At 18 months of age, his parents had concerns about language development as he had an expressive vocabulary of five words, inconsistent response to his name, and infrequent use of gestures. They consider him to be "independent" and somewhat "aloof" by nature. A developmental screening test had suggested a moderate risk for language development.

Four months later, his mother gave birth to his sister. Within days, he stopped speaking altogether. Now, his parents express more concern and ask if this is a possible reaction to his sibling's birth. He shows little interest in others and prefers to occupy himself with electronic media.

How do you approach the parents' concerns?
The parents' concerns about their child's language development and behavior are examined by developmental surveillance and screening in primary care settings. Developmental surveillance is a clinical assessment that includes addressing parents' concerns, documenting the developmental history, making observations of behavior, and identifying risk and protective factors.

When surveillance suggests concerns about a child's development, providers should use validated screening tools to examine the concerns further and assess risk for developmental problems. A comprehensive, multidisciplinary assessment of the child and a referral for intervention services are both indicated if an increased risk is found.

CLINICAL PEARL   STEP 2/3

Evaluation of development is done at each preventative care encounter by developmental surveillance and screening. These activities identify children at risk for developmental problems who need additional assessment.

Case Point 8.1

The child's past medical history is unremarkable. He has a cousin in special education for language problems. Both parents have steady jobs and a reliable social support network.

During the interview, the child wanders about the room ignoring most bids for his attention by the parents and physician. Sometimes, he looks to his parents but not in a meaningful way (e.g., when hearing another child cry or when approached by the physician). He settles briefly on play with a toy truck but does not share the experience with either parent, even when they comment on his activity. Occasionally, he flaps his hands for no apparent reason.

He is fearful during the physical examination and makes no effort to cooperate. The examination is otherwise unremarkable.

How does one interpret this child's story and observed behavior?
A variety of biologic and psychosocial influences can affect developmental processes, particularly language development. In this case, a family history of similar language difficulty suggests a hereditary factor. Additionally, the history suggests loss of language as a possible psychological reaction to a sibling's birth. Observation of the child suggests a lack of social interest and unusual motor behavior (i.e., hand flapping).

How does one know if these observations and events should be of concern?
One may consider the parents' concerns in terms of emerging motor, cognitive, language and/or social-emotional milestones for the child. However, the story highlights more than emerging milestones—the child appears to have problems with the normal emergence of social communication competence.

This social competency can be understood from a relationship-based perspective by considering the child's behavior in a social context. To make sense of parent-child interaction, consider child development from the perspective of this relationship—emphasizing its adaptive issues and challenges. Briefly, these challenges are:

- *Physiologic adaptation (birth to 3 months) to life ex-utero.* Activities such as sleep, waking, and crying undergo physiological organization in relation to circadian rhythms, feeding, and other caregiving activities.
- *Social reciprocity (3 to 6 months).* Infants learn to engage in turn-taking exchanges with caregivers where the adult responds contingently to the infant's increased social interest, smiling, changes in emotional states, and vocalizations.
- *Initiative (6 to 9 months).* Increasing control of posture and movement enables clearly intentional behavior (e.g., reaching and grasping). This also shifts the infant's focus toward the exploration of objects and provides a context for understanding that experience can be shared (joint attention).
- *Attachment (9 to 12 months).* The infant seeks caregiver proximity when under stress and displays fear of strangers and separation. Social referencing—looking to the parent's expression when unsure of safety—is seen. The infant uses gaze and pointing to engage the caregiver's attention.
- *Exploration and experimentation (12 to 18 months).* The toddler explores the wider surroundings using trial-and-error strategies to learn. Nonverbal communication skills predominate given slowly-emerging verbal skills.
- *Autonomy and self-awareness (18 to 30 months).* The toddler becomes aware of the self as a separate individual, asserts the self ("me, not you"), and acquires the capacity for mental representation of experience. Rapid expansion of language, pretend play, and greater social awareness—including sensitivity to rules and behavioral expectations—are seen.
- *Self-control and peer relationships (30 to 60 months).* The preschool child understands and internalizes social expectations for behavior (i.e., guiding and directing one's own behavior) while engaging peers in cooperative exchanges (e.g., conversation and play). Continuing advances in language and the ability to think about, represent, and understand the experience of another individual build on earlier nonverbal skills based on joint attention and social referencing.
  A hallmark of this period is the realization that others have their own thoughts, beliefs, intentions, and desires. This capacity for understanding others' minds is called a *theory of mind* mechanism.

The child's story and observed behavior indicate more than a reaction to a sibling birth or a feature of temperament; he is lacking specific skills such as social referencing, joint attention, and even proximity-seeking behavior to the caregiver. All these signs suggest lack of expected social communication competence.

CLINICAL PEARL	STEP 2/3

Observation of parent-child interaction is a recommended clinical assessment at each health-care encounter.

CLINICAL PEARL	STEP 2/3

Evaluation of developmental and behavioral concerns requires an understanding of the social context; observation of parent-child interaction with an understanding of how the relationship changes as the child matures is critical to this process.

Case Point 8.2

A developmental screening test was repeated along with a screening test for autism spectrum disorders. Both indicate increased risk. The physician referred the child for audiological testing, comprehensive developmental assessment, and early intervention services.

How is a developmental diagnosis made?

Children considered at risk for developmental and behavioral problems should be referred for a comprehensive clinical assessment of developmental delay or a specific developmental disorder by clinicians experienced in the assessment of developmental disabilities.

The process entails a thorough evaluation of the child across multiple domains of development (e.g., cognition, language, communication, adaptive function, social interaction, social communication, and play behavior). Direct observation of the child, parental interview, and the use of standardized diagnostic assessments are used. Standardized diagnostic assessments for autism spectrum disorder (ASD) should be used when the clinical history is suggestive of social communication problems.

At the same time, a referral should be made to early intervention services.

CLINICAL PEARL	STEP 2/3

Once the possibility of developmental delay is suspected, referral for multidisciplinary diagnostic evaluation and for early intervention services should be made simultaneously. The diagnosis of ASD is made clinically by specialists experienced in developmental disabilities.

Case Point 8.3

Diagnostic assessment of the child yields a diagnosis.

Diagnosis: Autism Spectrum Disorder.

What are the clinical features of autism spectrum disorder?

ASD is a neurodevelopmental disorder whose impairments affect social communication and social interaction with restricted, repetitive patterns of behavior, interests, and activities. Some children will present in the first year with language concerns, but most children present in the second year. About a third present with regression of language after achieving early milestones, similar to the child presented in the vignette.

CLINICAL PEARL   **STEP 2/3**

Language regression in ASD may be incorrectly attributed by caregivers to a stressor such as a hospitalization or the birth of a sibling.

Impairments in social communication and social interaction are the primary clinical features of ASD. The impairments are best viewed in terms of their social relevance as noted earlier, e.g., in *social reciprocity*, the capacity for engaging in a turn-taking exchange of visual gaze and vocalization, in *joint attention* (shared awareness or shared enjoyment); *social referencing* (using the emotional expression of others for communicative information), and eventually in the development of a theory of mind – the understanding that others are capable of different thoughts, beliefs, and intentions. Impairments in these behaviors impact children's abilities to form social relationships with peers and generally function in relationships effectively.

A variety of restricted and repetitive behaviors, interests, and activities complete the ASD profile. These include stereotyped behavior such as the hand-flapping motor mannerisms described earlier, lining up of toys and objects, and/or other behavior, such as an insistence on maintaining the same routine. More intense behavior may be seen, and such behavior may be self-injurious. Sensory perception peculiarities have been described to various degrees in children with ASD, including preoccupations with various stimuli, objects, or activities.

BASIC SCIENCE/CLINICAL PEARL   **STEP 1/2/3**

The symptoms of ASD most often become evident in the second year of life.

How is the diagnosis of ASD made? What is the differential diagnosis?

The diagnosis of ASD is a clinical assessment based on the history, physical examination, and observation of behavior. This determination is guided by the diagnostic criteria of the *Diagnostic and Statistical Manual,* Fifth Edition (DSM5; Box 8.1) in the United States. Assessments of severity level are specified for the domains of social communication/social interaction, and repetitive/restricted behaviors based upon an estimated level of support required to accommodate the impact of the behaviors on the child's function (guidelines are suggested for three levels – requires support, substantial support, or very substantial support; Table 8.1).

The differential diagnosis for ASD includes global developmental delay, intellectual disability, other language disorders, learning disability, hearing loss, Landau-Kleffner syndrome, Rett syndrome, anxiety disorder, and obsessive-compulsive disorder. Additional genetic testing and counseling are indicated to identify heritable conditions commonly associated with ASD such as Fragile X syndrome, Angelman syndrome, and tuberous sclerosis complex.

BASIC SCIENCE/CLINICAL PEARL   **STEP 1/2/3**

A comorbid genetic disorder is more likely when ASD is associated with global developmental delay or intellectual disability.

CLINICAL PEARL   **STEP 2/3**

Testing for Fragile X syndrome is indicated in all children with ASD.

Metabolic testing should be considered with symptoms that suggest an inborn error of metabolism such as lethargy, hypotonia, recurrent vomiting and dehydration, early seizures, dysmorphic features, intellectual disability, and/or developmental regression. Neuroimaging and EEGs are considered when the history and/or physical exam are suggestive of an intracranial abnormality.

BOX 8.1 ■ Diagnostic Criteria for Diagnosis of Autism Spectrum Disorder

- Persistent deficits in social communication and social interaction across multiple contexts, as manifested by all of the following, currently or by history (examples are illustrative, not exhaustive; see referenced text[±]):
  1. Deficits in social-emotional reciprocity, ranging, for example, from abnormal social approach and failure of normal back-and-forth conversation; to reduced sharing of interests, emotions, or affect; to failure to initiate or respond to social interactions.
  2. Deficits in nonverbal communicative behaviors used for social interaction, ranging, for example, from poorly integrated verbal and nonverbal communication; to abnormalities in eye contact and body language or deficits in understanding and use of gestures; to a total lack of facial expressions and nonverbal communication.
  3. Deficits in developing, maintaining, and understanding relationships, ranging, for example, from difficulties adjusting behavior to suit various social contexts; to difficulties in sharing imaginative play or in making friends; to absence of interest in peers.
  Specify current severity: Severity is based on social communication impairments and restricted, repetitive patterns of behavior (see Table 8.1)
- Restricted, repetitive patterns of behavior, interests, or activities, as manifested by at least two of the following, currently or by history (examples are illustrative, not exhaustive; see referenced text[±]):
  1. Stereotyped or repetitive motor movements, use of objects, or speech (e.g., simple motor stereotypies, lining up toys or flipping objects, echolalia, idiosyncratic phrases).
  2. Insistence on sameness, inflexible adherence to routines, or ritualized patterns of verbal or nonverbal behavior (e.g., extreme distress at small changes, difficulties with transitions, rigid thinking patterns, greeting rituals, need to take same route or eat same food every day).
  3. Highly restricted, fixated interests that are abnormal in intensity or focus (e.g., strong attachment to or preoccupation with unusual objects, excessively circumscribed or perseverative interests).
  4. Hyper- or hyporeactivity to sensory input or unusual interest in sensory aspects of the environment (e.g., apparent indifference to pain/temperature, adverse response to specific sounds or textures, excessive smelling or touching of objects, visual fascination with lights or movement).
  Specify current severity: Severity is based on social communication impairments and restricted, repetitive patterns of behavior (see Table 8.1)
- Symptoms must be present in the early developmental period (but may not become fully manifest until social demands exceed limited capacities, or may be masked by learned strategies in later life).
- Symptoms cause clinically significant impairment in social, occupational, or other important areas of current functioning.
- These disturbances are not better explained by intellectual disability (intellectual developmental disorder) or global developmental delay. Intellectual disability and autism spectrum disorder frequently co-occur; to make comorbid diagnoses of autism spectrum disorder and intellectual disability, social communication should be below that expected for general developmental level.

[±]Reprinted with permission from the *Diagnostic and Statistical Manual of Mental Disorders*, 5th ed. Copyright (©) 2013. American Psychiatric Association. All Rights Reserved.

What interventions are available to children with ASD?

Children with ASD should participate in therapeutic programs as early as possible. Successful programs should be individualized, involve the family, and be administered with sufficient intensity. Programs use strategies based on behavioral modification, targeting of relationship-based skills, or both. These are supported by interventions specific to communication, social skills, and specific maladaptive behaviors (e.g., sleep problems, self-injury).

TABLE 8.1 ■ Severity Levels for Autism Spectrum Disorder

Severity level	Social communication	Restricted, repetitive behaviors
Level 3 "Requiring very substantial support"	Severe deficits in verbal and nonverbal social communication skills cause severe impairments in functioning, very limited initiation of social interactions, and minimal response to social overtures from others. For example, a person with few words of intelligible speech who rarely initiates interaction and, when he or she does, makes unusual approaches to meet needs only and responds to only very direct social approaches.	Inflexibility of behavior, extreme difficulty coping with change, or other restricted/repetitive behaviors markedly interfere with functioning in all spheres. Great distress/difficulty changing focus or action.
Level 2 "Requiring substantial support"	Marked deficits in verbal and nonverbal social communication skills; social impairments apparent even with supports in place; limited initiation of social interactions; and reduced or abnormal responses to social overtures from others. For example, a person who speaks simple sentences, whose interaction is limited to narrow special interests, and who has markedly odd nonverbal communication.	Inflexibility of behavior, difficulty coping with change, or other restricted/repetitive behaviors appear frequently enough to be obvious to the casual observer and interfere with functioning in a variety of contexts. Distress and/or difficulty changing focus or action.
Level 1 "Requiring support"	Without supports in place, deficits in social communication cause noticeable impairments. Difficulty initiating social interactions, and clear examples of atypical or unsuccessful responses to social overtures of others. May appear to have decreased interest in social interactions. For example, a person who is able to speak in full sentences and engages in communication but whose to-and-fro conversation with others fails, and whose attempts to make friends are odd and typically unsuccessful.	Inflexibility of behavior causes significant interference with functioning in one or more contexts. Difficulty switching between activities. Problems of organization and planning hamper independence.

Reprinted with permission from the *Diagnostic and Statistical Manual of Mental Disorders*, 5th ed. Copyright © 2013. American Psychiatric Association. All Rights Reserved.

Case Point 8.4

Early intervention services are started. An individualized treatment plan is made with contributions from members of the multidisciplinary treatment team, as well as the family, as further manifestations of ASD are seen.

BEYOND THE PEARLS

- Most of what we know about intervention effectiveness for children with ASD comes from studies of preschool- and elementary school-age children. For children under 3 years of age, the general program for early intervention services is recommended.
- Children with ASDs are prone to develop other medical problems such as epilepsy, sleep disturbances, nutritional disturbances due to idiosyncratic food preferences or implementation of alternative diets and supplements, gastrointestinal disturbances (e.g., constipation, reflux), and maladaptive behaviors (e.g., self-injury, elopement, pica).
- Medications do not change the core symptoms of ASD. However, many children and adolescents with ASD have comorbid disorders (e.g., Attention Deficit Hyperactivity Disorder, Anxiety Disorders, and/or Depressive Disorders) and some children and adolescents with ASD can be prone to aggression and self-injurious behaviors. When behavioral interventions have not succeeded or are not feasible, it may be appropriate to use psychotropic medications to treat these comorbid conditions.
- The role of the primary care physician includes evaluation of developmental and behavioral concerns, referral as indicated for diagnostic evaluation and intervention services, and supervision of medical management in conjunction with specialists.
- Although there is no cure for children with ASD, early identification and services for the child and family can optimize function and adaptation.

Case Summary

Complaint/History: A 24-month-old boy presents with loss of speech after the birth of his younger sister.

Findings: He is fearful during the physical examination and makes no effort to cooperate. Occasionally, he flaps his hands for no apparent reason.

Labs/Tests: Comprehensive developmental assessment confirms the diagnosis.

Diagnosis: Autism spectrum disorder.

Treatment: Early intervention services followed by individualized multidisciplinary treatment plan.

Bibliography

American Academy of Pediatrics, Council on Children with Disabilities, Section on Developmental Behavioral Pediatrics, Bright Futures Steering Committee, Medical Home Initiatives for Children With Special Needs Project Advisory Committee. Identifying infants and young children with developmental disorders in the medical home: an algorithm for developmental surveillance and screening. *Pediatrics*. 2006;118(1):405–420.

Carver L, Chawarska K, Constantino J, et al. Clinical assessment and management of toddlers with suspected autism spectrum disorder: insights from studies of high-risk infants. *Pediatrics*. 2009;123:1383.

Committee on Children With Disabilities. Role of the pediatrician in family-centered early intervention services. *Pediatrics*. 2001;107(5):1155–1157.

Maglione Margaret A, Gans D, Das L, et al. Nonmedical interventions for children with ASD: recommended guidelines and further research needs. *Pediatrics*. 2012;130:S169.

Neurodevelopmental Disorders. In: *Diagnostic and Statistical Manual*, 5th ed. Washington, DC: American Psychiatric Association; 2013.

Regalado M, Schneiderman J, Duan L, Ragusa G. Preliminary validation of a parent-child relational framework for teaching child development assessment to pediatric residents. *Acad Pediatr*. 2017;17:74–78.

Volkmar F, Siegel M, Woodbury-Smith M, et al. Practice parameter for the assessment and treatment of children and adolescents with autism spectrum disorder. *J Amer Acad Child Adolesc Psychiatr*. 2014;53(2):237–257.

2-Year-Old Male With Pallor, Decreased Urine Output, and Edema

June Chapin ■ Richard Fine

A 2-year-old male presents to the emergency department with 2 days of decreased urine output and lower extremity edema. The patient's mother reports that he looks "pale" and has been less active over the last several days. He is eating and drinking less and the number of wet diapers he produces has decreased from a normal of six to only two in the last 24 hours. She states that his feet and eyelids look "puffy."

He developed a nonproductive cough and rhinorrhea, as well as a tactile fever 1 week ago, but these symptoms are resolving.

BASIC SCIENCE/CLINICAL PEARL	**STEP 1/2/3**

A decreased number of wet diapers may be a sign of dehydration in infants and toddlers.

Case Point 9.1

He is afebrile, with a pulse rate of 133/min and blood pressure of 118/77 mm hg (>99th percentile for age and height). On general observation, he is tired-appearing, although he cries and pushes you away during the examination. Petechiae are present on the skin under his eyes. He has a systolic II/VI murmur best heard at the apex, which has not been previously documented in this child. Pitting edema is noted in the dorsal feet, extending to the medial tibia bilaterally.

What is the differential diagnosis at this point?

A renal cause—rather than cardiac, hepatic, or inflammatory—for the patient's edema is suggested by the patient's hypertension and oliguria. Renal causes that must be considered include nephrotic and nephritic syndromes, which encompass many underlying causes but principally manifest with similar characteristics.

Nephrotic syndrome results from noninflammatory damage to the glomerular capillary wall, which increases glomerular permeability to plasma proteins, thus causing proteinuria (>50 mg/kg per day in children and >3.5 g/day in adults), hypoalbuminemia, edema, and hyperlipidemia. Minimal change disease would be the most likely underlying nephrotic cause in this child because it predominates in boys (2:1) from the ages of 2 to 6 years and may occur after viral infections, although the cause is generally idiopathic.

Nephritic syndromes are characterized by intraglomerular inflammation that results in hematuria, often with dysmorphic or misshapen urinary erythrocytes and erythrocyte casts, renal insufficiency, and variable levels of proteinuria. Hypertension and hematuria are more predominant in nephritic syndrome, whereas edema and proteinuria are more predominant in nephrotic syndrome. The most common nephritic syndromes in children are postinfectious glomerulonephritis and immunoglobulin A (IgA) nephropathy.

BASIC SCIENCE PEARL	**STEP 1**

Postinfectious glomerulonephritis, which typically develops after a streptococcal pharyngitis or skin infection, is the most common worldwide cause of glomerular disease in children from 5 to 15 years of age. IgA nephropathy is the most common cause of glomerular disease in developed countries and typically presents with episodic gross hematuria coinciding with viral infections (so-called synpharyngitic) rather than after infections.

Case Point 9.2

The peripheral blood count reveals a white blood cell count of 9.8×10^9/L with a normal differential, hemoglobin of 6.8 mg/dL, mean corpuscular volume of 80.4 fL, hematocrit of 20.2%, and platelet count of 38×10^9/L. Visual examination of his peripheral smear reveals schistocytes (Fig. 9.1).

What is the significance of schistocytes?

The presence of anemia and schistocytes as a predominant morphology suggests a microangiopathic hemolytic anemia, which, along with consumptive thrombocytopenia, defines the thrombotic microangiopathy (TMA) syndromes. Pathologically, these syndromes result from vascular damage in the endothelium and vessel wall, with arteriolar and capillary thrombosis.

Although TMA is seen in the setting of disseminated intravascular coagulopathy and may be secondary to medications or medical conditions, the two primary causes of TMA are thrombotic thrombocytopenic purpura (TTP) and hemolytic-uremic syndrome (HUS). TTP is characterized by TMA with fevers, significant neurologic symptoms and, to a lesser extent, renal disease. HUS, on the other hand, is characterized by TMA in the setting of significant renal disease.

Case Point 9.3

A chemistry panel shows levels of sodium, 135 mEq/L, potassium, 5.3 mEq/L, chloride, 101 mEq/L, bicarbonate, 19 mEq/L, urea nitrogen, 25 mg/dL, creatinine, 0.7 mg/dL, lactate dehydrogenase, 325 U/L, and haptoglobin, 7 mg/dL. A urine dipstick test is significant for the presence of gross protein and blood. Microscopy reveals hematuria (6–10 red blood cells/high-powered field) with hyaline and fine and coarse granular casts.

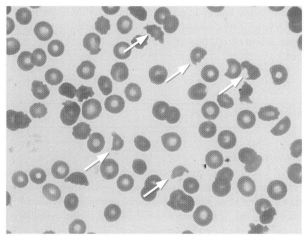

Fig. 9.1   Visual examination of the patient's peripheral blood reveals schistocytes and helmet and burr cells.

CLINICAL PEARL   **STEP 2/3**

In pediatric patients, it is essential to compare laboratory values to age- and gender-matched standards. Although a serum creatinine level of 0.7 mg/dL is normal in an adult, the same value for a 2-year-old is at the upper limit of normal, indicative of renal insufficiency. Additionally, determining the estimate glomerular filtration rate (eGFR) is helpful in determining the magnitude of renal impairment.

BASIC SCIENCE PEARL   **STEP 1**

Urine produced by a dehydrated individual may be concentrated, dark yellow in color, and have a strong odor of urea; specific gravity typically exceeds 1.025 on urinalysis. Gross hematuria is suggested by red-tinged urine or urine with blood clots, although not all red urine is due to hematuria. Microscopic hematuria, defined as two red blood cells or more per microliter of urine, is not visible to the naked eye. Hematuria from a glomerular cause is often described as brown or tea- or cola-colored, whereas that from lower in the urinary tract, such as the bladder and urethra, is more bright red in color. Proteinuria may be suggested historically by frothy or bubbly urine.

Case Point 9.4

The child is admitted to the hospital. Blood and sputum cultures are negative for *Streptococcus pneumoniae*. Stool culture and antigen testing are negative for *E. coli* and *Shigella*. ADAMTS13 activity level is normal at more than 10%. C3 is normal and C4 is low.

BASIC SCIENCE/CLINICAL PEARL   **STEP 1/2/3**

It is important when considering HUS as a diagnosis to be sure that the diagnosis is not TTP. Determining the ADAMTS13 activity level is therefore part of the workup for HUS.

What is the most likely diagnosis at this point?
An algorithm to differentiate the various primary TMA syndromes is presented in Fig. 9.2. TTP has been ruled out at this point by the normal ADAMTS13 activity level. Therefore, HUS, the most common cause of acute kidney injury in childhood, is the most likely diagnosis in this patient given his microangiopathic hemolytic anemia (presenting with pallor, tachycardia, new systolic flow murmur, schistocytes), thrombocytopenia (petechiae), and renal insufficiency (oliguria, hypertension).

Case Point 9.5

Diagnosis: Hemolytic-Uremic syndrome.

What is Hemolytic-Uremic syndrome?
HUS is a form of TMA common in children and is the most common cause of acute pediatric renal failure. It is characterized by the triad of microangiopathic hemolytic anemia, consumptive thrombocytopenia, and acute renal injury—hematuria, proteinuria, azotemia, oliguria or anuria, hypertension, volume overload. The presence of fragmented erythrocytes, elevated lactate dehydrogenase (LDH) level, and decreased haptoglobin level are all consistent with the intravascular origin of hemolysis.

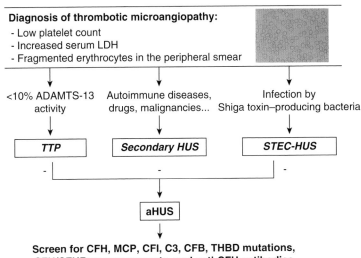

Fig. 9.2 An algorithm to assist in diagnosing suspected hemolytic uremic syndrome. *aHUS,* Atypical hemolytic-uremic syndrome; *HUS,* hemolytic-uremic syndrome; *LDH,* lactate dehydrogenase; *STEC-HUS,* Shiga-like toxin-producing *E. coli* HUS; *TTP,* thrombotic thrombocytopenic purpura. (From Noris M, Remuzzi G. Glomerular diseases dependent on complement activation, including atypical hemolytic uremic syndrome, membranoproliferative glomerulonephritis, and C3 glomerulopathy: core curriculum, 2015. *Am J Kidney Dis.* 2015;66[2]:359–375.)

Previously, cases were divided by causative factors into the categories of typical or diarrheal versus atypical or nondiarrheal cases. However, improved understanding of the underlying pathologic mechanisms of the latter cases has shifted classification schemes, and causes are better classified as either primary or secondary in nature. In children, secondary causes represent most cases, whereas primary or atypical HUS represents 5% to 10% of cases. The latter proportion has been growing due to better recognition of an underlying primary genetic complement-mediated mechanism in cases previously categorized as secondary.

What are the causes of secondary HUS?
Secondary cases of HUS in children are primarily caused by the effects of bacterial toxins. In diarrheal Shiga toxin-HUS (STEC-HUS), Shiga-like toxin produced by enterohemorrhagic *Escherichia coli* strains (O157:H7, O104:H4) and Shiga toxin produced by *Shigella dysenteriae* type 1, targets Gb3 on endothelial cells, renal mesangial cells, epithelial podocytes, and tubular cells, marking them for apoptosis. Shiga toxin is also prothrombotic by facilitating endothelial secretion of von Willebrand factor and proinflammatory by inhibiting complement factor H to activate the alternative complement pathway. Symptoms typically begin 2 to 5 days after consumption of contaminated food or water, with 3 to 5 days of crampy abdominal pain and bloody diarrhea, followed 2 to 5 days later by the development of pallor, bruising, weakness, and oligoanuria as gastrointestinal symptoms resolve.

Shiga toxin can be identified via stool antigen testing. Less than 5% of cases are fatal, although 50% of patients may require dialysis. Treatment is supportive, with management of hydration, blood pressure control, and dialysis. Antibiotics are not recommended because they cause additional toxin release. Once the acute illness resolves, end-stage renal disease and the need for continued dialysis are uncommon, although chronic kidney disease with hypertension and proteinuria may persist.

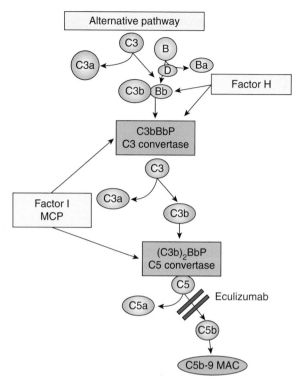

Fig. 9.3 The alternative complement pathway. Shown are inhibitors of the activated complement system and its action sites in the complement cascade. The inhibition site of the C5 antibody eculizumab, the first clinically available complement inhibitor, is indicated as well. (From Scheiring J, Rosales A, Zimmerhackl LB. Clinical practice: today's understanding of the haemolytic uraemic syndrome. *Eur J Pediatr.* 2010;169:7–13.)

Streptococcus pneumonia infections can also precipitate HUS by a different mechanism. Streptococcal neuraminidase exposes normally covered Thomsen-Friedenreich (TF) antigen on erythrocytes, platelets, glomerular endothelial cells, and hepatocytes. When this antigen is exposed, antibodies are formed, resulting in cell lysis. Although less common than Shiga toxin–mediated HUS, *S. pneumoniae*–induced cases have a higher morbidity rate, with 10% progressing to end-stage renal disease and a 12% mortality rate. Treatment includes antibiotics and supportive care.

Other secondary causes, less common in children, include human immunodeficiency virus (HIV) and influenza A infection, malignancy, pregnancy, and autoimmune diseases (e.g., systemic lupus erythematous, antiphospholipid antibody syndrome).

What characterizes primary (also known as atypical) HUS?

Complement-mediated HUS, also known as atypical HUS (aHUS), results from uncontrolled activation of the alternative complement pathway (Fig. 9.3). In the absence of normal regulation, the constitutively active alternative pathway produces the terminal membrane attack complex which injures normal cells. Dysregulation may be due to loss-of-function mutations in alternative pathway regulatory genes (*CFH, CFI, CD46*), gain-of-function mutations in effector genes (*CFB, C3*), or inhibitory antibodies against regulatory proteins. Approximately 60% to 70% of patients with aHUS carry identifiable mutations or antibodies.

In up to 80% of pediatric cohorts, an infectious event, mainly upper respiratory tract infection, diarrhea, or gastroenteritis, triggers the onset of aHUS, as seen in this case. Thus, complement-mediated HUS is a multifactorial disease with environmental triggers that initiate endothelial damage and genetic factors that determine the severity and progression of the disease. Disease onset varies by mutation and ranges from the neonatal period to adulthood, although 75% of children have the first episode before the age of 2 years. In childhood, there is equal distribution between the genders, although females slightly predominate (60%) in adulthood.

Although most cases of aHUS involve complement dysregulation, two less common recessive mutations may also cause aHUS independent of complement. Mutations in *DGKE*—which encodes a protein in the lipid kinase family expressed in the endothelium, platelets, and podocytes—result in a prothrombotic state, platelet activation, and aHUS occurring in the first year of life. Additionally, inborn errors of cobalamin absorption and metabolism, including methylmalonic aciduria and homocystinuria cause hyperhomocysteinemia that damages the glomerular endothelium, which precipitates HUS in neonates, presenting with anorexia, vomiting, lethargy, and failure to thrive.

What are the complications of HUS?

Acute complications of renal insufficiency or failure include hyperkalemia, hyponatremia, metabolic acidosis, and volume overload. Hypertension may induce posterior reversible encephalopathy syndrome (PRES). Central nervous system (CNS) involvement may be manifested by mental status changes, seizures, encephalopathy, vision changes, and hemiparesis or hemiplegia. Approximately 5% of patients may develop life-threatening multiorgan failure due to diffuse thrombotic microangiopathy, including cardiac ischemic events, pulmonary hemorrhage, CNS manifestations, and gastrointestinal ischemia.

What is the treatment for complement-mediated HUS?

Treatment and prognosis has changed dramatically in the last decade, prior to which plasma infusion was the mainstay of treatment, and prognosis was dismal. Eculizumab—a humanized monoclonal antibody against the C5 portion of the complement activation pathway—was approved for aHUS by the US Food and Drug Administration in 2011. Eculizumab results in terminal complement blockade by preventing the formation of the membrane attack complex. It is efficacious in genetic- and immune-mediated causes of complement dysregulation.

CLINICAL PEARL   STEP 2/3

Because eculizumab terminally blocks complement, it increases the risk for infection with encapsulated organisms, most notably *Neisseria meningitides*. All patients should be vaccinated against meningococcus.

Is any further workup indicated prior to initiating treatment?

Individuals should have no other associated disease that may contribute to secondary HUS. Shiga toxin–associated infections and *S. pneumoniae* infections should be ruled out. ADAMTS13 function should be normal to rule out TTP. Genetic testing may reveal mutations in *CFH, CD46 (MCP), CFI, C3, CFB,* and *THBD*, and serologic testing may identify anticomplement factor H antibodies (see Fig. 9.2.)

Case Point 9.6

Eculizumab is initiated on hospital day 2 as his renal function progressively worsens, with a creatinine level of 1.2 mg/dL. The platelet count and hemoglobin continue to drop, with persistent evidence of hemolysis on laboratory testing. Three days after the induction dose, creatinine and LDH levels have peaked and begin to return to normal levels without dialysis. Hemoglobin and platelets stabilize without transfusion. Genetic testing reveals a *CFH* mutation, so outpatient infusions of eculizumab are continued following discharge.

BEYOND THE PEARLS

- Red blood transfusions are often necessary for the treatment of severe hemolytic anemia. In pneumococcal-associated HUS, red blood cells should be washed prior to transfusion to remove residual plasma proteins. This is because a recipient's endogenous IgM directed against the revealed Thomsen-Friedenreich antigen on donor erythrocytes can accelerate pathogenesis of the disease.
- Genetic testing for abnormalities of the alternative complement pathway should parallel the workup for infectious causes if suspicion is high.
- The efficacy of eculizumab complement blockade can be monitored with CH50—a measure of total complement activity—before and after initiation of therapy. CH50 activity of 10% or less indicates near-complete terminal complement blockade.
- Families of patients receiving eculizumab must be educated about the signs and symptoms of meningitis and given a pocket card listing these warning signs, as provided by the drug manufacturer. They should seek immediate medical attention for any warning signs.

Case Summary

Complaint/History: A 2-year-old male presents with 2 days of decreased urine output and lower extremity edema.

Findings: Fatigue, pallor, petechiae, edema, systolic murmur.

Labs/Tests: Hemoglobin, 6.8 g/dL; platelet count, 38×10^9/L; creatinine, 0.7 mg/dL.

Diagnosis: Complement-mediated hemolytic-uremic syndrome.

Treatment: Eculizumab.

Bibliography

George JN, Nester CM. Syndromes of thrombotic microangiopathy. *N Engl J Med.* 2014;371.7: 654–666.

Loirat C, et al. An international consensus approach to the management of atypical hemolytic uremic syndrome in children. *Pediatr Nephrol.* 2016;31:15–39.

Loriat C, Frémeaux-Bacchi V. Atypical hemolytic uremic syndrome. *Orphanet J Rare Dis.* 2011;6:60.

Pan CG, Avner ED. Clinical evaluation of the child with hematuria. In: *Nelson Textbook of Pediatrics.* 20th ed. Philadelphia: Elsevier; 2016:2494–2496.

Why Van SK, Avner ED. Hemolytic-uremic syndrome. In: *Nelson Textbook of Pediatrics.* 20th ed. Philadelphia: Elsevier; 2016:2507–2510.

29-Weeks'-Gestation Fetus With Worsening Anemia

Loren Fox Yaeger ■ Rowena G. Cayabyab ■ Randall Y. Chan

The obstetric service is monitoring a 33-year-old G_9P_{2071} pregnant female with a history of a prior pregnancy ending in intrauterine fetal demise at 8 months of gestation. A prenatal ultrasound performed at 29 weeks of gestation shows worsening anemia, as evidenced by an elevated peak systolic velocity (PSV) through the middle cerebral arteries (MCA; Fig. 10.1).

CLINICAL PEARL   **STEP 2/3**

Doppler velocimetry of the fetal MCA has become the standard of care to screen for fetal anemia replacing amniotic fluid spectrophotometry. Although the most accurate method of determining the presence of fetal anemia is percutaneous umbilical cord sampling, it is an invasive procedure associated with a risk of fetal loss.

What is the differential diagnosis for fetal anemia?

Causes for anemia in the fetus can be categorized into three groups—ineffective production of red blood cells (RBCs), increased destruction of RBCs, and hemorrhage.

The most common cause of fetal anemia is increased destruction of RBCs secondary to red cell alloimmunization, in which the mother's antibodies destroy fetal RBCs; this is termed hemolytic disease of the fetus and newborn (HDFN). Other causes of hemolytic anemia are nonimmune-mediated hemolysis, such as red cell membrane defects, red cell enzyme defects, disorders in hemoglobin synthesis, and congenital TORCH (*t*oxoplasmosis, *o*ther, *r*ubella, *c*ytomegalovirus, *h*erpes virus, and *s*yphilis) infections.

The second most common cause of fetal anemia is fetal or neonatal hemorrhage. Important causes of prenatal hemorrhage leading to anemia include fetomaternal hemorrhage, placental abruption, and twin-twin transfusion syndrome. Intrapartum hemorrhage can result from rupture of the umbilical cord, placental laceration, as in vasa previa, and neonatal trauma resulting in visceral injury, such as hepatic rupture with breech delivery or subgaleal hemorrhage with vacuum extraction.

The third cause of fetal anemia (rare) is ineffective production of RBCs, including intrauterine infections (e.g., parvovirus B19), inherited bone marrow failure syndromes (e.g., Diamond-Blackfan anemia), megaloblastic anemia, and bone marrow replacement by leukemia, osteopetrosis, or mucopolysaccharidosis.

Case Point 10.1

Maternal anti-Rh(D) antibody titers are detected at a titer of 1:64.

Diagnosis: Hemolytic disease of the fetus and newborn due to Rh(D) alloimmunization.

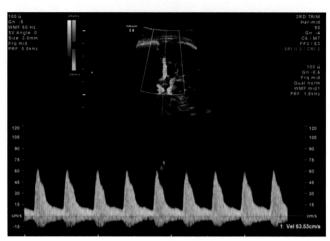

Fig. 10.1 Middle cerebral artery Doppler study showing elevated peak systolic velocity. (From Liley HG. Immune hemolytic disease. In: Orkin SH, Nathan DG, Ginsburg D (eds): *Nathan and Oski's Hematology and Oncology of Infancy and Childhood,* ed 8. Philadelphia: Elsevier; 2015:76–100.e6.)

What is the pathophysiologic mechanism behind hemolytic disease of the fetus and newborn?
HDFN occurs when antibodies produced by a pregnant mother against incompatible fetal RBC antigens cross the placenta and induce an immune hemolytic anemia. In general, prior maternal exposure to the incompatible blood antigen is necessary. This can occur in several ways, the most common of which is fetomaternal hemorrhage. Other mechanisms of alloimmunization include exposure to incompatible blood via a transfusion or via contaminated needles while needle sharing.

BASIC SCIENCE PEARL	**STEP 1**

Although many red blood cell antigens have been described as causing alloimmunization, the Rh(D) antigen is the most antigenic. Less than 0.5 mL of fetal blood at any time during pregnancy and/or repeated exposures to less than 0.05 mL of fetal blood can alloimmunize an Rh-negative mother.

BASIC SCIENCE/CLINICAL PEARL	**STEP 1/2/3**

Spontaneous, small, fetomaternal hemorrhages occur throughout pregnancy; most are too small to lead to alloimmunization. The largest amount of fetomaternal hemorrhage occurs at the time of delivery, and sensitization affects subsequent pregnancies.

After antigen exposure, mothers initially form immunoglobulin M (IgM) antibodies that cannot cross the placenta. Prolonged or repeated exposure leads to production of immunoglobulin G (IgG) antibodies that then cross the placenta and affect the fetus in subsequent pregnancies.

Can maternal Rh alloimmunization be prevented?
Prevention of Rh(D) alloimmunization in an Rh(D)-negative mother is achieved via the administration of anti-Rh(D) immunoglobulin. It is given routinely at 28 weeks gestation and again within 72 hours of delivery, and as needed in any situation in which a large fetomaternal hemorrhage is suspected.

BASIC SCIENCE/CLINICAL PEARL   STEP 1/2/3

In the absence of anti-Rh(D) immune prophylaxis, approximately 16% of Rh(D)-negative women will become sensitized in their first ABO-compatible, Rh(D)-positive pregnancy. After five Rh(D)-positive pregnancies, 50% will be sensitized.

BASIC SCIENCE/CLINICAL PEARL   STEP 1/2/3

The use of maternal anti-D prophylaxis has substantially reduced the role of Rh(D) in HDFN. After the introduction of anti-Rh(D) prophylaxis, the alloimmunization rate of at-risk mothers decreased from 16% to 2% with one dose and further decreased to 0.2% with the second dose administered after delivery of an Rh(D)-positive baby.

CLINICAL PEARL   STEP 2/3

Once alloimmunization has occurred, anti-Rh(D) prophylaxis no longer has a role in the management.

How is maternal alloimmunization managed?

A pregnant woman's blood group, Rh(D) type, and antibody screening is routinely checked at the first prenatal visit. In a patient who is found to be Rh(D)-negative but whose anti-Rh(D) antibody titers are positive, the paternal Rh(D) status should be determined to assess the risk of an Rh(D)-incompatible pregnancy. If it is not possible to obtain the Rh(D) status of the father, the fetal RBC genotype can be determined from fetal DNA isolated from a maternal peripheral blood sample.

Once the fetus has been determined to be at risk for developing HDFN due to Rh(D) incompatibility, the disease severity is determined using maternal antibody titers. In patients with low titers (<1:16) and no history of prior pregnancy affected by HDFN, monitoring of titers alone is sufficient. In pregnant women with high or increasing titers, serial Doppler ultrasound of the middle cerebral artery, peak systolic velocity (MCA PSV) in the fetus is used to screen for and monitor anemia. Ultrasound monitoring for the development of hydrops is also indicated.

An MCA PSV of more than 1.5 multiples of the median (MoM) for gestational age is predictive of moderate to severe fetal anemia. Percutaneous umbilical blood sampling is used to confirm fetal anemia in a fetus at less than 35 weeks' gestation prior to intrauterine transfusion; a fetus at 35 weeks gestation or more should proceed directly to delivery. Intrauterine fetal transfusion can be performed as early as 18 to 20 weeks gestation.

BASIC SCIENCE/CLINICAL PEARL   STEP 1/2/3

Intrauterine transfusions carry a risk of fetal loss of 1% to 2% per procedure. The overall survival rate for severely anemic fetuses that undergo intravascular transfusion is 90% to 95%.

BASIC SCIENCE/CLINICAL PEARL   STEP 1/2/3

One of the best predictors of severity of alloimmunization is a history of a previous hydropic baby. In the first pregnancy after alloimmunization occurs, the risk of hydrops is 8% to 10%. If a previous baby had hydrops, the risk of hydrops in subsequent pregnancies is 90%.

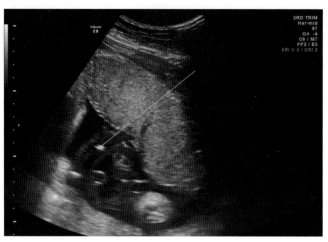

Fig. 10.2   Ultrasound view of umbilical vein catheterization for intrauterine transfusion. (From Liley HG. Immune hemolytic disease. In: Orkin SH, Nathan DG, Ginsburg D (eds): *Nathan and Oski's Hematology and Oncology of Infancy and Childhood,* ed 8. Philadelphia: Elsevier; 2015:76–100.e6.)

Case Point 10.2

An intrauterine RBC transfusion is performed at 30 weeks gestation (Fig. 10.2). The pre- and post-transfusion fetal hemoglobin values determined by umbilical cord blood sampling are 6.4 g/dL and 13.3 g/dL, respectively. A second intrauterine transfusion was planned at 33 weeks gestation; however, fetal distress was detected, and the mother went to immediate cesarean section delivery.

What problems can be anticipated in resuscitation of a neonate with anemia?

Most fetuses with HDFN tolerate induction of labor and delivery well; however, fetuses with severe anemia, high-output cardiac failure, and hydrops fetalis do not tolerate labor due to a higher risk for hypoxemic respiratory failure. It is imperative that an experienced neonatology team be present at the delivery room to perform all aspects of neonatal resuscitation, including but not limited to intubation, umbilical vein catheterization, and chest compressions. Group O Rh(D)-negative blood should be immediately accessible. Hydropic infants may need drainage of pleural and/or ascitic fluid to improve their respiratory status.

Optimal outcomes require careful prenatal management. Fetuses determined to have HDFN are monitored at least twice weekly starting at 32 weeks gestation until delivery, in addition to the serial MCA Doppler studies every 1 to 2 weeks starting at 18 weeks. Although a term delivery would be the goal of an affected pregnancy, a fetus determined to need additional intrauterine transfusions past 35 weeks will have a higher risk of fetal demise; therefore, delivery may be indicated. If delivery prior to 34 weeks gestation appears to be necessary, lung maturation can be accelerated by a 48-hour course of glucocorticoids.

Case Point 10.3

The infant cries immediately on delivery but then stops breathing within the first 30 seconds of life. He is noted to be pale, apneic, and bradycardic, with a heart rate of 60 beats/min, and he has poor muscle tone. The baby's heart rate improves to greater than 100 beats/min after initiation of positive-pressure ventilation via an endotracheal tube. His Apgar scores are 1 (+1 only for heart rate) at 1 minute of life and 7 (−1 for color, tone, and respirations) at 5 minutes of life.

BASIC SCIENCE/CLINICAL PEARL   **STEPS 1/2/3**

The Apgar score—named for Dr. Virginia Apgar—describes the condition of a newborn infant during initial resuscitation. Two points each are given for heart rate, respiratory effort, color of the skin, muscle tone, and response to physical stimulation, for a total possible score of 10.

BASIC SCIENCE/CLINICAL PEARL   **STEP 1/2/3**

Early delivery remains a cornerstone for severe HDFN with fetal hydrops.

After stabilization in the delivery room, the infant is admitted to the neonatal intensive care unit (NICU). The patient immediately underwent isovolemic partial exchange transfusion to increase hemoglobin to 10 g/dL. He is placed on intensive phototherapy for a total of 7 days, with serial bilirubin monitoring.

How is hemolytic disease of the fetus and newborn managed?

A detailed prenatal history, including review of records of any prior transfusions and/or hematologic workup, will provide an overview of the severity of HDFN. Pallor, hepatosplenomegaly, and intradermal erythropoiesis on examination—the latter of which will appear as purpuric skin lesions—indicate severe disease. Initial laboratory examinations should include assessment of the degree of anemia and hyperbilirubinemia, as well as determination of the infant's blood type, reticulocyte count, and direct antiglobulin test (Coombs test).

Infants with HDFN are at high risk for complications of hyperbilirubinemia, including bilirubin encephalopathy. To prevent these complications, intensive phototherapy should be started as soon as is feasible—immediately after resuscitation and admission to the NICU. For infants with rising total serum bilirubin (TSB), despite phototherapy, exchange transfusion may be required.

Immediate exchange transfusions at birth are indicated for severe anemia, severe hyperbilirubinemia, or early signs of bilirubin-induced encephalopathy. Immediate transfusion can remove a potential bilirubin load (i.e., antibody-coated erythrocytes) in addition to correcting anemia; once significant hemolysis has occurred, with distribution of bilirubin throughout the tissues, removal of bilirubin by exchange transfusion becomes more difficult.

Case Point 10.4

On discharge, the patient is followed in the hematology clinic. He is given one more transfusion after hospital discharge and ultimately becomes transfusion-free by 3 months of age.

CLINICAL PEARL   **STEP 2/3**

Infants with HDFN often require PRBC transfusion beyond the NICU stay due to transient erythroblastopenia (due to destruction of RBC precursors). This commonly resolves by 6 to 8 weeks as the antibodies are cleared from circulation. Hemoglobin usually stabilizes at around 12 weeks of postnatal age.

What is the ultimate prognosis of hemolytic disease of the fetus and newborn?

In children treated with intrauterine transfusion for fetal anemia due to alloimmunization, the vast majority have a normal neurodevelopmental outcome. In a landmark study, several factors were found to be associated with increased risk for neurodevelopmental impairment—fetal hydrops, number of intrauterine transfusions, parental education, and severe prematurity-associated morbidity.

BEYOND THE PEARLS

- There are variants of Rh(D), such as weak D or partial D. These Rh(D) variants may result in a patient requiring Rh(D)-negative blood when receiving a transfusion but whose own blood should only be given to Rh(D)-positive recipients. These Rh(D) variants can induce Rh(D) alloimmunization severe enough to cause HDFN.
- There may be a role for high-dose intravenous immunoglobulin (IVIG) to suppress maternal antibody production and/or plasmapheresis to filter maternal antibodies during pregnancy. These interventions are usually performed when percutaneous umbilical sampling and intravascular transfusion are not yet feasible. There is a lack of quality evidence supporting the use of these interventions.
- An ABO incompatibility between the mother and fetus can provide protection against Rh(D) incompatibility. The reduced risk of Rh sensitization with ABO incompatibility may result from the rapid clearance of incompatible red cells, thus reducing the overall exposure to D antigen.
- The risk of Rh(D) alloimmunization is not even across racial groups. In particular, the risk is highest for pregnancies from two parents of European descent, particularly the Basque population, where one in seven pregnancies will involve an Rh(D)-negative mother and Rh(D)-positive father.
- If intravascular transfusion into the umbilical cord is not feasible (e.g., because of insufficient cord size due to early gestation or hypoplasia, cord not accessible due to implantation site), transfusion can be performed by injection of RBCs into the peritoneal space. About 10% of intraperitoneal RBCs will be absorbed into systemic circulation daily.
- IVIG has been recently described as a potentially useful adjunct in HDFN with severe hyperbilirubinemia. Meta-analysis studies have shown a reduction in the need for exchange transfusion, although this finding was not confirmed, despite three randomized controlled trials.

Case Summary

Complaint/History: A 29-weeks'-gestation male fetus presents with anemia requiring transfusion.

Findings: Fetal ultrasound shows increased cerebral blood velocity consistent with anemia.

Labs/Tests: Maternal anti-Rh(D) antibody is detected.

Diagnosis: Hemolytic disease of the fetus and newborn due to Rh(D) alloimmunization.

Treatment: Isovolemic partial exchange blood transfusion and intensive phototherapy.

Bibliography

American Academy of Pediatrics Subcommittee on Hyperbilirubinemia. Management of hyperbilirubinemia in the newborn infant 35 or more weeks of gestation. *Pediatrics.* 2004;114(1):297.

Haas MD, et al. Haemolytic disease of the fetus and newborn. *Vox Sang.* 2015;109(2):99–113.

Liley HG, Gardener G, Lopriore E, Smits-Wintjens V. Immune hemolytic disease. In: Orkin SH, Fisher DE, Ginsburg D, et al., eds. *Nathan and Oski's Hematology of Infancy and Childhood.* Philadelphia: Saunders; 2015:76–100.

Lindenburg IT, Smits-Wintjens VE, Klink JM, et al. Long-term neurodevelopmental outcome after intrauterine transfusion for hemolytic disease of the fetus/newborn: the LOTUS study. *Am J Obstet Gynecol.* 2012;206(2). https://doi.org/10.1016/j.ajog.2011.09.024.

Turner RM, Lloyd-Jones M, Anumba DOC, et al. Routine antenatal anti-D prophylaxis in women who are Rh(D) negative: meta-analyses adjusted for differences in study design and quality. *PloS One.* 2012;7(2):e30711.

4-Year-Old Male With Abdominal Pain

Mark Sims ▦ Randall Y. Chan

A 4-year-old male presents to the emergency department with 3 weeks of abdominal pain, lower back pain, and increased fatigue.

What are the most common causes of abdominal pain in a child?
Causes of abdominal pain vary by anatomic location (Table 11.1). Although some of these causes are rare, they must be differentiated from more common (and benign) causes of abdominal pain, such as constipation and acute gastroenteritis. The absence of diarrhea should always prompt the provider to carefully reassess a child with presumed acute gastroenteritis because vomiting without diarrhea may be an early indicator of another insidious cause for the abdominal pain. Additionally, the presence of bilious vomiting suggests obstruction past the level of the ligament of Treitz and ampulla of Vater.

Atypical causes of abdominal pain should be considered when the cause of acute abdominal pain is unclear. Ovarian and testicular torsion may present with atypical pain. Genital and pelvic examination is essential. Streptococcal pharyngitis and lower lobe pneumonia are also notorious mimickers of acute appendicitis.

Case Point 11.1

An examination of the child reveals an anxious but cooperative child, ill-appearing, in mild distress. He has abdominal distension, with visible venous pattern over the skin. A firm, nontender mass—presumed to be the liver—is palpated in the right upper quadrant, with a span of 15 cm. No splenomegaly is appreciated.

What is your differential diagnosis for an abdominal mass in a young child?
The differential diagnosis for an abdominal mass in a young child includes anatomic abnormalities, as well as malignant and benign neoplasia. Infectious causes include appendicular abscesses and mononucleosis causing splenomegaly. Anatomic causes include hernia, intussusception, bladder neck obstruction, and kidney enlargement (from either hydronephrosis or congenital abnormality). Malignant abdominal neoplasia classically is either a Wilms tumor or neuroblastoma but may also include intestinal lymphoma (more common in older children) and soft tissue malignancy, such as rhabdomyosarcoma. Benign neoplasia includes focal nodular hyperplasia of the liver, choledochal cyst, and ovarian cyst.

TABLE 11.1 ■ Selected Differential Diagnosis of Abdominal Pain Categorized by Predominant Location

Location	Differential Diagnosis
Epigastric	Gastritis, esophagitis Peptic ulcer disease Pancreatitis Volvulus
Periumbilical	Appendicitis (early) Constipation
Right upper quadrant	Hepatitis Biliary tract disease (e.g., cholecystitis)
Right lower quadrant	Appendicitis (late) Mesenteric lymphadenitis Ovarian torsion
Left lower quadrant	Ovarian torsion

BASIC SCIENCE PEARL   **STEP 1**

There are multiple genetic syndromes that include Wilms tumor. WAGR syndrome presents with aniridia, genitourinary abnormalities, and growth retardation. Beckwith-Wiedemann syndrome presents with hemihypertrophy and organomegaly (notably of the tongue). Finally, Denys-Drash syndrome is characterized by the presence of mesangial sclerosis, which progresses to renal failure. Children with these syndromes should be screened for Wilms tumor, with an annual ultrasound in conjunction with a genetics specialist.

Case Point 11.2

Ultrasound imaging reveals a mass. Follow-up computed tomography performed for staging and surgical planning confirms the large, heterogeneous, necrotic mass arising from the right adrenal gland (Fig. 11.1). Diffuse osseous metastases are seen, with compression fractures noted in the T9, L1 and L3 vertebrae (Fig. 11.2). Regional lymph node metastases are seen.

What further testing may help elucidate the diagnosis?

These tumors may produce catecholamines, and their metabolic byproducts will accumulate in the urine. Norepinephrine and epinephrine metabolize to normetanephrine and metanephrine, respectively. Both are then metabolized to vanillylmandelic acid which may be detected in the urine. Dopamine is predominantly metabolized to homovanillic acid, which may be similarly measured in urine.

BASIC SCIENCE/CLINICAL PEARL   **STEP 1/2/3**

Urine catecholamine metabolites—vanillylmandelic acid and homovanillic acid—are measured by quantitative high-performance liquid chromatography in a young child and have a sensitivity of 84.2% and specificity of 99.9% for neuroblastoma. Despite the high specificity, the positive predictive value is only 21.1% when applied to a general population due to the rarity of the tumor; thus, the test should only be used when a patient is actually suspected to have neuroblastoma.

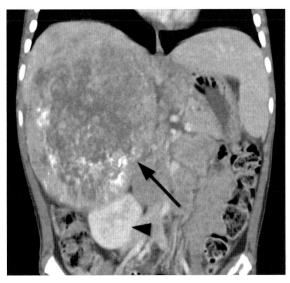

Fig. 11.1 A large, heterogeneous, necrotic mass *(arrow)* is seen arising from the right adrenal gland (above the right kidney; *arrowhead*).

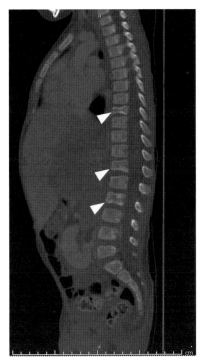

Fig. 11.2 Compression fractures are noted in the T9, L1, and L3 vertebrae *(arrowheads).*

Case Point 11.3

Laboratory analysis shows elevated concentrations of urine homovanillic acid and vanillylmandelic acid. Biopsy of the tumor confirms the diagnosis.

Diagnosis: Neuroblastoma, poorly differentiated.

BASIC SCIENCE PEARL	STEP 1

Neuroblastoma is the most common cancer in the first year of life.

BASIC SCIENCE PEARL	STEP 1

Neuroblastoma arises from the sympathoadrenal progenitor cells migrating from the neural crest. The tumors have a spectrum of histologic features, from highly undifferentiated to almost resembling nervous tissue. Tumors with an undifferentiated histology tend to be more aggressive and are more difficult to treat successfully.

What is the next step?

The next step is staging, or determining the risk of relapse and death, which allows for planning appropriate treatment and determining prognosis. Neuroblastoma risk classification is determined by localized versus metastatic presentation, age at diagnosis, and histologic and genetic features. Advanced stage (aside from stage Ms, previously known as 4S), older age, *MYCN* gene amplification, hyperploidy, higher serum lactate dehydrogenase and ferritin levels, and poor tumor differentiation are all associated with a risk of relapse. Patients with a combination of features indicating a higher risk of relapse will require more intensive therapy.

BASIC SCIENCE PEARL	STEP 1

Metaiodobenzylguanidine (MIBG) scanning is a unique imaging modality for staging and assessing the response to treatment in those with neuroblastoma. MIBG is a radioactive iodine compound bound to an aralkylguanidine that is structurally similar to norepinephrine. It is taken up by neuroblastoma cells and other cells of neuroendocrine origin. It is used as the predominant modality for assessing metastatic disease, although CT scanning may still be necessary because 10% of tumors do not take up MIBG.

BASIC SCIENCE PEARL	STEP 1

The most important somatic gene mutation is amplification of the *MYCN* gene, which infers a significantly worse prognosis. Essentially all tumors that are *MYCN*-amplified are considered to be high-risk tumors.

CLINICAL PEARL	STEP 2/3

Neonates may present with metastatic disease restricted to the skin, liver, and bone marrow (stage Ms, also formerly known as 4S). These patients have an excellent prognosis and often spontaneously go into remission without therapy.

What are the ways in which neuroblastoma can present?
Neuroblastoma can arise anywhere along the parasympathetic axis, given its origin from a neural crest cell. If the tumor presents in the paravertebral chain ganglion, it can invade the intervertebral foramen; the resulting mass may appear to be dumbbell-shaped, with part of the tumor in the vertebrae and part adjacent to the foramen. The spinal cord compression can result in a number of different focal neurologic deficits, depending on location.

Cervical and thoracic neuroblastoma may present with isolated cervical lymphadenopathy and/or a mediastinal mass, respectively. Nerve compression from a cervical tumor may result in Horner syndrome. Venous compression from a mediastinal mass may result in superior vena cava syndrome, with swelling and plethora in the face and upper chest.

A tumor arising in the adrenal gland is more likely to be discovered on physical examination as a large palpable mass. Such tumors may cause pain, irritability, and bowel and bladder symptoms due to direct compression. Pelvic neuroblastoma may arise from the organ of Zuckerkandl.

Distant metastases can present with bone marrow infiltration leading to pancytopenia, as well as bone pain. Orbital involvement can present with proptosis and periorbital hemorrhage, causing a so-called raccoon eyes presentation. Meningeal spread can lead to increased intracranial pressure.

CLINICAL PEARL   **STEP 2/3**

The most common cause of Horner syndrome in a child (in addition to an unknown cause) is neuroblastoma. Horner syndrome in a young child is neuroblastoma, unless otherwise proven.

What presentations of neuroblastoma are acutely an emergency?
If a mass is within the anterior mediastinum, rapid growth can result in airway compromise. The child will present with a widened mediastinum on a chest radiograph and upper airway stridor.

If a mass extensively invades the parasympathetic chain ganglion, it can cause acute spinal cord compression. Urgent neurosurgical decompression is required to avoid permanent neurologic dysfunction.

What paraneoplastic syndromes can present with neuroblastoma?
Opsoclonus-myoclonus-ataxia syndrome (OMAS) is an uncommon paraneoplastic syndrome associated with neuroblastoma. It is also known as *dancing eyes, dancing feet syndrome*. Opsoclonus is a rapid, multidirectional, nonrhythmic, conjugate, torsional movement of the eyes without a slow phase; it differs from nystagmus, which is a rhythmic pendular motion of the eyes with an intersaccadic interval or slow phase. OMAS is also characterized by myoclonic jerks and ataxia. An exhaustive search for neuroblastoma should be undertaken in all children confirmed to have OMAS.

Kerner-Morrison syndrome (KMS) is another neuroblastoma-associated paraneoplastic syndrome characterized by the production of vasoactive intestinal peptide (VIP). The VIP overproduction leads to secretory diarrhea, which is frequently chronic and copious enough to cause growth failure.

BASIC SCIENCE PEARL   **STEP 1**

OMAS and KMS are both associated with favorable tumor biology, with a better cancer prognosis, but OMAS often does not resolve, even with cure of the cancer.

Case Point 11.4

The child is started on neoadjuvant chemotherapy, with a plan for surgery following initial chemotherapy to resect the primary tumor. Future planned treatments include radiation, high-dose chemotherapy with hematopoietic stem cell rescue, and biologic and immunologic therapy.

BEYOND THE PEARLS

- Prognosis in neuroblastoma is more favorable in patients who are older, of a lower stage (less tumor spread), and have a more favorable histology and *MYCN*-nonamplified disease. Risk stratification into low-, intermediate-, and high-risk groups take all these factors into account. Survival is higher than 90% in those with low- or intermediate-risk disease, but less than 50% in those with high-risk disease.
- Treatment for low-risk disease is often surgery alone. Intermediate-risk disease warrants a short course of chemotherapy. High-risk disease is treated with a combination of chemotherapy, surgery, myeloablative consolidation chemotherapy, with autologous hematopoietic stem cell transplantation, radiation therapy, and biologic and immunologic therapy (in that order).
- Biologic therapy includes the use of 13-*cis*-retinoic acid, which is a differentiating agent that is also used for the treatment of severe acne. When used after consolidation chemotherapy and radiation, it reduces the risk of disease recurrence.
- One of the first uses of immunologic therapy against pediatric cancers was a monoclonal antibody targeted to the disialoganglioside GD2 expressed on the cell surface of neuroblastoma cells, in conjunction with immune growth factors and cytokines. The antibody coats the surface of the tumor cell and marks it for immune destruction.
- OMAS is caused by neuroblastoma but does not always resolve with cure of the cancer. Treatments that have been used for OMAS include ATCH, glucocorticoids, cyclophosphamide (low-dose) and IVIG.
- Neuroblastoma almost always occurs in a young child (median age, <2 years old) but has been described in adolescents and young adults. These tumors are often slow-growing and relatively chemotherapy-resistant.

Case Summary

Complaint/History: A 4-year-old male presents with abdominal pain, lower back pain, and increased fatigue.

Findings: A large abdominal mass is palpated on examination.

Labs/Tests: A CT scan shows a large mass arising from the adrenal gland; urine catecholamine levels are elevated.

Diagnosis: Neuroblastoma.

Treatment: Multimodality treatment, including chemotherapy, surgery, and radiation.

Bibliography

Brodeur AE, Brodeur GM. Abdominal masses in children: neuroblastoma, Wilms tumor, and others. *Pediat Rev.* 1991;12:196–206.

Maris JM, Hogarty MD, Bagatell R, Cohn SL. Neuroblastoma. *Lancet.* 2007;369(9579):2106–2120.

Monclair T, et al. The International Neuroblastoma Risk Group (INRG) staging system: an INRG task force report. *J Clin Oncol.* 2009;27.2:298–303.

Ross A, LeLeiko NS. Acute abdominal pain. *Pediat Rev.* 2010;31.4:135.

Yu AL, et al. Anti-GD2 antibody with GM-CSF, interleukin-2, and isotretinoin for neuroblastoma. *N Engl J Med.* 2010;363.14:1324–1334.

12-Month-Old Female With Picky Eating

Mayra Jones-Betancourt ■ Audrey Ahn ■ Randall Y. Chan

A 12-month-old female presents for a well-child care visit. The mother is concerned that the patient is a "picky eater." She was exclusively breast-fed until she was 6 months old and then switched to formula with the introduction of solids. At 12 months of age, the mother began giving her cow's milk. The mother states that the patient refuses to eat most vegetables and instead prefers milk. She drinks four 8-ounce bottles of whole cow's milk per day.

She is otherwise healthy and meeting all developmental milestones.

What screening interventions are recommended for healthy children at 12 months of age?
The following are recommended at all preventive pediatric visits by the American Academy of Pediatrics (AAP):
- An interval history
- Measurement of height, length, weight, weight for length, head circumference
- Physical examination
- Surveillance of developmental progress
- An assessment of behavior
- Administration of immunizations that are due
- Age-appropriate anticipatory guidance
- Assessment for anemia and lead poisoning

Case Point 12.1

The patient is well-appearing on examination, although pallor is noted. The patient's screening hemoglobin concentration is 7.8 g/dL. A confirmatory complete blood count (CBC) shows 5.6×10^9/L leukocytes, 7.6 g/dL hemoglobin, 25.1% hematocrit, and 363×10^9/L platelets. Her red blood cell count is 4.49×10^{12}/L with a mean corpuscular volume (MCV) of 55.7 fL, mean corpuscular hemoglobin concentration of 30.5 g/dL, and red cell distribution width of 22%. Her reticulocyte count is 42.2×10^9/L.

What is the differential diagnosis for her low hemoglobin concentration?
Anemia is defined as a hemoglobin concentration that is two standard deviations (SDs) or more below the mean for a healthy population of the same age (and gender and race). For her age, 11 g/dL of hemoglobin would be 2 SDs below the mean when using data from the World Health Organization global database on anemia. This patient is therefore anemic.

The use of red blood cell indices can narrow the differential diagnosis of anemia; a suggested algorithmic approach to anemia is presented in Fig. 12.1. She presents with a microcytic hypochromic anemia, and therefore the differential diagnosis primarily includes iron deficiency anemia and thalassemia trait. Other thalassemia syndromes and certain sideroblastic anemias are also in the differential, although these diagnoses are less likely given her good health.

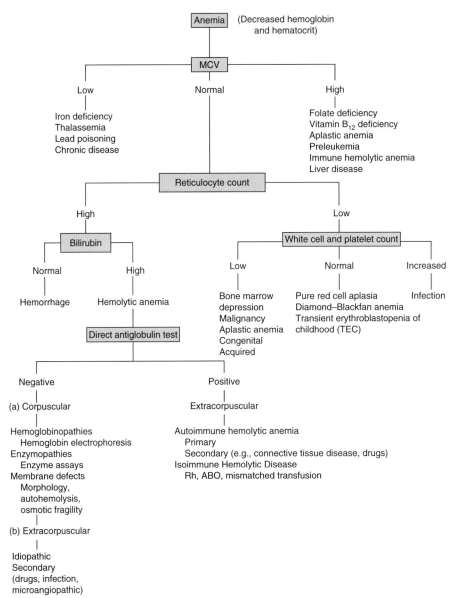

Fig. 12.1 An algorithm categorizing the causes of anemia based on mean corpuscular volume. (From Lanzkowsky P. Classification and diagnosis of anemia in children. In: Lanzkowsky P, Lipton J, Fish J, eds. *Lanzkowsky's Manual of Pediatric Hematology and Oncology*, 6th ed. New York: Academic Press; 2016: 32–41.)

BASIC SCIENCE/CLINICAL PEARL   **STEP 1/2/3**

The normal range for MCV changes with age. The lower limit of normal is approximately 70 fL during most of the first year of life after the immediate newborn period, slowly rises about 1 fL/year of life until the age of 10 years, and remains at 80 fL into adulthood.

What testing is indicated at this time, as recommended by the American Academy of Pediatrics?

The three tests recommended by the AAP for discriminating an iron-deficient state (from normal) include the serum ferritin concentration, the reticulocyte hemoglobin concentration (abbreviated CHr), and the soluble transferrin receptor 1 (STfR) concentration.

The serum ferritin level determination is the most widely used test of the three because it is available in most laboratories. A cutoff of less than 12 µg/L is used for adults and less than 10 µg/L is used for children to diagnose iron deficiency. Serum ferritin is an acute-phase reactant, however, and may be falsely elevated in iron-deficient states if the patient has chronic inflammation. Therefore the AAP recommends obtaining a C-reactive protein (CRP) level at the same time as the serum ferritin. If the CRP level is normal, the ferritin level may be used as a sensitive and specific marker for iron deficiency.

If the CRP level is high, then a normal or elevated serum ferritin level does not necessarily denote normal iron stores. (A low serum ferritin level is still indicative of iron deficiency, regardless of the CRP level.) In cases where both the CRP and serum ferritin levels are high, either CHr or STfR can be used to detect and/or rule out iron deficiency.

Case Point 12.2

The child's serum ferritin level is 5 ng/mL. Her CRP level is normal. Visual examination of her peripheral blood smear reveals markedly microcytic and hypochromic red blood cells, with anisocytosis and poikilocytosis (**Fig. 12.2**).

Diagnosis: Iron deficiency anemia (IDA).

What is the role of iron in cellular metabolism? What is its role in red blood cell physiology, and why would a deficient state lead to anemia?

Iron is incorporated, for example, within cytochromes, aconitases, and catalases due to its ability to participate in reduction-oxidation reactions easily. Iron is required for the function of all cells in the human body.

Most iron in humans is contained in hemoglobin, where it aids in the vital function of oxygen transport. Up to 1 quintillion (1×10^{18}) atoms of iron is incorporated into heme daily for new red blood cells in a healthy person. A deficiency in available iron thus rapidly results in the ineffective production of hemoglobin, ultimately leading to anemia.

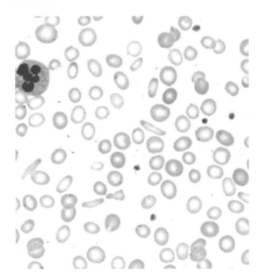

Fig. 12.2 Blood smear shows a microcytic hypochromic anemia consistent with iron deficiency. Both anisocytosis (varying size) and poikilocytosis (varying shape) are hallmarks of iron deficiency anemia. (From Brittenham GM, et al. Disorders of iron homeostasis: iron deficiency and overload. In: Hoffman R, Benz EJ, Jr, Silberstein LE, et al, eds. *Hematology: Basic Principles and Practice,* 6th ed. Philadelphia: Saunders/Elsevier; 2013:437–449.)

How is iron absorbed and metabolized?

After iron-containing food is ingested, iron is absorbed throughout the intestinal tract—primarily in the duodenum. The rate at which iron is absorbed is dependent on a number of factors, with total iron stores being the most prominent factor. Normally, only 10% of daily iron intake is absorbed, but the amount absorbed can increase dramatically in iron-deficient states.

BASIC SCIENCE PEARL   **STEP 1**

Absorption of iron across the basolateral membrane of the enterocyte is mediated by ferroportin and regulated by hepcidin. Hepcidin slows down iron absorption by blocking the function of ferroportin.

Daily absorbed iron only reflects a small percentage of iron that is used daily, however. Most of the iron used is recycled through the breakdown of aged red blood cells via the reticuloendothelial system; very little iron is actually excreted from the body. A small amount of iron is lost each day via sloughing of cells from the skin and mucosal surfaces in the lung and gastrointestinal tract, keeping the total body iron stores relatively constant.

As the body is progressively deprived of iron, iron deficiency will result sequentially in iron depletion (reduced stores), iron-deficient erythropoiesis (depleted stores but otherwise normal MCV and red cell morphology), and iron deficiency anemia (microcytic hypochromic anemia).

CLINICAL PEARL   **STEP 2/3**

Anemia is a late manifestation of iron deficiency. It is also the first manifestation to resolve with iron therapy; resolution of anemia, therefore, is not an adequate treatment endpoint.

What causes iron deficiency anemia?

Iron deficiency occurs when there is deficient intake, inadequate iron absorption from dietary sources, or when iron is lost from the body.

Deficient intake may be due to many different factors, depending on age. The primary cause of inadequate placental transfer of iron (and thus neonatal iron deficiency) would be prematurity. In toddlers, inadequate intake is the primary culprit (e.g., due to excessive consumption of cow's milk, which has a low iron content). Deficient intake can also be seen in older children and adolescents during periods of rapid growth.

Inadequate absorption can be seen for a variety of reasons. The most common reasons include a high gastric pH (e.g., due to antacid therapy), starch ingestion (due to avid iron binding), inflammatory bowel or celiac disease, or ingestion of metals that compete with iron for transport (e.g., lead).

The pathologic loss of iron from the body is almost exclusively due to blood loss. The most common cause seen in the pediatric population is menorrhagia. Perinatal hemorrhage, gastrointestinal hemorrhage (occult or overt), and other types of hemorrhage may also result in iron deficiency.

CLINICAL PEARL   **STEP 2/3**

The most common causes of IDA in the pediatric population in developed countries are excessive milk intake in toddlers and menorrhagia in teenagers. Worldwide, the most common cause is gastrointestinal blood loss due to parasitic infection.

What are the signs and symptoms of iron deficiency anemia?

Most children will be asymptomatic. When anemia is severe, infants will present with lethargy, pallor, irritability, cardiomegaly, poor feeding, tachycardia, and tachypnea, all symptoms of anemia that are not specific to IDA. Older children may present with pica (appetite for dirt or other nonfood substances), pagophagia (appetite for ice), and/or behavioral changes in addition to symptoms of anemia.

What is the recommended therapy for iron deficiency anemia?

Infants and children with iron deficiency should be prescribed iron replacement therapy. A reasonable starting dose is 3 to 6 mg/kg per day of elemental iron, depending on the severity of the IDA. Depending on the severity of the initial anemia, a CBC should be repeated within 4 weeks to determine if there was a response to therapy. A rise of approximately 1 g/dL of hemoglobin would be expected after 4 weeks of therapy.

Dietary modifications for toddlers include decreasing the amount of cow's milk to less than 20 oz/day and modifying the diet to include or increase consumption of both iron-fortified foods (e.g., infant cereals) and foods that contain vitamin C (ascorbic acid—e.g., citrus fruit).

Assuming that there are no ongoing losses, oral iron supplementation should then be continued after complete correction of anemia for an additional 2 to 3 months to replenish iron stores.

Case Point 12.3

The patient starts ferrous sulfate at 3 mg/kg of elemental iron daily. The mother is also instructed to decrease the amount of cow's milk in the patient's diet. At a visit 4 weeks later, the patient is visibly improved, with a decrease in pallor and reported improvement in energy level. Her hemoglobin level is now 9.6 g/dL.

What preventive measures can be taken to reduce the likelihood of developing iron deficiency anemia?

Preterm infants who are breast-fed should receive a supplement of elemental iron at 2 mg/kg per day by 1 month of age, extending through 12 months of age. Full-term infants who are exclusively breast-fed should receive 1 mg/kg per day of supplemental iron, starting at 4 months of age and continuing until the introduction of iron-rich foods. All infants who are formula-fed should use iron-fortified formulas exclusively unless medically contraindicated.

Screening should begin at 12 months of age for most children with a baseline hemoglobin level, although an assessment of risk factors is indicated at each well-child care visit. Early screening should be considered in patients who are born prematurely, born with a low birth weight, exclusively breast-fed past 6 months of age, have a history of bleeding, or have any other high-risk features.

What is the impact of iron deficiency anemia on the developing child?

Anemia, if severe enough, can lead to high-output cardiac failure and growth restriction. Because red blood cell production in iron-deficient states preferentially uses iron over other cells, however, other manifestations may be seen, even in the absence of anemia. Specifically, iron deficiency has been linked to cognitive and neurodevelopmental defects in children in multiple observational studies worldwide. Iron has also been shown to be essential for normal neurodevelopment in animal models, where iron has been shown to be critical to neuronal energy metabolism, metabolism of neurotransmitters, myelination, and memory function.

BEYOND THE PEARLS

- Iron deficiency is the most common nutritional disorder worldwide, particularly in resource-limited nations. Its incidence in the United States has fallen significantly with the introduction of iron-fortified formulas.
- The luminal DMT1 iron transporter protein also transports other divalent metal ions. The enhanced absorption of nonheme iron in iron-deficient states thus also results in the enhanced absorption of other metals with divalent states, such as lead and cobalt. This is the theorized reason as to why lead poisoning is more prevalent in iron-deficient individuals (as well as increased lead ingestion due to pica).
- Hepcidin—which regulates iron absorption—is upregulated in states of inflammation. The restriction on iron absorption eventually leads to anemia of chronic inflammation.
- Breast milk contains less iron than cow's milk. Breast milk iron is nearly 10-fold more readily absorbed, however.
- Iron deficiency from excessive cow's milk consumption is multifactorial. Whole milk has a low iron content. Additionally, excessive milk consumption reduces the caloric intake from solid food. Finally, proteins in cow's milk causes irritant damage to enterocytes in young children, leading to malabsorption of iron and even to chronic occult hemorrhage.
- Iron deficiency anemia is often accompanied by thrombocytosis.

Case Summary

Complaint/History: A 12-month-old female presents with picky eating and excessive milk consumption.

Findings: Pallor in an otherwise well-appearing child.

Labs/Tests: Hemoglobin, 7.6 g/dL; platelet count, 363×10^9/L; ferritin, 5 ng/mL.

Diagnosis: Iron deficiency anemia.

Treatment: Oral iron repletion, reduction of cow's milk consumption.

Bibliography

Baker D, Greer FR, The Committee on Nutrition. Diagnosis and prevention of iron deficiency and iron-deficient anemia in infants and young children (0-3 years of age). *Pediatrics*. 2010;126:1040–1050.

Gozzelino R, Arosio P. Iron homeostasis in health and disease. *Int J Mol Sci*. 2016;17:130.

McDonagh MS, et al. Screening and routine supplementation for iron deficiency anemia: a systematic review. *Pediatrics*. 2015;135:723–733.

Sills R. Iron deficiency anemia. *Nelson Textbook of Pediatrics*. 2016:2323–2326.

Siu AL. Screening for iron deficiency in young children: USPSTF recommendation statement. *Pediatrics*. 2015;136:746–752.

8-Day-Old Male Infant Presenting for Weight Follow-Up

Melissa Harada ▨ Laura Wachsman ▨ Merujan Uzunyan

An 8-day-old male infant, born at 38 weeks of gestation, presents to his pediatrician for weight follow-up.

He was born via normal spontaneous vaginal delivery to a 30-year-old mother who received prenatal care from 9 weeks of gestation. His birth weight was 2910 g. He had a normal physical examination. His hearing screen and critical congenital heart disease screens were passed prior to discharge. He was discharged home on day 2 of life with a weight of 2755 g.

CLINICAL PEARL   **STEP 2/3**

The critical congenital heart disease screen is a pulse oximetry–based screening tool administered after 24 hours of life. Pulse oximetry probes are placed on the right hand (preductal) and either foot (postductal). Any infant with oxygen saturation of less than 95% in either extremity or a more than 3% absolute difference between the upper and lower extremity is evaluated for causes of hypoxemia, which may include echocardiographic evaluation. The critical congenital heart disease screen is an important part of predischarge care, along with a hearing test, neonatal screening tests (varies by state), and administration of hepatitis B vaccine.

Case Point 13.1

He was first seen for scheduled posthospital discharge well-child care at 3 days old, at which time he had lost 7% of birth weight and was not latching well due to maternal flat nipples. The mother was seen by a lactation specialist who assisted her with breast feeding, and he was scheduled for a weight check in 5 days.

What are the American Academy of Pediatrics guidelines regarding newborn follow-up?
Bright Futures—a national health promotion and prevention initiative led by the American Academy of Pediatrics (AAP)—provides evidence-based guidelines for preventive and well-child visits. Based on its guidelines, newborn follow-up should occur within 3 to 5 days after birth and within 48 to 72 hours after discharge. For infants whose hospital stay is 96 hours or longer, follow-up should occur up to 1 week after discharge. These guidelines are based on common newborn health risks that evolve during the first week of life (e.g., jaundice, feeding difficulties, weight loss, sepsis, congenital anomalies).

Case Point 13.2

At his 8 days of life visit, mother reports that he is taking 2 ounces of formula every 2 to 4 hours. Mother is also pumping breast milk, giving 1 to 2 ounces of expressed breast milk three times a day. She wakes him every 2 hours to feed at night. Mother feels that her breast milk has come in. Baby is not having difficulty taking a bottle but will not latch on. He has six or seven wet diapers a day and three or four soft yellow stools a day.

What are the American Academy of Pediatrics guidelines regarding infant feeding?
Exclusive breastfeeding during the first 4 to 6 months of life is believed to provide the best nutrition for growth and development. Recommendations state that babies should breast-feed about 8 to 12 times in 24 hours. If a baby sleeps more than 4 hours, the baby should be wakened for a feeding during the first 2 weeks. As the mother's milk comes in, she will ordinarily produce enough milk to meet her baby's needs. A baby should have six to eight wet diapers in 24 hours once a mother's milk supply is in. Stools should be frequent, as often as with every feed. Parents should wait until 1 month of age to give a pacifier to a breast-fed infant.

CLINICAL PEARL   **STEP 2/3**

Breastfeeding imparts passive immunity and boosts maternal-infant bonding.

If mothers are unable to breastfeed or choose not to breastfeed, iron-fortified formula is recommended for the first year of life. Caloric needs for babies are 100 to 120 kcal/kg per day. Bottle propping should be discouraged because it increases the risk of choking, ear infections, and early childhood caries.

Case Point 13.3

At the 2-month-old visit, his mother asks about episodes of fast breathing that have been occurring with increasing frequency. She says that the baby has episodes of fast breathing lasting a few seconds before normal breathing resumes. He has no periods of sustained fast breathing, apnea, or cyanosis. These episodes happen at different times of day and are not related to specific activities or sleep. During feeding, he often pauses to take several breaths. He does not sweat with feeds and can finish 2 ounces in 5 minutes.

What is tachypnea in an infant, and what is the significance?
Tachypnea means rapid breathing. The World Health Organization (WHO) defines it as more than 60 breaths/min in infants younger than 30 days old, more than 50 breaths/min in 2- to 12-month-olds, and more than 40 breaths/min in 1- to 5-year-olds. Because tachypnea compensates for hypercarbia, hypoxemia, and metabolic and respiratory acidosis, it is a nonspecific finding that may indicate a respiratory, cardiovascular, metabolic, or systemic disorder.

What is the differential diagnosis of tachypnea in this child?
One way to approach a differential diagnosis is to consider disorders by anatomic location. Airway causes such as laryngeal or tracheal atresia (rapidly life-threatening at birth), airway hemangioma, or laryngomalacia would be accompanied by noisy breathing. Pulmonary causes to consider are infection (e.g., pneumonia, bronchiolitis, croup), pneumothorax, pleural effusion, bronchopulmonary sequestration, and congenital pulmonary airway malformation. Other respiratory problems after birth that could cause tachypnea are respiratory distress syndrome, transient tachypnea of the newborn, and meconium aspiration.

Cardiovascular causes include cyanotic and acyanotic congenital heart defects, neonatal cardiomyopathy, pericardial effusion or cardiac tamponade, fetal arrhythmia with compromised cardiac function, and high-output cardiac failure due to extracardiac arteriovenous malformations. Thoracic causes are pneumomediastinum, mass, skeletal dysplasia, and diaphragmatic hernia. Neuromuscular causes include effects of medications, meningitis, hydrocephalus, and congenital myopathies.

Other systemic causes to consider include sepsis, hypoglycemia, metabolic acidosis, inborn errors of metabolism, and anemia.

CLINICAL PEARL   **STEP 2/3**

Tachypnea is a sensitive symptom for congestive heart failure. Other symptoms include tachycardia, poor feeding, sweating profusely during feeds, failure to grow or gain weight, irritability or excessive sleepiness, hepatomegaly, cool extremities, and gallop rhythm. A heart murmur may or may not be present.

Case Point 13.4

His vitals are a temperature of 36.8°F, blood pressure of 78/46 mm Hg, pulse rate of 160/min, respiratory rate of 80 breaths/min, and oxygen saturation of 100% on room air.

BASIC SCIENCE/CLINICAL PEARL   **STEP 1/2/3**

The heart rates of newborns are rapid and have wide fluctuations. The average heart rate in newborns ranges from 120 to 140 beats/min and may increase to 170+ beats/min during crying. Persistent tachycardia (>200 beats/min in neonates and 150 beats/min in infants), bradycardia, or an irregular heartbeat should have further workup done.

On examination, he has subcostal retractions and clear lung sounds. A 3/6 holosystolic murmur is audible throughout the chest, although it is best heard at the left sternal border with radiation to the back. There is no click or rub. The brachial and femoral pulses are 2+. The rest of the physical examination is normal.

What is the most likely diagnosis? How would you proceed with the workup?
Given the findings of tachycardia, tachypnea, and no cyanosis in the setting of a significant systolic heart murmur, the highest on the differential diagnosis is acyanotic congenital heart disease (Table 13.1).

A chest radiograph (CXR) will help evaluate for cardiac enlargement and pulmonary vascularity. Traditionally, based on x-ray findings and clinical assessment, it is possible to classify a congenital heart defect. An electrocardiogram (ECG) then may be obtained to evaluate for arrhythmias or to elucidate a congenital heart defect further (Table 13.2).

CLINICAL PEARL   **STEP 2/3**

ECGs in the newborn period may be difficult to interpret without first familiarizing oneself with normal findings on a newborn's ECG. Additionally, although an ECG may provide an anatomic guide to a heart defect in the right clinical context, a normal ECG alone does not exclude congenital heart disease.

Ultimately, an echocardiogram will be needed to determine the anatomy of the heart and the specific cardiac lesion. Finally, if a child presents with tachypnea in the absence of increased work of breathing and cardiac findings, it would be reasonable to carry out laboratory studies to evaluate for metabolic derangements and/or sepsis.

Case Point 13.5

A CXR (Fig. 13.1), ECG, and echocardiogram (Fig. 13.2) are obtained. The ECG demonstrates sinus tachycardia, with a heart rate of 170 beats/min. A pro brain natriuretic peptide level is 9370 pg/mL.

Diagnosis: Ventricular septal defect (VSD).

TABLE 13.1 ■ **Cyanotic and Acyanotic Congenital Heart Disease by Age of Presentation**

Age	Cyanotic Lesions	Acyanotic Lesions
Birth to first week of life	Transposition of the great arteries	—
First week of life	Total anomalous pulmonary venous return	Hypoplastic left heart syndrome Coarctation of the aorta
First 2–3 weeks of life	—	Complete atrioventricular canal
1–4 weeks of life	Tricuspid atresia; severe pulmonic stenosis	Patent ductus arteriosus
1–12 weeks of life	Tetralogy of Fallot	Ventricular septal defect
Any time in infancy	Truncus arteriosus	—

TABLE 13.2 ■ **Differential Diagnosis of Heart Disease Based on Cyanosis, Chest Radiography and Electrocardiogram**

Examination	X-Ray (CXR)	ECG	Differential Diagnosis
Cyanosis	↑PBF	RVH	Transposition of the great arteries Total anomalous pulmonary venous return Hypoplastic left heart syndrome
		LVH/BVH	Truncus arteriosus Single ventricle
	↓PBF	RVH	Tetralogy of Fallot Pulmonic stenosis
		LVH	Tricuspid atresia Coarctation of the aorta Mitral regurgitation Hypoplastic right heart syndrome
No cyanosis	↑PBF	LVH, BVH	Patent ductus arteriosus Ventricular septal defect Endocardial cushion defect
		RAH	Atrial septal defect
	Normal PBF	RVH	Aortic stenosis Coarctation of the aorta
		LVH	Pulmonic stenosis

NOTE: Electrocardiographic changes can be age-dependent.
BVH, Biventricular hypertrophy; *CXR,* chest radiograph; *ECG,* electrocardiogram; *LVH,* left ventricular hypertrophy; *PBF,* pulmonary blood flow; *RAH,* right atrial hypertrophy; *RVH,* right ventricular hypertrophy.

BASIC SCIENCE PEARL   **STEP 1**

VSDs are associated with infants of diabetic mothers, as is truncus arteriosus.

BASIC SCIENCE/CLINICAL PEARL   **STEP 1/2/3**

VSDs are often heard as a holosystolic murmur.

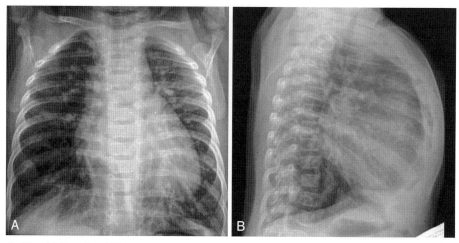

Fig. 13.1 (A) Frontal and (B) lateral chest radiographs reveal increased pulmonary vascularity, with a suggestion of left-to-right shunt. The cardiomediastinal silhouette is enlarged. (From Benson LN, Yoo SJ. Ventricular septal defects. In: Anderson R, et al (eds). *Paediatric Cardiology*. Philadelphia, PA: Churchill Livingstone/Elsevier; 2010:591–624.)

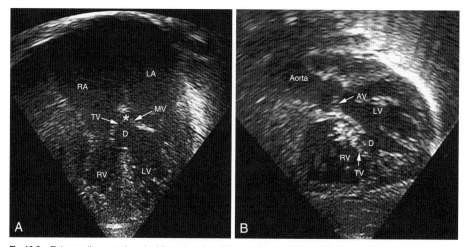

Fig. 13.2 Echocardiograms in apical four-chamber (A) and subcostal left ventricular outflow tract cut (B) show a moderate to large sized ventricular septal defect (D), primum and secundum atrial septal defects with left to right shunting. The defect is demarcated by the tricuspid and mitral valves that are in direct contact (asterisk). *AV*, Aortic valve; *LA*, left atrium; *LV*, left ventricle; *MV*, mitral valve; *RA*, right atrium; *RV*, right ventricle; *TV*, tricuspid valve. (From Benson LN, Yoo SJ. Ventricular septal defects. In: Anderson R, et al (eds). *Paediatric Cardiology*. Philadelphia, PA: Churchill Livingstone/Elsevier; 2010:591–624.)

What is the pathophysiology of a ventricular septal defect?

A VSD can occur along any part of the ventricular septum, although most are membranous in location (Fig. 13.3).

The amount of left-to-right shunting depends on the VSD size and the relative pulmonary and vascular resistance. Small (<5-mm) VSDs are pressure-restrictive—the high pressure in the left ventricle drives the direction of left-to-right shunting, whereas the right ventricle maintains normal pressure, and the size of the VSD limits the magnitude of the shunting.

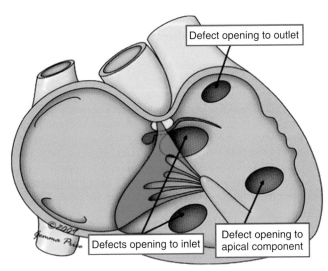

Fig. 13.3 Ventricular septal defects occur along any part of the ventricular septum. (From Benson LN, Yoo SJ. Ventricular septal defects. In: Anderson R, et al (eds). *Paediatric Cardiology*. Philadelphia, PA: Churchill Livingstone/Elsevier; 2010:591–624.)

In large (>10 mm) VSDs, the left and right ventricular pressures are equal, and the direction and magnitude of shunting are determined by the relative pulmonary and systemic vascular resistance. At birth, left-to-right shunting is limited due to elevated fetal pulmonary vascular resistance. However, as infants age and pulmonary vascular resistance decreases, the degree of left-to-right shunting increases, and clinical symptoms of heart failure arise.

CLINICAL PEARL   **STEP 2/3**

Loud murmurs often result from small defects and vice versa.

BASIC SCIENCE PEARL   **STEP 1**

Ventricular left-to-right shunting overloads the pulmonary circuit and the left side of the heart, which may lead left ventricular dilatation and much later left ventricular hypertrophy. If the VSD is large, the right ventricle will be subject to systemic pressure and will undergo hypertrophy. On the other hand, although an ASD is also a left-to-right shunt, which overloads the pulmonary circuit, it volume overloads the right ventricle rather than the left.

With time, individuals with VSDs may develop pulmonary vascular disease (obstructed pulmonary vessels and pulmonary hypertension), which results in shunt reversal with right-to-left shunting of blood, known as Eisenmenger syndrome. Symptoms typically develop in the second or third decade of life, with cyanosis, dyspnea, and fatigue. In later stages, heart failure, chest pain, headaches, and syncope may develop.

CLINICAL PEARL   **STEP 2/3**

Although irreversible pulmonary hypertension occurs by 2 years of age in most patients with VSDs and heart failure, survival into adulthood is common.

How would you proceed with treatment?

The size of the VSD affects treatment decisions; 30% to 50% of small defects will spontaneously close, typically during the first 2 years of life. Most children with small defects are asymptomatic and do not develop increased heart size, pulmonary arterial pressure, or resistance. These children can live normal unrestricted lives, and surgical repair is currently not recommended.

On the other hand, only 8% of moderate to large sized VSDs close spontaneously. Children with larger defects typically have recurrent respiratory infections, heart failure and failure to thrive and are at risk of developing Eisenmenger syndrome. Management of large VSDs focuses on controlling symptoms of heart failure and preventing pulmonary vascular disease. Medical management—diuretics and afterload reducing agents—are used as a temporizing measure to alleviate and control the symptom and allow growth while waiting for either spontaneous VSD closure or size reduction. However, if this is unsuccessful in a symptomatic patient, surgical correction should not be delayed.

Timely surgical closure within the first year of life typically prevents the development of pulmonary vascular disease. Indications for surgical closure of a VSD include patients with large defects, as well as clinical symptoms of heart failure and/or failure to thrive who are not able to be controlled by medical management. Such patients usually have large left-to-right shunts (defined as a ratio of pulmonary to systemic blood flow or Qp:Qs > 2:1).

Case Point 13.6

The patient is treated with furosemide to reduce symptoms of heart failure. He is closely followed by a pediatric nutritionist, and his formula is fortified to increase the caloric density in light of his poor weight gain. Ultimately, he undergoes surgical closure.

BEYOND THE PEARLS

- VSDs, as discussed in this chapter, are considered as isolated entities or in combination with atrial septal defects. They are completely different entities when they occur as part of a constellation of defects, such as in tetralogy of Fallot, common arterial trunk, or double-outlet ventricles.
- Based on the size, plane, and boundaries of the defect, VSDs may disrupt the conduction pathways of the heart and/or the seating of the cardiac valves. Surgeons must take these factors into account when planning closure surgeries.
- There are many ways to classify VSDs, but they can mostly be separated into four groups: perimembranous VSDs, muscular VSDs, AV canal type VSDs, and supracristal VSDs.
- Pulmonary outflow obstruction, if present, can be protective against pulmonary hypertension in patients with large VSDs and may limit left-to-right shunting and congestive heart failure symptomatology. The right ventricular pressure will be elevated, however, and in certain cases may even rise to levels above left ventricular pressure. At this point, the shunt will reverse to a right-to-left shunt, and cyanosis will result.
- In addition to pulmonary hypertension, two other VSD complications that may result in premature death in early adulthood are aortic regurgitation and infective endocarditis. Surgical closure early in life removes the risk of aortic regurgitation and if no residual shunt is present, minimizes the risk of infective endocarditis.
- If an infant requires surgical intervention early in life, and primary closure is not an option, pulmonary artery banding can be performed to decrease pulmonary blood flow. However, with modern surgical techniques for primary closure, this palliative procedure is no longer commonly performed.

Case Summary

Complaint/History: An 8-day-old male presents with poor feeding and 2 months later with tachypnea.

Findings: A 3/6 holosystolic murmur is audible throughout the chest.

Labs/Tests: Chest radiography reveals cardiomegaly. An echocardiogram reveals a ventricular septal defect.

Diagnosis: Ventricular septal defect.

Treatment: Surgical closure.

Bibliography

Benson LN, et al. Ventricular septal defects. In: *Paediatric Cardiology.* 2010:591–624.

Bernstein D. Acyanotic congenital heart disease: the left-to-right shunt lesions. In: Kliegman RM, Stanton BF, Schor NF, et al., eds. *Nelson Textbook of Pediatrics.* 19th ed. Philadelphia: Elsevier Saunders; 2011.

Bernstein D. Pulmonary hypertension. In: Kliegman RM, Stanton BF, Schor NF, et al., eds. *Nelson Textbook of Pediatrics.* 19th ed. Philadelphia: Elsevier Saunders; 2011.

Feigelman S. The first year. In: Kliegman RM, Stanton BF, Schor NF, et al., eds. *Nelson Textbook of Pediatrics.* 19th ed. Philadelphia: Elsevier Saunders; 2011.

Hagan JF, Shaw JS, Duncan P, eds. *Bright Futures: Guidelines for Health Supervision of Infants, Children, and Adolescents.* 3rd ed. Elk Grove Village, IL: American Academy of Pediatrics; 2008:271–302.

Sharieff GQ, Wylie TW. Pediatric cardiac disorders. *J Emerg Med.* 2004;26(1):65–79.

A Newborn With Hydrops Fetalis

Monika Alas-Segura ■ Tracey Samko ■ Priya Shastry ■ Rowena G. Cayabyab ■ Thomas C. Hofstra ■ Randall Y. Chan

A premature female neonate is born to a $G_1P_{0\rightarrow1}$ mother at 24 $^5/_7$ weeks gestation with a birth weight of 769 g via spontaneous vaginal delivery after preterm onset of labor. The infant requires immediate endotracheal intubation as she is noted to be markedly pale and edematous (hydropic; Fig. 14.1). Oxygen saturation is in the 60%–70% range. Apgar scores are 1 and 6 at 1 and 5 minutes, respectively.

What are the clinical manifestations of hydrops fetalis?

Hydrops fetalis is a condition that is manifested by extravascular fluid collections in two or more fetal compartments, including the fetal soft tissue and serous spaces: pleural space, peritoneal space, pericardial space, or placenta. It is often discovered incidentally on prenatal ultrasound or during workup for decreased fetal movement or polyhydramnios. Although the pathogenesis is incompletely understood, it is generally due to an imbalance in the fetal hydrostatic and oncotic pressures.

BASIC SCIENCE PEARL	STEP 1

Edema in general results from a mismatch between the hydrostatic and oncotic pressures of the capillary space and the interstitial space, as governed by Starling's law. In the fetus, impaired flow in the lymphatics and increased permeability of capillaries both aid in the susceptibility of the fetus to accumulating interstitial fluid.

What is the differential diagnosis of hydrops fetalis?

The differential diagnosis for hydrops fetalis is generally divided into immune and nonimmune causes.

Immune fetal hydrops develops when maternal antibody crosses the placenta to destroy fetal red blood cells, leading to severe anemia. The fetal bone marrow cannot produce sufficient red blood cells to outpace the hemolysis, so blood production is shifted to extramedullary sites, including the liver and spleen, leading to hepatosplenomegaly.

Nonimmune hydrops fetalis (NIHF) currently accounts for more than 90% of cases of hydrops fetalis, originally defined by a lack of circulating maternal red cell antibodies. The causes of NIHF are summarized in Table 14.1. The most likely cause varies depending on the ethnicity of the patient and the trimester in which NIHF is diagnosed. NIHF in the first trimester is more likely to be genetic in origin, whereas second- and third-trimester diagnoses are more likely to be cardiac.

What needs to be done if hydrops is detected prior to delivery?

If NIHF is diagnosed prenatally, the mother should be referred to a maternal fetal medicine specialist for a comprehensive ultrasound and investigation for potential causes. Depending on

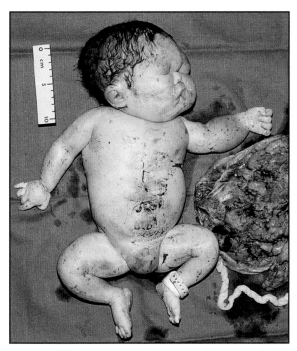

Fig. 14.1   Infant with severe hydrops. (From Immunopathology. In Damjanov, ed. *Pathology for the Health Professions*, 4th ed. Philadelphia: Saunders; 2012:40–66.)

the cause, the treating obstetrician may offer a variety of procedures to mitigate the hydrops and prevent its progression. Therapeutic maneuvers include intravascular fetal blood transfusion for anemia, repeated amniocentesis to prevent preterm labor, insertion of a shunt into an effusion when repeated pleurocentesis fails, antiarrhythmic drugs, or antithyroid drugs. Open fetal surgery or laser vessel ablation may be required for vascular mass or for twin-twin transfusion, respectively.

When NIHF presents prior to 24 weeks gestational age and structural anomalies are found, the prognosis is quite poor. Regardless of the time of presentation, without treatment the prognosis is also generally quite poor.

CLINICAL PEARL	STEP 2/3

Once NIHF is diagnosed and investigation for a cause has begun, the mother should be monitored for mirror syndrome—the development of maternal edema secondary to fetal hydrops, associated with preeclampsia.

How is hydrops managed in the delivery room?

Immediate intubation is recommended for infants with severe hydrops fetalis because of facial edema, decrease in respiratory system compliance, compression of the lungs by pleural fluid, limited mobility of the diaphragm secondary to ascites, and the possible presence of pulmonary hypoplasia. This is followed by surfactant administration and mechanical ventilator support. Drainage

TABLE 14-1 ■ Differential Diagnosis of Nonimmune Fetal Hydrops

Condition Type	Specific Conditions
Hemolytic anemias	Alloimmune, Rh, Kell, α-chain hemoglobinopathies (homozygous α-thalassemia) Red blood cell enzyme deficiencies (glucose phosphate isomerase deficiency, glucose-6-phosphate dehydrogenase)
Other anemias	Fetomaternal hemorrhage Twin-twin transfusion Diamond–Blackfan syndrome
Cardiac conditions	Premature closure of foramen ovale Ebstein anomaly Hypoplastic left or right heart Subaortic stenosis with fibroelastosis Cardiomyopathy, myocardial fibroelastosis Atrioventricular canal Myocarditis Right atrial hemangioma Intracardiac hamartoma or fibroma Tuberous sclerosis with cardiac rhabdomyoma
Cardiac arrhythmias	Supraventricular tachycardia Atrial flutter Congenital heart block
Vascular malformations	Hemangioma of the liver Any large arteriovenous malformation Klippel-Trénaunay syndrome Idiopathic infantile arterial calcification
Vascular accidents	Thrombosis of umbilical vein or inferior vena cava Recipient in twin-twin transfusion
Infections	Cytomegalovirus, congenital hepatitis, human parvovirus, enterovirus, other viruses Toxoplasmosis, Chagas disease Coxsackie virus Syphilis Leptospirosis
Lymphatic abnormalities	Congenital lymphatic dysplasia Lymphatic malformations Lymphangiectasia Cystic hygroma Noonan syndrome Multiple pterygium syndrome Congenital chylothorax Hereditary lymphedema type 1
Nervous system lesions	Absence of corpus callosum Encephalocele Cerebral arteriovenous malformation Intracranial hemorrhage (massive) Holoprosencephaly Fetal akinesia sequence
Pulmonary conditions	Cystic adenomatoid malformation of the lung Mediastinal teratoma Diaphragmatic hernia Lung sequestration syndrome Lymphangiectasia

TABLE 14-1 ■ Differential Diagnosis of Nonimmune Fetal Hydrops—cont'd

Condition Type	Specific Conditions
Renal conditions	Urinary ascites Congenital nephrosis Renal vein thrombosis Invasive processes and storage disorders Tuberous sclerosis Gaucher disease Mucopolysaccharidosis Mucolipidosis
Chromosome abnormalities	Trisomy 13, trisomy 18, trisomy 21 Turner syndrome 46, XX/XY chimerism
Bone diseases	Osteogenesis imperfecta Achondroplasia Asphyxiating thoracic dystrophy
Gastrointestinal conditions	Bowel obstruction with perforation and meconium peritonitis Small bowel volvulus Other intestinal obstructions Prune-belly syndrome
Tumors	Neuroblastoma Choriocarcinoma Sacrococcygeal teratoma Hemangioma or other hepatic tumors Congenital leukemia Cardiac tumors Renal tumors
Maternal or placental conditions	Maternal diabetes Maternal therapy with indomethacin Multiple gestation with parasitic fetus Chorioangioma of placenta, chorionic vessels, or umbilical vessels Toxemia Systemic lupus erythematosus
Miscellaneous	Neu-Laxova syndrome Myotonic dystrophy Hereditary lymphedema type 1
Idiopathic	

Adapted from Lorch SA and Mollen TJ. Nonimmune Hydrops. In: Gleason CA, Juul SE, eds. *Avery's Diseases of the Newborn,* 10th ed. Philadelphia: Elsevier; 2018:82–89.e2.

of fluid collections (i.e., pleural, peritoneal) may be necessary to help establish adequate lung expansion and achieve better ventilation and oxygenation.

Infants with hydrops are also at increased risk of cardiogenic shock or severe symptomatic anemia. Clinicians should be prepared for immediate placement of an umbilical venous catheter in the delivery room for the administration of intravenous fluids, inotropic support, and blood transfusion as needed. If severe anemia is anticipated, O-negative packed red blood cells should be available for immediate transfusion in the delivery room.

Case Point 14.1

Aggressive resuscitation begins with endotracheal intubation followed by the administration of three doses of surfactant. Dopamine is started for blood pressure support. Point-of-care testing at bedside in the delivery room reveals a hemoglobin level of 6.4 g/dL. The child receives a transfusion of packed red blood cells.

A review of prenatal records reveals that the mother had recently moved here from Hong Kong and began prenatal care 3 weeks ago. During prenatal workup, she was found to have a mild microcytic, hypochromic anemia.

What is the most likely diagnosis based on the mother's past medical history?

In the setting of fetal hydrops, the microcytic anemia in the mother suggests that she carries a *cis*-deletion of two α-globin genes, resulting in α-thalassemia trait. The clinical picture in the child suggests that the father also carries a *cis*-deletion and the most likely diagnosis would therefore be four-gene α-thalassemia. Other types of α-thalassemia mutations, including *trans*-deletion or carrier status in either parent, are much less likely to cause hydrops fetalis because the fetus should have inherited at least one, if not two or three functioning α-globin genes.

Severe γ-thalassemia (including large deletions of the β-cluster) have been described to cause hydrops as well. Other causes of maternal microcytosis would not lead to hydrops.

BASIC SCIENCE PEARL	STEP 1

β-Globin, γ-globin and δ-globin are all β-globin–like chains in the β-cluster of genes. β-Globin, γ-globin and δ-globin all form heterodimers with α-globin to form hemoglobin A, hemoglobin F, and hemoglobin A$_2$, respectively.

Case Point 14.2

Hemoglobin electrophoresis reveals the presence of Hemoglobin Barts. Genetic testing reveals a homozygous inheritance of the --$_{SEA}$ α-globin cluster mutation (large deletion).

Diagnosis: Four-gene deletion α-thalassemia (hydrops fetalis).

BASIC SCIENCE/CLINICAL PEARL	STEP 1/2/3

Whereas hemoglobin F is abundant in fetal life, hemoglobin A and A$_2$ are minimally present at birth. Hemoglobin A is the predominant hemoglobin (>95% of all hemoglobin) by the first year of life. α-Globin is in both hemoglobin F and A/A$_2$ and thus α-thalassemia presents early; β-thalassemia will not present until hemoglobin A is produced in large amounts during the first year of life.

What are the different α-thalassemia syndromes and how do they present?

α-Thalassemia is caused by the absence (or decreased production) of one or more genes encoding the α-chain of hemoglobin, located on chromosome 16. Two copies of the α-globin gene are on each chromosome, and thus each individual possesses four alleles in total—two inherited from the mother and two from the father. The phenotype expressed depends on the number of genes mutated/deleted.

Individuals who have only one α-globin gene deleted (-α/αα) are considered silent carriers, with no clinical manifestations.

Individuals with two α-globin gene deletions (-α/-α, or *trans*-deletion) or (- -/αα, or *cis*-deletion) are considered to have α-thalassemia trait. These individuals have microcytosis and a normal hemoglobin level or very mild anemia.

BASIC SCIENCE PEARL	STEP 1

Like most mild hemolytic anemias, α-thalassemia trait is thought to provide a protective effect against malaria.

Hemoglobin H disease is seen when three α-globin genes are mutated (- -/-α), leading to a hemolytic anemia. The relatively increased amounts of γ and β chains causes the formation of tetramers—γ_4 (hemoglobin Bart) and β_4 (hemoglobin H), respectively. These tetramers precipitate, leading to membrane damage and hemolysis.

BASIC SCIENCE/CLINICAL PEARL	STEP 1/2/3

Hemoglobin H disease tends to be mild. Inheriting the Constant Spring (α_{CS}) mutation—a mutation resulting in a longer, unstable α-globin chain—along with a *cis*-deletion (- -/$\alpha\alpha_{CS}$), however, results in a more severe form of hemoglobin H disease.

α-Thalassemia major (also known as hydrops fetalis or hemoglobin Barts disease) is a mutation of all four alpha chains (- -/- -) and most develop hydrops and die in utero. Homozygous inheritance of large deletions of the α-globin cluster is incompatible with life, but deletions that preserve the zeta (ζ) globin genes preserve the ability produce hemoglobin Gower 1 ($\zeta_2\varepsilon_2$) and hemoglobin Portland ($\zeta_2\gamma_2$). This allows for the pregnancy to continue through the first trimester, but the fetus will start to suffer from chronic hypoxia and anemia as production shifts to α-globin, eventually leading to high output cardiac failure. This in turn results in ascites, edema, heart failure, pleural and pericardial effusions and massive organomegaly, and eventually death.

CLINICAL PEARL	STEP 2/3

A hemoglobin level of 6.4 g/dL would normally not account for the severity of this child's clinical presentation. Her hemoglobins are exclusively hemoglobin Barts and hemoglobin H, however, and both are high-affinity hemoglobins that transport oxygen poorly.

How do the β-thalassemia syndromes present differently from the α-thalassemia syndromes? Why?
The β-thalassemia syndromes do not present in utero or in the neonatal period—as opposed to the α-thalassemia syndromes—because fetal hemoglobin (hemoglobin F, $\alpha_2\gamma_2$) predominates at birth. The absence of functioning β-globin clinically manifests around 6 to 12 months of age.

Case Point 14.3

The patient is started on chronic transfusion therapy with a pretransfusion hemoglobin goal of 9 to 10 g/dL.

How are the α-thalassemia syndromes treated?

A patient with α-thalassemia trait usually requires no treatment as the patient is generally asymptomatic, with normal hemoglobin but microcytosis. These patients should have genetic counseling because each patient is at risk of having a child with hemoglobin H disease or α-thalassemia major if his/her partner either has the trait or is a silent carrier, respectively.

Patients with hemoglobin H disease are managed primarily with supportive care. Patients should be started on folic acid supplementation and a non–iron-containing multivitamin as calcium and vitamin D deficiencies can develop. Patients may require periodic transfusions during hemolytic crises that may be precipitated by oxidative stress, infection, fever, and/or pregnancy.

α-Thalassemia major and subsequent hydrops fetalis requires in utero transfusions and/or immediate exchange transfusion at birth. Mortality is high. If the patient survives, s/he will be transfusion-dependent for life. Hematopoietic stem cell transplantation (HSCT) is the only curative option.

CLINICAL PEARL	STEP 2/3

Patients dependent on blood transfusions should be considered for hematopoietic stem cell transplantation.

What are the complications of chronic anemia?

In milder forms of overt thalassemia with anemia (e.g., hemoglobin H disease), the primary complications are a result of chronic hemolysis. Splenomegaly and biliary pigment gallstones are common. Folic acid deficiency may occur due to increased demand stemming from purine synthesis.

In severe thalassemia, bone abnormalities occur as a result of bone marrow expansion due to ineffective erythropoiesis. The resulting bony abnormalities lead to skeletal deformities (e.g., thalassemic facies), as well as osteoporosis and increased bone fragility. Vertebral bones are at particular risk. The ineffective erythropoiesis also leads to extramedullary erythropoiesis with evidence of production in the liver and spleen leading to hepatosplenomegaly.

What are the complications of chronic transfusion therapy?

In the era of chronic transfusions for thalassemia major, the main complication of chronic severe thalassemia is iron overload. Although primarily a concern in transfused patients, iron overload can occur in non–transfusion-dependent patients as well, due to increased intestinal absorption of iron in compensation for ineffective erythropoiesis.

Iron overload leads to free iron in the body which is toxic to cells and causes organ failure. Iron overload occurs most rapidly in the liver, ultimately leading to cirrhosis. Myocardial free iron uptake occurs more slowly than hepatic uptake, but with time cardiomyopathy and heart failure will also result. Endocrinopathies commonly seen include hypogonadotropic hypogonadism, diabetes mellitus, and hypothyroidism.

Generally, patients should be started on chelators no later than 2 to 3 years after repeated transfusions. Intermittent quantitative monitoring for iron overload—commonly achievable using magnetic resonance imaging of the heart and liver—is used to evaluate the efficacy of chelation.

BASIC SCIENCE/CLINICAL PEARL	STEP 1/2/3

Prior to iron chelation, death from iron cardiomyopathy would occur by the second decade of life.

BEYOND THE PEARLS

- Dozens of gene mutations and deletions have been described in both the α-globin gene cluster and the β-globin gene cluster, leading to a wide variety of thalassemia phenotypes.
- It is estimated that up to 40% of the population in China and Southeast Asia are α-thalassemia carriers. The *cis*-mutation is more common in the Asian population. In Southeast Asian populations, α-thalassemia accounts for up to 80% of cases of NIHF.
- Co-inheriting both α- and β-thalassemia gene mutations may actually lead to milder disease, as there is less imbalance in the α:β ratio.
- α-Thalassemia major is associated with congenital malformations, including hypospadias and musculoskeletal defects.
- α-Thalassemia major (and hydrops in general) is associated with significant placental hypertrophy, which can lead to major complications for the mother at birth, including toxemia and hemorrhage.
- Iron loading occurs much more rapidly in thalassemia patients than in those with other transfusion-dependent diseases, such as myelodysplastic syndrome or sickle-cell disease, due to the higher pretransfusion hemoglobin goals required to suppress extramedullary hematopoiesis, as well as decreased reutilization of iron in the bone marrow due to ineffective erythropoiesis.
- Survival into the fourth decade of life with thalassemia major has increased from less than 50% to greater than 90% since the introduction of iron chelators. Nonetheless, iron overload continues to account for 70% of deaths in patients with thalassemia major.

Case Summary

Complaint/History: A female neonate is born prematurely at 24 weeks of gestation with marked pallor and edema (hydrops).

Findings: Hypoxia, pallor, edema, hydrops.

Labs/Tests: Hemoglobin 6.4 g/dL. Hemoglobin electrophoresis reveals presence of hemoglobin Barts.

Diagnosis: Four-gene α-thalassemia.

Treatment: Red blood cell transfusion.

Bibliography

Bellini C, et al. Etiology of non-immune hydrops fetalis: an update. *Am J Med Genet A*. 2015;167(5):1082–1088.

Chmait RH, et al. Treatment of alpha (0)-thalassemia (−SEA/−SEA) via serial fetal and post-natal transfusions: can early fetal intervention improve outcomes? *Hematology*. 2015;20(4):217–222.

Kremastinos DT, Farmakis D. Iron overload cardiomyopathy in clinical practice. *Circulation*. 2011;124(20): 2253–2263.

Vichinsky EP. Alpha thalassemia major—new mutations, intrauterine management, and outcomes. *ASH Education Program Book*. 2009;2009(1):35–41.

9-Year-Old Female With Joint Pain and Swelling

Huynh Tran ▥ Stratos Christianakis

A 9-year-old female presents with joint swelling and pain for the past 4 months. Her symptoms started with morning stiffness in the joints of her hands, wrists, and elbows. Subsequently, she developed joint swelling and pain. Her past medical history is otherwise unremarkable.

What is the differential diagnosis?

The differential diagnosis for joint pain in a child is generally very large; thus, a thorough history is critical to allow narrowing of the differential diagnosis. Regardless of the reported course, infections should always be considered, given the gravity of a missed diagnosis. In this child, with several months of pain and swelling in multiple joints, inflammatory conditions and rheumatic diseases, malignancies, and metabolic diseases should also be considered.

Chronic infections may be associated with arthritis—joint inflammation characterized by pain and swelling. Reactive arthritis is generally accompanied by associated symptoms from the underlying infection. In rheumatic fever, arthritis would be migratory; in Lyme disease, it would be intermittent.

CLINICAL PEARL   **STEP 2/3**

Consideration of septic arthritis is critical in a child with joint pain and swelling, although a prolonged course and multiple joint involvement makes it less likely.

The primary malignancy to consider is acute lymphoblastic leukemia, which may infiltrate synovium. Inflammatory diseases to consider include inflammatory bowel disease and sarcoidosis, which would respectively be associated with abdominal symptoms (e.g., bloody diarrhea) or intrathoracic findings (e.g., hilar adenopathy).

BASIC SCIENCE PEARL   **STEP 1**

Sarcoid arthritis often occurs in association with hilar adenopathy and erythema nodosum; this triad together is known as Löfgren syndrome.

Rheumatic diseases include juvenile idiopathic arthritis (JIA), systemic lupus erythematosus (SLE), dermatomyositis, and scleroderma. In general, arthritis is erosive in JIA and nonerosive in SLE; antibody testing and associated symptomatology also help differentiate the two diagnoses. Patients with dermatomyositis would present with rash and muscle weakness. Scleroderma may initially mimic arthritis, but joint pain would be due to contractures, not arthritis.

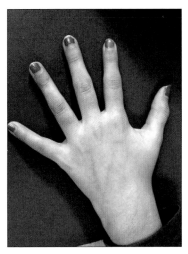

Fig. 15.1 Physical examination reveals painful swelling of the metacarpophalangeal and proximal interphalangeal joints. (From Nordal E, Rygg M, Fasth A. Clinical features of juvenile idiopathic arthritis. In: Hochberg MC, Silman AJ, Smolen JS, et al, eds. *Rheumatology,* 6th ed. Philadelphia: Elsevier Mosby; 2015: 833–844.)

Case Point 15.1

Her blood pressure is 108/60 mm Hg, pulse rate is 80/min, respiration rate is 18/min, and oxygen saturation is 98% on room air. On physical examination, the metacarpophalangeal (MCP) and proximal interphalangeal joints of her bilateral hands are swollen and tender (Fig. 15.1). The affected joints exhibit mildly decreased range of motion. She does not have a rash. The remainder of her musculoskeletal examination—including back and neck—is normal, as is the remainder of her physical examination.

What laboratory tests and imaging studies would be useful at this time?

Given the symmetric polyarthritis and absence of fever, chills, rash, and other systemic symptoms, polyarticular JIA is the most likely diagnosis. Laboratory analysis should be geared to evaluate for other diagnoses on the differential.

A complete blood count would be helpful to evaluate for malignant disease. A mild anemia in inflammatory polyarthritis is common, but pancytopenia should trigger further workup for malignancy or SLE.

Inflammatory markers such as the erythrocyte sedimentation rate (ESR) and/or C-reactive protein (CRP), may be helpful to evaluate inflammation, although they are nonspecific. Detection of antinuclear antibodies (ANAs) may help differentiate SLE from JIA, although many children with polyarticular JIA exhibit ANA positivity with low titer and homogeneous pattern. ANA positivity is associated with uveitis and early-onset disease in JIA.

Rheumatoid factors (RFs) are not necessarily useful in making a diagnosis of JIA because they may be positive or negative in both JIA and SLE. The RF status is important to ascertain in polyarticular JIA, however, because RF-positive and RF-negative polyarticular JIA are considered separate diseases. The detection of anticyclic citrullinated peptide antibodies (APCAs) is not diagnostic but may be prognostic.

Radiographs of the joints should be obtained to evaluate for joint space narrowing and erosion and to rule out other organic causes of articular symptoms, such as fracture or malignancy. Most

TABLE 15.1 ■ **Patient's Laboratory Test Results**

	Result
Leukocyte count	18×10^9/L with a normal differential
Hemoglobin	13 g/dL
Platelet count	540×10^9/L
Serum creatinine	1.1 mg/dL
Urinalysis	Normal
Erythrocyte sedimentation rate	56 mm/hour
C-reactive protein	11 mg/L
Antinuclear antibodies	Not detected
Rheumatoid factor	Not detected
Anticyclic citrullinated peptide antibodies	Not detected

patients with JIA will have normal radiographic findings early in the disease course, but nearly 50% will demonstrate joint space narrowing and erosion after 6 years. Other findings include soft tissue swelling, osteopenia, growth disturbances (epiphyseal overgrowth, or "ballooning"), and joint subluxation.

Synovial fluid analysis is generally not performed, except to rule out other conditions such as septic arthritis.

BASIC SCIENCE/CLINICAL PEARL   **STEP 1/2/3**

Be wary of relying on inflammatory markers (e.g., ESR, CRP) alone for the detection of inflammatory joint disease. Many JIA patients will have a normal ESR and CRP on initial presentation.

Case Point 15.2

Plain radiographs of the hands and wrists are unrevealing. Laboratory tests are performed (Table 15.1).

What is the most likely diagnosis?
This patient likely has JIA, based on histories, clinical symptoms, physical examination, and laboratories results. JIA is a disease of chronic inflammation affecting the synovium. The precise underlying causes are not known—and the term *juvenile idiopathic arthritis* itself actually stands for multiple subsets of disease with likely varying causes—but a pathologic autoimmune response is the common endpoint.

The International League of Associations for Rheumatology (ILAR) has defined JIA as arthritis without a known cause lasting at least 6 weeks and beginning prior to 16 years of age. ILAR recognizes seven distinct subtypes of JIA:

    1. Oligoarthritis (≤four joints)
    2. Polyarthritis (RF-negative)
    3. Polyarthritis (RF-positive)
    4. Systemic arthritis
    5. Psoriatic arthritis
    6. Enthesitis-related arthritis (ERA)
    7. Undifferentiated arthritis

Systemic arthritis separates itself from oligoarthritis and polyarthritis by the presence of systemic symptoms such as fever/chills, rash, weight change, lymphadenopathy, and pruritus. Psoriatic arthritis is associated with psoriasis, nail pitting, and/or dactylitis. ERA is associated with enthesitis (inflammation of tendon/ligament/fascia/joint capsule insertion sites into bone) and involvement of the axial skeleton and sacroiliac joints.

BASIC SCIENCE PEARL   **STEP 1**

Oligoarthritis—the most common JIA subtype—typically presents in young females, with involvement of the knees and/or ankles. ANA is typically detectable.

This patient meets the classification of RF-negative polyarthritis, which is defined as arthritis that affects five or more joints in the first 6 months of disease and without detectable RF; the other forms of JIA must be excluded.

BASIC SCIENCE/CLINICAL PEARL   **STEP 1/2/3**

The classification criteria for JIA do not include all clinical characteristics of that particular disorder, only those that distinguish the disorder from other joint diseases.

Case Point 15.3

Diagnosis: RF-Negative polyarthritis subtype of juvenile idiopathic arthritis

---

CLINICAL PEARL   **STEP 2/3**

Early diagnosis of JIA is critical because early treatment may be able to prevent long-term destruction and bony deformities.

What are the manifestations of RF-negative polyarthritis?

The arthritis in RF-negative polyarthritis generally has an insidious onset. Only a few joints may be involved initially, with the number of joints increasing over time to at least five joints in the first 6 months of disease. The affected joints may have intraarticular fluid accumulation and synovial hypertrophy from articular inflammation. Knees, wrists, and ankles are the joints most commonly affected; arthritis is characteristically symmetric in polyarthritis. The hip is involved in less than 20% of cases at initial presentation but may become involved over time, with significant morbidity.

The temporomandibular joint (TMJ) and/or the cervical spine are often involved in RF-negative polyarthritis. TMJ arthritis can lead to joint damage, resulting in malocclusion, micrognathia, and/or retrognathia—all of which can result in facial deformity (Fig. 15.2). Cervical spine arthritis may lead to cervical spine joint stiffness and/or even atlantoaxial subluxation (Fig. 15.3). Both TMJ and cervical spine arthritis are commonly asymptomatic and may require advanced imaging (e.g., magnetic resonance imaging) to detect in the early stages.

Ocular inflammation is commonly seen in patients with JIA (Fig. 15.4). Inflammation of the anterior uveal tract (anterior uveitis) is most common, and the adjacent ciliary body is often involved (iridocyclitis). Anterior uveitis–iridocyclitis characteristically presents in an asymptomatic manner in polyarthritis. Periodic screening with a slit lamp ophthalmic examination is recommended due to the irreversible vision damage that may accompany uncontrolled chronic ocular inflammation.

Systemic manifestations are uncommon in RF-negative polyarthritis, but growth failure may be seen. Abnormal growth velocity is associated with uncontrolled disease.

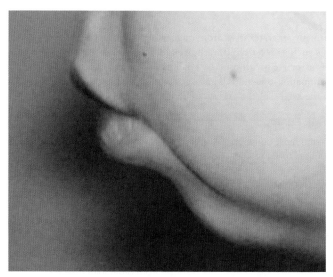

Fig. 15.2 Retrognathia seen 9 years after the onset of JIA. (From Rosenberg AM, Oen KG. Polyarticular juvenile idiopathic arthritis. In: Petty RE, Laxer RM, Lindsley CB, et al, eds. 7th ed. *Textbook of Pediatric Rheumatology*. Philadelphia: Elsevier; 2015:217–228.e6.)

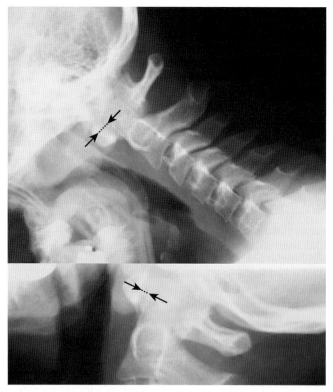

Fig. 15.3 Mild atlantoaxial subluxation on plain radiographs. The distance between the *arrows* indicates abnormal widening of the normal gaps between the vertebra. (From Rosenberg AM, Oen KG. Polyarticular juvenile idiopathic arthritis. In: Petty RE, Laxer RM, Lindsley CB, et al, eds. 7th ed. *Textbook of Pediatric Rheumatology*. Philadelphia: Elsevier; 2015:217–228.e6.)

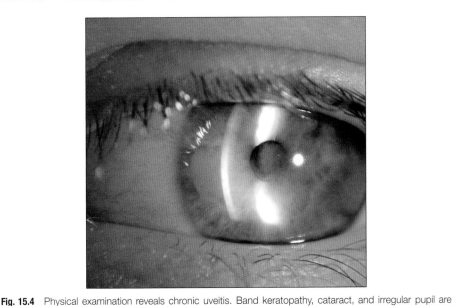

Fig. 15.4 Physical examination reveals chronic uveitis. Band keratopathy, cataract, and irregular pupil are seen. (From Nordal E, Rygg M, Fasth A. Clinical features of juvenile idiopathic arthritis. In: Hochberg MC, Silman AJ, Smolen JS, et al, eds. *Rheumatology,* 6th ed. Philadelphia: Elsevier Mosby; 2015: 833–844.)

CLINICAL PEARL   **STEP 2/3**

Patients with JIA are at increased risk of cardiovascular disease.

How do you approach treatment for juvenile idiopathic arthritis in accordance with American College of Rheumatology (ACR) guidelines?
A timely pediatric rheumatology referral is indicated for all patients with JIA. ACR guidelines for the treatment of JIA vary by the number of joints involved, systemic involvement, and sacroiliac involvement. A multidisciplinary approach is recommended, including prominent roles for occupational and physical therapy. In addition to inducing a remission of arthritis symptoms, the therapeutic plan should also include monitoring for growth failure, progressive joint damage, and loss of function.

BASIC SCIENCE/CLINICAL PEARL   **STEP 1/2/3**

Loss of joint function from arthritis may inhibit normal childhood development.

For initial therapy in a patient with arthritis in five or more joints without systemic or sacroiliac involvement, a nonsteroidal antiinflammatory drug (NSAID) may be started. NSAID monotherapy generally will not be continued more than 2 months prior to starting methotrexate (or leflunomide). Patients with high disease activity, or moderate activity with poor prognostic features—involvement of the hip or cervical spine, presence of RF or ACPA, or radiographic evidence of joint damage—should be started immediately on methotrexate. Patients who continue to have disease activity should be switched to tumor necrosis factor alpha (TNFα) inhibitors.

BASIC SCIENCE/CLINICAL PEARL	STEP 1/2/3

Disease-modifying antirheumatic drugs (DMARDs; e.g., methotrexate and leflunomide) play a critical role in inducing and maintaining remission status in JIA. The side effects of DMARDs can be substantial and require specific monitoring by experienced practitioners (e.g., pediatric rheumatologists).

Case Point 15.4

The patient is started on ibuprofen and referred to a pediatric rheumatologist. Her joint swelling and pain improve but do not resolve. Methotrexate is started along with folic acid to reduce bone marrow suppression. Her symptoms improve to the point where she is able to reduce her ibuprofen use substantially, and treatment of her disease is maintained on weekly oral methotrexate.

BEYOND THE PEARLS

- The age of onset of polyarticular JIA has a bimodal distribution with two peaks, between 2 and 5 years of age and between 10 and 14 years of age. JIA is more common in females than males at all ages.
- RF-positive disease is rarely seen in children younger than 10 years. Older children with RF-positive disease are more likely to be female and tend to have more severe disease.
- In systemic arthritis, systemic symptoms may precede the actual arthritis by up to 1 year.
- Intraarticular glucocorticoid injections are effective in JIA but are primarily recommended for patients with a history of arthritis in four or fewer joints only.
- Clinicians should have a high index of suspicion for avascular necrosis as a cause for new-onset joint pain in patients with JIA who have had long-term glucocorticoid exposure.
- Most JIA relapses occur within the first year after the cessation of immunosuppressive therapy and may or may not affect the same joints as the initial presentation.

Case Summary

Complaint/History: A 9-year-old female presents with joint swelling and pain with morning stiffness for 4 months.

Findings: Metacarpophalangeal (MCP) and proximal interphalangeal joints of her bilateral hands are swollen and tender, with mildly decreased range of motion.

Labs/Tests: Her erythrocyte sedimentation rate is 56 mm/hour; otherwise, laboratory test results and plain radiographs of her hands and wrists are unrevealing.

Diagnosis: Polyarthritis (RF-negative) subtype of juvenile idiopathic arthritis.

Treatment: Methotrexate.

Bibliography

Beukelman T, Patkar NM, Saag KG, et al. 2011 American College of Rheumatology recommendations for the treatment of juvenile idiopathic arthritis: initiation and safety monitoring of therapeutic agents for the treatment of arthritis and systemic features. *Arthritis Care Res.* 2011;63(4):465–482. (Also Clinician's Guide with treatment algorithms).

Gadkowski LB, Stout JE. Joint disease. *Clin Arthritis Rev.* 2008;21(2):305–333.

Petty RE, Southwood TR, Manners P, et al. International League of Associations for Rheumatology classification of juvenile idiopathic arthritis: Second Revision, Edmonton 2001. *J Rheumatol.* 2004;31(2):390–392.

Ravelli A, Martini A. Juvenile idiopathic arthritis. *Lancet.* 2007;369(9563):767–778.

Rosenberg AM, Oen KG. Polyarticular juvenile idiopathic arthritis. In: Petty RE, Laxer RM, eds. *Textbook of Pediatric Rheumatology.* Philadelphia: Elsevier; 2016:217–228.e6.

Saurenmann RK, Levin AV, Feldman BM, et al. Prevalence, risk factors, and outcome of uveitis in juvenile idiopathic arthritis: a long-term followup study. *Arthritis Rheum.* 2007;56(2):647.

11-Year-Old Male With Bruising

Tracey Samko ■ Randall Y. Chan

An 11-year-old male presents with scattered petechiae and increased bruising over 3 weeks, first on his legs, then spreading to his abdomen and arms. He cannot recall any trauma preceding the bruising but does report fever, cough, rhinorrhea, and headache 6 weeks prior that resolved over several days. He had a deciduous (baby) tooth fall out (shed) 3 days prior to presentation, without excess bleeding. He does not have gingival bleeding, nose bleeds, or joint swelling.

BASIC SCIENCE PEARL   **STEP 1**

Petechiae are pinpoint hemorrhages that do not blanch with pressure. They are caused by the extravasation of blood from the vasculature into the skin or mucous membranes.

What is in your differential diagnosis in children with petechiae?

Petechiae (Fig. 16.1) are usually caused by platelet disorders, which may be qualitative or quantitative in nature.

Qualitative platelet dysfunction may be due to a number of conditions. Congenital platelet dysfunction syndromes include conditions such as Glanzmann thrombasthenia (deficiency in glycoprotein IIb/IIIa) and Bernard-Soulier disease (deficiency in glycoprotein Ib/V/IX). Medications such as aspirin, nonsteroidal antiinflammatory drugs, furosemide, and heparin all interfere with platelet function. Uremia also results in platelet dysfunction, although resulting petechiae would be uncommon.

Endothelial damage and/or abnormalities may lead to the formation of purpuric lesions, including petechiae. Trauma is the most common endothelial cause of petechiae and purpura in children. Petechiae may be seen in various congenital endothelial disorders, such as hereditary hemorrhagic telangiectasia and Ehler-Danlos syndrome, and acquired endothelial disorders, such as vitamin C deficiency and IgA vasculitis (also known as Henoch-Schönlein purpura).

The most common cause of generalized petechiae, however, is a decrease in the number of circulating platelets (thrombocytopenia).

BASIC SCIENCE/CLINICAL PEARL   **STEP 1/2/3**

When an ill-appearing child has petechiae on physical examination, she or he should be rapidly evaluated for life-threatening disorders, including meningococcemia, disseminated intravascular coagulation secondary to sepsis, hemolytic-uremic syndrome, thrombotic thrombocytopenic purpura, and malignancy.

CLINICAL PEARL   **STEP 2/3**

Localized petechiae should trigger consideration for mechanical stressors that increase venous pressure, such as coughing, vomiting, or strangling.

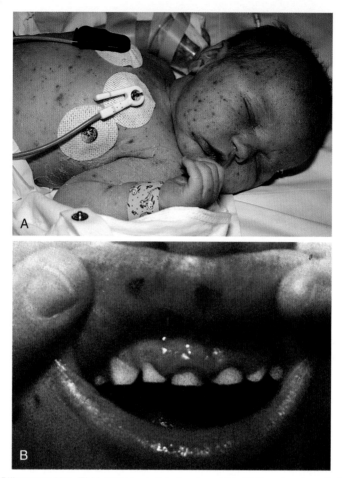

Fig. 16.1 (A) Diffuse petechiae. (B) Mucosal purpuric lesions in a child with thrombocytopenia. (From Cooper JD, Tersak JM. Hematology and oncology. In: Zitelli BJ, McIntire SC, Nowalk AJ, eds. *Zitelli and Davis' Atlas of Pediatric Physical Diagnosis,* 7th ed. 2018:419–454.)

Case Point 16.1

> On physical examination he is well-appearing. He has multiple areas of ecchymosis of variable stages of healing on his bilateral legs, bilateral arms, and abdomen. His largest ecchymosis is on his left lower flank and measures 10 cm in diameter. He also has buccal petechiae and scattered petechiae to the posterior hard palate. No lymphadenopathy or hepatosplenomegaly is noted. His examination is otherwise unremarkable.
>
> A blood count reveals a total white blood cell count of 6.9×10^9/L, hemoglobin of 12.8 g/dL, hematocrit of 36.9% and platelet count of 5×10^9/L with a mean platelet volume of 11.4 fL.

What are common causes of thrombocytopenia (decreased platelets)?
The common causes of thrombocytopenia are summarized in Fig. 16.2. Ultimately, increased platelet destruction from immune thrombocytopenia (ITP, previously known as idiopathic thrombocytopenic purpura) is the most common cause of thrombocytopenia in childhood.

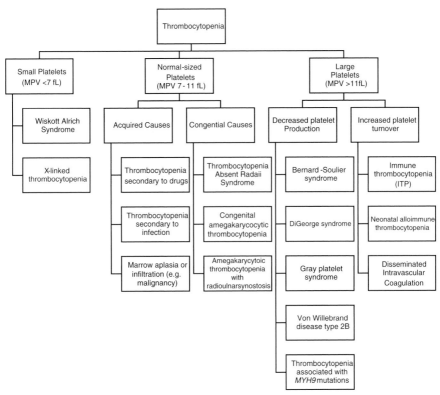

Fig. 16.2 Causes of thrombocytopenia, organized by mean platelet volume (MPV). *MYH9*, Nonmuscle myosin heavy chain 9 gene. (Adapted from McGuinn C, Bussel JB. Disorders of platelets. In: Lanzkowsky P, Lipton JM, Fish JD, eds. *Lanzkowsky's Manual of Pediatric Hematology and Oncology,* 6th ed. New York: Academic Press; 2016:239–278; and from Branchford B, Di Paola J. Approach to the child with a suspected bleeding disorder. In: Stuart H, Orkin SH, Nathan DG, Ginsburg D, eds. *Nathan and Oski's Hematology and Oncology of Infancy and Childhood*. Philadelphia: Elsevier; 2014:999–1009.e2.)

BASIC SCIENCE PEARL	STEP 1

Thrombocytopenia is defined as a platelet count of less than $150 \times 10^9/L$ at essentially any age.

CLINICAL PEARL	STEP 2/3

One of the most common causes of a low platelet count is pseudothrombocytopenia from platelet clumping. Another cause is platelet activation from traumatic blood draw.

BASIC SCIENCE/CLINICAL PEARL	STEP 1/2/3

Age changes the differential of thrombocytopenia substantially. NAIT/maternal ITP, TORCH infections, and congenital causes should be considered in the newborn, whereas acquired causes predominate in the older child. Drug-induced thrombocytopenia can occur at any age.

How does the severity of thrombocytopenia help narrow down the differential? How about the size of the platelet?

Severe thrombocytopenia (<20–50×10^9/L) often suggests an immune cause, whereas more moderate thrombocytopenia ($>50 \times 10^9$/L) suggests a nonimmune cause, such as sepsis, splenomegaly, or congenital thrombocytopenias, including syndromes involving mutations in the nonmuscle myosin heavy chain 9 (*MYH9)* gene.

Platelet size may also help determine the cause of thrombocytopenia (see Fig. 16.1). Tiny platelets (mean platelet volume [MPV] <7 fL) are seen in Wiskott-Aldrich syndrome and X-linked thrombocytopenia. Giant platelets (MPV >11 fL) are seen primarily in *MYH9* syndromes and Bernard-Soulier syndrome. Most other causes of thrombocytopenia will result in platelets with a normal platelet size and volume, although thrombocytopenia resulting from increased platelet turnover often results in a modestly increased MPV.

BASIC SCIENCE/CLINICAL PEARL   **STEP 1/2/3**

Platelets normally live for 9 to 10 days, and younger platelets are generally larger than older platelets. A mildly elevated mean platelet volume performed by an automated counter suggests a destructive process because a predominance of young platelets would increase the average size.

What laboratory tests are indicated at this point?

A visual examination of the peripheral smear should be performed. Abnormalities in the white blood cell population such as blasts or atypical lymphocytes would suggest leukemia or viral infection, respectively. Abnormalities in the red blood cell population such as fragmented red blood cells (RBCs; schistocytes) would suggest a thrombotic microangiopathy such as disseminated intravascular coagulation, hemolytic-uremic syndrome, or thrombotic thrombocytopenic purpura.

If the complete blood count is otherwise normal, and no other visual abnormalities are noted beyond a low platelet count, no further laboratory testing would be indicated in an otherwise normal, healthy-appearing child.

Case Point 16.2

Visual examination of the patient's peripheral smear reveals large (but not giant) platelets (Fig. 16.3). No platelet clumping is seen. White blood cell (WBC) morphology is normal.

Diagnosis: Immune thrombocytopenia (ITP).

BASIC SCIENCE/CLINICAL PEARL   **STEP 1/2/3**

The classic presentation of ITP is a 2- to 6-year-old otherwise healthy child with a history of sudden onset of bruising and/or petechiae. Overt bleeding (e.g., epistaxis, gum bleeding, gastrointestinal bleeding) is present on diagnosis in less than 50% of cases.

What is the pathophysiology of immune thrombocytopenia?

The pathogenesis of ITP is multifactorial. Primarily, ITP is caused by the production of autoantibodies against platelet antigens (specifically glycoprotein IIb/IIIa and Ib/IX). Platelet autoantibodies primarily mediate platelet destruction but have been shown to also impair platelet production by binding to megakaryocytes. Antigen-presenting cells (APCs; e.g., macrophages) and cytotoxic T cells may also play a role in the destruction of platelets as antibody-immune

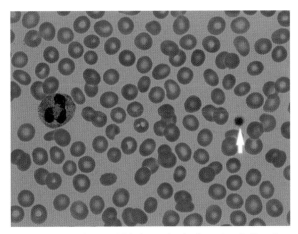

Fig. 16.3 Peripheral smear shows only one visible large platelet *(arrow)* and otherwise normal morphology.

complexes attached to platelets bind to and activate APCs. In turn, these APCs help stimulate the production of T cells, which stimulates the production of antiplatelet-antibody–producing B cells.

What infections are associated with immune thrombocytopenia?
In approximately two-thirds of cases, the onset of ITP is preceded by a viral illness, often a viral upper respiratory tract infection. Other viral infections that have been implicated include rubella, varicella, mumps, rubeola, parvovirus B19, Epstein-Barr virus, and cytomegalovirus (CMV). CMV in particular may present with severe refractory cases. Additionally, the chronic form of ITP has been associated with human immunodeficiency virus (HIV), hepatitis C virus, and *Helicobacter pylori*. ITP has also been associated with the measles-mumps-rubella (MMR) vaccine and the varicella vaccine.

What are the diagnostic criteria for immune thrombocytopenia?
Traditionally a diagnosis of exclusion, ITP has been defined by an International Working Group (IWG) consensus panel as a platelet count less than 100×10^9/L in the absence of another disorder known to cause thrombocytopenia. Practically, the diagnosis of primary ITP is made when a well-appearing, otherwise healthy child presents with acute-onset bleeding symptoms, such as petechiae, purpura, epistaxis and, rarely, severe hemorrhage, without other findings, such as congenital anomalies, clinically significant lymphadenopathy, hepatomegaly or splenomegaly, other cytopenias such as anemia or neutropenia, or other dysmorphic changes on visual examination of the peripheral smear. Secondary ITP can be diagnosed in a patient with isolated thrombocytopenia who is found to have an underlying associated condition such as HIV infection, hepatitis C virus (HCV) infection, or systemic lupus erythematosus (SLE).

BASIC SCIENCE/CLINICAL PEARL   **STEP 1/2/3**

Hepatosplenomegaly should point away from ITP and toward malignancy (e.g., acute leukemia). Congenital anomalies (particularly in the radius or thumbs) should point away from ITP and toward inherited bone marrow failure syndromes (e.g., thrombocytopenia–absent radii syndrome).

What is the time course of immune thrombocytopenia?
Of those with a platelet count of less than 20×10^9/L at diagnosis, 80% will have a persistently low count at 1 week, 20% will have a persistently low count at 2 months, 9% will have a persistently

low count at 6 months, 6% will have a persistently low count at 12 months, and 3% will have persistent disease at 2 years. Chronic ITP is defined by the IWG as counts less than $100 \times x \times 10^9/L$ for longer than 12 months.

What therapy is available for immune thrombocytopenia?

For most affected children, ITP is a benign, self-limited disease process, with low risk for serious bleeding. In children with no bleeding or skin manifestations only, observation is the recommended therapy, regardless of platelet count. If pharmacologic therapy is indicated, intravenous immunoglobulin (IVIG; 1 g/kg) or a short course of glucocorticoids is recommended as first-line treatment. Anti-Rh(D) immunoglobulin can be used in Rh-positive, nonsplenectomized children without evidence of autoimmune hemolysis or a decrease in hemoglobin due to bleeding. In the setting of acute hemorrhage or intracranial hemorrhage (ICH), platelet transfusion in addition to glucocorticoid therapy and IVIG should be given. High-dose dexamethasone can be given to those with ongoing significant bleeding that is not responding to the above therapies. Depot medroxyprogesterone acetate or its equivalent should be considered in women with menorrhagia.

CLINICAL PEARL	STEP 2/3

Platelet transfusions in ITP can transiently raise the platelet count in many patients with ITP. Platelets should not be routinely given in ITP, however, because most patients with ITP are not at risk for major hemorrhage, even without platelet support. In the event of life-threatening hemorrhage or intracranial hemorrhage (ICH), platelet transfusion may be used. It is unclear if prophylactic platelet transfusion in children who have very low platelet counts ($<10 \times 10^3$) is effective in preventing life-threatening hemorrhage.

BASIC SCIENCE/CLINICAL PEARL	STEP 1/2/3

The most feared complication of ITP is intracranial hemorrhage. The risk is very low, however; it has been estimated to be approximately 0.2%. No study has ever shown that platelet-raising therapy reduces the risk of ICH in ITP, and the platelet count alone also has never been shown to predict ICH in patients with ITP.

Case Point 16.3

The patient is treated with IVIG. He responds to therapy with complete resolution of his symptoms and normalization of his platelet count.

He ultimately relapses 4 years later. His second course of ITP is associated with mild normocytic anemia, and his platelet count does not respond to IVIG. The bone marrow examination is unremarkable, supporting a diagnosis of recurrent ITP.

What group of children is more likely to proceed to a chronic course?

Children who are older than 10 years at onset, those with insidious onset, and those with higher platelet counts are more likely to have chronic ITP. In addition, those with recurrent ITP are less likely to achieve a therapy-induced or spontaneous remission.

What therapeutic options are available for chronic immune thrombocytopenia?

As in acute ITP, the therapy of choice for children with asymptomatic or mildly symptomatic (skin manifestation only) is observation only. In children with symptomatic chronic ITP, second-line treatment options include rituximab, splenectomy, and thrombopoietin receptor agonists (e.g., eltrombopag, romiplostim). Splenectomy should be delayed for at least 12 months, if possible.

Vaccinations against *Haemophilus influenzae* type b, *Streptococcus pneumoniae*, and *Neisseria meningitidis* should be given prior to splenectomy.

Third-line therapies include immune modulators such as azathioprine, cyclophosphamide, danazol, vinca alkaloids, cyclosporine, dapsone, and mycophenolate mofetil or combination therapy.

Case Point 16.4

The patient undergoes a course of rituximab, which is unsuccessful. The patient is then started on eltrombopag, which successfully maintains a platelet count between 50 and 200 × 10^9/L.

BEYOND THE PEARLS

- Consider a bone marrow aspirate and biopsy in ITP that does not respond to platelet-raising therapy (e.g., anti-D or IVIG), although this is not required (see the American Society of Hematology 2011 guidelines). Also consider a bone marrow aspirate and biopsy in patients with atypical features (e.g., splenomegaly).
- Antiplatelet antibody testing is available but is neither sensitive nor specific enough to warrant routine clinical use in the diagnosis of ITP.
- Anti-D therapy will cause a mild hemolytic anemia, so it should probably not be used in patients with preexisting anemia due to bleeding.
- The MMR vaccine is associated with the development of ITP, although this is rare. Children with ITP prior to their first dose of MMR can receive the MMR vaccine, however. If children with ITP have already received at least one dose, then titers can be checked, and children who are already immune do not need to complete the remaining doses in the series.
- Chronic ITP should trigger a search for related autoimmune disease (e.g., check thyroid-stimulating hormone level for thyroiditis) and immunodeficiency (e.g., check IgG levels).

Case Summary

Complaint/History: An 11-year-old male presents with scattered petechiae and increased bruising over 3 weeks, first on his legs and then spreading to his abdomen and arms.

Findings: He has multiple areas of ecchymosis in variable stages of healing on his bilateral legs, bilateral arms, and abdomen.

Labs/Tests: A blood count reveals a total white blood cell count of 6.9 × 10^9/L, hemoglobin of 12.8 g/dL, hematocrit of 36.9%, and platelet count of 5 × 10^9/L, with a mean platelet volume of 11.4 fL.

Diagnosis: Immune thrombocytopenia (ITP).

Treatment: Intravenous immunoglobulin.

Bibliography

Khair K, Liesner R. Bruising and bleeding in infants and children—a practical approach. *Br J Haematol.* 2006;133(3):221–231.

Kuhne T, Berchtold W, Michaels LA, et al. Intercontinental Childhood ITP Study Group. Newly diagnosed immune thrombocytopenia in children and adults: a Comparative Prospective Observational Registry of the Intercontinental Cooperative Immune Thombocytopenia Study Group. *Haematologica.* 2011; 96(12):1831–1837.

Leung AK, Chan KW. Evaluating the child with purpura. *Am Fam Physician.* 2001;64(3):419–428.

Neunert C, et al. The American Society of Hematology 2011 evidence-based practice guideline for immune thrombocytopenia. *Blood.* 2011;117(16):4190–4207.

3-Year-Old Female With Cough and Purulent Sputum Production

Reza Ronaghi ▓ Kelly Fan ▓ Raj Dasgupta ▓ Ann Sahakian

A 3-year-old white female presents to the emergency department with 1 week of cough, purulent sputum production, dyspnea, fever, and failure to thrive. Her symptoms have been steadily worsening during this time period. The parents state that they suspect she has pneumonia, because she has already had pneumonia three times in the last 2 years. Seven months ago, she required a 2-week course of intravenous antibiotics when she presented to a different hospital with the same symptoms. The patient is admitted for further workup of both her acute and chronic symptoms.

What is the differential diagnosis for recurrent infections in this patient?

In a child with recurrent infections, one should consider three major categories, including immunodeficiency, underlying chronic illnesses that predispose to infections, and atopy.

Immunodeficiencies by definition render a child susceptible to a variety of uncommon infections. The types of infections would be dictated by the nature of the defect in the innate or adaptive immune system.

Chronic illnesses such as cystic fibrosis (CF), neurologic injury with chronic aspiration, autoimmune inflammatory disorders (e.g., inflammatory bowel disease), and congenital heart malformations may also predispose children to repeated infections. The child with a chronic illness will often present with failure to thrive, an overall sickly appearance, and examination findings specific to the specific illness.

Atopy may also predispose children to repeated infections, via inflamed respiratory epithelia and increased mucosal permeability. Recurrent upper respiratory infections such as sinusitis, rhinitis, and otitis media may be seen.

BASIC SCIENCE/CLINICAL PEARL   **STEP 1/2/3**

Recurrent infections may be a normal variation, particularly in young children with repeated viral upper respiratory tract infections. These children have normal growth patterns, respond to appropriate treatment, and are asymptomatic between infections. The average child has four to eight infections/year; tobacco smoke exposure may increase the risk of upper airway infections.

Case Point 17.1

Review of systems is positive for a chronic daily cough "since she was born," poor weight gain despite voracious appetite, and pale, loose, greasy, voluminous, and foul-smelling stools. When a birth history is elicited, the parents state that the patient was born at home with minimal medical intervention. They are unable to confirm if state-mandated newborn screening for hereditary disorders was performed.

Both height and weight are at the second percentile for age. Vitals signs are notable for a temperature of 37.5°C, blood pressure of 90/50 mm Hg, heart rate of 110/min, respiratory rate of 38/min, and 92% oxygen saturation on room air. On physical examination, the patient appears thin, malnourished, and in mild respiratory distress. The chest examination is significant for diffuse bilateral rales on auscultation and subcostal retractions.

What is the most likely diagnosis?

The loose, foul-smelling greasy stools suggest steatorrhea due to fat malabsorption, generally seen in exocrine pancreatic insufficiency. Although pancreatic insufficiency may be seen in diseases such as Shwachman-Diamond syndrome (SDS), which also would present with recurrent infections and failure to thrive, the combination of pancreatic insufficiency and pulmonary infections should raise suspicion for CF.

BASIC SCIENCE PEARL   **STEP 1**

The triad of fatty diarrhea, repeated infections, and failure to thrive suggest CF and SDS. Pulmonary manifestations would indicate CF, whereas hematologic and skeletal anomalies would indicate SDS.

What is the next step?

The sweat chloride test is the screening test of choice for CF. In patients with CF, a defective membrane adenosine triphosphate (ATP)–gated chloride channel prevents normal chloride transport, which can be detected as high levels of chloride in sweat. Genetic testing would be required for a definitive diagnosis.

BASIC SCIENCE PEARL   **STEP 1**

Parents often note a saltier taste to the child's sweat in children with CF.

Case Point 17.2

The patient has a positive sweat chloride test. Cystic fibrosis transmembrane conductance regulator gene *(CFTR)* sequencing ultimately reveals a homozygous three base pair deletion resulting in a missing phenylalanine residue at position 508 (delta-F508 deletion).

Diagnosis: Cystic fibrosis.

BASIC SCIENCE PEARL   **STEP 1**

Although the phenylalanine deletion at position 508 is the most common mutation for cystic fibrosis, there are many more mutations that cause different structural and functional abnormalities in the ATP-gated chloride channel. These various mutations are important to keep in mind as new treatment medications (discussed below) target specific defects caused by specific mutations.

What is cystic fibrosis?

CF is a hereditary (autosomal recessive) disease that results in progressive organ damage and eventually premature death. Multiple organ systems, including the sinuses, upper and lower respiratory tracts, pancreas, bowels, hepatobiliary system, reproductive tract, and sweat glands on the skin are affected. Infants and children often present with meconium ileus, recurrent pneumonias, and failure to thrive. Pulmonary symptoms tend to predominate, stemming from an inability to clear airway secretions that lead to recurrent infections, which in turn eventually leads to bronchiectasis and progressive loss of lung function.

BASIC SCIENCE PEARL   **STEP 1**

CF also results in upper respiratory epithelial damage. Nearly all patients with CF will have chronic rhinosinusitis.

CF is caused by a defect in the *CFTR* gene on chromosome 7. *CFTR* encodes an ATP-gated chloride channel that secretes chloride in the lungs and gastrointestinal (GI) tract and reabsorbs chloride in the sweat glands. Usually, a deletion of the amino acid phenylalanine causes protein misfolding and degradation; the protein never reaches the cellular membrane. Loss of this channel results in thick mucus secretions in the lungs and GI tract. Abnormally thick mucus, in addition to abnormal mucous clearance and mucosal defense, contribute to ongoing damage that culminates in pulmonary failure (Fig. 17.1).

BASIC SCIENCE PEARL   **STEP 1**

CF is an autosomal recessive disease affecting primarily the white population, with a frequency of 1/2500 to 3500 live births. Screening at birth is mandated throughout the United States, and thus a diagnosis is often made within the first few weeks of life.

BASIC SCIENCE PEARL   **STEP 1**

In fewer than 10% of patients with CF, diagnosis is not made until adulthood. These patients often have unusual genetic mutations leading to less severe disease phenotype and equivocal sweat chloride test results. Presenting symptoms may include indigestion, infertility, and new-onset diabetes mellitus. Pulmonary symptoms may be subclinical.

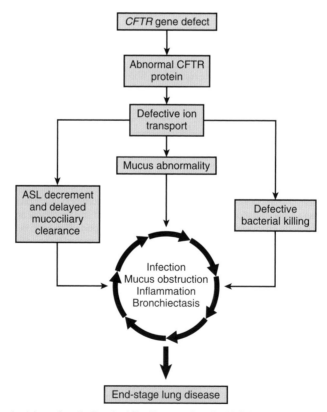

Fig. 17.1 Pathophysiology of cystic fibrosis. *ASL,* Airway surface liquid. (Adapted from Rowe SM, Hoover W, Solomon GM, Sorscher EJ. Cystic fibrosis. In: Mason RJ, Broaddus VC, Ernst JD, King TE Jr, eds. *Murray and Nadel's Textbook of Respiratory Medicine.* Philadelphia: Elsevier/Saunders; 2016;822–852.e17.)

What are the extrapulmonary manifestations of cystic fibrosis?
Table 17.1 summarizes the extrapulmonary complications of CF.

Case Point 17.3

Radiographs and computed tomography scans of the chest are obtained (Figs. 17.2 and 17.3, respectively). Empiric broad-spectrum intravenous antibiotics are initiated. Sputum cultures grow *Staphylococcus aureus* after 48 hours of incubation.

What is a cystic fibrosis exacerbation, and how is it treated?
Ongoing respiratory mucosal damage in the lower respiratory tract results in bronchial inflammation and a chronic cough. An acute infection, chemical irritant (e.g., tobacco smoke), or other factor that worsens the bronchial inflammation enough to cause symptomatic decompensation is termed a *cystic fibrosis exacerbation.* Common symptoms include dyspnea, tachypnea, malaise, and a loss of appetite.

There are multiple different considerations for the treatment of CF exacerbation. Antibiotics remain the forefront of acute CF management, along with aggressive measures to increase pulmonary mucous clearance. The goal of therapy is to restore lung function, reduce the burden of bacterial infection, and eradicate the causative organism whenever possible.

BASIC SCIENCE/CLINICAL PEARL	STEP 1/2/3

Regardless of culture results, antipseudomonal antibiotics should always be part of an antibiotic regimen for CF exacerbation. These antibiotics help improve pulmonary function, because most of the pulmonary symptoms in cystic fibrosis exacerbation are thought to be caused by *Pseudomonas aeruginosa.*

TABLE 17.1 ▓ **Extrapulmonary Complications in Cystic Fibrosis**

System	Complication
Pancreatic	Pancreatic insufficiency leads to fat and protein malabsorption, water-insoluble vitamin (A, D, E, and K) deficiency, and a failure to thrive presentation. Endocrine disorders lead to CF-related diabetes mellitus in 50% of CF (cystic fibrosis) patients by adulthood.
Gastrointestinal tract	Meconium ileus is the presenting problem in 10%–20% of infants with CF. Distal intestinal obstructive syndrome is seen in patients with more advanced lung disease. Rectal prolapse is rare and is more likely to present in patients not adequately treated for pancreatic insufficiency.
Hepatobiliary	Thickened bile ducts most often lead to asymptomatic liver disease. A minority of patients can develop cirrhosis; CF is the third leading cause of liver transplantation in the pediatric population.
Reproductive tract	Most men with CF are infertile due to the absence of the vas deferens. Reduced fertility in women, on the other hand, is secondary to malnutrition and production of thick cervical mucosa.
Musculoskeletal	The inability to absorb vitamin D adequately and glucocorticoid therapy predisposes CF patients to decreased bone mineral density and increased rates of fractures and kyphoscoliosis.
Renal	Hyperoxaluria due to fat malabsorption and hypocitraturia increase the risk of renal stones threefold compared to age-matched controls.

CLINICAL PEARL   **STEP 2/3**

Although initial antibiotic regimens should be broad-spectrum, antibiotics should be tailored to culture results when available.

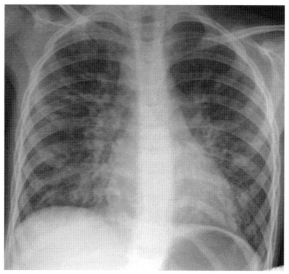

Fig. 17.2 Chest radiograph reveals bronchiectasis, bronchial wall thickening, and mild hyperinflation. (Courtesy Michael Gotway, MD. From Rowe SM et al. Cystic fibrosis. In *Murray and Nadel's Textbook of Respiratory Medicine*. 2016; 822–852.e17.)

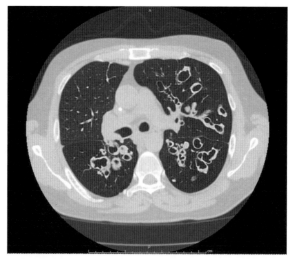

Fig. 17.3 Computed tomography scan of the chest confirms severe bronchiectasis, with mucous impaction. (Courtesy Raj Dasgupta.)

Should intravenous, oral, or inhaled antibiotics be started?

Mild exacerbations can be treated with oral antibiotics. Indications for intravenous antibiotics include severe exacerbations, failure to respond to oral antibiotics, documented antibiotic resistance, or drug allergy. Inhaled antibiotics are generally not used in the treatment of acute exacerbations due to nonhomogeneous distribution within the lungs and low bioavailability. An inhaled antibiotic may be used in conjunction with oral and/or intravenous antibiotics when it provides specific coverage for a colonizing organism. If the patient is on oral prophylactic or inhaled antibiotics at home, these should be continued during the acute exacerbation.

What is the role of airway clearance in a cystic fibrosis exacerbation?

CF patients have high-viscosity sputum filled with mucous glycoproteins, denatured deoxyribonucleic acid (DNA), and protein polymers. Often, sputum is purulent (contains inflammatory granulocytes) as well.

Several medications may assist in sputum clearance. DNase (dornase alfa) decreases the viscosity of secretions via cutting DNA polymers that cause cellular clumping. Hypertonic saline draws water from the airway to help establish an aqueous surface. Hypertonic saline is usually not recommended for children younger than 6 years.

Airway clearance is also enhanced via chest physiotherapy. There are multiple options to increase clearance of the large airways (e.g., vest therapy, manual percussion).

CLINICAL PEARL   **STEP 2/3**

All cystic fibrosis patients should be started on at least one form of airway clearance/chest physiotherapy. Chest physiotherapy helps improve secretions, partially alleviates symptoms, and reduces exacerbations.

Case Point 17.4

The patient is started on vest therapy twice a day, along with dornase alfa for airway clearance. Oral pancreatic enzyme replacement is started, improving her steatorrhea. High-dose supplementation of fat-soluble vitamins (A, D, E, and K) are also started to correct and prevent further deficiencies. These therapies are continued on discharge home.

What is the role of chronic antibiotic therapy for prophylaxis?

Chronic infections with multiple organisms eventually lead to pulmonary function decline; therefore, prophylactic oral antibiotics have been trialed to prevent these infections. No benefit has been shown, however, and prophylactic oral antibiotics increase colonization by antibiotic-resistant organisms. Prophylactic azithromycin is an exception and has had occasional chronic use in patients with CF, used more for its antiinflammatory effects rather than its antibiotic effects.

Inhaled antibiotics targeted against *Pseudomonas aeruginosa* have been shown to be beneficial and improve lung function, however, and are used more routinely in patients in CF.

Case Summary

Complaint/History: A 3-year-old female presents with 1 week of cough, purulent sputum production, dyspnea, and fever.

Findings: Thin, malnourished child in mild respiratory distress.

Labs/Tests: Homozygous *CFTR* gene mutation.

Diagnosis: Cystic fibrosis.

Treatment: Vest therapy, dornase alfa for airway clearance, oral pancreatic enzyme replacement, fat-soluble vitamins (A, D, E, and K); antibiotics for her infection.

BEYOND THE PEARLS

- Infants may present with meconium ileus. This is pathognomonic for CF. Without intervention, intestinal perforation, peritonitis, and death may ensue.
- In addition to pulmonary function decline, other pulmonary complications commonly seen in CF include pneumothorax, hemoptysis, and allergic bronchopulmonary aspergillosis.
- As pulmonary function decline advances, chronic hypoxia will result in pulmonary hypertension, which will in turn result in right-sided heart failure (cor pulmonale). Digital clubbing is often present as a sign of chronic hypoxia.
- CFTR modulators—a new class of drugs that help improve the function of the defective CFTR protein—are available to patients with the G551D mutation and the delta F508 gene deletion.
- Lung transplantation is the only curative treatment for patients with cystic fibrosis but carries a high morbidity rate. The decision to pursue transplantation is based on the rate of decline of lung function, quality of life, and social support.

Bibliography

Farrell PM, et al. Diagnosis of cystic fibrosis: consensus guidelines from the Cystic Fibrosis Foundation. *J Pediatr.* 2017;181S:S4–S15. e1.

Ramsey BW, et al. A CFTR potentiator in patients with cystic fibrosis and the G551D mutation. *N Engl J Med.* 2011;365(18):1663–1672.

Rehman A, et al. Lumacaftor-ivacaftor in patients with cystic fibrosis homozygous for Phe508del CFTR. *N Engl J Med.* 2015;373(18):1783.

Rowe SM, et al. Cystic fibrosis. *N Engl J Med.* 2005;352(19):1992–2001.

Rowe SM, et al. Cystic Fibrosis. In: *Murray and Nadel's Textbook of Respiratory Medicine.* 2016;822–852. e17.

VanDevanter DR, et al. Cystic fibrosis in young children: A review of disease manifestation, progression, and response to early treatment. *J Cyst Fibros.* 2016;15(2):147–157.

Zemanick ET, et al. Highlights from the 2016 North American Cystic Fibrosis Conference. *Pediatr Pulmonol.* 2017;52(8):1103–1110.

4-Year-Old With Fever and a Rash

Ann Sahakian ■ Lindsey Miller ■ Merujan Uzunyan

A 4-year-old fully immunized male presents with 2 days of fever and irritability. His examination is normal. He is presumed to have a viral syndrome and discharged with reassurance and instructions to bring him back if his fever continues or if any other symptoms of concern develop.

Three days later, the patient is brought back. His fevers have persisted, rising as high as 103°F. He has been particularly irritable, and new symptoms include red eyes and a rash. There has been no recent travel or known animal exposures. He has been on no medications other than intermittent acetaminophen and ibuprofen for the fever.

What is the differential diagnosis of a child with fevers and a rash?

There are a few important pieces of information in the history so far that can help narrow down the differential. Measles may be at the top of the differential in nonimmunized children, but it is much less likely in this patient as by the age of 4 years, most children have received the complete measles vaccine series.

Other emergent things to consider are meningococcal infection and toxic shock syndrome, especially if the patient is ill appearing. Meningococcal infections may present with maculopapular rash and irritability. This rash may disappear quickly or the patient may develop a petechial rash. Toxic shock syndrome can also present with fever and a rash, and there is often conjunctival involvement. The rash is often a subtle, diffuse, macular erythema resembling a sunburn in the setting of a group A *Streptococcus* infection or *Staphylococcus aureus* infection.

Scarlet fever caused by group A *Streptococcus* causes a blanching, erythematous, papular "sandpapery" (scarlatiniform) rash over the trunk. Adenovirus can cause fever and rash, along with conjunctivitis, pharyngitis, and coryza. Roseola due to human herpes virus 6 or 7 (HHV-6 or -7) results in a fever and rash, but the fever typically resolves before the rash appears. Parvovirus B19 infection presents with red "slapped" cheeks followed by a reticular rash on the trunk, arms, and legs.

Geography and travel history is also important to consider. For instance, Rocky Mountain spotted fever—a tick-borne illness that can cause fever, headache, and a rash in a patient with a history of a tick bite—is primarily seen in the southeastern and south central United States.

Noninfectious causes to consider include Kawasaki disease (KD) and systemic juvenile idiopathic arthritis (JIA). KD is an acute vasculitis that has specific diagnostic criteria but would include several of this patients' symptoms, including the fever of 5 days or more, rash, and conjunctival injection. Systemic JIA may present with fever, arthritis, rash, and lymphadenopathy.

BASIC SCIENCE/CLINICAL PEARL STEP 1/2/3

Maculopapular rashes are both common and nonspecific. Such rashes are most commonly associated with viral infections in children.

CLINICAL PEARL STEP 2/3

Measles may be mistaken for Kawasaki disease and should be considered in nonimmunized children.

Case Point 18.1

His blood pressure is 118/70 mm Hg, pulse rate is 140/min, respiration rate is 20/min, oxygen saturation is 99% on room air, and temperature is 102.3°F.

On physical examination, the child is irritable but mostly consolable by his mother when not being examined. The bulbar conjunctiva of his eyes are injected bilaterally, with noted limbic sparing (Fig. 18.1A). His lips are erythematous, with a dry, cracked appearance (see Fig. 18.1B). A palpable 2 cm lymph node is noted in his left anterior cervical chain. His trunk is covered in a diffuse, blanching maculopapular rash (see Fig. 18.1C). His hands are swollen and red.

What is the most likely diagnosis at this time?

Clinical findings that help narrow the differential diagnosis include exudative conjunctivitis (suggestive of bacterial infection), exudative pharyngitis (group A *Streptococcus*), ulcerative oral lesion, bullous or vesicular rash, generalized adenopathy, or splenomegaly (JIA).

Of the list of possibilities discussed above, the patient's presentation is most consistent with KD.

What are the diagnostic criteria of Kawasaki disease? What other clinical features can be seen in Kawasaki disease?

The diagnostic criteria for KD are listed in Box 18.1.

KD is an acute systemic inflammatory inflammation in all medium-sized arteries which affects multiple organs and tissues, leading to several other associated clinical findings. The diagnostic criteria exist to distinguish KD from other infectious or inflammatory disorders, and do not include the many other manifestations seen, which are summarized in Box 18.2.

BASIC SCIENCE/CLINICAL PEARL	STEP 1/2/3

Exudative conjunctivitis or pharyngitis are almost never Kawasaki disease. Viral and bacterial infections should be considered instead (group A *Streptococcus* pharyngitis, for example).

Supportive laboratory tests can help confirm the diagnosis if a patient does not meet the strict clinical criteria. Infants in particular may present with fever and no other clinical criteria.

In children with persistent fever (5+ days) and at least two clinical criteria, OR in infants with at least 7 days of fever without an identifiable source, a C-reactive protein (CRP) level of 3 mg/dL or higher and/or an erythrocyte sedimentation rate of 40mm/hr or higher, either a positive echocardiogram OR any three (or more) of the following laboratory findings is an indication to presumptively treat: white blood cell count $15 \times 10^9/L$ or higher, anemia, platelet count of $450 \times 10^9/L$ or higher after the seventh day of fever, albumin level of 3 g/dL or less, elevated serum alanine aminotransferase (ALT) and/or 10/hpf or more urine leukocytes (sterile pyuria).

Case Point 18.2

The child is admitted to the hospital. An echocardiogram is performed, revealing dilation of the right coronary artery (Fig. 18.2).

Diagnosis: Kawasaki disease, classic.

CLINICAL PEARL	STEP 2/3

Cardiac presentations in Kawasaki may range from no cardiac manifestations to severe presentations including myocardial infarction and/or cardiogenic shock. The initial echocardiogram is typically normal in the first week of illness, however, and a normal echocardiogram should not delay therapy to prevent late cardiac complications.

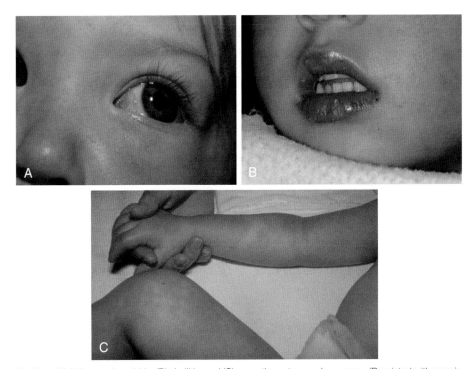

Fig. 18.1 (A) Bulbar conjunctivitis, (B) cheilitis, and (C) an erythematous rash are seen. (Reprinted with permission from Burns JC, et al. Kawasaki syndrome. *Lancet.* 2004;364(9433):533–544.)

BOX 18.1 ■ Diagnosis of Classic Kawasaki Disease

Classic KD is diagnosed in the presence of fever for at least 5 days (the day of fever onset is taken to be the first day of fever) together with at least four of the five following principal clinical features. In the presence of ≥4 principal clinical features, particularly when redness and swelling of the hands and feet are present, the diagnosis of KD can be made with 4 days of fever, although experienced clinicians who have treated many patients with KD may establish the diagnosis with 3 days of fever in rare cases:

1. Erythema and cracking of lips, strawberry tongue, and/or erythema of oral and pharyngeal mucosa
2. Bilateral bulbar conjunctival injection without exudate
3. Rash: maculopapular, diffuse erythroderma, or erythema multiforme-like
4. Erythema and edema of the hands and feet in acute phase and/or periungual desquamation in subacute phase
5. Cervical lymphadenopathy (≥1.5 cm diameter), usually unilateral

A careful history may reveal that ≥1 principal clinical features were present during the illness but resolved by the time of presentation.

Patients who lack full clinical features of classic KD are often evaluated for incomplete KD. If coronary artery abnormalities are detected, the diagnosis of KD is considered confirmed in most cases.

Laboratory tests typically reveal normal or elevated white blood cell count with neutrophil predominance and elevated acute-phase reactants such as C-reactive protein and erythrocyte sedimentation rate during the acute phase. Low serum sodium and albumin levels, elevated serum liver enzymes, and sterile pyuria can be present. In the second week after fever onset, thrombocytosis is common.

KD, Kawasaki disease.

Reprinted with permission. *Circulation.* 2017;135(17):e927–e999. (c) 2017 American Heart Association, Inc.

BOX 18.2 ■ Associated Clinical Findings in Classic Kawasaki Disease

Other clinical findings may include the following:
Cardiovascular
   Myocarditis, pericarditis, valvular regurgitation, shock
   Coronary artery abnormalities
   Aneurysms of medium-sized noncoronary arteries
   Peripheral gangrene
   Aortic root enlargement
Respiratory
   Peribronchial and interstitial infiltrates on CXR
   Pulmonary nodules
Musculoskeletal
   Arthritis, arthralgia (pleocytosis of synovial fluid)
Gastrointestinal
   Diarrhea, vomiting, abdominal pain
   Hepatitis, jaundice
   Gallbladder hydrops
   Pancreatitis
Nervous system
   Extreme irritability
   Aseptic meningitis (pleocytosis of cerebrospinal fluid)
   Facial nerve palsy
   Sensorineural hearing loss
Genitourinary
   Urethritis/meatitis, hydrocele
Other
   Desquamating rash in groin
   Retropharyngeal phlegmon
   Anterior uveitis by slit lamp examination
   Erythema and induration at BCG inoculation site
   The differential diagnosis includes other infectious and noninfectious conditions, includ-
      ing the following:
Measles
Other viral infections (e.g., adenovirus, enterovirus)
Staphylococcal and streptococcal toxin-mediated diseases (e.g., scarlet fever and toxic shock
   syndrome)
Drug hypersensitivity reactions, including Stevens Johnson syndrome
Systemic onset juvenile idiopathic arthritis
With epidemiologic risk factors:
   Rocky Mountain spotted fever or other rickettsial infections
   Leptospirosis

BCG, Bacillus Calmette-Guérin; *CXR,* chest radiography.
From McCrindle BW, et al. Diagnosis, treatment, and long-term management of Kawasaki disease:
   a scientific statement for health professionals from the American Heart Association. *Circulation.*
   2017;135(17):e927–e999, Table 3.

BASIC SCIENCE/CLINICAL PEARL   **STEP 1/2/3**

Although Kawasaki disease affects children of all races and ethnicities, it is more common in
those of Asian, particularly Japanese, descent.

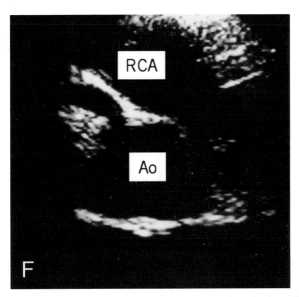

Fig. 18.2 Right coronary dilatation, which evolved into an aneurysm over time. *Ao,* Aorta; *RCA,* right coronary artery. (From Kato H. *Cardiology.* 2010:1613–1626.)

What is the pathophysiology of Kawasaki disease?

The exact cause of KD is unknown but is thought to involve both a hereditary predisposition and environmental triggers.

The pathophysiology of arterial damage involves three processes: (1) a necrotizing arteritis within the first 2 weeks of illness in mid-sized arteries that results in saccular aneurysms that may potentially thrombose or rupture; followed by (2) a subacute chronic vasculitis that may continue for months to years; and finally (3) progressive arterial stenosis over months to years (Fig. 18.3).

All layers of the heart may be affected from the pericardium to the myocardium to the endocardium. Small pericardial effusions are common. Valvular dysfunction—especially that of the mitral valve—may occur in up to 25% of patients. Arrhythmia, prolonged PR interval, non-specific ST and T wave changes, as well as low voltage due to myocardial or pericardial involvement, may all be seen on an electrocardiogram.

BASIC SCIENCE/CLINICAL PEARL	STEP 1/2/3

Tachycardia out of proportion to the fever, a flow murmur, and/or a gallop rhythm all suggest decreased compliance or diastolic dysfunction. Tachycardia is often a sign of myocardial inflammation in Kawasaki disease.

What is the initial management of Kawasaki disease?

A single dose of intravenous immunoglobulin (IVIG) 2 g/kg should be administered together with an antiinflammatory dose of acetylsalicylic acid (ASA, aspirin). IVIG should be started within the first 10 days of illness marked by the onset of fever if at all possible, as delayed therapy puts the child at a higher risk of coronary artery abnormalities. The exact mechanism of action of IVIG is not known but thought to be antiinflammatory in nature.

ASA does not decrease the incidence of coronary abnormalities but is used for its antiinflammatory and antiplatelet effects. For children that do go on to develop coronary artery aneurysms, ASA is continued indefinitely.

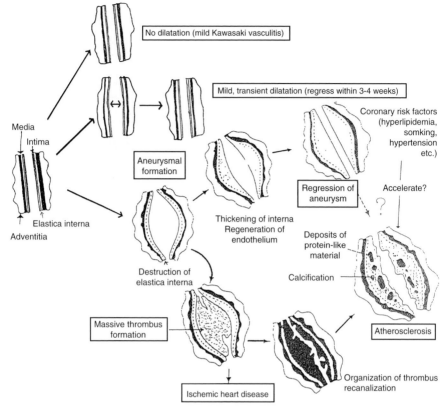

Fig. 18.3   Theorized progression of vasculitic events in Kawasaki disease. (From Kato H. Cardiovascular complications in Kawasaki disease: coronary artery lumen and long-term consequences. *Prog Pediatr Cardiol.* 2004;19(2):137–145.)

Case Point 18.3

The patient is treated with high-dose IVIG and ASA. His fever resolves over the next 24 hours, and the ASA dose is reduced to a low dose (antiplatelet dose) after resolution of the fever.

What instructions should be given to the family upon discharge?

It is important to note that some patients will have complications despite IVIG therapy. Therefore, it is important to instruct the patient to return to the hospital for evaluation if the fever recurs. Additionally, parents should be warned of the desquamating rash that typically occurs 2 to 3 weeks after the onset of fever, starting under the nails of the fingers and toes, and potentially spreading to involve the palms and soles.

For uncomplicated patients, an echocardiogram should be repeated within 1 to 2 weeks. ASA therapy should continue for at least 4 to 6 weeks after the onset of illness, and another echocardiogram will be performed at that time. For any patient with evolving coronary artery abnormalities during the acute illness, echocardiography should be performed twice a week until the coronary artery luminal dimensions have stabilized.

What is the prognosis for children with Kawasaki disease?

The patients at highest risk for coronary abnormalities are those who are less than 1 year old, those whose diagnosis and treatment were delayed beyond 10 days, patients who are IVIG-resistant, patients with recurrent KD, male gender, and those with prolonged fever, high CRP levels, low albumin levels, and anemia.

Long-term management is focused on preventing thrombosis and maintaining optimal cardiovascular health. The extent of cardiology care will depend on the level of risk as defined by coronary artery luminal dimensions.

For any patients with a small, medium or large aneurysm, follow-up with cardiology may include stress echocardiography, stress electrocardiography, or stress magnetic resonance perfusion imaging.

ASA should be continued in those with current or persistent aneurysm(s). Additionally, long-term anticoagulation may be considered, as well as dual-antiplatelet therapy with ASA and clopidogrel. A β-blocker may be considered in a patient with a large aneurysm. Statin therapy may be considered in any patient with an aneurysm as well.

BASIC SCIENCE/CLINICAL PEARL   **STEP 1/2/3**

Without IVIG therapy, up to 25% of children will develop coronary artery abnormalities. With high-dose IVIG, the risk is reduced to approximately 4%.

BEYOND THE PEARLS

- Although Kawasaki disease is uncommon in children under 6 months of age or over 5 years of age, these two groups are at higher risk for coronary artery complications than children between 6 months and 5 years of age.
- Some vaccine considerations: Measles-mumps-rubella and varicella vaccines should be deferred for 11 months after IVIG. Only inactivated flu vaccine can and should be given to those on ASA therapy.
- The cause of Kawasaki is not known but is likely to be a combination of genetic risk and infectious cause Siblings of patients appear to be at higher risk of developing Kawasaki disease.
- The 10%–20% of patients whose fevers do not resolve after administration of IVIG have disease termed *IVIG-resistant.* Such patients often have a poorer prognosis, with more cardiac complications.
- Second-line agents used in IVIG-resistant patients include glucocorticoids and antiinflammatory biologic therapy (e.g., infliximab).
- Ibuprofen should be avoided in patients on ASA therapy as it antagonizes the irreversible platelet inhibition induced by ASA.
- ASA is rarely used in pediatrics due to the increased risk of Reye Syndrome, a rapidly progressive encephalopathy due to hepatic dysfunction, especially in the setting of influenza or varicella infection. The low dose (antiplatelet) therapy has not been shown to lead to Reye syndrome.

Case Summary

Complaint/History: A 4-year-old fully immunized male presents with 5 days of fever and irritability.

Findings: Bulbar conjunctivitis, cheilitis, lymphadenopathy, and a rash.

Labs/Tests: Echocardiogram reveals mild coronary artery dilation.

Diagnosis: Kawasaki disease.

Treatment: Intravenous immunoglobulin and aspirin.

Bibliography

Holve TJ, et al. Long-term cardiovascular outcomes in survivors of Kawasaki disease. *Pediatrics*. 2014;133(2):e305–e311.

McCrindle BW, Rowley AH, Newburger JW, et al. Diagnosis, treatment, and long-term management of Kawasaki disease: a scientific statement for health professionals from the American Heart Association. *Circulation*. 2017;135(17):e927–e999.

Newburger JW, Takahashi M, Beiser AS, et al. A single intravenous infusion of gamma globulin as compared with four infusions in the treatment of acute Kawasaki syndrome. *N Engl J Med*. 1991;324:1633–1639.

Orenstein JM, Shulman ST, Fox LM, et al. Three linked vasculopathic processes characterize Kawasaki disease: a light and transmission electron microscopic study. *PLoS One*. 2012;7:e38998.

2-Week-Old Female Infant With Vomiting, Diarrhea, and Poor Feeding

Asma Hasan ▓ Caroline T. Nguyen

A 2-week-old female infant is seen for a follow-up visit. She was born at term after an uncomplicated vaginal delivery. Over the past week, she has developed recurrent vomiting, diarrhea, and poor feeding. She has not been able to gain weight and appears less interactive. Her blood pressure is 70/40 mm Hg, pulse rate is 165 beats/min, respiration rate is 18 breaths/min, and oxygen saturation was 95% on room air. On physical examination, she appears lethargic. She has sunken fontanelles, dry mucous membranes, and decreased capillary refill. On genitourinary examination, there is significant clitoromegaly and fusion of the labiosacral folds. There is also slight hyperpigmentation of the skin that is more prominent in the skin creases and genital area (Fig. 19.1).

What should you consider when faced with ambiguous genitalia at birth? What are the basics of sexual differentiation?

The term *ambiguous genitalia* refers to external genitalia that do not appear completely male or female. Sexual differentiation is the process whereby male or female phenotypes develop. A defect in this pathway can lead to ambiguous genitalia. In utero, gonadal cells have the potential to differentiate into a testicular or ovarian cell from wolffian and mullerian ducts, respectively. The Y chromosome has a gender-determining region on the *SRY* gene. By week 8, testicular cells secrete testosterone and antimullerian hormone (AMH). Testosterone initiates virilization of the wolffian duct into the epididymis, vas deferens, and seminal vesicle. Dihydrotestosterone (DHT), produced from circulating testosterone, is necessary to fuse genital folds to form the penis and scrotum, thus forming the external genitalia. AMH causes regression of mullerian ducts. In the absence of AMH, the mullerian ducts persist as the uterus, fallopian tubes, cervix, and upper vagina. Without the presence of DHT, the clitoris, labia majora, minora, and lower vagina form the external female genitalia.

What are the basics of steroid formation, and what are the functions of different steroid hormones?

Steroid hormones are synthesized in the adrenal gland. The inner part of the gland is the medulla, which synthesizes catecholamines. The outer cortex is responsible for steroidogenesis. There are three zones of the cortex, starting from the periphery—zona *g*lomerulosa, zona *f*asciculata, and zona *r*eticularis (GFR). Each zone is responsible for producing their respective hormones: aldosterone, cortisol, and androgens (Fig. 19.2).

Cholesterol is the substrate for all steroid hormones. The steroidogenic acute regulatory protein (stAR) regulates transport of cholesterol into the mitochondria of cells, where it is cleaved to form pregnenolone, which then undergoes various processes in each adrenal cortex zone.

The outer zone of the cortex is the zona glomerulosa, which is responsible for the formation of mineralocorticoids. These are the hormones that influence salt and water balance, with the principal hormone being aldosterone. The most important action is on receptors in the

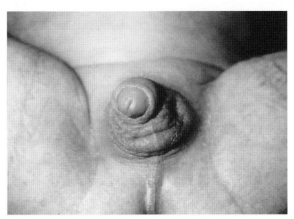

Fig. 19.1   Newborn ambiguous genitalia with cliteromegaly. (From Cummings E, Salisbury S. *Pediatric Clinical Skills*. Philadelphia: Elsevier Saunders; 2010.)

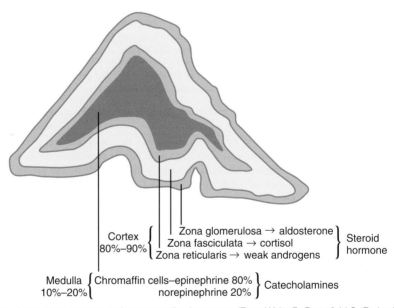

Fig. 19.2   Adrenal cortex zones and corresponding hormones. (From White B, Porterfield S. *Endocrine and Reproductive Physiology*. Philadelphia: Elsevier Mosby; 2013.)

distal convoluted tubules and collecting ducts of the kidney, where they induce reabsorption of sodium and excretion of potassium and also influence water retention. A deficiency would result in hypotension, hyponatremia, and hyperkalemia. This zone is primarily regulated by angiotensin II.

In the zona fasciculata, pregnenolone is converted by enzymatic action to form glucocorticoids, principally cortisol. This is regulated by adrenocorticotropic hormone (ACTH). Glucocorticoids have multiple targets for action. They are important for stress reactions and can increase glucose production, insulin resistance, and cardiac contractility and output. They also play an important role in growth and development and immune function.

In the zona reticularis, pregnenolone is converted in a series of steps to dehydroepiandrosterone sulfate (DHEAS), which is further converted to androstenedione. These hormones are then converted in peripheral tissues to testosterone, dihydrotestosterone, estrone, or estradiol.

CLINICAL PEARL	STEP 1/2/3

Androgens are steroid hormones responsible for the activity of the male sex organs and secondary male characteristics (Fig. 19.3). The most common causes of ambiguous genitalia typically arise from an imbalance in androgens. The differential diagnosis for ambiguous genitalia includes virilizing congenital adrenal hyperplasias, androgen insensitivity syndrome, mixed gonadal dysgenesis, clitoral anomalies, and hypogonadotropic hypogonadism.

Case Point 19.1

In addition to the ambiguous genitalia, the newborn has now developed recurrent vomiting and poor feeding.

What are common causes of poor feeding in a newborn?
Failure to feed is a common symptom seen in most ill newborn infants and includes a wide differential. Infections remain a frequent cause of neonate morbidity and, if severe enough, can manifest along with other symptoms, including hypotension, lethargy, and irritability. Central nervous system (CNS)–related disorders should also be considered in the setting of seizures, weak tone, or central cyanosis. Poor feeding coupled with frequent vomiting can be due to congenital gastrointestinal (GI) tract defects, such as hypertrophic pyloric stenosis or necrotizing enterocolitis. When poor feeding is found in the setting of hypotension and ambiguous genitalia, adrenal insufficiency must be considered.

What is the pathophysiology of congenital adrenal hyperplasia?
Congenital adrenal hyperplasia (CAH) refers to a group of inherited disorders characterized by abnormal steroidogenesis due to enzymatic defects. As discussed earlier, cholesterol in the adrenal cortex is catalyzed by various enzymes to produce the steroid hormones. CAH encompasses multiple different enzymatic defects, but 95% of cases involve a 21-hydroxylase deficiency. This enzyme is responsible for the conversion of 17-hydroxyprogesterone (17-OHP) to 11-deoxycortisol, a step in the cortisol synthesis pathway. 21-Hydroxylase is also responsible for the conversion of progesterone to deoxycorticosterone, which is the precursor to mineralocorticoids. Deficiency of the enzyme leads to a deficiency in glucocorticoids, as well as an excess of accumulated precursors proximal to the 21-hydroxylation step.

Decreased negative feedback inhibition leads to an increase in ACTH production and more stimulation on the adrenal gland, causing hyperplasia and increased androgen production. Precursors are shunted to this pathway because they do not require the 21-hydroxylase enzyme. The result is high levels of androstenedione, which are then converted to testosterone. Affected females are exposed to high levels of androgens in utero and, as a result, have masculinized external genitalia. Inability of the adrenal glands to produce cortisol leads to adrenal insufficiency.

There are several distinct variants of 21-hydroxylase deficiency. Some may have the simple virilizing form, but approximately 75% will have the classic salt-wasting form due to a deficiency in aldosterone production as well. These patients will present with salt wasting and hypotension, usually after the first 2 weeks of life.

CLINICAL PEARL	STEP 2/3

In CAH, male patients usually have unaffected genitalia. In female patients, the external genitalia are virilized. Internal genitalia will be unaffected.

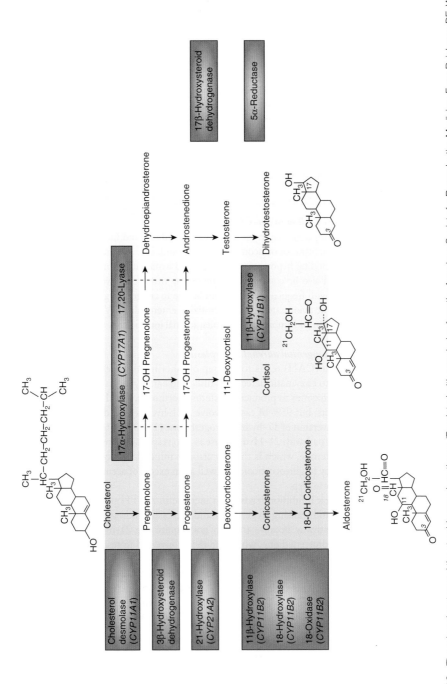

Fig. 19.3 The adrenal cortex and the steroidogenesis pathway. (Reprinted with permission from the American Society for Reproductive Medicine. From Reichman DE, White PC, New MI, Rosenwaks Z. Fertility in patients with congenital adrenal hyperplasia. *Fertil Steril.* 2014;101(2):301–309.)

TABLE 19.1 ■ **Patient's Laboratory Results**

Parameter	Result
Basic Metabolic Panel	
Sodium	126 mmol/L
Chloride	88 mmol/L
Potassium	6.5 mmol/L
Bicarbonate	15 mmol/L
Blood urea nitrogen	30 mg/dL
Creatinine	0.8 mg/dL
Endocrinologic Laboratory Tests	
17-Hydroxyprogesterone (17-OHP)	41,000 ng/dL
Adrenocorticotropin hormone (ACTH)	40 pg/mL
Androstenedione	2,200 ng/dL
Total cortisol	0.8 µg/dL

What are classic signs and symptoms of acute adrenal crisis and salt wasting in the newborn?
Signs of salt wasting can include poor feeding, vomiting, failure to thrive, lethargy, and sepsis-like syndromes. Acute adrenal crisis can present with these signs, as well as unresponsiveness, dry mucous membranes, hyperpigmentation, hyponatremia, hyperkalemia, hypoglycemia, metabolic acidosis, and hypotension.

CLINICAL PEARL	**STEP 1**

Because male patients usually have unaffected genitalia, salt wasting seen in a newborn male can be a clue to a diagnosis of CAH.

What is an appropriate laboratory workup?
In an evaluation for adrenal crisis, the initial workup should include glucose, complete metabolic panel, and arterial blood gas. The most characteristic laboratory abnormality is an elevated 17-OHP, which is the main substrate for the 21-hydroxylase enzyme. Serum values are higher than 3500 ng/dL and usually exceed 10,000 ng/dL up to 100,000 ng/dL with the salt-wasting form. Other hormones in the adrenal axis can be determined, including cortisol, ACTH, and androstenedione levels, and plasma renin activity. Diagnosis should be confirmed with ACTH stimulation testing. However, in the setting of acute adrenal crisis, treatment should not be delayed. Poor feeding is often a late sign and is indicative of crisis.

In the evaluation of ambiguous genitalia, an ultrasound to identify internal structures and karyotype can be obtained as well.

Case Point 19.2

The patient's laboratory test results indicate hyponatremia, hyperkalemia, hypoglycemia, hypochloremia, metabolic acidosis, uremia, and elevated serum creatinine levels. Serum 17-hydroxyprogesterone (OHP) levels are elevated, at 41,000 ng/dL, with an androstenedione level of 2,200 ng/dL. Total cortisol was low, at 0.8, with an elevated ACTH level of 40 pg/mL (Table 19.1). Ultrasound revealed a uterus and ovaries.

CLINICAL PEARL   **STEP 2/3**

In the setting of acute adrenal crisis, prompt treatment is indicated. Fluid resuscitation should be started immediately because patients are severely volume-depleted. The initial bolus should be with 20 mL/kg of 0.9% normal saline, with repeated boluses as needed. Intravenous fluids should be continued to replace fluid loss with dextrose-containing isotonic fluids at a rate 1.5 to 2 times that of maintenance. Along with the intravenous fluid treatment, a stress dose of glucocorticoids should be given. This is usually done with an IV bolus of hydrocortisone of 50 to 100 mg/m^2, followed by 50 to 100 mg/m^2 per day divided every 6 hours. Frequent monitoring of vital signs and electrolytes should be done to ensure adequate response to treatment.

What are the main goals for the long-term treatment of classic congenital adrenal hyperplasia?

All patients with classic CAH should be on maintenance glucocorticoid replacement, with the goal of androgen suppression. By replacing the deficient hormones, the aim is to suppress excessive ACTH secretion and therefore decrease the production of androgens. Glucocorticoid replacement will also prevent adrenal crisis. By preventing further virilization, this allows for normal growth and development. In patients with salt wasting, the sodium content in breast milk or formula is insufficient, and they should be treated with fludrocortisone and sodium chloride supplements in the newborn period and early infancy.

CLINICAL PEARL   **STEP 1**

Hydrocortisone is the preferred glucocorticoid in childhood because its short half-life minimizes adverse side effects. More potent and long-acting glucocorticoids, such as dexamethasone and prednisolone, have been shown to suppress growth. After completion of linear growth has occurred, a longer acting glucocorticoid can be used. Dexamethasone may be preferred because it can be given once daily.

CLINICAL PEARL   **STEP 1/2/3**

In times of acute stress, such as febrile illness, dehydration, trauma, or surgery, the dose of glucocorticoid replacement needs to be increased in patients with classic CAH. These patients are unable to produce an appropriate cortisol response in times of physical stress. High doses of glucocorticoids often act on mineralocorticoid receptors and therefore do not need a change in dosage of mineralocorticoid replacement. They should also wear medical alert identification indicating that they have adrenal insufficiency.

How should therapy be monitored?

Long-term monitoring requires a balance between hyperandrogenism and hypercortisolism. The goal is not to suppress adrenal androgen production completely because this can lead to complications of overtreatment of glucocorticoids. 17-OHP, androstenedione, and testosterone levels are the best indicators of adequacy of treatment. Adrenal androgen secretion should not be suppressed. Normal 17-OHP levels usually indicate overtreatment. A target range of a 17-OHP level of 500 to 1000 ng/dL can prevent overtreatment. Dose adjustments of glucocorticoids should be based on clinical symptoms rather than on any certain laboratory value. Signs of inadequate treatment can be virilization, advanced bone age, premature bone maturation, or accelerated height velocity. Regular monitoring should include height, weight, and a physical examination. Annual bone age assessment is indicated after the age of 2 years, along with careful monitoring of linear growth.

CLINICAL PEARL   STEP 2/3

Signs of iatrogenic Cushing syndrome in young children can include rapid weight gain, poor growth velocity, hypertension, pigmented striae, and osteopenia.

What is the long-term outcome for reproductive health?

Most females with CAH will achieve menarche if properly treated. Those with inadequate treatment usually go through menarche at a later age than others. Symptoms similar to those of polycystic ovarian syndrome can often be seen, including irregular bleeding, anovulation, and hyperandrogenic symptoms. Breast development is suppressed but is reversible with treatment. Females can become pregnant with treatment. Males infrequently have impaired gonadal function.

What is nonclassic congenital adrenal hyperplasia?

Partial deficiency in 21-hydroxylase activity can result in milder symptoms of the disease. It may be one of the most common autosomal recessive disorders in humans. The presentation is usually later in life due to androgen excess. Females may present with abnormal menses and increased virilization. Males may present with accelerated pubertal growth. Both genders may develop problems in bone development such as advanced bone age, which can result in short stature. These patients do not usually develop adrenal crisis.

What is the role of surgery in congenital adrenal hyperplasia?

This may be important for patients presenting with ambiguous genitalia. Different surgical options include clitoral or perineal reconstruction for severely virilized females. Consideration of surgery is suggested in infancy but may be done in adolescence as well. Adrenalectomy should only be considered in cases of failed treatment with glucocorticoids, especially adult women with salt wasting.

In what situation would screening tests be the most helpful?

As noted, males with 21-hydroxylase deficiency present with a normal phenotype at birth. If not recognized, they can develop adrenal insufficiency and salt wasting. Screening can identify these situations before the potentially fatal salt wasting develops. Current guidelines recommend screening for 21-hydroxylase deficiency in all newborns. The main goal is for early prevention and diagnosis of salt wasting. Screening can also assist with correct gender assignment if there are ambiguous genitalia present. The standard test measures 17-OHP levels in a dried blood spot used for other screening newborn tests. Cutoff levels are typically set very low. Therefore, the test is sensitive but poorly specific with a high false-positive rate. 17-OHP levels can be elevated in premature or sick infants. Mild elevations should have repeat spot testing. If significantly elevated, electrolytes and serum 17-OHP levels should be checked. Confirmatory testing can be done with an ACTH stimulation test.

Case Point 19.3

The patient is discharged home with oral hydrocortisone, fludrocortisone, and sodium chloride supplements. During a 6-month follow-up visit, her mother reports that she is interacting well and feeding appropriately. She has had appropriate weight gain for her age. Her 17-OHP Level is 830 ng/dL. The family considers surgical reconstruction for the external genitalia but wants to defer the decision to a later time.

BEYOND THE PEARLS

- CAH can be caused by enzyme deficiencies other than 21-hydroxylase deficiency. The next most common form is caused by 11β-hydroxylase deficiency, the enzyme that converts 11-deoxycortisol to cortisol and deoxycorticosterone to corticosterone in the pathway of aldosterone synthesis. In addition to being virilized, these patients often have hypertension as a result of deoxycorticosterone' s mineralocorticoid effects.
- All cases of CAH must be confirmed with an ACTH stimulation test. This is important because 17-OHP may be elevated in the setting of other enzymatic defects (e.g., 11β-hydroxylase deficiency). Levels of 17-OHP, cortisol, deoxycorticosterone, 11- deoxycortisol, 17-OH-pregnenolone, androstenedione, and DHEA should be obtained at 0 and 60 minutes after the administration of cosyntropin. Without a complete profile, other enzymatic deficiencies may be incorrectly diagnosed as 21-hydroxylase deficiency.
- Current methods of oral glucocorticoid replacement do not act in the same manner as physiologic glucocorticoid secretion in the body. The secretion of cortisol peaks in the morning and decreases during the rest of the day. Studies have evaluated the use of continuous glucocorticoid infusion that would mimic natural physiologic secretion. Different formulations of oral glucocorticoids are also being developed.
- Studies have been carried out looking at the relationship between CAH and sexual orientation, but this remains controversial.
- Treatment should be continued during pregnancy for females with CAH. Hydrocortisone and prednisone do not cross the placenta, so these glucocorticoids are preferred. Dosages need to be increased due to alterations in steroid metabolism and clearance. Placental aromatase also prevents androgens from effecting the fetus.
- Benign ATCH-dependent testicular tumors, referred to as *testicular adrenal rest tumors,* are common in males with classic CAH. These are often seen in inadequately treated patients. They are usually bilateral and decrease in size with treatment. If untreated, they can lead to gonadal dysfunction and infertility.

Case Summary

Complaint/History: A 2-week-old female infant has vomiting, diarrhea, and poor feeding.

Findings: The examination reveals an infant who is lethargic, with poor perfusion and signs of dehydration. The genitourinary examination shows cliteromegaly and fusion of the labiosacral folds. Her skin shows hyperpigmentation in areas with flexion creases and genital regions.

Labs/Tests: Laboratory test results indicate hyponatremia, hypochloremia, hyperkalemia, metabolic acidosis, uremia, hypoglycemia, and elevated serum creatinine level. Serum 17-hydroxyprogesterone (17-OHP) level is elevated, at 41,000 ng/dL, and the androstenedione level is 2200 ng/dL. Total cortisol was low, at 0.8, with an elevated ACTH level of 40 pg/mL. Ultrasound revealed a uterus and ovaries.

Diagnosis: Congenital adrenal hyperplasia (CAH).

Treatment: Acute adrenal crisis—intravenous fluid resuscitation and stress dose of hydrocortisone (50-mg/m^2 bolus, followed by 50 mg/m^2/day divided in six doses). The long-term maintenance regimen consists of hydrocortisone, fludrocortisone, and sodium chloride supplementation.

Bibliography

Antal Z, Zhou P. Congenital adrenal hyperplasia: diagnosis, evaluation, and management. *Pediatr Rev.* 2009;30(7):e49–e57.

Kliegman R, et al. *Nelson Textbook of Pediatrics.* 20th ed. Philadelphia: Elsevier; 2016.

Speiser PW, et al. Congenital adrenal hyperplasia due to steroid 21-hydroxylase deficiency: an endocrine society clinical practice guideline. *J Clin Endocrinol Metab.* 2010;95(9):4133–4160.

Sperling M. *Pediatric Endocrinology.* 4th ed. Philadelphia: Elsevier/Saunders; 2014.

White PC, Speiser PW. Congenital adrenal hyperplasia due to 21-hydroxylase deficiency. *Endocr Rev.* 2000;21(3):245–291.

A 3-Year-Old Female With Nausea, Vomiting, and Progressive Abdominal Pain

Patricia Lorenzo ▪ Caroline T. Nguyen

A 3-year-old female presents to the emergency department with a 1-day history of nausea, vomiting, and progressive abdominal pain. Her parents state that she has not been her usual self for the past week. She has felt more tired and is taking longer naps. Although previously bathroom-trained, she has urinated on the bed for the past several nights. Parents deny any fevers or recent illness. The pregnancy was normal, and the patient was delivered via spontaneous vaginal birth. She is up to date on all her immunizations. On physical examination, blood pressure is 105/56 mm Hg, heart rate is 130 beats/min, respiratory rate is 20 breaths/min, temperature is 98.8°F, and oxygen saturation is 94% on room air. The patient is found to be irritable but responsive. Her mucous membranes are dry. Cardiac examination revealed tachycardia. The abdominal examination shows diffuse tenderness to palpation. The remainder of the examination is normal.

What are some causes of changes in mood and behavior, nausea, vomiting, polyuria, abdominal pain, and tachycardia in an otherwise previously healthy child?
An infection such as gastroenteritis, pyelonephritis, or appendicitis should be considered. The presence of polyuria is suggestive of diabetic ketoacidosis (DKA).

What further history would be useful to obtain?
You would want to know if there was a history of autoimmune conditions, including diabetes mellitus type 1 in the patient or patient's family and whether there was a precipitating event such as an infection.

In general, when should you consider diabetic ketoacidosis as a diagnosis?
A diagnosis of DKA should be considered in a child when the patient presents with nonspecific symptoms such as nausea, vomiting, fatigue, lethargy, and abdominal pain or is simply ill-appearing. Patients younger than 5 years are difficult to assess because they cannot provide a detailed history. DKA at the time of diagnosis of type 1 diabetes mellitus is most common in children younger than 5 years and children of lower socioeconomic status. Biochemical evidence may also be taken into account for the diagnosis of DKA.

CLINICAL PEARL   **STEP 2/3**

The criteria for the diagnosis of DKA is hyperglycemia (blood glucose > 200 mg/dL, venous pH < 7.3, and/or bicarbonate < 15 mmol/L). There may be associated glycosuria, ketonemia, and ketonuria. Based on the laboratory values and clinical picture, the diagnosis can be classified as mild, moderate, or severe (see Table 20.1).

What is the pathophysiology of diabetic ketoacidosis?
DKA is due to insufficient circulating insulin in association with increased levels of counter-regulatory hormones, such as glucagon, cortisol, catecholamines, and growth hormone. These hormones contribute to rising serum glucose levels by increasing glycolysis and gluconeogenesis in the liver and kidneys. Hyperglycemia causes osmotic diuresis, electrolyte loss, dehydration, and impaired glomerular filtration. Despite having increased circulating glucose, uptake of the glucose is impaired due to insufficient insulin. Lipolysis results in the release of free fatty acids used in ketogenesis to produce ketones, an alternative source of energy. Ultimately, metabolic acidosis ensues. The progressive dehydration, hyperosmolarity, acidosis, and electrolyte imbalance exaggerate the stress hormone response propagating the cycle.

Case Point 20.1

Laboratory analysis of DKA are listed in Table 20.1. The patient meets criteria for DKA given the elevated glucose and low bicarbonate levels, ketonuria, elevated anion gap, and low pH.

How is the anion gap calculated and used?
The anion gap is used to estimate the retained anions, which are usually β-hydroxybutyrate and acetoacetate. A normal anion gap is approximately 12 ± 2 mmol/L. Patients with DKA typically have a higher anion gap due to increased ketones. Ketones are produced as a source of energy for the brain. The anion gap can be used to follow the treatment of diabetic ketoacidosis. As the DKA resolves, the anion gap will normalize.

BASIC SCIENCE/CLINICAL PEARL   **STEP 1/2/3**

The anion gap is the difference between the measured cations (sodium and potassium) and the measured anions (chloride and bicarbonate) in the serum. The normal value is approximately 10 to 14 mEq/L.
   In DKA, there is an increased anion gap due to retained anions; major ions are β-hydroxybutyrate and acetoacetate.
   Anion gap = $[Na^+] - ([Cl^-] + [HCO_3^-])$

What is the first step in the management of diabetic ketoacidosis in this patient?
The severity of DKA may be determined based on the physical examination and laboratory data. The physical examination includes assessing for the duration of symptoms. A longer duration is associated with more severe disease, compromised circulation, depressed level of consciousness, and risk for cerebral edema. Laboratory analysis includes assessing the degree of acidosis and bicarbonate (Table 20.2). Patients in DKA should be admitted to the intensive care unit. Intravascular resuscitation should be started as soon as the diagnosis is made. There are three major components of DKA management—fluids, electrolytes, and insulin (Fig. 20.1). Volume expansion is obtained with an isotonic solution such as 0.9% normal saline or lactated Ringer's solution (LR). The initial rate is 10 to 20 mL/kg over 1 to 2 hours. Frequent reassessment of the patient is required. The serum glucose concentration is known to decrease with fluid resuscitation. Therefore, after the initial fluid bolus, 5% dextrose should be added to the intravenous fluids if the serum glucose level is less than 300 mg/dL. It may be necessary to increase the dextrose concentration to prevent hypoglycemia, which will allow continuous insulin infusion to correct the metabolic acidosis.

TABLE 20.1 ■ **Laboratory Tests**

Test	Results
Sodium	128 mmol/L
Potassium	3.8 mmol/L
Chloride	100 mmol/L
Bicarbonate	9 mmol/L
Blood urea nitrogen	15 mg/dL
Creatinine	0.8 mg/dL
Glucose	328 mg/dL
Urinalysis	Positive for ketones
pH	7.16
pco_2	26 mm Hg
po_2	87 mm Hg

TABLE 20.2 ■ **Severity of Diabetic Ketoacidosis Based on pH and Bicarbonate Levels**

Parameter	Severity		
	Mild	Moderate	Severe
pH	<7.3	<7.2	<7.1
Bicarbonate	<15 mmol/L	<10 mmol/L	<5 mmol/L

How is insulin administered?

Initially, intravenous hydration can decrease the glucose concentration but, overall, insulin is required to correct the glucose level to the normal range and suppress lipolysis and ketogenesis. Insulin therapy should be initiated 1 to 2 hours after fluid resuscitation. Currently, the standard of care is to start insulin infusion at a dose of 0.1 unit/kg per hour and should be continued until resolution of the DKA episode, which is defined as a pH higher than 7.3, bicarbonate level higher than 15 mmol/L, and/or closure of the anion gap.

CLINICAL PEARL	STEP 2/3

Infusion with intravenous insulin is the standard of care for the treatment of diabetic ketoacidosis in adults and children, although there have been successful reports of treatment with subcutaneous rapid-acting insulin administered every 4 hours.

How are electrolytes followed and managed?

Potassium. Overall, patients who present with DKA have a total body potassium deficit, ranging from 3 to 6 mmol/kg. Potassium is mostly intracellular, and there is a shift to the extracellular fluid as a result of hypertonicity, insulin deficiency, and buffering of the hydrogen ions in the cell. Potassium is also lost during vomiting and osmotic diuresis. Volume depletion exacerbates the urinary potassium loss by causing a secondary hyperaldosteronism. Despite total body loss of potassium, the patient may present with hyperkalemia, hypokalemia, or normal potassium levels. Hyperkalemia may be present due to

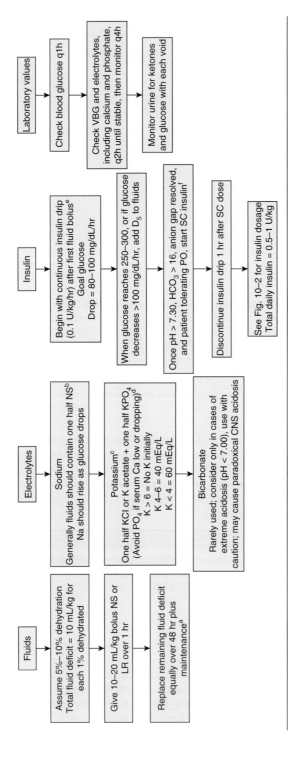

Fig. 20.1 The comprehensive management of diabetic ketoacidosis (DKA). *LR,* Lactated Ringer's; *NS,* normal saline; *SC,* subcutaneous; *VBG,* venous blood gases. (Modified from Cooke DW, Plotnick L. Management of diabetic ketoacidosis in children and adolescents. *Pediatr Rev.* 2008;29:431–436.)

[a]Additional fluids may be needed if there is a large negative fluid balance in the first hours of treatment due to the osmotic diuresis when serum glucose is high.
[b]Some DKA protocols recommend using NS rather than half NS during part of the replacement period in an effort to further decrease risk of cerebral edema.
[c]Patients with DKA are total body K[+] depleted and are at risk for severe hypokalemia during DKA therapy. However, serum K[+] levels may be normal or elevated as a result of the shift of K[+] to the extracellular compartment in the setting of acidosis.
[d]Phosphate is depleted in DKA and will drop further with insulin therapy. Consider replacing half of K as KPO_4 for first 8 hr, then all as KCl. Excessive phosphate may induce hypocalcemic tetany.
[e]Lower dose insulin infusions can be considered in very young patients.
[f]Some protocols recommend also waiting for urine ketones to decrease or clear before starting SC insulin.

renal dysfunction, which decreases potassium excretion. Treatment with insulin will lead to a decreased level of serum potassium by correcting the acidosis and causing an intracellular shift.

Potassium replacement is essential in the treatment of DKA. Potassium replacement is recommended if the serum potassium level is normal or decreased. If the patient is hypokalemic, it is important to replete potassium before insulin administration to prevent acute hypokalemia. If the patient is hyperkalemic, potassium supplementation can be delayed until the urine output is increased. The maximum rate of potassium replacement is 0.5 mmol/kg per hour.

BASIC SCIENCE PEARL	STEP 1

Potassium and phosphate are the main ions found in the intracellular fluid. Therefore, low serum levels represent a total body depletion. Sodium and chloride, on the other hand are mostly found in the extracellular fluid.

Phosphate. Osmotic diuresis leads to a depletion of total body phosphate. Insulin administration will further decrease serum phosphate levels due to intracellular shifts. In prospective studies, administration of phosphate has not shown clinical benefit. Severe hypophosphatemia—phosphate level less than 1 mg/dL—has been shown to cause muscle weakness, which can be concerning in patients with respiratory failure. If phosphate is administered, calcium must be monitored carefully because there is a risk for hypocalcemia due to calcium-phosphate binding. Phosphate repletion should be discontinued in the setting of hypocalcemia. Hypophosphatemia may persist for several days after resolution of the DKA.

Case Point 20.2

The patient is given intravenous fluids and insulin infusion. She weighs 29 kg, and intravenous insulin infusion was started at 2.9 U/hr, with close monitoring of her electrolyte and serum glucose levels. During treatment, the patient starts to become more irritable, and repeat vitals at this time show that her blood pressure is 127/74 mm Hg, heart rate is 66 beats/min, and respiratory rate is 19 breaths/min.

What are the risk factors for cerebral edema, and how does it present?
Cerebral edema occurs in 0.5% to 1% of pediatric patients who present with DKA. Given that cerebral edema has a mortality of 21% to 24%, recognizing this complication is crucial to the treatment of the patient. The risk factors for cerebral edema include increases in serum sodium levels during treatment, severe hypocapnia, severe acidosis, and an elevated blood urea nitrogen (BUN) at presentation, which represents the degree of dehydration.

Patients typically present with cerebral edema 4 to 12 hours after treatment is initiated but may develop this at any time during treatment. Frequent assessments of the patient to monitor for signs and symptoms of cerebral edema, which include headache, decreasing level of consciousness, increases in blood pressure, inappropriate slowing of the heart rate, decreased oxygen saturation, and recurrence of vomiting are essential. The presence of the Cushing triad—hypertension with widened pulse pressure, bradycardia, and irregular respiration—signaling cerebral edema is a late sign and denotes impending cerebral herniation.

What is the treatment of cerebral edema?
Given that cerebral edema during the treatment of DKA in children is a rare occurrence, the evidence behind treatment is limited. Treatment should be initiated as soon as the diagnosis is suspected. Case reports have shown that IV mannitol, 0.25 to 1 g/kg over 20 minutes, may be beneficial. This treatment can be repeated after 2 hours if there is no response. Hypertonic saline (3% sodium chloride) at a rate of 5 to 10 mL/kg over 30 minutes can be used as an alternative. It has been noted that hyperventilation in patients diagnosed with cerebral edema can lead to poorer neurologic outcomes and therefore should be avoided.

BASIC SCIENCE PEARL	STEP 1

The mechanism of cerebral edema is poorly understood. The current theory is that cerebral edema may be related to cerebral hypoperfusion prior to treatment and to vasogenic edema during DKA treatment as a result of the reperfusion of ischemic brain tissue. Mannitol and hypertonic saline reduce blood viscosity and improve cerebral blood flow.

Case Point 20.3

The patient is started on intravenous mannitol at a rate of 14.5 g over 20 minutes. The dose was calculated as 29 kg × 0.5 g/kg = 14.5 g. The patient's mental status improves slowly over the next hour.

The patient is doing well, and she has a growing appetite. Her clinical examination and laboratory analysis show resolution of the DKA. She is weaned off the insulin drip and transitioned to subcutaneous insulin.

What is the evidence for the resolution of diabetic ketoacidosis?

Normalization of the blood glucose concentration is one of the first signs of improvement in DKA, but is not a sign of resolution of DKA. DKA is considered resolved when the pH is higher than 7.30, bicarbonate level is higher than 15 mmol/L, and/or the anion gap is closed.

How is subcutaneous insulin calculated and administered?

Prepubertal total daily dose (TDD) insulin should be approximately 0.75 to 1 U/kg. Half or slightly more of the TDD should be long-acting basal insulin. To calculate the initial carbohydrate coverage ratio, divide 450 by the TDD; this is equivalent to the grams of carbohydrates per unit of insulin for rapid-acting insulin.

CLINICAL PEARL	STEP 2/3

Smaller proportions of insulin prior to meals, such as one-quarter or one-third of the total daily dose of insulin, is required for infants, toddlers, and preschool age children. Children tend to require more intermediate or longer acting basal insulin than adolescents or adults.

Prior to discharge, what is essential for the patient, as well as the parents?

Parents and patients, if they are old enough to comprehend, should be educated on the signs and symptoms of DKA. They should also be educated by a trained diabetes educator on insulin administration, checking glucose levels by fingerstick, signs and symptoms of hypoglycemia, and troubleshooting problems with insulin administration. All patients should have a medical alert bracelet stating "type 1 diabetes."

Case Point 20.4

The patient and her parents received thorough diabetes mellitus and DKA education through a trained educator. The parents are given the emergency contact line for the pediatric endocrinology clinic, which is available 24 hours/day, 7 days/week.

How can diabetic ketoacidosis be prevented in the future?

Families with a history of type 1 diabetes mellitus should be educated about the signs and symptoms of diabetes and therefore could assist in the diagnosis of the condition prior to an episode of DKA. Once a patient has experienced an episode of DKA, it is important to have an inpatient consultation with a diabetes educator. Patients also should have access to a 24-hour helpline for emergency situations. It is also essential to recognize that diabetes education is an ongoing process and should be continued in the outpatient setting. Insulin omission is one of the main causes for DKA in young patients with an established diagnosis of diabetes. DKA prevalence is reduced 10-fold if a responsible adult administers insulin.

Case Summary

Complaint/History: A 3-year-old female presents with nausea, vomiting, and progressive abdominal pain for 1 day.

Findings: The patient exhibited tachycardia and dry mucous membranes.

Labs/Tests: Laboratory analysis revealed an anion gap of 19 mEq/L, glucose level of 328 mg/dL, and bicarbonate level of 9 mmol/L, with a pH of 7.16. Urinalysis confirmed ketones.

Diagnosis: Diabetic ketoacidosis complicated by cerebral edema.

Treatment: The patient received intravenous fluids, intravenous insulin, and electrolyte repletion and was transitioned to a subcutaneous insulin regimen once the patient's mental status and symptoms of nausea and abdominal pain improved, the anion gap normalized, the pH was higher than 7.30, and the bicarbonate level improved to above 15 mmol/L. She suffered a mild case of cerebral edema, which improved after the administration of intravenous mannitol. She and her parents received diabetes education prior to discharge, with close follow-up with a pediatric endocrinologist.

BEYOND THE PEARLS

- Diabetic ketoacidosis (DKA) is the leading cause of morbidity and mortality in children with type 1 diabetes mellitus. Mortality in these patients is strongly linked to cerebral edema, which occurs in 0.3% to 1% of all episodes of DKA.
- The inciting event that precipitates DKA is usually insulin omission in patients with known type 1 diabetes mellitus but can be the initial presentation of type 1 diabetes mellitus at diagnosis.
- Patients at increased risk for DKA include children with poor metabolic control, previous episodes of DKA, psychiatric disorders, peripubertal and adolescent females or those from lower socioeconomic status who lack appropriate health insurance.
- Severe acidosis is reversible with fluid repletion and insulin. Insulin administration allows the ketones to be metabolized, allowing bicarbonate production.
- Routine bicarbonate treatment is not recommended because it has not shown clinical benefit. Patients with severe acidemia (pH < 6.9) may benefit from cautious administration.
- Intravenous administration of insulin is the standard of care for the treatment of DKA, but subcutaneous administration of insulin every 3 to 4 hours has been used and can be performed if a location has limited resources and access to ICU level care.
- Further investigation into the classification of diabetes is required once the patient has been stabilized. Types 1 and 2 diabetes mellitus are most common, but other forms of diabetes need to be investigated, such as monogenic diabetes and maturity-onset diabetes of the young (MODY). The classification can affect the long-term treatment course.
- Clinicians should be aware that caring for a pediatric patient with diabetes mellitus requires a multidisciplinary approach, which also includes the patient, patient's caregiver, nutritionist, diabetes educator, and social worker.

Bibliography

Dunger DB, Sperling MA, Acerini CL, et al. European Society for Paediatric Endocrinology/Lawson Wilkins Pediatric Endocrine Society Consensus Statement on Diabetic Ketoacidosis in Children and Adolescents. *Pediatrics.* 2004;113(2):e133–e140.

Lavoie ME. Management of a patient with diabetic ketoacidosis in the emergency department. *Pediatr Emerg Care.* 2015;31(5):376–380.

Marks T. Diabetes. *The Harriett Lane Handbook: A Manual for Pediatric House Officers.* 20th ed. In: Engorn B, Fleriage J, eds. Philadelphia: Saunders/Elsevier; 2015.

Watts W, Edge JA. How can cerebral edema during treatment of diabetic ketoacidosis be avoided? *Pediatr Diabetes.* 2014;15:271–276.

Wolfsdorf J, Glaser N, Sperling MA. Diabetic ketoacidosis in infants, children, and adolescents. A consensus statement from the American Diabetes Association. *Diabetes Care.* 2006;29(5):1150–1159.

An 8-Year-Old Child With Snoring and Behavioral Difficulty in School

David T. Kent ▦ Raj Dasgupta

An 8-year-old child presents for outpatient evaluation of loud snoring and pauses in his breathing during sleep that have been observed by his parents. He has snored lightly for at least 5 years, but over the past year and a half his snoring has become significantly louder, and he has had occasional pauses in his breathing while asleep that have worried his parents.

Should snoring be considered abnormal? What are causes of snoring in a child this age? How concerned should parents be with these symptoms?
Snoring is a sign of partial airway obstruction and falls under the category of sleep-disordered breathing (SDB). Snoring can occur on its own but can also be associated with hypopnea (decrease in airflow resulting in oxygen desaturations and/or arousal from sleep) or apnea (cessation in breathing that may result in oxygen desaturations and/or arousal from sleep). The two main categories of sleep apnea are central sleep apnea (CSA) and obstructive sleep apnea (OSA). Central apnea and hypopnea are caused by aberrations in central nervous system (CNS) respiratory control mechanisms, whereas obstructive apnea and hypopnea are due to mechanical obstruction of the upper airway. Habitual snoring occurs in almost all cases of pediatric OSA.

Most cases of SDB are due to OSA. During sleep, the body becomes atonic, with the greatest degree of atonicity occurring in the rapid eye movement (REM) sleep stage. Relaxation of the pharyngeal musculature results in partial or complete collapse of the upper airway during inspiration due to the negative pressure in the airway. CSA results from pathology in the CNS respiratory drive centers. It is generally caused by congenital abnormalities, neurologic injury, or cardiopulmonary pathology affecting oxygen and carbon dioxide chemoreceptors in the CNS. Epidemiologic studies have estimated that approximately 4% to 11% of children have pathologic breathing during sleep.

What are some risk factors for sleep-disordered breathing?
For obstructive sleep apnea, it is helpful to visualize the skeleton of the upper airway as a box into which the soft tissues of the upper airway, including the nasal airway, soft palate, tongue, epiglottis, and pharynx, must fit. Any condition that makes the box smaller, increases the volume of soft tissues within the box, or increases the risk of tissue collapse (e.g., lack of muscle tone) will restrict the available airway space and increase the risk of obstruction. In children, adenotonsillar hypertrophy is a common condition and the most common cause of SBD. A wide variety of craniofacial malformations also increase the risk of SBD because of pathologic development of the upper airway skeleton. Examples include Treacher Collins syndrome, Pierre Robin sequence, and isolated cleft palate. Neuromuscular disorders such as

Duchenne muscular dystrophy or mucopolysaccharidoses result in decreased airway muscle tone and increased risk of OSA.

Obesity leads to increased fat deposition in the tissues surrounding the upper airway and can create or exacerbate preexisting OSA. It has other more complex effects on the pulmonary system and respiratory control. The prevalence of OSA due to obesity is expected to increase due to the current obesity epidemic.

CNS pathology due to developmental abnormalities, tumor growth, or injury can lead to aberrations in respiratory control. This can manifest as CSA caused by an abnormal respiratory drive or as OSA caused by poor coordination or tone in the upper airway musculature. Down syndrome is an example of a disease process with both central and obstructive sleep pathology. Many children with Down syndrome have relative macroglossia (enlarged tongue), which increases the risk of upper airway obstruction. These children also frequently suffer from muscle hypotonicity, which further increases the risk of airway obstruction from the tongue falling backward during sleep.

Case Point 21.1

His mother lies down with him until he falls asleep in the evening because he will not go to sleep without her present.

What behavior does this represent? Should the mother be concerned that he will not go to sleep without her present?
This child is displaying behavior consistent with behavioral insomnia of childhood (BIC) due to sleep onset association. He has accommodated himself to the presence of his mother before falling asleep and is unable to soothe himself to sleep. This problem may also manifest as periods of long wakefulness at night, in which the child awakens and is unable to self-soothe back to sleep without the presence of the mother. Although not central to this case, BIC is a common condition, with a prevalence of approximately 25%. It should always be considered within the differential and treatment plan when a parent complains of a child's sleeping problems.

Case Point 21.2

After he falls asleep, she reports that it looks like he is "trying to breathe, but he's not moving any air." She has not seen him turn blue.

BASIC SCIENCE PEARL   **STEP 1**

Pharyngeal muscle tone is maintained during sleep by the pharyngeal dilator muscles. The primary pharyngeal dilator is the genioglossus muscle, which is innervated by the hypoglossal nerve.

Why does it matter that the patient appears to be "trying to breathe"?
This observation implies that the patient is attempting to breathe against an obstruction, which increases the clinical suspicion for OSA. However, studies have shown that caregiver observation and clinical history are not sensitive enough to differentiate adequately between primary snoring and OSA. The definitive diagnosis of the type and severity of sleep apnea requires a multichannel diagnostic study of sleep called *polysomnography.*

TABLE 21.1 ▪ National Sleep Foundation: Recommended Hours of Sleep Across Different Age Groups

Age	Hours of Sleep
Newborn (0–3 mo)	14–17
Infant (4–11 mo)	12–15
Toddler (1–2 yr)	11–14
Preschool (3–5 yr)	10–13
School Age (6–13 yr)	9–11
Teenager (14–17 yr)	8–10
Adult (18–64 yr)	7–9
Older adult (≥65 yr)	7–8

Case Point 21.3

The patient sleeps from 10 PM until 6 AM, when his parents awaken him for school. Over the last several months, he has become much more difficult to arouse from bed, especially on school days. He seemed less tired when he was able to take scheduled naps in preschool. He now frequently comes home from school and sleeps 30 to 60 minutes in the afternoon. He has gotten in some trouble at school for "not paying attention," and his teacher has told his parents that he may have attention deficit hyperactivity disorder (ADHD). His academic performance is mediocre.

CLINICAL PEARL	STEP 2/3

If a child has been previously diagnosed with ADHD, be aware that prescription stimulant medications may mask the symptoms of excessive daytime sleepiness.

What are the normal sleep requirements for children?
It is important to be aware of sufficient sleep requirements in children. The National Sleep Foundation has reported that the average adult requires 6 to 10 hours of sleep per night, with the majority needing between 7 and 9 hours per night. However, it is recommended that an 8-year-old child should get 7 to 12 hours of sleep per night, with most children needing between 9 and 11 hours per night (Table 21.1). This child may be getting an insufficient amount of sleep for his age.

What are some signs indicating that a child may not be obtaining adequate sleep?
Several large studies have suggested an association between OSA in children and behavioral problems, as well as poor academic performance. Children are occasionally misdiagnosed with ADHD when the true cause of their symptoms is poor sleep. This child's combination of insufficient sleep and poor sleep quality may be causing excessive daytime sleepiness and impairing academic performance, and it warrants further investigation.

What are the causes of excessive daytime sleepiness in children?
The differential diagnosis for excessive daytime sleepiness in children is broad, including, but not limited to, OSA or CSA, insufficient sleep, primary and secondary insomnia, circadian rhythm sleep disorders, hypothyroidism, restless leg syndrome, and periodic leg movement disorder. The search for causes of sleepiness in a child should not end once SBD has been ruled out.

Case Point 21.4

His mother notes that he has "a healthy appetite." He frequently has juice and snacks while watching television in the afternoon before dinner. He has gained a significant amount of weight over the last 2 years.

How do dietary habits affect sleep?

Obesity is frequently associated with poor dietary habits in children. Failure to develop good dietary habits at a young age may increase the risk of obesity and comorbid diseases, including OSA, from childhood into adulthood. There is a large body of evidence supporting the health benefits of regular exercise; however, parents should be counseled that exercise alone is unlikely to counteract poor dietary choices completely.

Healthy eating requires portion control in addition to healthy food choices. Many parents are not aware of the caloric density of fruit juices and soft drinks. Consider eliminating juice, soft drinks, and calorie-dense snacks from the diet of overweight children and transitioning to less calorie-dense foods, such as lean meats and high-fiber vegetables, as a first step toward healthier eating choices.

Case Point 21.5

The patient was born full term and had no perinatal complications. He was diagnosed with mild intermittent asthma last year which is well controlled with an albuterol inhaler, and he is not exposed to tobacco smoke at home. He does not take any other medications. He has not had issues with persistent mouth breathing or recurrent pharyngitis. His father snores as well. The remainder of his review of systems (ROS) is negative.

Why is it important to assess a prenatal and perinatal history when evaluating a child with sleep problems?

It is important to assess for any significant prenatal and perinatal history when evaluating young children to assess for other possible causes of breathing problems and build a comprehensive differential diagnosis. For example, a history of respiratory distress or intubation at birth would raise suspicion for a primary pulmonary cause unrelated to OSA that could contribute to breathing difficulties, such as bronchopulmonary dysplasia or tracheal stenosis.

Why is it important to assess for a history of asthma and tobacco smoke exposure?

Obesity, family history of OSA, poorly controlled asthma, and exposure to tobacco smoke at home have all been associated with an increased risk for OSA. African American ancestry is an additional risk factor, but the underlying pathophysiology has not been well defined.

Why is it important to assess for a history of persistent mouth breathing or recurrent pharyngitis?

All these symptoms are suggestive of possible adenotonsillar hypertrophy, the leading cause of pediatric OSA. Mouth breathing may be secondary to adenoid hypertrophy, with resultant obstruction of the nasopharynx. Recurrent pharyngitis is associated with adenotonsillar hypertrophy, although these conditions frequently occur independently of one another. A history of recurrent pharyngitis is an indication for adenotonsillectomy, independent of sleep history.

BASIC SCIENCE PEARL	STEP 1

The nasopharyngeal tonsil (adenoid) and palatine tonsils make up two-thirds of Waldeyer's lymphatic ring, the annular configuration of lymphoid tissue in the pharynx. The remainder of Waldeyer's ring is comprised of the lingual tonsil. These lymphoid tissues frequently swell and hypertrophy during childhood as part of the robust pediatric immunologic response to novel environmental pathogens and antigens. The pediatric upper airway is smaller than its final adult conformation and is therefore more susceptible to obstruction by lymphatic tissue hypertrophy. Rapid or asymmetric lymphoid tissue hyperplasia in an adult should raise suspicion for neoplastic, infectious, or autoimmune pathologies (e.g., squamous cell carcinoma, lymphoma, human immunodeficiency virus).

Case Point 21.6

On physical examination, the patient's body mass index (BMI) is 19.5 kg/m^2, blood pressure is 120/80 mm Hg, pulse rate is 70/min, respiration rate is 20/min, and oxygen saturation is 97% on room air. No concerning craniofacial deformities are noted, but the patient does have a 2-mm overjet. His modified Mallampati score is III, and his tonsils are 2 to 3+ in size. There are no abnormalities on cardiac auscultation, with normal S1 and S2 heart sounds, and no audible murmurs or gallops. His lung fields are clear to auscultation bilaterally. Capillary refill is normal, and no pallor is noted.

CLINICAL PEARL	STEP 2/3

Palatine tonsil size is most commonly graded on physical examination using the Brodsky grading scale:
1. Tonsils occupy 25% or more of the oropharyngeal airway.
2. Tonsils occupy 26% to 50% of the oropharyngeal airway.
3. Tonsils occupy 51% to 75% of the oropharyngeal airway.
4. Tonsils occupy 75% or more of the oropharyngeal airway.

What is the modified Mallampati score?

The modified Mallampati score is an anatomic assessment made by an examiner of an upright patient who is protruding the tongue from the mouth as far as possible (Fig. 21.1). A class I score indicates that the soft palate, uvula, fauces (opening into the oropharynx), and tonsillar pillars are visible. A class II score has a greater degree of obstruction by the tongue, with only the soft palate, uvula, and fauces visible. The soft palate and only the base of the uvula are visible in a class III score. The hard palate is the only visible structure in class IV occlusion due to obstruction by the tongue.

How do you interpret this child's physical examination? Does this change your assessment?

Recognize that children are not just "little adults." Although the above documented vital sign measurements are benign in an adult, a blood pressure of 120/80 mm Hg in an 8-year-old child is concerning for borderline hypertension. He is just under the 95th percentile for weight at his age, with a BMI of 19.5 kg/m^2, making him overweight and almost obese. His moderately enlarged tonsils, relatively small mandible, and higher modified Mallampati score are all considered anatomically normal but, in combination, they decrease the available size of his upper airway and increase the suspicion for OSA.

What is the next best step in management?

It depends on who you ask! The accepted first-line therapy for children with OSA is adenotonsillectomy. However, there is no clear consensus on whether a clinical suspicion of OSA is sufficient

Class I   Class II

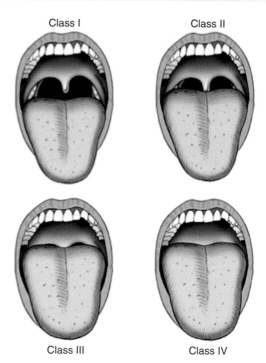

Class III   Class IV

Fig. 21.1   Modified Mallampati classification: class I—fully visible uvula and soft palate; class II—hard and soft palate and upper portion of uvula are visible; class III—soft and hard palate and base of uvula are visible; class IV—only hard palate visible. (From Islam S, Selbong U, Taylor CJ, Ormiston CW. Does a patient's Mallampati score predict outcome after maxillomandibular advancement for obstructive sleep apnoea? *Br J Oral Maxillofac Surg.* 2015;53(1):23–27.)

or whether polysomnography is required in all cases prior to surgery. Clinical practice guidelines from the American Academy of Otolaryngology–Head and Neck Surgery (AAO-HNS) have recommended that polysomnography be completed prior to adenotonsillectomy in children with any of the following comorbidities: obesity, Down syndrome, craniofacial abnormalities, neuromuscular disorders, sickle cell disease, or mucopolysaccharidosis.

Additionally, the clinician should advocate for polysomnography in children for whom the need for surgery is uncertain or when there is a discordance between tonsillar size on physical examination and the reported severity of SDB. The American Academy of Sleep Medicine (AASM) is more conservative and has recommended polysomnography for all patients in whom clinical assessment suggests the diagnosis of OSA. An otolaryngologist would therefore be following established clinical practice guidelines for this child by recommending surgery without prior diagnostic testing. Definitive diagnosis of OSA is never discouraged, and polysomnography is frequently recommended by otolaryngologists when parents would like additional information before electing for surgery.

Case Point 21.7

An overnight polysomnography study is ordered. The patient has loud snoring and frequent obstructive hypopnea, resulting in arousals from sleep. His apnea-hypopnea index (AHI) is 4.5 events/hr. Sleep is fragmented, and the patient awakens frequently overnight. His oxygen level nadir overnight is 86%. His central apnea index (CAI) is normal, at 1.7 events/hr.

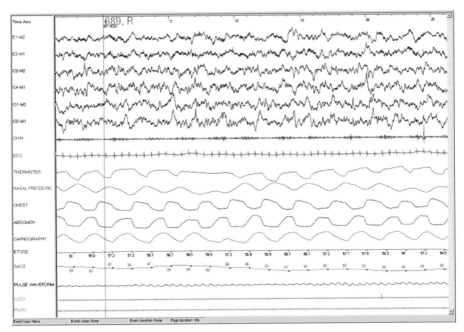

Fig. 21.2 Pediatric polysomnography. This polysomnography of a pediatric patients shows obstructive hypoventilation with overall perserved nasal airflow with paradoxical chest and abdominal wall motion, elevated end tidal carbon dioxide (CO2), and prolonged oxygen desaturation. *Chin*, chin electromyography (EMG); *E1-M2, E2-M1,* electro-oculogram; *C3-M2, C4-M1, O1-M2, O2-M1,* electroencephalogram (EEG); *ETCO2*, end tidal PCO2 (mm Hg); *SaO2*, arterial oxygen saturation (%). (From Beck S, Marcus S. Pediatric polysomnography. *Sleep Med Clin.* 2009;4(3):393-406.)

What is monitored during polysomnography?

Type I polysomnography is performed in a laboratory and monitored by a technician. Standard measurement modalities include encephalography, electrooculography, electrocardiography, electromyography (of the chin and lower limb muscles), pulse oximetry, airflow measurements using a nasal thermistor and/or pressure transducer, and monitoring of respiratory effort at the thorax and abdomen (Fig. 21.2).

What is the importance of his AHI and CAI?

The AHI and CAI are the average number of obstructive and central events that occur per hour of sleep, respectively. The AHI is a commonly used measure of OSA severity that has been correlated with various health risks. In adults, mild OSA is defined as 5 to 15 events/hr, moderate OSA is 15 to 30 events/hr, and severe OSA is 30 events/hr or more. In children, mild OSA is defined as 1.5 to 5 events/hr, moderate OSA is 5 to 10 events/hr, and severe OSA is 10 events/hr or more. Despite having an AHI in the normal range for an adult, this child has mild OSA and is on the border for moderate OSA.

Case Point 21.8

Diagnosis: Obstructive sleep apnea.

CLINICAL PEARL   **STEP 2/3**

Obstructive sleep apnea is a sleep-related breathing disorder characterized by intermittent partial or complete airway obstruction that disrupts normal sleep patterns and ventilation. The International Classification of Sleep Disorders coding manual has defined polysomnography criteria sufficient for diagnosing OSA: I, one or more obstructive events per hour of sleep, or II, obstructive hypoventilation with $Paco_2 > 50$ mm Hg for >25% of observed sleep together with snoring, paradoxic thoracoabdominal movement, or flattening of the nasal airway pressure waveform measurement. Most sleep centers define mild OSA as an AHI >1 but ≤5, moderate OSA as an AHI >5 but ≤10, and severe OSA as an AHI >10.

How do you counsel his parents regarding further management?

The patient's polysomnography results are consistent with mild OSA. Adenotonsillectomy is the recommended first-line therapy for pediatric OSA. In patients for whom surgery is not an option, medical therapies should be considered, such as lateral positioning during sleep, nasal steroids and montelukast to reduce upper airway inflammation, and continuous positive airway pressure (PAP).

Recent evidence has suggested that a significant percentage of pediatric patients may see normalization of AHI through watchful waiting over a period of at least 7 months, presumably by allowing the airway lumen to increase in size as the child grows. Adenotonsillectomy does, however, improve AHI more rapidly and dramatically. Watchful waiting is less likely to be successful in obese children, African American children, and children with more severe disease.

Case Point 21.9

The child undergoes an uneventful adenotonsillectomy and is seen in your office 2 months after surgery. His parents are happy to report that his snoring and excessive daytime sleepiness have resolved.

Is repeat polysomnography required to confirm resolution of obstructive sleep apnea?

Absence of clinical symptoms after adenotonsillectomy for mild OSA does not require postoperative polysomnography. The AASM has recommended repeat polysomnography if OSA symptoms persist postoperatively, or if there is a history of moderate to severe OSA, obesity, craniofacial anomalies that obstruct the upper airway, or neurologic disorders.

Case Summary

Complaint/History: An overweight 8-year-old child presents with a history of loud snoring, witnessed apneas, daytime fatigue, and behavioral problems.

Findings: BMI is 19.5 kg/m², 2-mm overjet, modified Mallampati score of III, and his tonsils are 2 to 3+ in size on examination.

Labs/Tests: AHI is 4.5 during overnight polysomnography.

Diagnosis: Mild obstructive sleep apnea.

Treatment: Adenotonsillectomy, after which his snoring and excessive sleepiness resolves.

BEYOND THE PEARLS

- Weight loss should always be recommended for obese children with OSA. Obesity is a risk factor for residual OSA after adenotonsillectomy, and weight loss can reduce or cure pediatric OSA.
- Rapid-onset obesity with hypothalamic dysfunction, hypoventilation and autonomic dysregulation (ROHHAD syndrome) is an extremely rare disease with a heterogeneous presentation. It is not associated with *PHOX2B,* the gene linked to earlier presentations of congenital central hypoventilation syndrome. Rapid increases in weight, hyperphagia (overeating), and dramatically worsening SBD in preadolescent children should raise suspicion for this potentially lethal disease.
- PAP therapy is a highly efficacious medical therapy for OSA in children, but there is generally a long learning curve for therapy acceptance and mask tolerance. If a child has residual OSA after adenotonsillectomy, consider referral to a pediatric pulmonology service with experience in pediatric PAP therapy.
- Consider evaluation for reconstructive skeletal surgery options for children with OSA and congenital craniofacial development disorders (e.g., cleft lip and/or palate, Pierre Robin sequence, midface hypoplasia, hemifacial macrosomia) prior to adenotonsillectomy and other soft tissue surgeries because craniofacial surgery may relieve or cure OSA. Select children with severe OSA may benefit from perioperative PAP therapy to minimize anesthesia risks.
- Upper airway soft tissue surgery for children with residual OSA after adenotonsillectomy can be effective in select cases and is an area of active research. Drug-induced sleep endoscopy (DISE) is a diagnostic technique used for assessing specific sites of collapse in the upper airway in patients with OSA. DISE may be useful in guiding surgical decision making for pediatric patients with residual OSA after adenotonsillectomy.
- Tonsil sizes between 2+ (extending medially beyond the anterior and posterior tonsillar pillars) and 4+ (complete oropharyngeal obstruction) have not been correlated with AHI severity. Children with 2+ tonsils are just as likely to have severe OSA as children with 4+ tonsils.
- The odds of having OSA in a child increases by more than sixfold for each point increase in the modified Mallampati score.
- A high incidence (20%–30%) of OSA has been reported in children diagnosed with full syndromal ADHD.

Bibliography

Aurora RN, Zak RS, Karippot A, et al. Practice parameters for the respiratory indications for polysomnography in children. *Sleep.* 2011;34(3):379–388.

Galluzzi F, Pignataro L, Gaini RM, Garavello W. Drug induced sleep endoscopy in the decision-making process of children with obstructive sleep apnea. *Sleep Med.* 2015;16(3):331–335. Epub 2015 Jan 20.

Marcus CL, Moore RH, Rosen CL, et al. A randomized trial of adenotonsillectomy for childhood sleep apnea. *N Engl J Med.* 2013;368(25):2366–2376.

Marcus CL, Moore RH, Rosen CL, et al. Childhood Adenotonsillectomy Trial (CHAT). A randomized trial of adenotonsillectomy for childhood sleep apnea. *N Engl J Med.* 2013;368(25):2366–2376.

Roland PS, Rosenfeld RM, Brooks LJ, et al. Clinical practice guideline: polysomnography for sleep-disordered breathing prior to tonsillectomy in children. *Otolaryngol Head Neck Surg.* 2011;145(suppl 1):S1–S15.

Tang A, Benke JR, Cohen AP, Ishman SL. Influence of tonsillar size on OSA improvement in children undergoing adenotonsillectomy. *Otolaryngol Head Neck Surg.* 2015;153(2):281–285.

Wootten CT, Chinnadurai S, Goudy SL. Beyond adenotonsillectomy: outcomes of sleep endoscopy-directed treatments in pediatric obstructive sleep apnea. *Int J Pediatr Otorhinolaryngol.* 2014;78(7):1158–1162.

A 3-Year-Old Male With Lower Extremity Edema, Abdominal Distention, and Discomfort

Joseph Meouchy ▪ Cynthia Hayek ▪ Hui Yi Shan

A 3-year-old Native American male, previously healthy, is brought to your office for worsening swelling of his feet, legs, and thighs. His mother reports an episode of upper respiratory tract infection 2 weeks prior followed by progressive worsening of a lower extremity swelling. She also noticed abdominal distention and diffuse abdominal discomfort. The male denies any dysuria, hematuria, urinary frequency, and urgency but his mother mentions that his urine appears foamy lately.

What is the significance of foamy urine?
Foaming occurs because protein has a soap-like effect that reduces the surface tension of urine. It is generally thought that foamy urine may be an early sign of renal disease, and thus patients with this condition should be further evaluated. Note that foamy urine is subjective and is not always pathologic.

Case Point 22.1

The family history is unremarkable for any renal disease. The male has gained about 4 pounds since his illness. His vital signs show blood pressure of 100/60 mm Hg. The examination is notable for mild periorbital edema, bilateral +1 pitting edema of his hands, feet, legs, and thighs and a slightly distended abdomen, with minimal discomfort to palpation. The rest of the physical examination is within normal limits.

What is the differential diagnosis of generalized edema and anasarca?
The differential diagnosis includes the following:
1. Congestive heart failure (peripheral edema generally less commonly observed in children than in adults)
2. Renal disease (as a result of sodium and water retention)
3. Decreased capillary oncotic pressure:
   - Protein malnutrition (severe protein malnutrition or kwashiorkor).
   - Protein-losing enteropathy (hypertrophic gastritis—Ménétrier disease, milk protein allergy, celiac disease, inflammatory bowel disease, giardiasis, intestinal lymphangiectasia, and right-sided heart dysfunction; post–Fontan procedure).
4. Increased capillary hydrostatic pressure:
   - Venous obstruction—causes localized swelling
5. Liver cirrhosis: uncommon in children, mainly caused by the following:
   - Genetic disorders (e.g., alpha-1 antitrypsin deficiency, cystic fibrosis, Wilson disease)
   - Infectious causes
   - Structural problems of the biliary tree (e.g., biliary atresia, Alagille syndrome).
6. Increased capillary permeability: angioedema

What is an easy and quick test to perform to evaluate for proteinuria?
Dipstick urinalysis is a convenient and quick method to detect proteinuria, but false-positive and false-negative results are not unusual. The main causes for a false-positive test result are alkaline and concentrated urine. A false-negative test result can be seen with acidic or dilute urine. Because the dipstick only detects albumin, nonalbumin protein will not cause a positive dipstick test result.

Case Point 22.2

The urinary dipstick assay is performed and shows 3+ protein, negative glucose, negative leukocyte esterase and nitrates, and negative blood.

What is the significance of 3+ protein on urinary dipstick, and what is the best way to quantify the amount of protein excreted?
Dipstick tests for trace amounts of protein. It becomes positive at concentrations of around 5 to 10 mg/dL, lower than the threshold for clinically significant proteinuria. A result of 1+ corresponds to approximately 30 mg of protein/dL and is considered positive, 2+ corresponds to 100 mg/dL, and 3+ corresponds to 300 mg/dL. Nephrotic-range proteinuria typically corresponds to dipstick proteinuria of 3+ to 4+. Measurement of the protein content in a 24-hour urine sample is the definitive method of establishing the presence of abnormal proteinuria. However, the process of urine collection is cumbersome. Studies have shown a strong correlation between spot urine protein-creatinine ratio and 24-hour urine total protein excretion in proteinuria levels from 300 to 3499 mg/day.

BASIC SCIENCE/CLINICAL PEARL   **STEP 1/2/3**

The reagent on most dipstick tests is sensitive to albumin but may not detect low concentrations of γ-globulins and Bence Jones proteins. In patients with monoclonal gammopathy, the dipstick may be negative despite high amounts of nonalbumin protein excretion.

Case Point 22.3

Urine microscopy shows 0 to 1 white blood cells; 2 to 3 red blood cells; 1 to 5 epithelial cells; 0 casts, and 24-hour urine collection of 6.2 g of protein.

What is the definition of nephrotic syndrome?
The clinical triad of edema, nephrotic-range proteinuria, and hypoalbuminemia (<2.5g/dL) defines nephrotic syndrome. In children, nephrotic-range proteinuria means that there is more than 1 g/m^2 per 24 hr (40 mg/m^2 per hr) of protein or a spot protein-creatinine ratio of more than 2. This triad is typically accompanied by dyslipidemia, with elevated plasma cholesterol and triglyceride levels. You can detect lipid-laden casts in urine microscopy from a patient with nephrotic syndrome (Fig. 22.1).

What is the pathophysiology of nephrotic syndrome?
- Nephrotic-range proteinuria. Normally, the kidneys do not excrete high amounts of protein (<150 mg/day). The mechanism of proteinuria in nephrotic syndrome is a defective glomerular filtration barrier. This barrier (Fig. 22.2) is normally impermeable to protein due to the large size of proteins and its net negative charge. The appearance of significant proteinuria heralds a disruption of the normal barrier function of the glomeruli and glomerular disease. Nephrotic syndrome is defined by a protein excretion over 20 times the upper limit of normal.

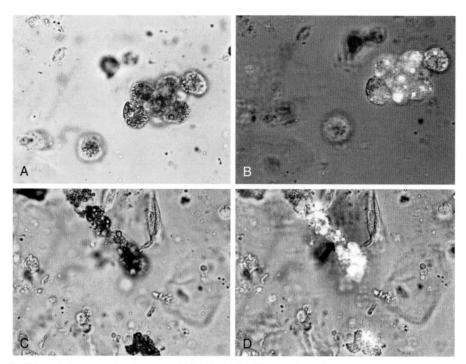

Fig. 22.1   Urinalysis and urine microscopy. (A) Oval fat bodies. (B) Same field as in A, viewed under polarized light. (C) Lipid-laden cast, bright field illumination. (D) Same field as in C, viewed under polarized light. (From Gilbert S, Weiner D. *National Kidney Foundation's Primer on Kidney Disease.* 6th ed. Philadelphia: Elsevier/Saunders; 2014.)

- Hypoalbuminemia. Hypoalbuminemia is a result of urinary loss of albumin and failure of the liver to compensate fully by increasing the hepatic synthesis of albumin.
- Edema. A fall in oncotic pressure from hypoalbuminemia leads to a redistribution of fluid from the intravascular space to the interstitial compartment. The subsequently reduced effective blood circulating volume in the intravascular space causes renal sodium and water retention and further contributes to edema formation.

Case Point 22.4

Laboratory examination reveals a serum creatinine (SCr) level of 0.6 mg/dL and serum albumin level of 2.9 mg/dL.

What is the differential diagnosis of nephrotic syndrome?
Nephrotic syndrome in children can be congenital or acquired. Congenital disease may be due to a genetic mutation. It occurs in children younger than 1 year of age. Acquired nephrotic syndrome can be divided into primary (idiopathic) and secondary (associated with systemic diseases) types. Examples of idiopathic nephrotic syndrome include minimal change disease (MCD) and focal segmental glomerular sclerosis.

Table 22.1 summarizes the causes of secondary nephrotic syndrome. The patient's history, presence or absence of hypertension, renal failure, and urine sediments can help narrow down the differential diagnosis.

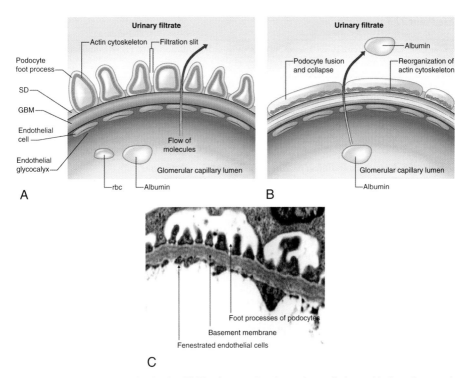

Fig. 22.2 The glomerular filtration barrier. (A) Blood enters the glomerular capillaries and is filtered across the endothelium and glomerular basement membrane (GBM) and through the filtration slits between the podocyte foot processes to produce the primary urine filtrate. In healthy glomeruli, this barrier restricts the passage of macromolecules. The proteins that form the slit diaphragm are essential for the normal functioning of the filtration barrier. (B) Loss of these proteins, either genetically or acquired, leads to foot process effacement and breakdown of the barrier and leakage of albumin. (C) Electron micrograph of normal filtration barrier. (From Kumar PJ, Clark M. *Kumar and Clark's Clinical Medicine.* 8th ed. Philadelphia: Elsevier/Saunders; 2012.)

TABLE 22.1 ▦ **Causes of Secondary Nephrotic Syndrome**

Cause	Examples
Infection	Hepatitis B, hepatitis C, HIV/AIDS, malaria, syphilis, toxoplasmosis
Systemic disease	Systemic lupus erythematosus, Henoch-Schönlein purpura, sickle cell disease, IgA nephropathy, postinfectious glomerulonephritis
Drugs, toxins	Penicillamine, gold, nonsteroidal antiinflammatory drugs (NSAIDs), pamidronate, interferon, mercury, heroin, lithium, sirolimus
Immune and allergic disorders	Castleman syndrome, Kimura disease, bee stings
Malignancy	Lymphoma, leukemia

CLINICAL PEARL   **STEP 2/3**

Two-thirds of nephrotic syndrome cases that occur during the first year of life and as many as 85% of cases that occur during the first 3 months of life have a genetic basis and a poor outcome.

Case Point 22.5

> The C-reactive protein (CRP) level, erythrocyte sedimentation rate (ESR), and complement components C3 and C4 are within normal limits.

What is the most likely diagnosis in this case?

Idiopathic nephrotic syndrome is the most common form of childhood nephrotic syndrome. It accounts for more than 90% of cases in those from 1 to 10 years of age and 50% of cases after 10 years of age. The most common idiopathic nephrotic syndrome in children younger than 6 years is MCD.

What are the characteristic clinical findings of minimal change disease?

1. Generalized edema develops during days to weeks, and fluid retention often exceeds more than 3% of the body weight.
2. Up to two-thirds of initial presentations and relapses follow an infection, most often in the upper respiratory tract, but whether these are of causative significance is uncertain.
3. Ascites is common in children with MCD, who may present with abdominal pain, a symptom that may suggest peritonitis.
4. Hepatomegaly is common in children but may be overlooked in the presence of ascites.
5. Microscopic hematuria is rare in MCD.
6. Although hypertension is not typical in children, higher than normal blood pressure has been described in 14% to 21% of children. Hypertension usually resolves during remission, especially in children.
7. Pulmonary embolism can be present and may be overlooked in children because of a lack of suspicion. Pulmonary symptoms in children also may not be obvious because children may compensate better than adults.
8. Renal function is generally preserved. Serum creatinine concentrations are usually low in children.
9. Vitamin D deficiency—urinary loss of vitamin D–binding proteins—may lead to reduced intestinal calcium absorption.

CLINICAL PEARL   **STEP 2/3**

The clinical findings that are more predictive of MCD are as follows:
- Age younger than six years
- Absence of hypertension
- Absence of hematuria
- Normal complement levels
- Normal renal function

CLINICAL PEARL   **STEP 2/3**

There is an increased susceptibility to thrombosis in patients with nephrotic syndrome. Increased urinary loss of endogenous anticoagulants, particularly antithrombin III, protein C, and protein S, may account for the hypercoagulable state.

What is the next step in management?

Due to the geographic prevalence of MCD, renal biopsy is unnecessary for children from the Northern Hemisphere who are 2 to 12 years of age unless the patient does not respond to a standard prednisone treatment. In Africa and South America, the prevalence of MCD is lower. The decision to give a trial course of corticosteroids might depend on the frequency of MCD in that particular region.

MCD is usually associated with selective proteinuria of smaller molecules, including albumin and transferrin, but not of larger molecules, such as immunoglobulins and ferritin.

$$\text{Selectivity index} = [(IgG)_u(albumin)_s]/[(IgG)_s(albumin)_u]$$

If the selectivity index is less than 0.1, the proteinuria is highly selective and, if more than 0.2, is nonselective. Highly selective proteinuria, when present, does indicate that MCD is more likely to be the diagnosis

What is the treatment of choice for a first episode of minimal change disease?

Corticosteroids are the initial treatment of choice. According to the International Study of Kidney Disease in Children (ISKDC) guidelines, children 2 to 12 years of age with a first episode of nephrotic syndrome should be treated with oral prednisone (or prednisolone), 60 mg/m^2/day (maximum dose, 80 mg/day), in three divided doses (calculated on the basis of estimated dry weight) for 4 to 6 weeks. This daily dose should be followed by an alternate-day dose of 40 mg/m^2/48 hr for an additional 4 to 6 weeks.

Case Point 22.6

Your patient responded to initial steroid treatment but comes back 1 month after completing his regimen with the same presentation.

How would you proceed with management?

Although MCD is still high on your differential diagnosis, a renal biopsy can be considered in patients with frequent relapses and in patients with relapse while being tapered off prednisone.

What are the characteristic findings of minimal change disease on kidney biopsy?

Typically, MCD is associated with normal-appearing glomeruli by light microscopy and is negative for immunoglobulins and complement by immunofluorescence staining. Extensive podocyte (epithelial cell) foot process effacement is observed with electron microscopy (Fig. 22.3) and is the only abnormality, but this is a nonspecific finding. The tubulointerstitium will show an absence of inflammation. Hyaline casts obstructing tubules, rare foam cells, and occasionally appearances consistent with those of acute tubular necrosis may be seen, especially if acute kidney injury is present at the time of biopsy.

On occasion, a renal biopsy may histologically appear similar to that of MCD, but there is another cause. In patients with nephrotic syndrome, this may be caused by FSGS, in which the sclerotic glomeruli are not sampled. In young children, it could result from a hereditary nephrotic syndrome resembling MCD. Rarely, early membranous nephropathy will have a light microscopy appearance of normal glomeruli, but immunofluorescence will reveal immune deposits. In non-nephrotic subjects, diseases such as thin basement membrane disease can appear histologically normal but can be diagnosed by the demonstration of the thin GBM on electron microscopy.

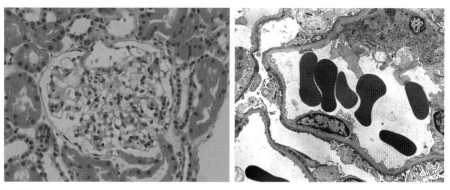

Fig. 22.3 Minimal change nephrotic syndrome. *Left,* The glomerulus appears normal to light microscopic examination, with normal mesangial matrix and cellularity. Capillary loops are dilated with normal thin capillary walls (H&E stain, ×400). *Right,* Low-power electron photomicrograph indicates a capillary loop with extensive effacement of foot processes, accompanied by swelling and microvillarization of podocytes. The glomerular basement membranes appear normal, and no dense deposits are noted. (From Niaudet P. Minimal change nephrotic syndrome. In Johnson R, Feehally J, Floege J, eds. *Comprehensive Clinical Nephrology,* 5th ed. Philadelphia: Elsevier/Saunders; 2014.)

Case Point 22.7

The kidney biopsy shows normal glomeruli on light microscopy, a negative immunofluorescence staining, and extensive foot process effacement on electron microscopy.

How would you treat a relapsing MCD?
Fig. 22.4.

Case Summary
Complaint/History: A 3-year-old Native American male presents with worsening swelling of his feet, legs, and thighs over a few weeks after an upper respiratory tract infection.

Findings: His examination shows periorbital edema, bilateral +1 pitting edema of his hands, feet, legs, and thighs, and a slightly distended abdomen, with minimal discomfort to palpation.

Labs/Tests: The urinary dipstick assay shows 3+ protein, negative glucose, negative leukocyte esterase and nitrates, and negative blood. A 24-hour urine collection has shown an estimated 6.2 g of protein.

Diagnosis: Minimal change disease.

Treatment: Oral prednisone (or prednisolone), 60 mg/m^2 per day (maximum dose, 80 mg/day), in three divided doses (calculated on the basis of estimated dry weight) for 4 to 6 weeks followed by an alternate-day dosage of 40 mg/m^2/48 hr for an additional 4 or 6 weeks.

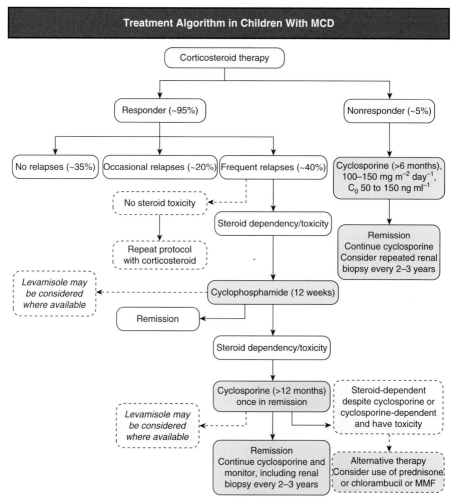

Fig. 22.4 Algorithm for the treatment of childhood minimal change disease (minimal change nephrotic syndrome). The patient or parents should be involved in the decision after the potential side effects of the second-line treatment are considered (*boxes with interrupted lines* show alternative options). In the rare patient who is a nonresponder to standard corticosteroid therapy and is by definition "corticosteroid resistant," a trial with cyclosporine may be considered. *MMF,* Mycophenolate mofetil. (From Niaudet P. Minimal change nephrotic syndrome. In Johnson R, Feehally J, Floege J, eds. *Comprehensive Clinical Nephrology,* 5th ed. Philadelphia: Elsevier/Saunders; 2014.)

BEYOND THE PEARLS

- The physical examination of patients with nephrotic syndrome may reveal white nail bands known as Muehrcke lines, which correlate with periods of clinical relapse (Fig. 22.5).
- There is an increased incidence of infection in patients with nephrotic syndrome due to the loss of immunoglobulins in the urine. Peritonitis remains a major cause of mortality in the developing world, mainly in children. *Streptococcus pneumoniae, Haemophilus influenzae,* and other encapsulated bacteria are implicated. Children with frequently relapsing nephrotic syndrome should be immunized against *S. pneumoniae* and *H. influenzae* during remission and given prophylactic oral penicillin in relapse.
- The classic drugs associated with MCD are NSAIDs, particularly fenoprofen. This is an idiosyncratic reaction associated with chronic NSAID use. Unlike classic MCD, this syndrome is usually associated with massive nephrotic syndrome with impaired renal function, and renal biopsy shows MCD with features of an acute interstitial nephritis with T cell infiltration. Other causes of secondary MCD, such as the use of interferon alfa or interferon beta, or MCD observed in Hodgkin disease, may appear clinically identical to idiopathic MCD.
- MCD is associated with selective proteinuria of smaller molecules, including albumin and transferrin, but not of larger molecules such as immunoglobulins and ferritin.
- About 75% of children with MCD respond within 2 weeks, and almost all who are corticosteroid-sensitive respond within 4 weeks. Patients who do not respond within this period are termed *nonresponders*. Whereas the International Study of Kidney Disease in Children (ISKDC) has recommended continuing the daily dose for 4 weeks, later studies have recommended 6 weeks. Extending the duration of corticosteroid treatment to at least 3 months reduces the 1- to 2-year risk of relapse.
- Congenital nephrotic syndrome can be due to genetic mutations affecting podocyte proteins such as nephrin and podocin. Children with these genetic mutations are resistant to corticosteroids, and currently the only curative treatment is renal transplantation.

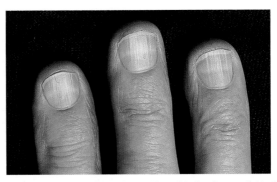

Fig. 22.5 Muehrcke lines (bands) in nephrotic syndrome. The *white line* lies parallel to the lunula (half-moon). They are associated with hypoalbuminemia caused by nephrotic syndrome. (From Floege J, Feehally J. Introduction to glomerular disease: clinical presentations. In Johnson R, Feehally J, Floege J, eds. *Comprehensive Clinical Nephrology*, 5th ed. Philadelphia: Elsevier/Saunders; 2014)

Bibliography

Gilbert S, Weiner D, et al. *National Kidney Foundation's Primer on Kidney Disease.* 6th ed. Philadelphia: Elsevier/Saunders; 2014.

Hodson E, Alexander S, Graf N. Steroid-sensitive nephrotic syndrome. In: Geary DF, Schaefer F, eds. *Comprehensive Pediatric Nephrology.* Philadelphia: Elsevier; 2008.

Hull RP, Goldsmith DJ. Nephrotic syndrome in adults. *BMJ.* 2008;336(7654):1185–1189.

Kang KK, Choi JR, Song JY, et al. Clinical significance of subjective foamy urine. *Chonnam Med J.* 2012;48(3):164–168.

Kumar P, Clark M. *Kumar and Clark's Clinical Medicine.* 8th ed. Philadelphia: Elsevier/Saunders; 2012.

Lennon R, Watson L, et al. Nephrotic syndrome in children. *Paediatrics and Child Health.* 2010;20(1):36–42.

Maarten T, Chertow G, Marsden P, et al. *Brenner and Rector's The Kidney.* 9th ed. Philadelphia: Elsevier/Saunders; 2012.

Niaudet P, Mason P, Hoyer P. Minimal change nephrotic syndrome. *Comprehensive Clinical Nephrology.* 5th ed.

Simerville JA, Maxted WC, Pahira JJ. Urinalysis: a comprehensive review. *Am Fam Physician.* 2005;71(6): 1153–1162.

A 10-Year-Old Female With Recurrent Dysuria, Urinary Incontinence, and Increased Urinary Frequency

Hui Yi Shan

A 10-year-old female presents to clinic reporting recurrent episodes of burning pain during urination, urinary incontinence, and increased urinary frequency. She has a history of recurrent urinary tract infections (UTIs). The present urinary symptoms started 2 days ago. She denies having fever, chills, nausea, vomiting, abdominal pain, or flank pain. In between these episodes, the child denies having urinary urgency, hesitancy, and incontinence. She has one bowel movement per day and reports no history of constipation.

What is the differential diagnosis of this child's urinary symptoms?

Dysuria, urinary frequency, urgency, and new onset of incontinence are typical symptoms of UTIs. However, nonspecific vulvovaginitis, chemical or irritant urethritis related to bath products (e.g., bubble bath), vaginal foreign body, and bladder dysfunction can also present with these urinary symptoms. Children with urethral strictures often present with lower urinary tract symptoms in addition to difficulty urinating and an abnormal urine stream. Finally, nephrolithiasis and urethritis secondary to sexually transmitted diseases should be considered as well.

What is the significance of recurrent urinary tract infections in a child?

About 8% to 30% of children with a UTI experience recurrent infections. The main risk factors for the development of recurrent UTIs include primary vesicoureteral reflux (VUR) and an underlying bowel or bladder dysfunction.

CLINICAL PEARL **STEP 2/3**

The bacteria that cause UTIs originate from gut flora. The ability of bacteria to cause UTIs depends on host factors as well as bacterial virulence factors. Due to the presence of specific virulence factors that enable them to attack the uroepithelium, the most common type of bacteria causing UTIs is *Escherichia coli*. It accounts for 70% to 90% of community-acquired UTIs in children.

What is a primary vesicoureteral reflux?

A primary VUR is a congenital anomaly of the vesicoureteral junction, affecting 1% to 2% of children. VUR describes the retrograde flow of urine from the bladder to the ureter and kidney. The ureteral attachment to the bladder is normally oblique, and it creates a flap valve mechanism that prevents the retrograde flow of urine. Urinary reflux occurs when the submucosal tunnel between the bladder mucosa and detrusor muscle is short or absent

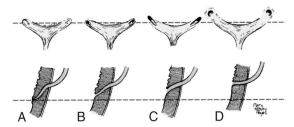

Fig. 23.1 Normal (A) and abnormal configurations (B–D) of the ureteral orifices. *Left to right,* Progressive lateral displacement of the ureteral orifices and shortening of the intramural tunnels. *Top,* endoscopic appearance. *Bottom,* Sagittal view through the intramural ureter. (From Kliegman RM, Stanton BF, St. Geme J, Schor N. *Nelson's Textbook of Pediatrics.* 20th ed. Philadelphia: Elsevier/Saunders; 2016.)

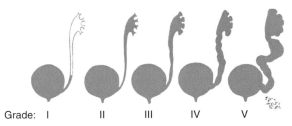

Grade: I   II   III   IV   V

Fig. 23.2 Grading of vesicoureteral reflux (VUR). Grade I: VUR into a nondilated ureter. Grade II: VUR into the upper collecting system without dilation. Grade III: VUR into dilated ureter and/or blunting of calyceal fornices. Grade IV: VUR into a grossly dilated ureter. Grade V: Massive VUR, with significant ureteral dilation and tortuosity and loss of the papillary impression. (From Kliegman RM, Stanton BF, St. Geme J, Schor N. *Nelson's Textbook of Pediatrics.* 20th ed. Philadelphia: Elsevier/Saunders; 2016.)

(Fig. 23.1). This condition predisposes to kidney infection (pyelonephritis) by facilitating the transport of bacteria from the bladder to the upper urinary tract. The severity of VUR is graded using the International Reflux Study Classification (Fig. 23.2) and is based on the appearance of the urinary tract on a contrast voiding cystourethrogram (VCUG; Fig. 23.3). With bladder growth and maturation, VUR often resolves or improves. Grades I to III generally improve with time, and this is attributed to the lengthening of the submucosal segment of the ureter. Spontaneous resolution is more common in non-Caucasians, lower grades of reflux, absence of renal damage, and lack of voiding dysfunction. The mean age of VUR resolution is 6 years.

VUR is usually discovered during evaluation for a UTI. Among these children, 80% are female, and the average age at diagnosis is 2 to 3 years. This condition may also be discovered during evaluation for antenatal hydronephrosis. In this select population, 80% of affected children are male, and they usually have high-grade reflux.

CLINICAL PEARL	STEP 2/3

Bladder and bowel dysfunction should be part of the initial and ongoing patient evaluation in children presenting with VUR and UTIs because they are frequently present. Treatment of bowel and bladder dysfunction reduces UTI recurrence. Direct questioning about a child's micturition and bowel symptoms when the child is well (in between UTIs) is essential. These questions include frequency of micturition, presence of urinary urgency, diurnal or stress incontinence, and constipation.

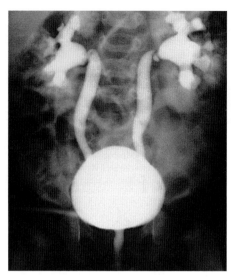

Fig. 23.3 A voiding cystourethrogram showing grade V vesicoureteral reflux and intrarenal reflux. (From Richard J, Feehally J, Floege J. *Comprehensive Clinical Nephrology*. 5th ed. Philadelphia: Elsevier/Saunders; 2015.)

Case Point 23.1

The physical examination is notable for blood pressure of 110/60 mm Hg, pulse rate of 100/min, and temperature of 37°C (98.6°F). She is thin and is not in acute distress. The examination is significant for mild suprapubic tenderness, no costovertebral angle tenderness, and a normal genitourinary examination.

What tests would you order initially?

Urinalysis and urine culture should be ordered first because this child's history and presentation highly suggest a UTI. Given a history of recurrent UTIs, ordering a basic metabolic panel would be a reasonable choice to detect potential renal scarring and compromised renal function from past infections.

Case Point 23.2

A urinary dipstick assay is performed and shows 3+ protein, large blood, 3+ leukocyte esterase, and positive nitrite. A 24-hour urine collection shows 2 g of protein. Urine culture is positive for *Escherichia coli*.

BASIC SCIENCE PEARL   **STEP 1**

The nitrite test in the urinary dipstick assay is a screening test for bacteriuria. It relies on the ability of gram-negative bacteria to convert urinary nitrate to nitrite, which activates the chromogen.

Laboratory testing reveals a serum creatinine level of 2.1 mg/dL and serum blood urea nitrogen level of 32 mg/dL.

TABLE 23.1 ■ **Primary and Secondary Glomerulonephritis in Children**

Primary Glomerulonephritis	Secondary Glomerulonephritis
Immunoglobulin A (IgA) nephropathy	Poststreptococcal glomerulonephritis
Membranoproliferative glomerulonephritis	Lupus nephritis
Anti–glomerular basement membrane disease	Henoch-Schönlein purpura
Thin basement membrane disease	Granulomatosis with polyangiitis (formerly Wegener granulomatosis)
	Microscopic polyangiitis

What is the differential diagnosis of her renal failure?
This child has a significant impairment of renal function, as well as proteinuria of 2 g. Kidney scarring from prior pyelonephritis is a likely cause. Her history of recurrent UTIs also highly suggests the presence of VUR, with the development of renal scarring known as *reflux nephropathy*. Finally, although her microscopic hematuria is most likely a result of a UTI, a glomerulonephritis workup is warranted in the setting of impaired renal function and proteinuria. Glomerulonephritides in children are divided into primary glomerulonephritis (disease process isolated to the kidney) or secondary glomerulonephritis (renal disease is a component of a systemic disorder). Table 23.1 summarizes primary and secondary glomerulonephritis in children.

What laboratory and imaging studies would be useful at this point?
An immunologic workup for glomerulonephritis that includes serum complement levels (C3 and C4), antinuclear antibody (ANA), anti–double-stranded DNA antibody, anti–neutrophilic cytoplasmic antibody (ANCA), anti–glomerular basement membrane antibody, anti–streptolysin O antibody, and hepatitis B and C panel should be ordered. A renal ultrasound is performed to look at the structure of the kidneys and evaluate for the presence of hydronephrosis.

Case Point 23.3

Serum complement levels (C3 and C4), ANA testing, anti–double-stranded DNA antibodies, ANCA, anti–glomerular basement membrane antibody, anti-streptolysin O antibody, and hepatitis B and C serologies are all within normal limits.
    On renal ultrasound, the right kidney is 2 cm smaller as compared to the left. The parenchyma are echogenic bilaterally and there is hydronephrosis on the left side.

What further testing needs to be performed to help establish a diagnosis?
A discrepancy in the length of the two kidneys on ultrasound should raise suspicion of renal scarring. Together with the presence of hydronephrosis, proteinuria, and impaired renal function, VUR with reflux nephropathy is the most likely diagnosis. A VCUG should be obtained to evaluate for the severity of VUR, followed by a dimercaptosuccinic acid (DMSA) renal scintigraphy scan to detect renal scarring (Fig. 23.4).

CLINICAL PEARL   **STEP 2/3**

The gold standard to establish the diagnosis of reflux nephropathy is from a renal biopsy. However, this procedure is invasive and is not always performed. Reflux nephropathy is more typically diagnosed via a dimercaptosuccinic acid (DMSA) scan, which involves the intravenous injection of DMSA that is taken up and filtered by the kidneys. When a region of reduced uptake is observed, this can represent a congenital absence of nephrons or an acquired loss secondary to a renal scar (see Fig. 23.4).

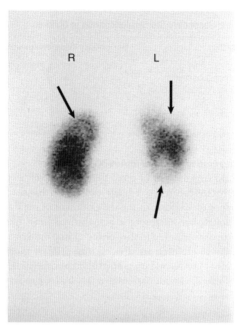

Fig. 23.4   Dimercaptosuccinic acid (DMSA) scintigraphy demonstrating upper and lower pole scarring *(arrows)* in the left kidney and scarring of the right upper kidney. (From Richard J, Feehally J, Floege J. *Comprehensive Clinical Nephrology*. 5th ed. Philadelphia: Elsevier/Saunders; 2015.)

Case Point 23.4

Left VUR grade III is demonstrated with a VCUG. DMSA renal scintigraphy demonstrates scars in both kidneys.

Diagnosis: Primary vesicoureteral reflux with reflux nephropathy.

What is the pathogenesis of reflux nephropathy?

Reflux nephropathy is categorized into two types, congenital and acquired reflux nephropathy. Congenital reflux nephropathy may be described as follows:

- Renal injury occurs prenatally. The injury has been postulated to be secondary to the so-called water hammer effect of high-grade reflux and occurs in the absence of infection. This typically causes renal dysplasia.
- Commonly noted in infants with high-grade urinary reflux.
- More common in males.

Acquired reflux nephropathy may be described as follows:

- Renal injury is due to a combination of VUR and repeated UTIs. The upper UTI and reflux lead to renal inflammation and permanent renal scarring (Fig. 23.5).
- More common in females.

How do you proceed with treatment?

The goals of treatment for VUR are to prevent pyelonephritis and reflux nephropathy. The decision to recommend observation, medical therapy, or surgery is based on the risk of VUR to the

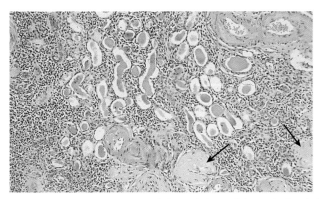

Fig. 23.5 Histologic changes in reflux nephropathy. Sclerosed glomeruli *(arrows)*, chronic inflammatory cell infiltration, and atrophic tubules with eosinophilic casts are present (hematoxylin-eosin; original magnification ×40). (From Richard J, Feehally J, Floege J. *Comprehensive Clinical Nephrology*. 5th ed. Philadelphia: Elsevier/Saunders; 2015.)

patient, the likelihood of spontaneous resolution, and the parents' and patient's preferences. The family should understand the risks and benefits of each treatment approach.

Long-term antimicrobial prophylactic therapy is indicated for children at greatest risk for VUR-related renal injury, such as those younger than 1 year, those with bladder and bowel dysfunction, and those with a febrile UTI. Surgical correction of VUR is generally recommended for patients with high-grade VUR (IV and V), patients with ineffective antimicrobial prophylaxis (as demonstrated by breakthrough UTIs), patients who are allergic to antimicrobials, patients with poor compliance, worsening of scars, and sometimes because of parents' preference. The main surgical approaches are ureteric reimplantation or the injection of a bulking agent below the ureteric orifice. Although surgical options have high success rates (80%–90%) of correcting VUR, studies have shown no benefits of surgery over prophylactic antibiotics in terms of prevention of renal scarring.

BASIC SCIENCE/CLINICAL PEARL	STEP 1/2/3

VUR appears to be an autosomal dominant inherited trait, with variable penetrance. Approximately 35% of siblings of children with VUR also have this condition. In addition, 50% of children born to women with a history of VUR have VUR. In 2010, the American Urological Association Vesicoureteral Reflux Guidelines Panel stated that in siblings of individuals with VUR, a voiding cystourethrogram or radionuclide cystogram is recommended if there is evidence of renal cortical abnormalities or renal size asymmetry on sonography, or if the sibling has a history of UTI. Otherwise, screening is optional.

Case Point 23.5

The child is treated with long-term trimethoprim-sulfamethoxazole (TMP-SMZ). A low-dose angiotensin-converting enzyme (ACE) inhibitor is also initiated to reduce proteinuria and limit the progressive loss of renal function. After receiving counseling on the treatment options for VUR, which include daily antimicrobial prophylaxis and surgical therapies, the parents and patient choose to be treated with long-term antimicrobial prophylaxis first before considering surgical options.

CLINICAL PEARL   **STEP 2/3**

The treatment of uncomplicated lower urinary tract infection in children consists of 3 to 7 days of oral antibiotic therapy. Pyelonephritis should be treated for 10 to 14 days. Quinolones are not recommended for children younger than 16 years because of its potential adverse effects on cartilage.

BEYOND THE PEARLS

- The proteinuria test on the urinary dipstick assay can yield false-positive reactions in the setting of highly alkaline urine and very concentrated urine. Therefore, quantification of proteinuria is essential with either a 24-hour urine protein collection or a random urine protein-to-creatinine ratio.
- Hematuria may arise from anywhere between the glomerular capillaries and the tip of the distal urethra. It can be macroscopic or microscopic. The presence of more than three erythrocytes per high power field is usually pathologic. Red blood cells of a glomerular origin usually change urine to brown, tea-colored, or cola-colored, whereas bleeding from the lower urinary tract changes urine to pink or red.
- In glomerular hematuria, there are small breakages in the integrity of the glomerular capillaries, which lead to leakage of both erythrocytes and protein into the urinary space. The erythrocytes acquire a dysmorphic shape during their passage across the glomerular capillaries. Glomerular hematuria is also associated with a significant amount of proteinuria (>1 g/24 hr). In nonglomerular hematuria (e.g., those originating in the collecting system), the erythrocytes retain their uniform shape, and there is absence of significant proteinuria.
- Primary VUR occurs in association with several congenital urinary tract abnormalities. Of children with multicystic dysplastic kidney or renal agenesis, 15% have VUR into the contralateral kidney and 10 % to 15% of children with ureteropelvic junction obstruction have VUR into the hydronephrotic kidney or contralateral kidney.
- Reflux nephropathy belongs to a group of diseases known as *chronic tubulointerstitial nephritides,* which are characterized by the presence of prominent interstitial fibrosis and tubular atrophy. Clinical features of chronic tubulointerstitial nephritis include indolent nature of the disease and renal failure that tends to progress slowly over years rather than weeks. Tubular defects such as renal tubular acidosis, nephrogenic diabetes insipidus, and Fanconi syndrome are common. Urinalysis in chronic interstitial nephritis is usually unremarkable. However, low-grade proteinuria and a few red blood cells or white blood cells may be seen.
- Hypertension occurs in 10% to 30% of children and young adults with reflux nephropathy. It is believed to be caused by impaired sodium excretion resulting from renal injury. Proteinuria may also be present. The presence of proteinuria may suggest a histologic diagnosis of secondary focal segmental glomerular sclerosis, which can be confirmed by renal biopsy.
- Of children on dialysis, 3.5% had reflux nephropathy, which makes it the fourth most common cause of end-stage renal disease in children after focal segmental glomerular sclerosis, renal aplasia or hypoplasia, and obstructive uropathy.

Case Summary

Complaint/History: A 10-year-old female is evaluated for recurrent episodes of burning pain during urination, urinary incontinence, and increased urinary frequency.

Findings: She is afebrile. The physical examination reveals mild suprapubic tenderness. There is no costovertebral angle tenderness.

Labs/Tests: The serum creatinine level is 2.1 *mg/dL*; a 24-hour urine collection shows 2 g of protein. Urine culture is positive for *Escherichia coli*. A smaller right kidney and a left-sided hydronephrosis are detected on renal ultrasound. A voiding cystourethrogram reveals left-sided grade III VUR. DMSA renal scintigraphy demonstrates scars in both kidneys.

Diagnosis: Primary VUR with reflux nephropathy.

Treatment: The child is prescribed long-term daily TMP-SMZ as prophylactic therapy for UTIs as well as a low-dose ACE inhibitor for proteinuria reduction.

Bibliography

Gilbert S, Weiner D, et al. *National Kidney Foundation's Primer on Kidney Diseases.* 6th ed. Philadelphia: Elsevier/Saunders; 2014.

Jadresic LP. Diagnosis and management of urinary tract infections in children. *Paediatr Child Health.* 2010; 20(6):274–278.

Kliegman RM, Stanton BF, et al. *Nelson's Textbook of Pediatrics.* 20th ed. Philadelphia: Elsevier/Saunders; 2016.

Mattoo TK. Vesicoureteral reflux and reflux nephropathy. *Adv Chronic Kidney Dis.* 2011;18(5):348–354.

Richard J, Feehally J, et al. *Comprehensive Clinical Nephrology.* 5th ed. Philadelphia: Elsevier/Saunders; 2015.

Tullus K. Vesicoureteric reflux in children. *Lancet.* 2015;385:371–379.

An 8-Month-Old Male With Chronic Intermittent Cough

Pranay Parikh ▓ Raj Dasgupta ▓ Ann Sahakian

An 8-month-old infant male is brought to the pediatrician for a cough, occurring intermittently for the past 6 months. He was initially diagnosed with viral bronchiolitis and has since been diagnosed with three more upper respiratory tract infections. His coughing episodes occur several times per week, and he has woken up coughing twice at night in the last month.

What is the differential diagnosis?

Chronic cough has a wide differential, summarized in Table 24.1. Coughing at night, in particular, raises suspicion for conditions such as sinusitis, gastroesophageal reflux (GER), or asthma. Sinusitis can lead to increased postnasal drainage, especially at night when the child is recumbent, leading to a cough. GER is a common cause of discomfort in infants that often self-resolves by 12 months of age, but could cause more significant problems such as aspiration in children with underlying neurologic or muscular disorders.

BASIC SCIENCE/CLINICAL PEARL   **STEP 1/2/3**

GER in infants is a physiologic process due to lower tone of the lower esophageal sphincter that worsens slightly over the first 4 to 6 months of life and generally improves by 12 months of life without treatment. Although commonly associated with cough in adults, there is limited evidence that GER is a significant trigger of cough in otherwise healthy children.

Asthma, a disease of airway hyperreactivity due to small airway inflammation, is also worsened at night. The reasons are multifactorial, thought to be due to pulmonary function variance, which is worse at night, as well as reduced glucocorticoid receptor affinity, lung volume, and distal airway inflammation at night. Nocturnal allergen exposures such as dust mites, rhinitis or sinusitis, gastroesophageal reflux, and obstructive sleep apnea can also contribute to nocturnal symptoms.

BASIC SCIENCE PEARL   **STEP 1**

Eosinophils are the main inflammatory cell in the airways of patients with asthma, whereas macrophages are the main antigen-presenting cells in the airways to initiate the immune response.

Case Point 24.1

Nothing worsens or improves the cough, and no other children are currently sick. The cough is present inside and outside the house and is not affected by the temperature. The family does not have any pets. The patient's father smokes but only outside the house.

TABLE 24.1 ■ Differential Diagnosis for Chronic Cough

System/Disorder	Diagnosis
Pulmonary	Asthma
	Allergic rhinitis
	Irritants (e.g., smoke, pollutants, gases)
	Cystic fibrosis
	Primary ciliary dyskinesia
	Bronchopulmonary dysplasia
	Bronchiolitis obliterans
	Interstitial lung disease
	Hemosiderosis
Infectious	Immunodeficiency
	Bronchiolitis
	Bacterial tracheitis
	Whooping cough–like syndrome (*Bordetella pertussis, Chlamydia, Mycoplasma*)
	Tuberculosis
	Protracted Bacterial Bronchitis
	Sinusitis
Structural	Bronchomalacia, tracheomalacia
	Vascular ring, sling
	Cystic lesion
	Tumor or mediastinal mass
	Lymphadenopathy causing tracheal or bronchial compression
	Vocal cord dysfunction
	Obstructive sleep apnea
Aspiration	Gastroesophageal reflux
	Foreign body, tracheal or esophageal
	Chronic aspiration due to swallowing dysfunction or tracheoesophageal fistula
Cardiac	Congestive heart failure causing pulmonary edema (multiple causes; e.g., cardio-myopathy, congenital heart disease)
	Left-to-right shunt leading to volume overload
	Pulmonary venous outflow obstruction (e.g., total anomalous pulmonary venous return)

BASIC SCIENCE PEARL	STEP 1

Tobacco smoke is a respiratory irritant. Although an infant may not be exposed directly, smoke residue can linger on surfaces (e.g., clothes) long after the cigarette has been extinguished and may still cause respiratory symptoms.

The family denies any fevers or chills. He does not have any choking or gagging with feeds and is gaining appropriate weight. He has been previously diagnosed with atopic dermatitis of the face (eczema). The family history is positive for the father with asthma.

On physical examination, the baby is afebrile, well appearing, and in no acute distress. Blood pressure is 90/50 mm Hg, pulse rate is 105/min, respiratory rate is 30/min, and oxygen saturation is 98% on room air. His atopic dermatitis is evident on his face and body (Fig. 24.1). The pulmonary examination is notable for wheezes in all lung fields but no stridor or accessory muscle use. He has no focal findings on the pulmonary examination.

What is the significance of our patient having wheezing, but no stridor?

A wheeze is a high- or low-pitched musical oscillatory sound and can be inspiratory or expiratory. Wheezes suggest airway narrowing, seen in conditions such as asthma or bronchiolitis, for example. Stridor is a high-pitched monophonic sound best heard in the upper airway. Conditions with large airway narrowing, such as laryngomalacia or croup, would result in stridor.

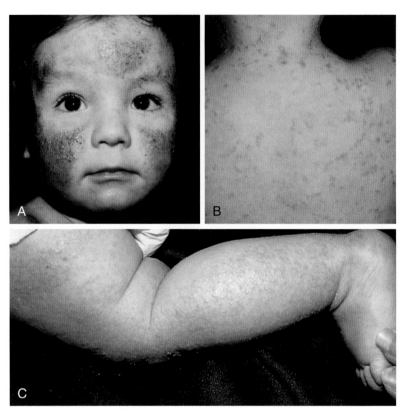

Fig. 24.1   (A–C) Infantile eczema seen on the face, trunk, and limbs, respectively. (From Gehris RP. Dermatology. In: Zitelli BJ, McIntire SC, Nowalk AJ, eds. *Zitelli and Davis' Atlas of Pediatric Physical Diagnosis*. 7th ed. Philadelphia: Elsevier; 2017:275–340.)

What is the next step?

Asthma is the most likely diagnosis at this time, given the patient's dry cough, nocturnal cough, diffuse wheezing on examination, atopic dermatitis, and positive family history. Asthma is defined by the National Heart, Lung, and Blood Institute (NHLBI) of the National Institutes of Health as episodic, partially or fully reversible airway obstruction due to airway inflammation and hyperreactivity. The hyperreactivity may be caused by a variety of stimuli, such as allergens, infection, and cold or dry air. Family history also plays a role; in particular, a history of atopy in the patient or family implies a possibility of asthma.

BASIC SCIENCE/CLINICAL PEARL	**STEP 1/2/3**

Atopy is a predisposition to allergic disease that is mediated by IgE immunoglobulins. Such diseases include atopic dermatitis (eczema), allergic rhinitis, asthma, and eosinophilic esophagitis.

According to recommendations from the expert panel review of the NHLBI, spirometry—a measurement of airflow over time—is recommended to demonstrate the reversible airway obstruction characteristic of asthma. Reversibility is defined as improvement in bronchial hyperreactivity, measured as an increase in the forced expiratory volume in 1 second (FEV_1) of at least 200 mL and at least a 12% increase from baseline after the administration of a short-acting β-agonist (SABA).

BOX 24.1 ■ Key Symptom Indicators of Asthma[a]

Wheezing—high-pitched whistling sounds when breathing out—especially in children. A lack of wheezing and a normal chest examination do not exclude asthma.

History of any of the following:
- Cough (worse particularly at night)
- Recurrent wheeze
- Recurrent difficulty in breathing
- Recurrent chest tightness

Symptoms occur or worsen in the presence of the following:
- Exercise
- Viral infection
- Inhalant allergens (e.g., animal dander, house dust mites, mold, pollen [which can be seasonal])
- Irritants (e.g., tobacco or wood smoke, airborne chemicals)
- Strong emotional expression (laughing or crying hard)
- Stress

Symptoms occur or worsen at night, awakening the patient.

---

[a]The probability of asthma as the correct diagnosis increases with multiple key indicators.

From National Asthma Education and Program Prevention. Expert Panel Report 3 (EPR-3): Guidelines for the Diagnosis and Management of Asthma—Summary Report 2007. *J Allergy Clin Immunol.* 2007;120(Suppl):S94–S138.

BASIC SCIENCE PEARL	STEP 1

Inhaled β-agonist drugs are sympathomimetics that directly induce bronchodilation.

Although described in infants and young children, spirometry is generally performed in children 5 years of age and older. In a patient with likely asthma who is too young to undergo spirometry reliably, it is reasonable to treat the child presumptively with a bronchodilator and an inhaled corticosteroid, if indicated. The NHLBI provides a number of key indicators that can guide a clinical diagnosis of asthma (Box 24.1).

Case Point 24.2

Diagnosis: Asthma.

What are the next steps?

A clinician should assess impairment and risk to determine the severity of a patient's asthma. Impairment reflects the frequency and intensity of symptoms and the functional limitations that the patient has experienced recently, such as wheezing, cough, chest tightness, shortness of breath, nocturnal awakening, frequency of use of rescue medications (e.g., an inhaled SABA), and difficulty or inability performing normal activities, including exercise. Consideration of risk involves looking at the last year for the likelihood of asthma exacerbations and progressive decline in lung function (or, for children, reduced lung growth), and consideration of risk of adverse effects from medication in the next year.

The overall picture from the impairment and risk assessments are combined to place a patient into an initial severity category: intermittent, or mild/moderate/severe persistent. The criteria are summarized in Fig. 24.2. Medications should then be started, and the patient and family should be taught proper use of inhalers and spacers. Finally, a clinician should create an asthma action plan and a plan for follow-up.

CLINICAL PEARL   **STEP 2/3**

All patients with asthma should be given an asthma action plan with a list of medications, when and how to give rescue and controller medications, and when to seek medical attention. Anticipatory guidance for asthma exacerbations can be lifesaving.

BASIC SCIENCE/CLINICAL PEARL   **STEP 1/2/3**

Intermittent asthma can be remembered by the rule of 2s—use of an inhaled SABA 2 days/ week or longer, symptoms 2 days/week or less, and nighttime awakenings twice each month or less.

Which medications should be started in this patient?

Six levels of therapeutic intensity are defined by the NHLBI guidelines, summarized in Fig. 24.3. All patients are started on an inhaled SABA (e.g., albuterol) as needed (step 1). The

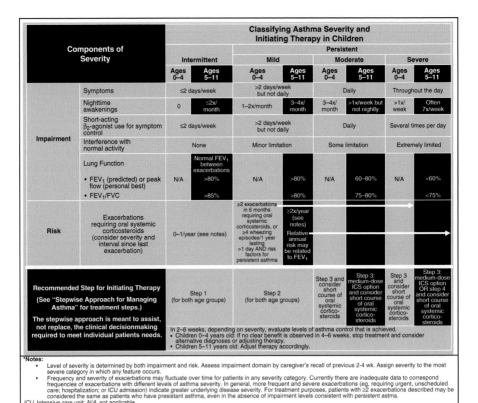

Fig. 24.2 Assessment of asthma severity at the time of diagnosis. (From National Asthma Education and Program Prevention. Expert Panel Report 3 [EPR-3]: Guidelines for the Diagnosis and Management of Asthma—Summary Report 2007. *J Allergy Clin Immunol.* 2007;120(Suppl):S94–S138.)

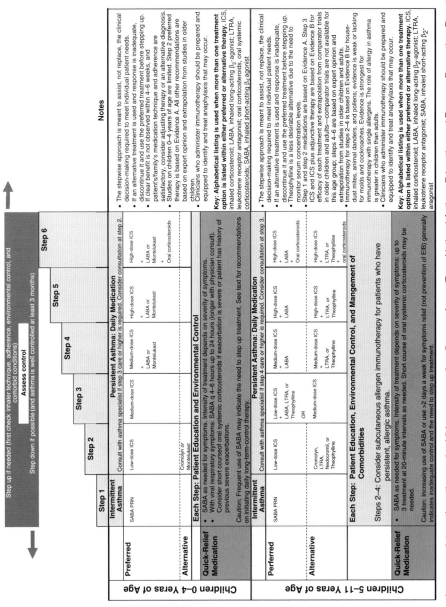

Fig. 24.3 Stepwise approach to asthma therapy in children younger than 5 years of age. (From National Asthma Education and Program Prevention. Expert Panel Report 3 [EPR-3]: Guidelines for the Diagnosis and Management of Asthma—Summary Report 2007. *J Allergy Clin Immunol.* 2007;120(Suppl):S94–S138.)

frequent use of SABA may indicate the need for more intensive therapy, however. In patients with severe or persistent symptoms, a controller medication such as an inhaled glucocorticoid (inhaled corticosteroid [ICS]) with or without a long-acting β-agonist (LABA) should be initiated (steps 2–4).

BASIC SCIENCE PEARL   **STEP 1**

Inhaled glucocorticoids modulate multiple inflammatory cells in the airway, resulting in decreased airway inflammation. Systemic glucocorticoids have the same airway effects but with more undesired systemic effects; thus, they are generally reserved for exacerbations.

CLINICAL PEARL   **STEP 2/3**

LABA should not be used as monotherapy because it may increase the risk of asthma-related deaths, first noted in the Salmeterol Multicenter Asthma Research Trial (SMART). A subgroup analysis suggested that the risk may be greater in African Americans.

Case Point 24.3

The family states that patient is symptomatic 2 to 5 days a week, with one or two nighttime awakenings per month. He is diagnosed with mild persistent asthma and is started on daily low-dose fluticasone and as-needed albuterol (ICS and SABA, respectively).

At his follow-up visit, his parents report that his symptoms have decreased to less than 1 day a week, without any nocturnal awakenings. He has needed his albuterol two times total in the last month, and he has not required oral corticosteroids.

How are medications titrated over time?

The same symptoms used to determine the severity at diagnosis in the impairment and risk domains are used to determine adequacy of symptom control. The level of control is determined using the guidelines outlined in Fig. 24.4, and a patient's medication regimen is stepped up or down (see steps in Fig. 24.3). Stepping up a patient's medication regimen is done if the disease is not adequately controlled after checking for medication adherence, environmental factors, and other possible comorbid conditions. If the patient's asthma is adequately controlled for 3 months, a step-down should be considered. The goal is always to have the patient on the lowest step needed for adequate control.

CLINICAL PEARL   **STEP 2/3**

Several terms commonly used in asthma are distinct, despite similar definitions. *Severity* is the intrinsic intensity of the disease used as a guideline to initiate therapy. *Control* is the degree to which symptoms are minimized and the goals of therapy are met, and it is used as a guide to adjust or maintain therapy. Finally, *responsiveness* is the ease with which asthma control is achieved by therapy.

His parents would like to know about his long-term prognosis. What are the chances that this patient will still have asthma symptoms at 10 years of age?

Not all young children who wheeze with viruses will go on to have asthma later in life. The asthma predictive index (API) is a clinical scoring system available to predict the risk of an asthma diagnosis in later childhood. Approximately 60% of children with at least one

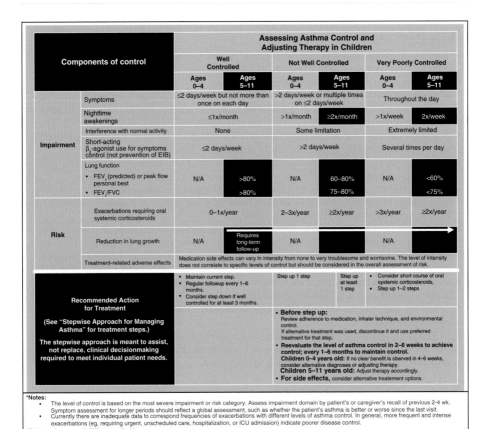

Fig. 24.4 Assessment of asthma control at the time of follow-up visits. (From National Asthma Education and Program Prevention. Expert Panel Report 3 [EPR-3]: Guidelines for the Diagnosis and Management of Asthma—Summary Report 2007. *J Allergy Clin Immunol.* 2007;120(Suppl):S94–S138.)

TABLE 24.2 ■ **Criteria for Prediction of Diagnosis of Active Asthma Later in Life**

Major Criteria	Minor Criteria
Clinician-diagnosed eczema	Clinician-diagnosed allergic rhinitis
Parental asthma	Wheezing apart from colds
	Eosinophilia ≥4%

Adapted from Castro-Rodriguez JA, Holberg CJ, Wright AL, Martinez FD. A clinical index to define risk of asthma in young children with recurrent wheezing. *Am J Respir Crit Care Med.* 2000;162:1403–1406.

major criterion or two minor criteria, summarized in Table 24.2, and parental report of any wheezing by a child of 3 years of age were found to have asthma later in life. The positive predictive value increased to approximately 75% in the subset of those with reported frequent wheezing.

BEYOND THE PEARLS

- Exercise-induced bronchospasm is common in asthmatics. Pretreatment with an inhaled SABA 15 to 20 minutes prior to activity can help prevent symptoms.
- A bronchoprovocation test may be done for patients who have a history and physical examination that is atypical for asthma. Diagnostic results are either indeterminate or negative. Methacholine, cold air, and exercise have all been used to demonstrate an increase in airway obstruction.
- Spirometry is used not only to diagnose asthma, but also to measure the response to controller medications, along with the history and physical examination.
- Vocal cord dysfunction is often misdiagnosed as asthma and should be considered when a patient has a diagnosis of asthma but does not respond to traditional treatments.
- Although parents often believe that medications delivered via nebulizer are more effective than the same medications delivered via a metered-dose inhaler with spacer, the latter has proven to be as effective in randomized trials.
- Although there is a greater body of evidence that inhaled corticosteroids are beneficial for mild persistent asthmatics in all age groups, oral leukotriene receptor antagonists are an alternative that may also be beneficial to those with comorbid allergic rhinitis. In practice, the ease of oral administration and parent preference may improve compliance as well.
- Cromolyn, a mast cell stabilizer, is mentioned as an alternative treatment for persistent asthma. However, it is an historic drug that is not practical in pediatrics due to its four times/day dosing schedule. It is not useful for the quick relief of symptoms once an asthma attack has begun.
- In patients 6 years of age and with persistent asthma who have poor control of their asthma despite standard therapy, one may consider omalizumab, which is a monoclonal antibody that prevents IgE from binding to mast cells.

Case Summary

Complaint/History: An 8-month-old infant male presents with an intermittent cough for the past 6 months.

Findings: Eczema and audible wheezes in all lung fields on chest auscultation.

Labs/Tests: None. Spirometry is deferred until 5 years of age.

Diagnosis: Asthma.

Treatment: Daily inhaled fluticasone and as-needed albuterol.

Bibliography

Castro-Rodriguez JA, et al. A clinical index to define risk of asthma in young children with recurrent wheezing. *Am J Respir Crit Care Med*. 2000;162:1403–1406.

Dicpinigaitis PV. Chronic cough due to asthma: ACCP evidence-based clinical practice guidelines. *Chest*. 2006;129(suppl 1):75S–79S.

Martinez FD, Wright AL, Taussig LM, et al. Asthma and wheezing in the first six years of life. The Group Health Medical Associates. *N Engl J Med*. 1995;332:133.

National Asthma Education and Program Prevention. Expert Panel Report 3 (EPR-3): guidelines for the diagnosis and management of asthma-summary report 2007. *J Allergy Clin Immunol*. 2007;120(5)(suppl):S94.

Nelson HS, et al. The salmeterol multicenter asthma research trial: a comparison of usual pharmacotherapy for asthma or usual pharmacotherapy plus salmeterol. *Chest J*. 2006;129(1):15–26.

Rubilar L, Castro-Rodriguez JA, Girardi G. Randomized trial of salbutamol via metered-dose inhaler with spacer versus nebulizer for acute wheezing in children less than 2 years of age. *Pediatr Pulmonol*. 2000;29:264.

Vonk JM, Postma DS, Boezen HM, et al. Childhood factors associated with asthma remission after 30 year follow up. *Thorax*. 2004;59:925.

5-Year-Old Kindergartener Who Failed a School Vision Screen

Steven M. Naids

A 5-year-old healthy male and his mother present with school papers indicating that he failed his most recent, first-time vision screen. He was born full-term gestational age to an otherwise healthy mother, and the pregnancy was uncomplicated. He has met his developmental milestones to date. His mother believes that the child sees well and has not noticed any abnormal deviations of either eye.

How do we begin to determine the cause of this child's poor vision?

Amblyopia is defined as unilateral or bilateral reduction of best-corrected visual acuity in the presence of a structurally sound eye and visual pathway. The prevalence in the North American population is 2% to 4% and is the most common cause of unilateral visual impairment in adults younger than 60 years. Depending on the maturity level of the child, the ease of determining the cause of visual dysfunction is variable. The most crucial components of the examination are the alignment of the eyes, motility in all directions of gaze, refractive error, and structure of the eye as seen under the slit lamp or with a handheld magnifier. For the ophthalmologist, this includes an assessment of the retina, optic nerve, and vasculature through the dilated pupil. Vision loss in children at any age may be multifactorial, so a thorough examination in trained hands (with tremendous patience!) is imperative (Fig. 25.1).

Case Point 25.1

The school documents indicate that his right eye, without any correction, read the 20/400 line of the Snellen acuity chart at best, but his left eye read the 20/40 line. He knows the alphabet, and visual acuity testing repeated in the office confirms the school's findings at both distance and near.

BASIC SCIENCE PEARL	**STEP 1**

Amblyopia signals a failure of neural development in the visual pathway in the absence of structural damage. In a functional pathway, light entering the eye stimulates the retinal photoreceptors, which ultimately relay their input to retinal ganglion cells. The fibers of these ganglion cells form the optic nerve (cranial nerve I), which leave the eye and travel to the optic chiasm. Fibers supplying the nasal visual field decussate, whereas those servicing the temporal field remain ipsilateral. All fibers then travel through their respective optic tracts to the lateral geniculate body of the thalamus. The fibers are then transmitted to the visual cortex of the occipital lobe by the optic radiations leaving the lateral geniculate body.

How do we screen for visual abnormalities in the United States?

While there are no standardized criteria, most states begin vision screenings at the time the child enters preschool or kindergarten. Children who fail a vision screen at school, their

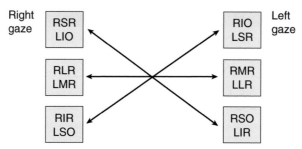

Fig. 25.1 A diagrammatic representation of the yolk muscles that allow for the various directions of gaze. Abnormalities of eye movement may help explain the cause of amblyopia. (From Trattler W, Kaiser PK, Friedman NJ. *Review of Ophthalmology.* 2nd ed. Edinburgh: Saunders Elsevier; 2012.)

pediatrician's office, or health fairs are then referred to an ophthalmologist for further exploration. In some cases, the child may not comprehend the examination, and the visual system is structurally intact and developing normally. In a recent study of 11,260 preschool children 3–5 years of age, 1007 children failed a vision screen and were examined by an ophthalmologist. 740 of those examined were prescribed glasses, and amblyopia attributed to the need for glasses was discovered in 9%.

Case Point 25.2

The child is very well behaved for his age. He sits upright in the examination chair with his hands folded and follows commands appropriately. On examination, you note that his ocular motility is full, there is no deviation of either eye on primary gaze and with cover-uncover testing. There is no head tilt. He has limited stereoacuity. The anterior segment is normal on slit lamp examination.

What is the most important next step in evaluation?
As mentioned previously, the most likely reason for poor vision in the child's right eye is refractive error. The next step is evaluation of the refractive state of the eye under cycloplegic conditions. By eliminating accommodation of the lens, we are able to measure the true refractive error. In addition, we can visualize the retina, optic nerve, and retinal vessels and determine if there is a structural cause for the vision loss.

CLINICAL PEARL	STEP 2/3

All causes of decreased vision in a child need to be explored. These include, for example, congenital abnormalities of the eye as a result of failure of complete fusion of the embryonic fissure, known as a *coloboma*. A coloboma may involve the optic disc alone or be part of a more extensive chorioretinal coloboma. They may be unilateral or bilateral and can be associated with the CHARGE syndrome (**c**oloboma, **h**eart defects, choanal **a**tresia, mental **r**etardation, **g**enitourinary abnormalities, and **e**ar abnormalities).

Case Point 25.3

The visualized retina, optic nerve, and vessels appear structurally normal. Retinoscopy is performed, and trial lenses are used to fine-tune the prescription. The right eye refraction is +3.50 +3.00 × 170. The left eye is +1.75 +0.50 × 150. The best-corrected acuity using this prescription is 20/100 in the right and 20/30 in the left (Table 25.1).

TABLE 25.1 ■ **Various Classifications of Astigmatism and Lenses Used for Correction**

Type	Location of Focal Lines	Corrective Lens	
		Notation	Refers To
Compound myopic	Both in front of retina	−sph −cyl; −sph +cyl	−Sphere regardless of notation
Simple myopic	One in front, one on retina	−sph +cyl; piano −cyl	−Sphere or piano
Mixed	One in front, one behind	−sph +cyl; +sph −cyl	−Sphere or +sphere, depending on notation
Simple hyperopic	One on retina, one behind	+sph −cyl; piano +cyl	+Sphere or piano
Compound hyperopic	Both behind retina	+sph +cyl; +sph −cyl	+Sphere regardless of notation

Adapted from Trattler W, Kaiser PK, Friedman NJ. *Review of Ophthalmology*. 2nd ed. Edinburgh: Saunders Elsevier; 2012.

CLINICAL PEARL   **STEP 2/3**

Retinoscopy is a technique to determine refractive error by neutralizing the movement of light in the dilated pupillary axis with spherical and cylindrical lenses. To get the most accurate measurement of the overall power of the eye, cycloplegic eye drops are administered. When the eye is given cycloplegic eye drops, accommodation is inhibited, and therefore the eye (and in particular the lens) loses its ability to adjust to the incoming light rays, which makes the retinoscopic measurement more precise.

How do we classify the reason for this child's vision loss, and what are the next best steps in treatment?

There is a larger refractive error in the right eye when compared to the left. The right eye also has much greater astigmatism. Thus, this child is considered to have anisometropic amblyopia of the right eye. He needs glasses, and quickly! The most reasonable next step is to prescribe the full cycloplegic refraction in eyeglasses for full-time wear. Due to the severe discrepancy in best-corrected visual acuity, the child should have follow-up within a few weeks to ensure that the glasses were obtained, the prescription is accurate, and the patient is able to tolerate full-time wear. Patching the left eye in conjunction with glasses is indicated when glasses alone are not improving vision. If the child does not tolerate patching the left eye, some clinicians recommend atropine penalization of the better seeing eye as an alternative.

BASIC SCIENCE/CLINICAL PEARL   **STEP 1/2/3**

Atropine is an antimuscarinic (anticholinergic) that can be administered topically to the better seeing eye as an alternative to patching. Its primary mechanism of action is to paralyze accommodation—the phenomenon that allows for near vision—so that the good eye sees a blurred image at near; therefore, the brain will preferentially select the image seen by the amblyopic eye. This has been shown to be as effective as patching in some cases. The half-life of atropine is about 2 weeks and is therefore less controlled than patching. Sometimes, this can cause weakening of vision in the better eye, a process known as *reverse amblyopia*. Additionally, the family should be warned of systemic adverse reactions that may occur, such as fever, dry mouth, flushing, tachycardia, nausea, and vomiting. Treatment is discontinuation of the medication or, if severe, physostigmine.

How should this child be followed?

First and foremost, it is important to make sure that the child has been given the correct glasses prescription. Regardless of how compliant the child is with wearing glasses, if the prescription is wrong, we have wasted precious time. Laboratory error happens, parents can forget to fill the prescription, and glasses break! Therefore, the patient should be seen within a few weeks of the initial visit. Vision at distance and near, eye alignment, and stereovision should be checked at each visit. If the child is progressing nicely, then follow-up in 4 to 6 weeks is appropriate. If the vision is not improving, patching or atropine penalization should again be considered.

BEYOND THE PEARLS

- The causes of amblyopia can be divided into three categories—refractive, strabismic, and sensory. These categories are not mutually exclusive of one another. For example, a plexiform neurofibroma of the upper lid in a child with neurofibromatosis type 1 may cause drooping of the upper lid (possibly into the pupillary axis), and compression of the globe from the lid mass will cause astigmatism. In addition, a child with strabismus likely has an underlying refractive cause.
- Not all amblyopia is correctable, may be unresponsive, and may need a repeat examination looking for subtleties; it also may require neuroimaging.
- A newborn with unilateral or bilateral cataracts is at risk for developing amblyopia. For optimal visual development, it is recommended that a visually significant unilateral cataract be removed before 6 weeks of age, and bilateral cataracts should be removed before 10 weeks of age.
- In amblyopia, the so-called crowding phenomenon can occur, in which objects on the eye chart are easier to recognize when presented singly rather than when surrounded by close similar objects; that is, it is easier to read one letter on the Snellen chart by itself rather than with other letters on the line.

Case Summary

Complaint/History: A 5-year-old male with decreased vision in the right eye.

Findings: High refractive error in the right eye compared to the left. Otherwise, a structurally normal eye examination.

Diagnosis: Anisometropic amblyopia of the right eye.

Treatment: He is given glasses with his full cycloplegic refraction for full-time wear.

Bibliography

Ferris, JD. Amblyopia: Atropine. American Academy of Ophthalmology. Available at: https://www.aao.org/pediatric-center-detail/amblyopia-atropine.

Hendler K, et al. Refractive errors and amblyopia in the UCLA Preschool Vision Program; first year results. *Am J Ophthalmol.* 2016;172:80–86.

Lueder, GT. et al. Basic and Clinical Science Course: Section 6. Pediatric Ophthalmology and Strabismus. *American Academy of Ophthalmology.* 2015-2016:33.

12-Month-Old Male With a White Pupillary Reflex

Steven M. Naids

A 12-month-old male is brought in to his pediatrician for a well-child visit. The parents eagerly show off recent holiday photographs; in one of the photograph, a white pupillary reflection is seen in the patient's right eye, whereas the left pupillary reflection is red (Fig. 26.1). The right optic disc is not able to be visualized with an ophthalmoscope; the remainder of the physical examination is normal.

What is the most concerning feature of this child's presentation?

This child has been found to have a white pupil, referred to as *leukocoria*. The differential diagnosis for leukocoria is wide, summarized in Box 26.1. The leading diagnosis until proven otherwise is retinoblastoma, given its potential lethality. Other causes to consider include cataracts, Coats disease (a vascular disorder of the retina leading to subretinal exudates), persistent fetal vasculature, and retinoblastoma. Severe retinopathy of prematurity and other causes of retinal detachment should be considered as well. Although each of these diagnoses may present with leukocoria, all of them have distinct appearances under direct retinal examination, and thus a definitive diagnosis can generally be made without imaging or laboratory testing.

Given the high possibility of retinoblastoma, leukocoria warrants immediate ophthalmologic evaluation.

Case Point 26.1

The patient is referred to a pediatric ophthalmologist and undergoes an examination under anesthesia. A tumor is seen in the right eye (**Fig. 26.2**). The left eye is normal.

Diagnosis: Retinoblastoma.

What is retinoblastoma?

Retinoblastoma is the most common malignant intraocular tumor of childhood and one of the most common pediatric solid tumors, with an incidence of 1 in 14,000 to 20,000 live births. It is equally common in both genders and has no racial predilection. Bilateral involvement is seen in 30% to 40% of cases. Approximately 90% of cases are diagnosed by 3 years of age. It is estimated that 250 to 300 new cases are diagnosed in the United States each year, and 5000 cases are diagnosed worldwide.

Retinoblastoma presents with leukocoria in over two-thirds of patients. Strabismus and nystagmus are also important presenting symptoms of early intraocular retinoblastoma. As the tumor grows, the patient may develop glaucoma (increased intraocular pressure), buphthalmos (increase in globe size), and even periorbital cellulitis. Proptosis is an ominous sign because it indicates spread of the tumor beyond the eye. Distant metastases are rare, although a bilateral retinoblastoma may present with a brain tumor in the location of the pineal gland, the so-called trilateral retinoblastoma).

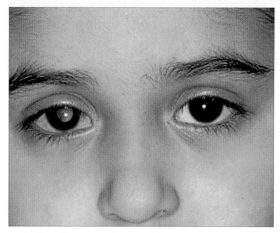

Fig. 26.1 A photograph using flash illumination shows a white pupillary reflex in the right eye. (From Lissauer T, Caroll W. Illustrated textbook of pediatrics. 5th ed. Philadelphia: Elsevier; 2018:385–400.)

BOX 26.1 ■ Differential Diagnosis of Leukocoria

- Angiomatosis retinae
- Cataracts
- Coats disease
- Colobomas
- Congenital retinal fold
- High myopia
- Incontinentia pigmenti
- Medulloepithelioma
- Myelinated nerve fibers
- Persistent hyperplastic primary vitreous (PHPV)
- Retinal detachment
- Retinal dysplasia
- Retinoblastoma
- Retinopathy of prematurity (ROP)
- Toxocariasis
- Uveitis
- Vitreous hemorrhage

Adapted from Cheng KP. Ophthalmology. In: Zitelli BJ, Nowalk AJ, McIntire SC, eds. *Zitelli and Davis' Atlas of Pediatric Physical Diagnosis.* 7th ed. Philadelphia: Elsevier; 2018:691–732.

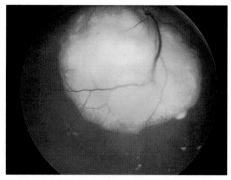

Fig. 26.2 A large exophytic tumor is seen on the retina, with subretinal fluid and tumor seeding. (From Rodriguez-Galindo C, Wilson MW, Dyer M. Retinoblastoma. In: Orkin S, Nathan D, Ginsburg D, et al., eds. *Nathan and Oski's Hematology and Oncology of Infancy and Childhood.* Philadelphia: Elsevier/Saunders; 2014:1747–1778.)

CLINICAL PEARL	STEP 1/2/3

Leukocoria is the most common initial finding in a patient with retinoblastoma.

CLINICAL PEARL	STEP 2/3

Patients with a neuroectodermal tumor of the pineal gland in addition to retinoblastoma are termed to have *trilateral retinoblastoma*. The tumor may arise in a synchronous or metachronous manner—that is, at the same time or different times, respectively. The prognosis for trilateral disease is poor.

What is the next step?

Once a diagnosis is established with direct visual examination, along with the remainder of a comprehensive examination, including intraocular pressure measurements, the extent of tumor spread must be determined; this process is known as *cancer staging*. The contralateral eye must be evaluated for involvement because one-quarter to one-third of patients present with bilateral tumors. Imaging of the orbits and brain with magnetic resonance imaging (MRI) is performed to evaluate for extraocular tumors. Certain patients will also require examination of the bones, bone marrow, and cerebrospinal fluid for metastatic tumor.

The tumor(s) within the eye are also staged according to size, location, and seeding into five prognostic groups known as the International Classification of Retinoblastoma (Table 26.1).

Case Point 26.2

The tumor is determined at the time of examination to be group C. MRI of the brain and orbits does not reveal extraocular tumor.

What is the next best step in the management of this patient?

Today, the management of retinoblastoma is much different than just a decade ago, although the general principles remain the same. Preservation of life is the primary goal, followed by eye salvage and preservation of vision. Lower risk groups (e.g., groups A and B) are more likely to respond to ocular salvage, whereas patients with higher risk group tumors may be better served with up-front enucleation due to the higher risk of extraocular spread and lower vision salvage potential.

CLINICAL PEARL	STEP 1/2/3

The extraocular spread of retinoblastoma can prove fatal. The primary goal of therapy in advanced cases is to preserve life first and the eye second.

Ocular salvage techniques include localized and systemic therapies. Small tumors can often be treated with laser photocoagulation or cryotherapy. Systemic chemoreduction has been used for large tumors and bilateral cases (Fig. 26.3), followed by local consolidation. One common regimen consists of intravenous vincristine and carboplatin, with or without etoposide. Intravitreal chemotherapy has also been used for refractory cases and for those that have seeded the vitreous.

Intraarterial chemotherapy, usually with melphalan, has become increasingly more common as first-line treatment. Chemotherapy is delivered via cannulation of the ophthalmic artery, thereby decreasing the amount absorbed systemically. This has provided higher

TABLE 26.1 ■ **International Classification of Retinoblastoma**

Group and Risk	Features
A; very low	Small discrete intraretinal tumors away from the fovea and optic disc All tumors ≤3 mm in greatest dimension, confined to the retina All tumors located > 3 mm from the fovea and 1.5 mm from the optic disc
B; low	All remaining discrete retinal tumors without seeding All tumors confined to the retina not in group A Any tumor size and location with no vitreous or subretinal seeding Small cuff of subretinal fluid allowed (3 mm from tumor border)
C; moderate	Discrete local disease with minimal focal subretinal or vitreous seeding Tumor(s) must be discrete Subretinal fluid involving up to one quadrant of the fundus Local subretinal or vitreous seeding, <3 mm from the tumor
D; high	Diffuse disease with significant vitreous and/or subretinal seeding Tumor(s) are massive or diffuse. Subretinal fluid, one quadrant of the fundus to total retinal detachment Diffuse subretinal seeding; may include subretinal plaques or tumor nodules Diffuse or massive vitreous disease may include greasy seeds or avascular tumor masses
E; very high	Presence of one or more of these poor prognosis features: • Neovascular glaucoma and/or buphthalmos • Tumor anterior to anterior vitreous face involving ciliary body or anterior segment on clinical examination or ultrasound biomicroscopy (i.e., tumor touching the lens) • Diffuse infiltrating retinoblastoma • Opaque media from hemorrhage • Tumor necrosis with aseptic orbital cellulitis • Phthisis bulbi

From Kim JW, Mansfield NC, Murphree AL. Retinoblastoma. In: Schachat AP, Wilkinson CP, Hinton DR, eds. *Ryan's Retina*. 5th ed. Philadelphia: Elsevier; 2018:2375–2420.

rates of globe salvage as primary therapy and has been effective in cases that have failed other means. Intraarterial chemotherapy, in conjunction with intravenous systemic chemotherapy, has been shown to be an alternative to enucleation in select advanced cases of retinoblastoma.

CLINICAL PEARL   **STEP 2/3**

More aggressive attempts at ocular salvage are indicated for patients with bilateral tumors because bilateral enucleation will universally result in blindness. Despite aggressive disease, some form of vision preservation is successfully achieved in over two-thirds of patients with bilateral tumors.

CLINICAL PEARL   **STEP 2/3**

Although enucleation of unilateral tumors results in cure in over 80% of cases, with excellent vision potential in the unaffected eye, concern for metachronous tumors arising in the contralateral eye after enucleation justifies ocular salvage therapy in low-risk group unilateral disease.

The basic approach to therapy is outlined in Fig. 26.4.

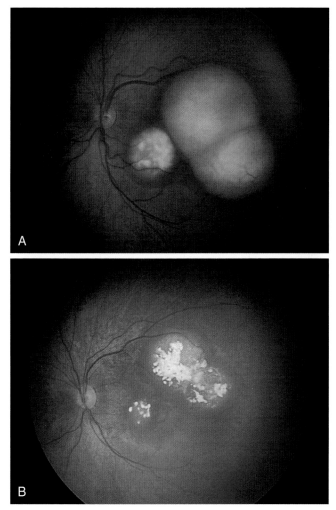

Fig. 26.3 Results of ocular salvage using systemic chemotherapy in a group B retinoblastoma tumor. (A) Before therapy. (B) After therapy. (From Rodriguez-Galindo C, Wilson MW, Dyer M. Retinoblastoma. In: Orkin S, Nathan D, Ginsburg D, et al., eds. *Nathan and Oski's Hematology and Oncology of Infancy and Childhood.* Philadelphia: Elsevier/Saunders; 2014:1747–1778.)

Case Point 26.3

The patient undergoes intraarterial chemotherapy with melphalan. The family asks about the risk of developing retinoblastoma in future children.

How does genetics play a role in the formation of retinoblastoma? What is the risk of retinoblastoma in siblings of a patient with retinoblastoma?
Retinoblastoma is most often due to loss of a potent tumor suppressor gene, *RB1*. The *RB1* gene is localized to the q14 band of chromosome 13 and encodes for pRB, a protein that suppresses tumor formation. Both *RB1* genes must have a mutation for retinoblastoma to occur, as described by Knudson's two-hit hypothesis.

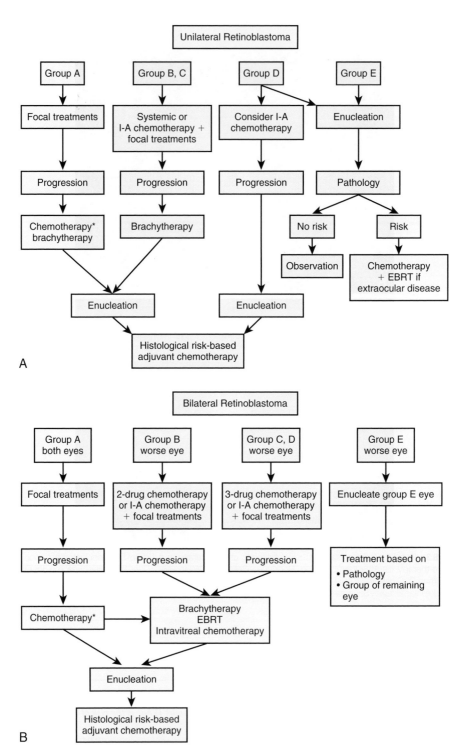

Fig. 26.4 Approach to therapy in (A) unilateral and (B) bilateral retinoblastoma. *EBRT,* External beam radiation therapy; *I-A,* intraarterial. (From Rodriguez-Galindo C, Wilson MW, Dyer M. Retinoblastoma. In: Orkin S, Nathan D, Ginsburg D, et al., eds. *Nathan and Oski's Hematology and Oncology of Infancy and Childhood.* Philadelphia: Elsevier/Saunders; 2014:1747–1778.)

TABLE 26.2 ■ **Risk of Retinoblastoma in Family Members of a Child With Retinoblastoma**

History	Unilateral Disease	Bilateral Disease
Positive family history	Subsequent Pregnancies – 40% Patient's Future Offspring – 40% Normal Sibling's Future Offspring – 7%	
Negative family history	Subsequent Pregnancies – 1% Patient's Future Offspring – 8% Normal Sibling's Offspring – 1%	Subsequent Pregnancies – 6% Patient's Future Offspring – 40% Normal Sibling's Offspring – 1%

Adapted from Lanzkowsky P. Retinoblastoma. In: Lanzkowsky P, ed. *Manual of Pediatric Hematology-Oncology*. 5th ed. London: Elsevier; 2011:759–775.

Although all tumors have two mutated *RB1* genes, 15% of patients with unilateral retinoblastoma and 100% of patients with bilateral retinoblastoma carry a mutated *RB1* gene in their germline genomes. The germline mutation thus allows for the development of tumor with only a single (additional) mutation. Germline mutation carriers develop tumors earlier in life and often present with multifocal (more than one tumor in a single eye) and/or bilateral (tumor[s] in both eyes) disease.

The penetrance for a carrier of a germline *RB1* mutation exceeds 90%; therefore, siblings and future offspring are both at a very high risk for developing retinoblastoma. The risk of developing retinoblastoma in family members is summarized in Table 26.2.

Case Point 26.4

Genetic testing of the patient does not reveal a germline mutation in *RB1*. The tumor involutes with intraarterial chemotherapy, and no progression is noted on serial examinations under anesthesia.

How should this patient be monitored?

A patient with a unilateral tumor as a result of somatic mutations is at low risk for the development of additional tumors after curative therapy is successfully administered. Patients presenting with bilateral tumors or those with unilateral tumors that arise in the setting of a germline mutation are at high risk. The risk of subsequent tumors decreases with time; the risk is highest in the first 3 years from diagnosis.

Patients with germline mutations must also be monitored for the development of nonocular tumors, known as *second malignant neoplasms* (SMNs). The most common secondary tumors that develop in patients with germline mutations are pinealoma, bone and soft tissue sarcomas (especially osteosarcoma), melanoma, and carcinomas (e.g., breast and lung cancers). The incidence of SMN is higher among patients treated with external beam radiation before 1 year of age.

Case Summary

Complaint/History: A 12-month-old male presents with a white pupillary reflection in the right eye.

Findings: A white retinal tumor of the right eye.

Labs/Tests: MRI of the brain without evidence of intracranial lesion. Genetic testing is negative for a germline mutation.

Diagnosis: Unilateral retinoblastoma of the right eye.

Treatment: Intraarterial chemotherapy.

BEYOND THE PEARLS

- The next most common presentation of retinoblastoma, after leukocoria, is strabismus. Less common presentations include vitreous hemorrhage, hyphema, glaucoma, proptosis, and pseudohypopyon.
- Reflection of light off the optic nerve at just the correct angle can simulate leukocoria.
- During primary enucleation of the eye for poor-prognosis tumors, a long segment of the optic nerve is taken to minimize the potential for extraocular spread.
- The characteristic histologic feature of retinoblastoma is the Flexner-Wintersteiner rosette. Less commonly, fleurettes are present.
- The incidence rate of SMNs in patients with germline *RB1* mutations is 1%/year of life.
- The retinoblastoma gene is located on the long arm of chromosome 13 (13q). Patients with the 13q deletion syndrome may exhibit characteristic features of microcephaly, broad prominent nasal bridge, hypertelorism, microphthalmos, ptosis, imperforate anus, and genital malformations. The midface is also notable for a prominent brow, large mouth, thin upper lip, and bulbous tipped nose.

Bibliography

Lueder GT, et al. Basic and clinical science course: Section 6. Pediatric Ophthalmology and Strabismus. *American Academy of Ophthalmology.* 2015–2016;338.

Rodriguez-Galindo C, et al. *Retinoblastoma. Nathan and Oski's Hematology and Oncology of Infancy and Childhood.* Philadelphia: Elsevier/Saunders; 2014:1747–1778.

Shields CL, Shields JA. Diagnosis and management of retinoblastoma. *Cancer Control.* 2004;11(5):317–327.

Shields CL, et al. Management of advanced retinoblastoma with intravenous chemotherapy then intra-arterial chemotherapy as alternative to enucleation. *Retina.* 2013;33(10):2103–2109.

13-Year-Old Male With Hematemesis

Arathi Lakhole ■ Michelle Pietzak

A 13-year-old male presents to the pediatric emergency department for hematemesis. He has had 2 months of upper abdominal discomfort worsening over time and associated with a mild (5-lb) weight loss. In the last week, he has had severe abdominal pain in the epigastric region that is dull in nature, nonradiating, and worse after food consumption. Bismuth subsalicylate and ranitidine does not relieve the pain. His pain is associated with nausea and occasional vomiting without any blood until today. He denies smoking cigarettes and drinking alcohol.

How does his described pain inform the differential diagnosis?

Chronic epigastric pain is usually due to gastroesophageal reflux disease (GERD), peptic ulcer disease (PUD), or functional dyspepsia—the latter being a diagnosis of exclusion because the pathology is not identifiable. Significant weight loss would suggest malignancy, although upper gastrointestinal malignancy is exceedingly rare in children. Epigastric pain that radiates to the back is suggestive of pancreatitis; although chronic pancreatitis is rare in children, it may explain the acute worsening. Gallstones should be considered in particular if the pain localizes more to the right upper quadrant (RUQ). Dyspepsia due to the use of drugs that can cause upper gastrointestinal (GI) pathology (e.g., nonsteroidal antiinflammatory drugs [NSAIDs]) corticosteroids, antiepileptic drugs, cigarettes, alcohol) should be ruled out.

BASIC SCIENCE/CLINICAL PEARL	STEP 1/2/3

GERD is exacerbated by several dietary and lifestyle components. Alcohol, nicotine, and caffeinated foods and beverages decrease lower esophageal tone, allowing gastric contents to reflux more easily into the esophagus. Fatty foods delay gastric emptying, giving the food bolus more time to sit in the stomach and reflux. Eating a large meal and then lying flat also increases GERD, especially in obese individuals. Spicy and acidic foods do not increase GERD or PUD but are felt more in the esophagus during GERD.

The acute presentation of emesis with bright red blood indicates a recent upper GI bleed, such as one from esophageal varices or from a gastric ulcer (e.g., in PUD). Coffee ground (dark brown to black)–colored emesis would suggest that the blood has stayed in the stomach for some hours, long enough to coagulate.

CLINICAL PEARL	STEP 2/3

Hematemesis with bright red blood can also be from non-GI causes, such as the oral cavity (e.g., trauma, loose tooth, dental infection), sinuses (e.g., sinusitis, polyps, hemangioma) and the lungs (e.g., hemoptysis can easily be confused for hematemesis in young children).

Case Point 27.1

On further history, he notes that his stools appear black, with a tar like consistency. Family history reveals that his father was recently diagnosed with a stomach ulcer.

What is the significance of the black tarry stools?

Upper GI (UGI) bleeding can cause melena (black tarry stools). This color occurs due to the digestion of red blood cells by various GI enzymes. The stools are often sticky and foul-smelling. If the amount of blood loss from the UGI tract is rapid, frank (undigested) blood may be seen in the stool. Bismuth and iron-containing medications can also make the stool appear black.

Conversely, rectal bleeding usually indicates a lower GI bleed, as seen in infections, polyps, cancer, ulcerative colitis, Crohn disease, and vascular malformations.

What are important physical examination findings to look for with hematemesis?

When a child presents with hematemesis, a careful physical examination needs to be done to rule out systemic illness. Oral aphthous ulcers can point to Crohn disease. Dental enamel erosions may suggest chronic gastroesophageal reflux, bulimia, or celiac disease. A large liver and/or spleen should suggest possible portal hypertension and the need for urgent intervention from esophageal variceal bleeding. The rectal examination is also important because it can reveal perianal lesions due to Crohn disease, and a quick test for occult blood in the stool can be performed.

Case Point 27.2

On physical examination, he is seen to be in moderate discomfort. He is afebrile. His pulse rate is 100/min, respiratory rate is 18/min, blood pressure is 115/75 mm Hg, and oxygen saturation is 99% on room air. His weight, height, and body mass index are average for age. He has pale conjunctiva, which are anicteric. He has mild tenderness in the epigastric region with an otherwise soft abdomen, without guarding or rigidity. The rest of his physical examination is normal.

What are the most likely diagnoses at this point?

Highest on the differential at this point would be PUD. The most common reason for PUD in a child is infection with *Helicobacter pylori (H. pylori)*. Other causes include medications, alcohol, physiologic stress, and other infections. Crohn disease should be ruled out because it can present with weight loss, abdominal pain, and GI erosions and ulcers. The patient does not have any stigmata of chronic liver disease, making esophageal variceal bleeding less likely.

What laboratory evaluation is important in a child with hematemesis?

A complete blood count may reveal anemia if the ulcer has been bleeding intermittently. If a microscopic anemia is detected, it is important to order an iron panel because *H. pylori* infection often leads to iron deficiency anemia, which is refractory to treatment. Serum chemistry analyses may show a hypokalemic, hypochloremic, metabolic alkalosis if the vomiting (of hydrochloric acid) has been severe. Serum transaminase, alkaline phosphatase, and bilirubin levels may be abnormal in chronic liver and biliary tract diseases. A stool test may be occult blood–positive because of UGI bleeding. Serum amylase and lipase levels can be considered to screen for pancreatitis.

CLINICAL PEARL   **STEP 2/3**

In children with a first-degree relative with a gastric ulcer, duodenal ulcer, or gastric cancer, testing for *H. pylori* may be considered.

Case Point 27.3

Laboratory testing reveals microcytic anemia with a hemoglobin of 10 g/dL and a mean corpuscular volume (MCV) of 70 fL (normal, 80–96 fL). Stool examination is positive for fecal occult blood.

BASIC SCIENCE/CLINICAL PEARL   **STEP 1/2/3**

Iron deficiency anemia, as demonstrated by this patient, is common in those with *H. pylori* infection. This is due to a combination of occult blood loss by the patient and iron scavenging by the microbe in the stomach. In children with refractory iron deficiency anemia in which other causes have been ruled out, testing for *H. pylori* may be considered.

What is the next step? When should esophagogastroduodenoscopy be performed? How is **Helicobacter pylori** *infection diagnosed?*

Although patients with chronic epigastric pain can be often be treated empirically, esophagogastroduodenoscopy (EGD) should performed in patients with alarming symptoms such as unexplained iron deficiency anemia, weight loss, evident bleeding, persistent vomiting, and/or jaundice. EGD can also be therapeutic to stop bleeding, such as when medications are injected into an ulcer or bands are placed over esophageal varices.

In patients with active *H. pylori* infection, EGD may reveal a nodular appearing stomach (so-called gooseflesh skin (Fig. 27.1). There may be frank gastritis, or single or multiple gastric and duodenal ulcers may be found. Other nonspecific signs of infection may be seen, such as erosions, erythema, and mucosal friability.

It is recommended that the initial diagnosis of *H. pylori* be based on positive histopathology from gastric biopsies and not from serum antibody, stool antigen, or urease breath tests (described later). Histopathology of active infection shows signs of inflammation, such as increased numbers of neutrophils, eosinophils, and lymphocytes. Special stains (Giemsa or silver stains) may be applied to improve the detection rates of the bacteria.

In children with suspected *H. pylori* infection, it is recommended to take one biopsy for rapid urease testing and culture, if possible, because this increases the sensitivity of the biopsies. Positive culture is 100% specific and is therefore sufficient to diagnose *H. pylori* infection.

BASIC SCIENCE PEARL   **STEP 1**

The *H. pylori* bacterium can survive in the acidic gastric environment due to its containing urease. Urease catalyzes the hydrolysis of urea into ammonia and carbon dioxide, which is detected by a change in color of the pH indicator in the rapid urease test.

Noninvasive tests for *H. pylori* include the urease breath test (UBT), stool antigen detection test, and serologic antibody tests. Urease breath testing and stool antigen detection are used to test for eradication of the organism posttreatment but not for diagnosis. IgG testing for *H. pylori* in children is not reliable and only indicates past exposure, not current infection.

Case Point 27.4

Due to the hematemesis, tachycardia, anemia, and black stools, an EGD with biopsies is performed. Visually, the gastric mucosa appears nodular and erythematous and a bleeding gastric ulcer is seen (see Fig. 27.1). A rapid urease test from the biopsy is positive. Histopathology is consistent with *H. pylori* infection (Fig. 27.2).

Diagnosis: PUD associated with *H. pylori* infection.

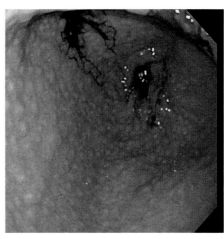

Fig. 27.1   Nodular antrum and bleeding gastric ulcer seen on esophagogastroduodenoscopy.

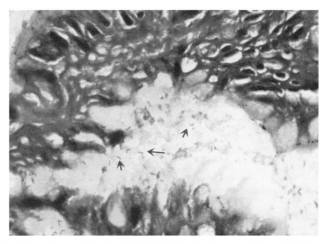

Fig. 27.2   Gastric biopsy with gastritis showing *Helicobacter pylori* colonization within the superficial mucus overlying the foveolar epithelial cells (*arrows;* Giemsa stain, ×400). (From Hassan TMM, Al-Najjar SI, Al-Zahrani IH. *Helicobacter pylori* chronic gastritis; updated Sydney grading in relation to endoscopic findings and *H. pylori* IgG antibody: diagnostic methods. *J Microsc Ultra Structure.* 2016;4(4):167–174.)

BASIC SCIENCE PEARL	STEP 1

H. pylori is a slow-growing, gram-negative, microaerophilic bacterium that colonizes the gastric mucosa. Risk factors for infection include lower socioeconomic status, higher residence density, and poor sanitary conditions. Co-infection among family members is common. Transmission occurs from direct person-to-person contact.

What is peptic ulcer disease?

PUD is an acid-related disorder that leads to injury to the mucosal barrier, penetrating the submucosa and deeper layers. It can affect any part the upper GI tract, including the esophagus, stomach, and duodenum. There are a variety of causes of PUD in children, including *H. pylori* infection (most common), physiologic stresses (e.g., trauma, sepsis, head injury), medications (e.g., NSAIDs), and hypersecretory states (e.g., Zollinger-Ellison syndrome)

BASIC SCIENCE PEARL	STEP 1

Zollinger-Ellison syndrome is a rare condition in which a tumor, usually in the duodenum or pancreas, produces large amounts of gastrin. These gastrinomas present with diarrhea, abdominal pain, GERD, and upper GI bleeding due to multiple peptic ulcers.

Many children have asymptomatic *H. pylori* infection, which may never lead to clinically evident disease. Others develop chronic gastritis without PUD and can also remain asymptomatic. A minority of children develop gastric and/or duodenal ulcers, which is more likely with specific strains. *H. pylori* has also been classified as a group 1 carcinogen associated with gastric adenocarcinoma, which is extremely rare in the pediatric population. Chronic *H. pylori* has also been implicated in causing mucosa-associated lymphoid tissue (MALT) lymphoma of the stomach.

BASIC SCIENCE PEARL	STEP 1

Risk for gastric cancer is increased in individuals with a positive family history of gastric cancer, smoking, alcohol ingestion, and CagA strain of *H. pylori* and in individuals with polymorphisms in interleukin-1, tumor necrosis factor-alpha, and interleukin-10.

How is Helicobacter pylori *infection treated?*

Children with PUD and *H. pylori* infection should receive treatment. First-line eradication regimens are as follows, with antibiotics given for 7 to 14 days and proton pump inhibitor for 2 months:

■ Triple therapy with proton pump inhibitor + amoxicillin + clarithromycin, *or* an imidazole

or

■ Proton pump inhibitor + bismuth salts + amoxicillin + an imidazole

CLINICAL PEARL	STEP 2/3

Proton pump inhibitors should ideally be given 0.5 to 1 hour before eating to prevent high postprandial gastric acid production.

Antibiotic susceptibility of the *H. pylori* to clarithromycin is recommended in areas with known high resistance rates. A noninvasive test for eradication is recommended at least 4 to 8 weeks following completion of therapy. If treatment has failed, one of these four options is recommended:

1. EGD with biopsy and culture of the *H. pylori* for antibiotic susceptibility
2. Fluorescence in situ hybridization (FISH) on previous paraffin-embedded biopsies, if clarithromycin susceptibility has not been performed before
3. Modification of therapy by adding an antibiotic or bismuth, or increasing the dose and duration of therapy
4. Repeat course of treatment if the *H. pylori* load seen to be high on pathology

Case Point 27.5

The patient is treated with 2 weeks of amoxicillin, clarithromycin, and metronidazole and 8 weeks of omeprazole to eradicate the *H. pylori* and heal the ulcer, respectively. Two months after finishing treatment, repeat EGD demonstrates healing of the ulcer and resolution of the nodular gastritis.

BEYOND THE PEARLS

- A trial of histamine-2 (H2)-receptor blockers or proton pump inhibitors may be offered for 4 to 6 weeks for dyspepsia without alarming symptoms. Lack of improvement of symptoms or relapse should be evaluated with EGD.
- The only indication for testing and treatment for *H. pylori* is demonstrated ulcer disease. Treatment can also be considered for those with iron deficiency anemia refractory to treatment or a first-degree relative with gastric cancer.
- *H. pylori* is not a cause of chronic abdominal pain. Patients with chronic abdominal pain should not be tested nor treated for *H. pylori* infection.
- Gastric biopsies for *H. pylori* should be obtained from both the antrum and body of the stomach. Normally, the highest bacterial count is found in the antrum, but in cases of low gastric acidity, the bacteria may be present only in the body or cardiac portion of the stomach. This can occur with the use of acid-blocking mediations, such as histamine-2 receptor antagonists and proton pump inhibitors.
- Predictors of failure to *H. pylori* treatment include poor patient compliance with the multidrug regimen, drug resistance of the organism, short duration of therapy, proton pump inhibitor pretreatment, and high bacterial load pretreatment.
- *H. pylori* has been implicated in immune thrombocytopenic purpura (ITP). There is cross-reactivity between the antiplatelet antigen and the CagA antigen of *H. pylori*. Studies from Japan, Italy, and Spain have shown improvements in chronic ITP after the eradication of *H. pylori*.
- In China, an oral recombinant vaccine against *H. pylori* prevented 72% of infections after the first year of vaccination and continued reduced risk for infection for up to 3 years.

Case Summary

Complaint/History: A 13-year-old male presents to the emergency room for hematemesis. He has had nausea, vomiting, and pain in his epigastric region, worsening in the past week. He notes black stools and a 5-lb unintentional weight loss over the past 2 months.

Findings: His physical examination is significant for tachycardia, moderate abdominal pain on palpation, and heme-positive stool in the rectal vault.

Labs/Tests: His laboratory tests are significant for a microcytic anemia. Esophagogastroduodenoscopy shows gastritis with a nodular antrum and a bleeding gastric ulcer. Histopathology demonstrates gastritis, with S-shaped, gram-negative rods in the mucus layer of the antral biopsies.

Diagnosis: Peptic ulcer disease due to *Helicobacter pylori* infection.

Treatment: He is treated with triple antibiotics for 2 weeks and a proton pump inhibitor for 2 months, with resolution of his disease.

Bibliography

Chelimsky G, Czinn S. Peptic ulcer disease in children. *Pediatr Rev.* 2001;22(10):349–355.

Hassan TMM, Al-Najjar SI, Al-Zahrani IH. *Helicobacter pylori* chronic gastritis updated Sydney grading in relation to endoscpic findings and *H. pylori* IgG antibody: diagnostic methods. *JMAU.* 2016;4(4):167–174.

Koletzko S, Jones NL, Goodman KJ, et al. Evidence-based guidelines from ESPGHAN and NASPGHAN for *Helicobacter pylori* infection in children. *J Pediatr Gastroenterol Nutr.* 2011;53:230–243.

Koletzko S. Noninvasive diagnosis tests for *Helicobacter pylori* infection in children. *Can J Gastroenterol.* 2005;19:433–439.

Talley NJ, Vakil NB, Moayyedi P. American gastroenterological association technical review on the evaluation of dyspepsia. *Gastroenterology.* 2005;129(5):1756–1780.

Veneri D, Bonani A, Franchini M, et al. Idiopathic thrombocytopenia and *Helicobacter pylori* infection: platelet count increase and early eradication therapy. *Blood Transfus.* 2011;9(3):340–342.

Zeng M, Mao XH, Li JX, et al. Efficacy, safety, and immunogenicity of an oral recombinant *Helicobacter pylori* vaccine in children in China: a randomised, double-blind, placebo-controlled, phase 3 trial. *Lancet.* 2015;386:1457–1464.

19-Year-Old Female With Chronic Diarrhea

Christine Kassissa-Mourad ■ Michelle Pietzak

A 19-year-old female presents with 4 months of diarrhea. She describes the diarrhea as three to four, yellow, small-volume, nonbloody stools per day. She also has abdominal pain that is not relieved by defecation. She describes the pain as cramping in nature and constant. She denies recent travel, human immunodeficiency virus (HIV) infection, use of antibiotics and nonsteroidal antiinflammatory drugs (NSAIDs), and consumption of potentially contaminated drinking water or foods.

What is the differential diagnosis for chronic diarrhea?

Chronic diarrhea, in the absence of risks for common infections, raises suspicion for inflammatory bowel disease (IBD). IBD encompasses Crohn disease (CD) and ulcerative colitis (UC). The hallmark of CD is chronic diarrhea that is associated with poor growth, abdominal pain, and weight loss, whereas UC is typically associated with grossly bloody stools and lower abdominal cramping that is relieved with defecation.

Other causes of diarrhea include infectious causes, which can be associated with both bloody and nonbloody stools; however, symptoms rarely last for months unless the patient has an underlying immunodeficiency. Recent travel, history of HIV infection, use of antibiotics and NSAIDs, and consumption of contaminated water, raises suspicion for infectious causes of chronic diarrhea. Enteric infections with *Shigella*, *Salmonella*, *Campylobacter*, *Mycobacterium*, and *Yersinia* spp., *Escherichia coli*, parasites, and amoebic pathogens should all be in the differential. *Clostridium difficile* infection should be considered, especially in patients recently treated with antibiotics. In this patient, however, the 4 months of diarrhea without a history of travel, immunosuppression, and antibiotic use is more concerning for a chronic inflammatory process.

BASIC SCIENCE/CLINICAL PEARL   **STEP 1/2/3**

Also on the differential is colitis due to *Mycobacterium tuberculosis*, which is more common in persons from endemic areas and the immunocompromised. Only 25% of patients will have a chest radiograph showing evidence of active or healed pulmonary infection with an enteric mycobacterial infection.

Case Point 28.1

The patient reports a recent 15-pound weight loss, fatigue, intermittent fever, mouth sores, ankle pain and swelling, and a rash on her bilateral shins. She denies cough, shortness of breath, chest pain, hematuria, night sweats, hemoptysis, chills, and changes in vision.

Does the review of systems narrow the differential diagnosis?
Fatigue, weight loss, abdominal pain, and fever are hallmark symptoms for IBD. She also has several complaints concerning for extraintestinal manifestations of IBD, including arthritis, skin manifestations (erythema nodosum), and oral involvement (aphthous ulcers). She does not complain of eye involvement (uveitis), although this may be asymptomatic.

CLINICAL PEARL	**STEP 2/3**

Chronic respiratory symptoms should alert the clinician to a possible mycobacterial infection. Acute onset of symptoms is more consistent with an infectious cause.

Case Point 28.2

The family history is significant for CD in her father.

CLINICAL PEARL	**STEP 2/3**

Children of patients with IBD have a greater risk of developing the condition in comparison to the general population. A family history of autoimmune diseases and gastrointestinal cancers should also be elicited.

Case Point 28.3

On physical examination, she is a thin-appearing female in no acute distress, but she appears chronically ill. She has pale conjunctiva. Her oral examination is notable for multiple 0.5-mm ulcers on the tongue, and upper and lower interior lips. Her abdomen is diffusely tender to palpation without rebound or guarding. She has no hepatosplenomegaly and no masses.

She has an anal fissure, a 3-cm perianal skin tag, and prolapsed rectal mucosa. No obvious fistula was seen. Her skin examination is significant for multiple small, tender erythematous nodules on both lower legs and swollen ankles, with pitting edema (Fig. 28.1). The remainder of her physical examination is normal.

What is the significance of the rectal examination?
The rectal examination findings suggest CD, which has many perianal complications, such as fissures, fistulas, abscesses, and skin tags. Symptoms can vary from anal pain and discharge, to frank bleeding and/or incontinence. This can severely impact on the quality of life. Approximately one-third of Crohn's patients develop these complications. Risk factors include an age of less than 40 years and being of non-Caucasian race.

BASIC SCIENCE/CLINICAL PEARL	**STEP 1/2/3**

Anal fissures, tears in the lining of the anal canal distal to the dentate line, can be seen in approximately 20% of patients with CD. They can be asymptomatic or can cause pain and bleeding.

BASIC SCIENCE/CLINICAL PEARL	**STEP 1/2/3**

One of the hallmarks of autoimmune disease is multisystem involvement. In our patient, there is involvement of her gastrointestinal tract, skin, and joints.

Case Point 28.4

Laboratory testing reveals an elevated erythrocyte sedimentation rate (ESR) and C-reactive protein (CRP) level. Complete blood count (CBC) reveals a microcytic anemia and thrombocytosis (elevated platelet count). Serum chemistries were notable for an albumin of 2.5 g/dL (normal, 3.5–5.5 g/dL). Stool cultures are negative, with negative acid-fast-bacilli (AFB) for mycobacterial spp., as well as ova and parasites. *Clostridium difficile* toxin is negative. Anti–*Saccharomyces cerevisiae* antibodies (ASCAs—immunoglobulin [Ig]G and IgA) are elevated. The perinuclear antineutrophil cytoplasmic antibody (pANCA) is negative. Colonoscopy reveals friable mucosa with cobblestoning and exudates, with histopathology showing the presence of noncaseating granulomas (Fig. 28.3). Biopsy is negative for AFB.

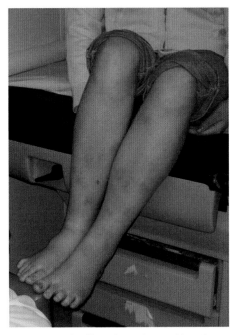

Fig. 28.1 Bilateral ankle swelling and a skin rash consistent with erythema nodosum are shown.

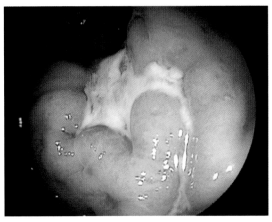

Fig. 28.2 Crohn disease of the colon showing colitis, exudate and deep ulcerations. (From Canard JM, Letard J-C, Penman I. Diagnostic colonoscopy. In: Canard JM, Letard J-C, Palazzo L, et al, eds. *Gastrointestinal Endoscopy in Practice.* Edinburgh: Churchill Livingstone/Elsevier; 2011:101–122, Fig. 11.5.)

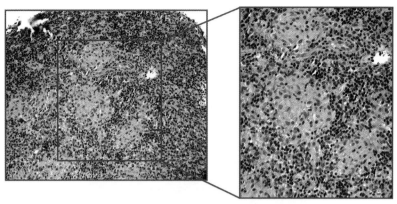

Fig. 28.3 Microscopic examination of a colonic biopsy reveals lymphocytic inflammation with granuloma formation.

Diagnosis: Crohn disease.

What is Crohn disease?

CD is a transmural inflammatory process that can involve the gastrointestinal tract anywhere from the mouth to the anus. The most common site for CD is the terminal ileum, which is involved in approximately 70% of pediatric patients. Patients with IBD classically have an abnormal CBC, with a microcytic anemia and thrombocytosis. The microcytosis is due to iron deficiency from low iron absorption in the duodenum (if involved in CD) and chronic occult blood loss. Thrombocytosis, with platelet counts exceeding 450×10^9/L of circulating blood, is common in inflammatory conditions.

BASIC SCIENCE/CLINICAL PEARL	**STEP 1/2/3**

Platelet counts exceeding 1000×10^9/L have been described in patients with IBD.

A low albumin level is a marker for protein losses in the stool. High levels of calprotectin and α_1-antitrypsin in stool tests can also indicate protein-losing enteropathy from intestinal inflammation. ASCA is more likely to be positive in CD, whereas pANCA is more likely to be positive in UC. However, either autoantibody can be seen in either condition, so antibody testing should be used as an adjunct to aid your clinical diagnosis and should not be used for a definitive diagnosis. Endoscopy with biopsy is the gold standard for the diagnosis of IBD.

How are Crohn disease and ulcerative colitis differentiated?

In CD, the inflammation is transmural. There is often perianal disease, internal rectal mucosal sparing, and skip areas (normal areas between inflamed areas of mucosa), and the terminal ileum is often involved. Endoscopy can show edema, hemorrhage, aphthous ulcers, cobblestoning, pseudoexudates, and discontinuous lesions. Pathologic examination will show a chronic mixed inflammation, with lymphocytes, eosinophils, and sometimes neutrophils in crypt abscesses. Noncaseating granulomas with multinucleated giant cells are pathognomonic for CD (see Fig. 28.3).

In UC, the rectum is usually involved, and the inflammation is continuous. Common findings on colonoscopy include erythema, edema, loss of vascular pattern, friability, spontaneous bleeding, granularity of mucosa, pseudopolyps, erosions, and ulcers. Crypt abscesses and granulomas are not characteristically present in the histology of UC. Of note, tuberculous colitis can visually appear similar to IBD; however, histology typically shows caseating granulomas. Biopsies can also be stained specifically for AFB.

CLINICAL PEARL	STEP 2/3
Colonoscopy is contraindicated in cases of severe inflammation with increased risk for bowel perforation. Flexible sigmoidoscopy (with biopsy) and/or magnetic resonance enterography (MRE) are alternative procedures.	

How would you initiate treatment?
The choice of medications for the induction of disease remission is based on the severity of the presenting symptoms. For mild disease, aminosalicylates are the drug of choice, with antibiotics (metronidazole or ciprofloxacin) given for any perianal involvement. For moderate to severe disease, glucocorticoids, 6-mercaptopurine or exclusive enteral nutrition (EEN)—providing all nutritional needs via an elemental, antigen-free liquid formula—can be used. EEN is preferred for patients with growth failure given the adverse effects of glucocorticoids on growth. Other than diarrhea, EEN does not have any of the major side effects seen with glucocorticoids or other immunosuppressants. Severe disease can be treated with anti–tumor necrosis factor-α (TNFα) antibodies, cyclosporine, methotrexate, and intravenous steroids.

CLINICAL PEARL	STEP 2/3
For high-risk patients—defined as those with extensive small bowel disease, growth failure in mid to late puberty, severe perianal disease, or glucocorticoid unresponsive disease—early treatment with anti–tumor necrosis factor-α (TNFα) antibodies (e.g., infliximab) should be considered.	

Once disease remission is achieved, maintenance therapy is given. Maintenance generally starts with aminosalicylates if they were effective in controlling symptoms and reducing relapses. There are two options for moderate to severe disease: one is a "step-up" approach which starts with thiopurines or methotrexate, and the other is a "top-down" approach which starts with anti-TNFα agents, thiopurines, cyclosporine, or methotrexate.

CLINICAL PEARL	STEP 2/3
The top-down approach of starting maintenance therapy is associated with an increased risk of complications; however, the risk of short-term relapse and need for surgery is lower.	

Case Point 28.5

The patient is classified as having moderate disease given her systemic symptoms and extraintestinal manifestations. She is started on prednisone for induction therapy, along with metronidazole for the perianal involvement. Her diarrhea improves and she achieves adequate weight gain. She is started on infliximab for maintenance therapy and is being followed closely by a pediatric gastroenterologist.

How should this patient be monitored?
In addition to gastrointestinal symptomatology, all patients should be monitored for extraintestinal manifestations, with routine eye, liver, joint, and skin examinations. Growth failure is common in those with IBD, especially CD, and should be closely tracked in addition to nutritional status. Although some studies have shown low levels of vitamin A, E, D, zinc, and selenium in patients with moderate to severe disease, there is no consensus on the recommendations for screening. Iron deficiency is very common. Bone mineral density is often reduced in IBD, so many patients require vitamin D and calcium supplementation. There are no widely accepted recommendations for the

use of bone densitometry to screen for osteopenia; however, the presence of risk factors, such as prolonged use of glucocorticoids, growth failure, and/or a history of fractures, would be reasonable indications.

BASIC SCIENCE/CLINICAL PEARL   **STEP 1/2/3**

Liver diseases associated with IBD include primary sclerosing cholangitis (PSC), autoimmune hepatitis, steatosis, and amyloid deposition. Additionally, patients with UC are at increased risk of developing colon cancer and require annual colonoscopies starting at 7 to 10 years after the initial diagnosis.

BEYOND THE PEARLS

- In CD, some studies have demonstrated that aminosalicylates are no better than placebo for induction and maintenance therapies.
- The use of infliximab as early treatment in children with newly diagnosed CD has been associated with high rates of remission when compared to immunomodulators (e.g., 6-mercaptopurine), as well as improvement in linear growth—thought to be due to reduced glucocorticoid exposure—and fewer complications, including bowel surgery.
- All patients should be assessed for latent tuberculosis prior to starting glucocorticoids and anti-TNFα antibody therapy. Immunity to hepatitis B, varicella, and measles viruses should also be assessed.
- Patients with IBD are at increased risk of developing nutritional complications, other autoimmune diseases, and colon cancer and require long-term follow-up with specialists familiar with this disease.

Case Summary

Complaint/History: A 19-year-old female presents with 4 months of diarrhea, abdominal pain, weight loss, mouth sores, ankle swelling, and a painful rash on her lower legs. Colonoscopy with biopsies confirms CD.

Findings: On physical examination, she is noted to be pale and thin. She has oral aphthous ulcers, lower extremity edema and erythema nodosum on her anterior shins. A rectal examination demonstrated an anal fissure and perianal skin tag.

Labs/Tests: Laboratory tests are significant for an elevated sedimentation rate and C-reactive protein level, low albumin level, and a microcytic anemia. ASCA IgG and IgA are elevated. Colonoscopy reveals friable mucosa with cobblestoning and exudates. Histopathology shows a predominantly lymphocytic inflammation and the presence of noncaseating granulomas.

Diagnosis: Crohn disease.

Treatment: Induction with metronidazole and prednisone; maintenance therapy with infliximab.

Bibliography

Kleinman RE, Baldassano RN, Caplan A, et al. Nutrition support for pediatric patients with inflammatory bowel disease: a clinical report of the north american society for pediatric gastroenterology, hepatology and nutrition. *J Pediatr Gastroenterol Nutr.* 2004;39:15.

North American Society for Pediatric Gastroenterology, Hepatology, and Nutrition, Colitis Foundation of America, Bousvaros A, et al. Differentiating ulcerative colitis from crohn disease in children and young adults: report of a working group of the north american society for pediatric gastroenterology, hepatology, and nutrition and the crohn's and colitis foundation of america. *J Pediatr Gastroenterol Nutr.* 2007;44:653.

Platell C, Mackay J, Collopy B, et al. Anal pathology in patients with crohn's disease. *Aust N Z J Surg.* 1996;66:5.

Rankin GB, Watts HD, Melnyk CS, et al. National cooperative crohn's disease study: extraintestinal manifestations and perianal complications. *Gastroenterology.* 1979;77:914.

Ruemmele FM, Veres G, Kolho KL, et al. Consensus guidelines of ECCO/ESPGHAN on the medical management of pediatric Crohn's disease. *J Crohns Colitis.* 2014;8:1179.

16-Month-Old Female With Foul-Smelling Diarrhea

June Chapin ▪ Michelle Pietzak

A 16-month-old female presents with her foster mother to clinic with the chief complaint of loose, foul-smelling stools.

What is the most likely diagnosis?

In this age group, the most common cause of diarrhea is so-called toddler's diarrhea, also known as chronic nonspecific diarrhea of childhood. This is due to excessive juice consumption. These children typically pass frequent, loose bowel movements without mucus or blood. Bowel movements typically become looser over waking hours, due to the ingestion of offending beverages, with the most formed stool occurring in the morning. It is common to see small, partially digested food particles in the stool. Growth should not be affected in a child with toddler's diarrhea, and the child should appear healthy with normal appetite and activity level. Symptoms may also include mild abdominal discomfort and distention. The pathophysiology of this condition relates to increased intestinal motility and osmotic effect from intraluminal solutes, including sorbitol and fructose, in juices, sweetened beverages, and sports drinks. Treatment includes reassurance and minimizing the intake of the offending beverages.

BASIC SCIENCE/CLINICAL PEARL   **STEP 1/2/3**

It is important to ask the child's caretaker about the specifics of the diarrhea. To some, increased frequency of formed stools represents diarrhea. Diarrhea is strictly defined as a stool volume >10 g/kg/day in infants and toddlers, >200 g/day in older children, and >300 g/day in adults. Chronic diarrhea is defined as diarrhea lasting for more than 14 days.

Case Point 29.1

The foster mother reports that since entering her care 1 month ago, bowel movements are "rotten" smelling with a tan, paste-like consistency. She has three bowel movements per day, typically occurring 1 to 2 hours after each meal. There are small undigested food particles in the stool, which often leak out of the diaper and onto her clothing. She is a "picky eater" and will only eat small amounts of food several times per day. The foster mother feels like she has to "force her to sit down and eat." Abdominal distention occurs frequently after meals and resolves after a bowel movement. Loud flatus often precedes her bowel movements. The foster mother denies hard stools, straining with evacuation, and blood, mucous or pus in stools. The stool floats in the toilet when she empties it out of the diaper. The foster mother knows very little about the child's past medical history, except that her biologic mother was homeless, leading to removal of the toddler from her care.

What is the differential diagnosis at this point?

A well-appearing child with normal growth parameters and chronic diarrhea, in the setting of prior homelessness, should be evaluated for chronic infectious diarrhea. The most common causes for diarrhea in all age groups are viruses and bacteria. In the toddler age group, other forms of malabsorption must be considered, such as food allergies, celiac disease, and inflammatory bowel disease. Although many infectious causes of diarrhea, including viruses such as Norwalk virus, rotavirus, and enteric adenoviruses, may cause acute diarrhea with short courses, bacteria and parasites are more likely to cause chronic diarrhea, particularly in the immunodeficient host. Chronic infectious diarrhea is suggested historically by bloating, nonbloody diarrhea, bulky or foul-smelling stools, and potentially the development of suboptimal growth in a previously healthy and normally growing child. Risk factors include daycare attendance, drinking well water, exposure to bodies of fresh water including streams or lakes, or living in an undeveloped region with poor sanitation.

BASIC SCIENCE/CLINICAL PEARL STEP 1/2/3

Steatorrhea, diarrhea with excessive fat in the stool, causes it to look pale, float, and be exceptionally malodorous. Oil droplets, which represent undigested fat, may also be seen on the surface of the toilet water. Fat malabsorption in pediatrics may be due to chronic cholestatic liver disease (e.g., biliary atresia), pancreatic insufficiency (e.g., cystic fibrosis), and abnormal lymphatic drainage of the intestine (e.g., mycobacterial infections, lymphangiectasias).

It is important to note if the child with chronic diarrhea was born in, or had recent visitors from, a developing country. In this patient's case, her homeless living situation may have exposed her to unchlorinated water or many other sick cohorts in daycare or a shelter. As noted in Table 29.1, the prevalent agents differ widely between industrialized and developing nations.

CLINICAL PEARL STEP 2/3

A detailed diet history, including a 24-hour dietary recall or a 3-day prospective diet history, is imperative when evaluating a child with chronic diarrhea. It is important to focus on the timing of food introduction and any subsequent change in stooling habits, as well as the number of sweetened beverages, such as fruit juice and sports drinks. Symptoms that start with the introduction of solid foods may suggest food allergy or celiac disease. Diarrhea with rapid transit and gassiness can be due to cow's milk allergy and/or lactase deficiency.

TABLE 29.1 ■ **A Comparative List of Prevalent Agents and Conditions in Children With Persistent Infectious Diarrhea in Industrialized and Developing Countries Indus**

Most Common Agents Causing Persistent Diarrhea in Childhood	
Industrialized Countries	**Developing Countries**
Clostridium difficile	Enteroaggregative E. coli
Enteroaggregative Escherichia coli	Atypical E. coli
Astrovirus	Shigella
Norovirus	Heat stable/heat labile enterotoxin-producing E. coli
Rotavirus	Rotavirus
Small intestinal bacterial overgrowth	Cryptosporidium
Postenteritis diarrhea syndrome	Giardia lamblia
	Tropical sprue

From Guarino A, Branski D, Winter HS. Chronic Diarrhea. In: Kliegman R, Stanton B, Behrman RE, et al, eds. *Nelson Textbook of Pediatrics*, 20th ed. Philadelphia: Elsevier, 2016:1875–1882.

Case Point 29.2

Vital signs are within normal parameters for age. Anthropometrics include a weight of 9 kg (10% for age), length of 77 cm (50% for age), weight for length 10%, and head circumference of 46 cm (50% for age). These are identical to her visit 1 month ago. Physical examination reveals a thin, well-kempt, active toddler, with nondysmorphic features. Her abdomen is mildly distended and tympanitic. A digital rectal examination reveals soft stool in the rectal vault and normal rectal tone. She has decreased subcutaneous fat stores in her extremities. Her examination is otherwise normal.

Is the child's growth pattern concerning?

Failure to thrive (FTT) is a term signaling that a child is receiving inadequate nutrition for optimal growth and development. It can be defined in several ways for a child of less than 2 years: a decrease in weight below the third or fifth percentile for age on two consecutive measurements; deceleration of weight crossing two major percentiles on the growth chart; weight less than 80% of the ideal body weight for age; or weight below the third or fifth percentiles for age. Examination of growth curves may show growth deceleration, primarily beginning with weight, then later deceleration in height, stagnant growth, or weight loss. Head circumference is usually preserved except in severe cases of FTT.

CLINICAL PEARL   **STEP 2/3**

Examination of serial growth measurements is an essential aspect of all well-child care visits, and particularly for visits in which there is a concern for sub-optimal growth.

In our case, the child does not meet these FTT criteria. However, because she is in foster care, we do not have her prior anthropometrics for comparison. Her weight for length of 10%, at this one isolated point in time, is concerning in the context of her chronic diarrhea. The physical examination of a distended abdomen and decreased subcutaneous fat stores and muscle bulk also point to protein-calorie malnutrition.

CLINICAL PEARL   **STEP 2/3**

Protein-calorie malnutrition occurs when there is inadequate caloric or protein intake to meet essential needs. In children, caloric and protein requirements are higher than in adults to promote growth. It can be divided into two types: marasmus, when the child is not eating enough calories; and kwashiorkor, when protein intake is low, resulting in edema, thinning hair, and dermatitis.

The underlying cause of FTT is often multifactorial and must include psychosocial as well as medical issues. Causes of FTT can be divided into categories of inadequate nutritional intake, malabsorption, and increased metabolic demand, as outlined in Box 29.1.

How should a child with FTT be evaluated?

When evaluating a child with potential failure to thrive, it is essential to complete a detailed history, including dietary intake, family and prenatal history, assessment of family psychosocial dynamics, and a complete physical examination, including observation of development and parent-child interaction. The psychosocial assessment should evaluate for: who lives in the home; who cares for the child; history of depression or other mental illness in caretakers; caretaker stressors, support, and fatigue; history of intimate partner violence; financial support of family, including government aid; and queries regarding parental perception of child's temperament and behavior.

BOX 29-1 ■ Major Causes of Failure to Thrive

Decreased Caloric Intake

Aversive feeding disorders
Impaired swallowing
　Neurological (e.g., brainstem lesions, Arnold-Chiari malformation)
　Dysphagia (e.g., eosinophilic esophagitis)
Injury to mouth and esophagus
　Trauma and burns – physical, chemical, or radiation
　Oropharyngeal or esophageal inflammation
Congenital anomalies affecting oropharyngeal and upper gastrointestinal tract
Chromosomal abnormalities
Genetic diseases
Diseases leading to anorexia (e.g., systemic illness, psychological, acquired immunodeficiency
　syndrome, neglect or abuse, chemotherapy or radiation therapy)
Accidental or inadvertent
　Difficult lactation
　Improper formula preparation or feeding technique
　Poor diet/bizarre diet
Psychosocial
　Maternal and/or infant related factors
Iatrogenic
　Restrictive or elimination diets
　Special diets from misdiagnosis

Increased Requirements

Sepsis/febrile states
Trauma
Burns
Acquired or congenital chronic cardiorespiratory disease
Hyperthyroidism
Diencephalic syndrome
Excessive involuntary movement or poorly controlled seizure
Chronic systemic diseases including chronic infections

Impaired Utilization

Inborn errors of metabolism

Excessive Caloric Losses

Persistent vomiting (e.g., gastric outlet obstruction, gastroesophageal reflux)
Malabsorptive states due to mucosal or luminal etiology (e.g., celiac disease, protein-losing en-
　teropathy, enzyme deficiency, inflammatory or allergic enteropathy)
Pancreatic insufficiency (e.g., cystic fibrosis, Shwachman-Diamond syndrome)
Congenital gut lesions or short gut syndrome leading to intestinal failure
Chronic immunodeficiency
Chronic enteric infections or parasitic infestations
Postenteritis syndrome
Chronic liver disease with cholestasis

From Shashidhar H, Tolia V. Failure to Thrive. *Pediatric Gastrointestinal and Liver Disease.* Robert
　Wyllie R, ed. Philadelphia: Elsevier; 2011:136–145.e3

CLINICAL FINDINGS OF MALNUTRITION

SPECIFIC DIAGNOSES AND ASSOCIATED FINDINGS

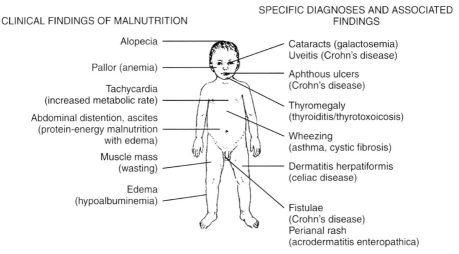

Alopecia

Pallor (anemia)

Tachycardia (increased metabolic rate)

Abdominal distention, ascites (protein-energy malnutrition with edema)

Muscle mass (wasting)

Edema (hypoalbuminemia)

Cataracts (galactosemia)
Uveitis (Crohn's disease)

Aphthous ulcers (Crohn's disease)

Thyromegaly (thyroiditis/thyrotoxicosis)

Wheezing (asthma, cystic fibrosis)

Dermatitis herpatiformis (celiac disease)

Fistulae (Crohn's disease)
Perianal rash (acrodermatitis enteropathica)

Fig. 29.1 Examples of relevant findings during the physical examination for failure to thrive. (From Maqbool A. Failure to thrive. In: Liacouras C, Piccoli D, eds. *Pediatric Gastroenterology: The Requisites in Pediatrics.* Philadelphia: Mosby/Elsevier; 2007:48–63.)

Growth parameters, including height, weight, and head circumference for children younger than 2 years, should be plotted serially on a growth curve. Children older than 2 years should also have body mass index (BMI) plotted. Careful physical examination (Fig. 29.1 and Box 29.2) may reveal phenotypic features characteristic of syndromes or underlying medical conditions associated with poor growth.

CLINICAL PEARL	STEP 2/3

Symmetric growth failure (low percentiles for weight, length, and head circumference evenly) from birth is suggestive of a prenatal (in utero) insult. Common reasons for this include
infection, teratogen exposure, and chromosomal abnormalities.

Case Point 29.3

Complete blood count and serum chemistries are normal. Stool is sent for bacterial culture and microscopic examination for ova and parasites (O+P).

BASIC SCIENCE/CLINICAL PEARL	STEP 1/2/3

Leukocytosis (high white blood cell count) can be seen with infections, malignancies, allergies, and as a stress response to trauma or surgery. Iron deficiency, one of the most common micronutrient deficiencies in toddlers, would demonstrate a microcytic (small red blood cell) anemia. Thrombocytosis (high platelet count) is seen as an acute-phase reactant to infection, inflammation, and stress. Pancytopenia may indicate malignancy with bone marrow infiltration or suppression of production by medications or infections (usually viral).

BOX 29-2 ■ Directed Physical Examination

Vital signs
  Bradycardia, hypothermia (indicative of critical malnutrition)
General
  Height, weight, head circumference, and body mass index plotted on growth chart
  Midparental height[a]
  Subcutaneous fat
  Poor hygiene, dental caries, other signs of possible neglect
  Dysmorphic features
Head, eyes, ears, nose, and throat
  Markedly enlarged tonsils
Stridor
  Craniofacial anomalies
Chest
  Increased work of breathing
  Chest wall deformities
Cardiovascular
  Signs of increased cardiac work (tachycardia, hyperdynamic precordium)
  Pathologic murmur
Abdomen
  Hepatomegaly or jaundice
Extremities
  Clubbing
Skin
  Pallor
  Cyanosis
  Unusual rashes
Neurologic
  Abnormal tone or reflexes
  Developmental delay
  Abnormal affect or social interactions

---

[a] Midparental height calculation: boys = (maternal height + paternal height + 13 cm)/2; girls =
  (maternal height + paternal height − 13 cm)/2.
From Wilson S. Failure to Thrive. *Comprehensive Pediatric Hospital Medicine.* Zaoutis LB, Chiang
  VW, eds. Philadelphia: Mosby; 2007:153–157

BASIC SCIENCE/CLINICAL PEARL   **STEP 1/2/3**

Serum chemistries in chronic diarrhea may reveal hypokalemia and acidosis, due to excessive
loss of potassium and bicarbonate from the gastrointestinal tract. Elevated transaminases,
bilirubin, or alkaline phosphatase levels can indicate a hepatic cause for the diarrhea, or an
infection such as hepatitis A.

Is imaging indicated?
The value of radiologic studies in chronic diarrhea is limited. Plain abdominal radiographs (a
KUB: kidney/ureter/bladder imaging) may show constipation (indicating overflow incontinence
rather than diarrhea) or dilated loops of small bowel with an infection. If concerned for inflammatory bowel disease or infectious colitis, computed tomography (CT) or magnetic resonance
imaging (MRI) of the abdomen could demonstrate bowel wall thickening.

Is endoscopy indicated?
Endoscopy is primarily indicated when there is high suspicion for inflammatory causes that can be visualized in the mucosa and require biopsy. Diseases that require endoscopic confirmation include inflammatory bowel disease (Crohn disease, ulcerative colitis), celiac disease, food allergies, gastroesophageal reflux disease (GERD), peptic ulcer disease, and eosinophilic diseases. Endoscopy may also be considered if highly suspicious for an infectious cause, but initial stool testing is negative and therefore mucosal biopsy specimens, or aspirations of intestinal fluid, are required.

Case Point 29.4

Microscopic examination of the stool demonstrates *Giardia lamblia*.

Diagnosis: Chronic giardiasis.

What is **Giardia lamblia?**
Giardia lamblia is a microscopic protozoan that can infect the small intestine of humans. It is the most commonly identified parasite (in O+P) in the United States. However, it is much more common in developing nations than in westernized nations because it is usually transmitted via drinking unchlorinated water contaminated with raw sewage. Person to person transmission can also occur, such as through household members, unprotected anal sex, and institutions (e.g., nursing homes, daycare centers).

BASIC SCIENCE/CLINICAL PEARL	STEP 1/2/3

Chronic giardiasis is also known as *beaver fever* because it can be contracted by drinking the water from lakes and streams where beavers or muskrats reside.

The incubation period for *G. lamblia* is about 1 to 2 weeks after exposure. Symptoms can include diarrhea, gas, bloating, vomiting, abdominal distention, anorexia, fever, and headache. Infection can cause chronic diarrhea with weight loss in healthy children, although this is more common in immunodeficient patients, particularly those with immunoglobulin A (IgA) deficiency. Chronic giardiasis can cause FTT, with malabsorption of vitamins A and B_{12}, lactose, and fat.

BASIC SCIENCE/CLINICAL PEARL	STEP 1/2/3

Symptoms of vitamin A deficiency include nyctalopia (night blindness), keratinization of the conjunctiva, xerosis (dry skin), xerophthalmia (dry eyes with lack of tear production), recurrent infections, osteoporosis, and poor tooth development in young children.

BASIC SCIENCE/CLINICAL PEARL	STEP 1/2/3

Symptoms of vitamin B_{12} deficiency include fatigue (due to a macrocytic anemia), muscle aches, and depression, and higher risks for infertility, heart disease, multiple sclerosis, and rheumatoid arthritis. About half of vegans and vegetarians are deficient in B_{12}.

BASIC SCIENCE/CLINICAL PEARL	STEP 1/2/3

Lactase is the enzyme which digests the milk sugar disaccharide lactose into the monosaccharides glucose and galactose. Malabsorption of lactose in the small bowel leads to its fermentation in the colon, resulting in flatulence, diarrhea, and abdominal pain and distention.

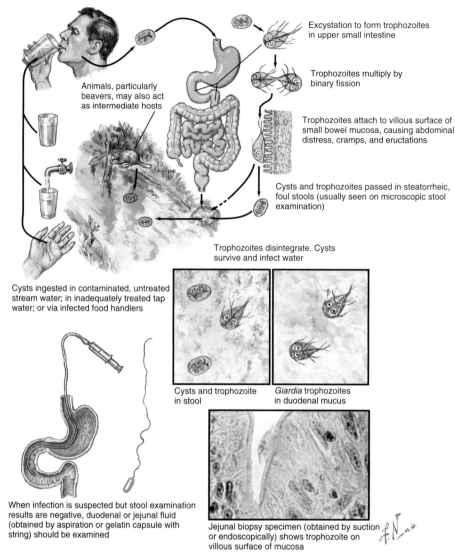

Fig. 29.2 The life cycle of *Giardia lamblia*. (Netter medical illustration used with permission of Elsevier. All rights reserved.)

Diagnosis of *G. lamblia* can be made in several ways. Traditionally, the organism is seen, in either the cyst or trophozoite form, when stool is sent for an O+P examination under the microscope. If the organism cannot be detected noninvasively, identification of the trophozoite can also be made microscopically from an endoscopic small bowel biopsy or duodenal fluid aspiration. Fecal antigen testing via an enzyme-linked immunosorbent assay (ELISA) is more rapid and has a higher sensitivity and specificity for giardiasis. However, O+P should still be ordered to check for the presence of other parasites, especially in those with a compromised immune system. The life cycle of *G. lamblia* is depicted in Fig. 29.2.

BASIC SCIENCE/CLINICAL PEARL   **STEP 1/2/3**

Ideally, three separate samples should be sent for O+P. Three stool samples can increase the detection rate for *Giardia lamblia* to over 90%, as opposed to one sample which has a detection rate of 60%–80%. Lack of discovery of this protozoan via O+P can be due to low levels or intermittent shedding of the organism.

How should the patient be managed?

G. lamblia can be treated with nitroimidazoles, nitazoxanide, and paromomycin. Nitroimidazoles, which include metronidazole, ornidazole, secnidazole, and tinidazole, are highly effective against *G. lamblia* and other protozoal infections. Metronidazole enters the trophozoite, interfering with respiration and causing DNA damage, leading to death. Another benefit of this drug is its rapid absorption and penetration into tissue and mucosal secretions. Nitazoxanide can be considered for patients with multiple types of enteric infections as it has a broad spectrum of activity not only against protozoans, but also against some bacteria and helminths. Paromomycin, an aminoglycoside, is a proposed treatment for *G. lamblia* in cases of pregnant patients and resistance to the previously-mentioned drugs. It also has activity against *Entamoeba histolytica* and *Trichomonas*.

Other symptomatic household members should be checked for the presence of the organism. Reinfection can be prevented by careful hand washing and avoidance of ingesting unchlorinated water (from pools, lakes, wells, hot tubs, and countries with poor sanitation).

Case Point 29.5

The patient is treated with a 10-day course of metronidazole, with resolution of her foul-smelling diarrhea. When she is seen back in clinic 1 month later, she has improved appetite and has gained 1 kg.

BEYOND THE PEARLS

- Failure to thrive should be managed by a multidisciplinary team, including a primary care physician, appropriate sub-specialists, dietician, social worker, mental health providers, and occupational therapists as indicated.
- Following acute gastrointestinal illnesses, children can typically resume their normal diet after the vomiting phase has ended. However, post-infectious malabsorption may occur, particularly after prolonged diarrhea persisting past 1 week. Inflammatory or infectious mucosal damage causes loss of enzyme producing brush border enterocytes, thus producing secondary malabsorption, which is particularly common for lactose.
- Up to 40% of patients experience lactose intolerance post-*Giardia* treatment. This can be confused for continued symptoms due to chronic giardiasis. If repeat stool testing is negative for the parasite, the child should be put on a lactose-free diet for several weeks.
- Infection with *Cryptosporidium* spp. protozoans can present similarly to chronic giardiasis. It can also cause chronic infectious diarrhea in primarily immunocompromised hosts, including those with human immunodeficiency virus. In immunocompetent children, infections are generally acute, although fluid and electrolyte losses can be profound. Exposure history may include contact with contaminated uncooked food or water. Diagnosis is made by identification of the organism in the stool under microscopy or in biopsies from the proximal small bowel. Like giardiasis, treatment includes anti-parasitic agents, such as nitazoxanide.
- Celiac disease should be considered in children with chronic diarrhea, particularly in those who exhibit symptoms after the introduction of gluten-containing foods. Gastrointestinal manifestations of celiac disease include FTT, chronic diarrhea, and abdominal pain and distention due to lactase deficiency. Extraintestinal manifestations include short stature, delayed puberty, rashes, and nutritional deficiencies (iron and fat-soluble vitamins).

Case Summary

Complaint/History: A 16-month-old female presents with her foster mother to clinic with a 1-month history of loose, foul-smelling stools which leak out of her diaper and onto her clothing. The stools are brown, nonbloody and are noted to float in the toilet.

Findings: On examination, she has normal vital signs but is underweight for age. She is noted to be a thin, well-kempt, active toddler with nondysmorphic features. Her abdomen is mildly distended and tympanitic. Digital rectal examination reveals soft stool in the rectal vault and normal rectal tone. She has decreased subcutaneous fat stores in her extremities. Her examination is otherwise unremarkable.

Labs/Tests: Laboratory workup includes normal complete blood count and serum chemistries. Her stool is sent for bacterial culture, and microscopic examination for ova and parasites. Stool antigen testing is positive for *G. lamblia.*

Diagnosis: Chronic giardiasis.

Treatment: The patient is treated with a 10-day course of metronidazole with resolution of her foul-smelling diarrhea. When she is seen back in clinic 1 month later, she has improved appetite and has gained 1 kg.

References

Branski DD. Chapter 338: Disorders of Malabsorption. *Nelson Textbook of Pediatrics.* 20th ed. Philadelphia: Elsevier; 2016:1831–1850.

Gardner TB, Hill DR. Treatment of giardiasis. *Clin Microbiol Rev.* 2001;14(1):114–128.

Garrett ZC, Israel EJ. Chronic diarrhea in children. *Pediatr Rev.* 2012;33(5):207–218.

Guarino A, Branski D, Winter HS, et al. Chapter 341: Chronic Diarrhea. *Nelson Textbook of Pediatrics.* 20th ed. Philadelphia: Elsevier; 2016:1875–1882.

Jaffe AC. Failure to thrive: current clinical concepts. *Pediatr Rev.* 2011;32(3):100–108.

McLean HS, Price DT. Chapter 41: Failure to Thrive. *Nelson Textbook of Pediatrics.* 20th ed. Philadelphia: Elsevier; 2016:249–252.

Pietzak MM, Thomas DW. Childhood malabsorption. *Pediatr Rev.* 2003;24(6):195–206.

Schwartz DI. Failure to thrive: an old nemesis in the new millennium. *Pediatr Rev.* 2000;21(8):257–264.

3-Week-Old Male With Resected Bowel

Amrita Narang   Mohammad Jami   Michelle Pietzak

A male is born prematurely at 29 weeks gestational age due to preterm labor. He is started on parenteral nutrition (PN) support during the initial few weeks of life through central venous access. He is slowly started on nasogastric (NG) tube feeds with a preterm formula at a slow rate. At 3 weeks of life (corrected age 32 weeks), he develops lethargy and abdominal distention with bloody diarrhea. An abdominal radiograph reveals pneumatosis intestinalis (Fig. 30.1). The patient is diagnosed with necrotizing enterocolitis (NEC).

Despite antibiotic treatment and supportive care, his clinical status worsens. He is taken to the operating room by pediatric surgery for an exploratory laparotomy. In the operating room, his small bowel and proximal colon appear dusky and distended. The nonviable bowel is resected: 100 cm of ileum, the ileocecal valve (ICV), and 30 cm of the colon. An end-ileostomy is created to the abdominal wall. The pathology of the bowel is consistent with severe NEC, showing necrosis, ischemia, and bacteria in the mucosa and submucosa Fig. 30.2).

Will this child be able to meet expected nutritional goals without parenteral nutrition?
It is highly unlikely that this child will be able to meet his nutritional goals enterally, given his bowel resection. His end-ileostomy will likely produce about 40 to 60 mL/kg per day of watery stool into the ostomy bag. The loss of half of his colon will also result in decreased water absorption, also generating diarrhea when he has reanastomosis surgery.

BASIC SCIENCE PEARL   **STEP 1**

A term infant is born with approximately 240 cm of small bowel and 40 cm of colon; and at 1 year of age, the average small bowel length is about 380 cm.

Case Point 30.1

At 2 months of age (corrected age 37 weeks), he is taken back to the operating room for takedown of his ileostomy, primary anastomosis of the remaining ileum to the transverse colon, placement of a gastrostomy tube (GT), and placement of a subclavian central venous catheter (CVC) for more permanent access for PN. Over the next 2 months, he continues to have watery diarrhea and acidosis and is unable to be weaned from PN. Ultimately, he is discharged home on partial PN given over 24 hours and trophic GT feeds over 12 hours.

CLINICAL PEARL   **STEP 2/3**

Prognostic factors to advancing to full enteral feeds and off of PN include length of small bowel remaining, presence of ICV, amount of colon remaining, ability to use continuous drip feeds, and primary disease progression.

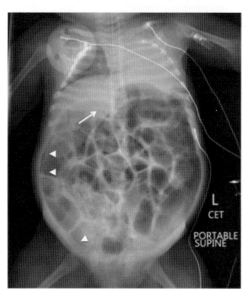

Fig. 30.1 Supine abdominal plain film taken 45 minutes after symptom onset, showing diffuse bowel dilation, pneumatosis intestinalis *(arrowheads),* and portal venous gas *(arrow).* (From Riggle KM, Davis JL, Drugas GT, et al. Fatal Clostridial necrotizing enterocolitis in a term infant with gastroschisis. *J Pediatr Surg Case Rep.* 2016;14:29–31.)

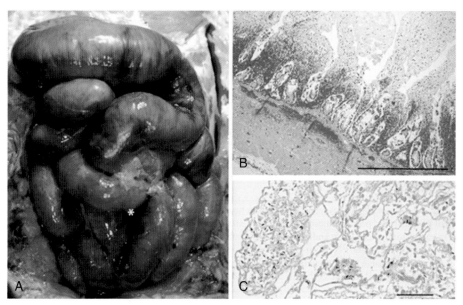

Fig. 30.2 (A) Small bowel, in situ, with diffuse distention and dusky discoloration consistent with ischemia. *Area of perforation. (B) Microscopic image with severe mucosal necrosis and ischemic changes (hematoxylin and eosin; 500μm). (C) Collections of rod-shaped gram-positive bacilli present within the mucosa and submucosa (Brown and Brenn [Gram stain], 100μm). (From Riggle KM, Davis JL, Drugas GT, et al. Fatal Clostridial necrotizing enterocolitis in a term infant with gastroschisis. *J Pediatr Surg Case Rep.* 2016;14:29–31.)

Diagnosis: Short bowel syndrome (SBS) secondary to NEC with intestinal failure.

What is short bowel syndrome? What nutritional deficiencies arise from loss of the proximal small intestine, distal small intestine and/or the colon?
SBS is a form of intestinal failure in which the patient is unable to absorb necessary fluids and nutrients to grow and maintain homeostasis. It can occur when the absolute length of bowel is short (such as in bowel resection for NEC, trauma, or inflammatory bowel disease) or when the bowel has intrinsic dysmotility (such as in intestinal pseudo-obstruction syndromes).

CLINICAL PEARL   **STEP 2/3**

Most nutrients are absorbed in the proximal small bowel; the exceptions are vitamin B_{12} and bile acids, which are absorbed in the terminal ileum.

The ICV is essential as a "brake" between the small intestine and colon, slowing the transit time of foods and secretions. It is thought to prevent colonic bacteria from ascending into the small bowel, leading to bacterial overgrowth. The colon mainly functions as a salvage organ, absorbing water, and maintaining most of the gut microbiome. The probiotic bacteria in the colon produce vitamin K, deconjugate bile acids, and digest plant matter in the diet.

BASIC SCIENCE/CLINICAL PEARL   **STEP 1/2/3**

Bowel adaptation—an evolutionary process of the remainder of the bowel to fulfill the function of the full length by cellular hyperplasia, villus hypertrophy, increased crypt depth, and bowel dilation—allows for some adaptation to SBS. This process begins immediately and can last for months to years. Enteral nutrition and other factors, such as growth factors and hormones, are key to this process.

Case Point 30.2

Three months after discharge, he is noted in clinic to have jaundice and scleral icterus. Laboratory testing reveals elevated serum levels of aspartate aminotransferase (AST), alanine aminotransferase (ALT), and total and conjugated bilirubin. He is started on ursodeoxycholic acid (UDCA).

What are the long-term complications of short bowel syndrome and receiving parenteral nutrition? Why does he have conjugated hyperbilirubinemia?
Long-term complications of SBS include intestinal failure–associated liver disease (IFALD) and catheter-related blood stream infections (CRBSIs). Long-term PN use is associated with the development of IFALD, also known as total parenteral nutrition–associated cholestasis (TPNAC). Mild liver injury leads to cholestasis, whereas severe forms can ultimately lead to portal hypertension and liver failure requiring transplantation.
Host factors that increase the risk for liver damage include prematurity, immature bile secretory mechanisms, bile stasis due to fasting, and repeated sepsis episodes leading to endotoxemia. Factors associated with PN formulation thought to predispose for liver injury include excessive glucose, which can result in hepatosteatosis and possibly hepatic fibrosis; excessive protein, which decreases bile flow; and direct oxidant damage due to phytosterols present in intravenous lipids (IL).

To minimize risk for IFALD, the PN should be formulated to provide enough calories for appropriate growth, but to otherwise avoid excessive calories. The introduction of enteral nutrition as soon as possible, with trophic feeds, is important to avoid bile stasis. Other interventions that can reduce IFALD include decreasing the IL to <1 g/kg body weight, cycling the lipids for several hours off per day, preventing septic events, and prevention of small intestinal bacterial overgrowth.

Case Point 30.3

The patient improves on UDCA with partial resolution of his jaundice. He continues to gain weight and grow while on a mix of enteral and PN. He does not successfully wean from PN. His parents would like to know if there are other options available besides lifelong PN because they are concerned about its long-term complications.

What are the long-term options for patients who are not able to achieve independence from parenteral nutrition?

Patients who cannot achieve enteral autonomy or develop IFALD can be helped with surgical procedures, such as longitudinal intestinal lengthening and tapering (LILT), the Bianchi procedure, or serial transverse enteroplasty (STEP), as seen in Figs. 30.3–30.5. Patients with treatment failure or treatment-associated complications, such as IFALD or venous thrombosis (with no site left for CVC), have the option to undergo small bowel transplant; however, the 5-year survival post–small bowel transplantation is only 50%. Patients with SBS and IFALD often require listing for both a liver and small bowel transplantation. The mortality on the waiting list for these two organs is also around 50%.

- UDCA is the synthetic form of bear bile acids. Despite gorging on high-fat salmon, and then hibernating and fasting, bears do not develop cholestasis and gallstones. Use of UDCA is to promote bile acid–dependent bile flow in the patient with SBS. It is also used in other diseases where there is cholestasis, such as primary biliary cirrhosis (PBC), cystic fibrosis, and Alagille's syndrome.
- The surgical intestine lengthening procedures, such as LILT, STEP, and the Bianchi procedure, must be performed on dilated bowel. The goal is not only to increase the length of the bowel, but also to slow down intestinal transit, allowing more time for the absorption of gut nutrients.
- The human growth hormone used in SBS is the same as that used for short stature in children. In combination with glutamine and specialized diets, growth hormone has been shown to promote weight gain and intestinal absorption of nutrients. However, these benefits do not continue once the hormone is stopped. Common side effects include peripheral edema and carpal tunnel syndrome.
- Gut hormone teduglutide, a 33-amino acid analogue of glucagon-like peptide-2 (GLP-2), promotes repair and normal growth of the intestine and increases absorption in patients with SBS. It was approved by the Food and Drug Administration (FDA) for PN-dependent SBS in 2012. It is given subcutaneously once daily. Common side effects include headache, nausea, and abdominal pain. It may also increase the risk of intestinal polyps and cancers.

BEYOND THE PEARLS—cont'd

- GLP-2 is secreted endogenously from enteroendocrine L cells, mainly located in the terminal ileum and colon. Its effects include intestinal growth, enhancement of intestinal function, reduction in osteoclastic activity, and neuroprotection. GLP-2 analogues are being studied as treatments not only for SBS, but also for Crohn disease, osteoporosis, and adjuvant therapy during chemotherapy.
- Tissue engineering has arisen from the improved understanding of normal intestinal stem cells. It is hoped that autologous transplantation, from the patient's own tissue engineered small intestine, will replace cadaveric small bowel transplantation in the future.
- New research is being done on fish-oil based lipid solutions to prevent liver damage in patients dependent on PN.

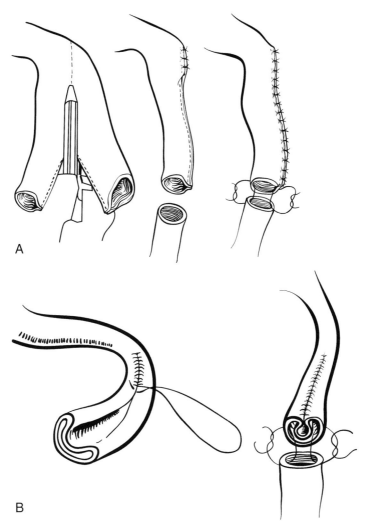

Fig. 30.3 Intestinal tapering can be achieved by either (A) longitudinal excision or (B) imbrication. (From Thompson J, Sudan D. Intestinal lengthening for short bowel syndrome. *Adv Surg.* 2008;42:49–61.)

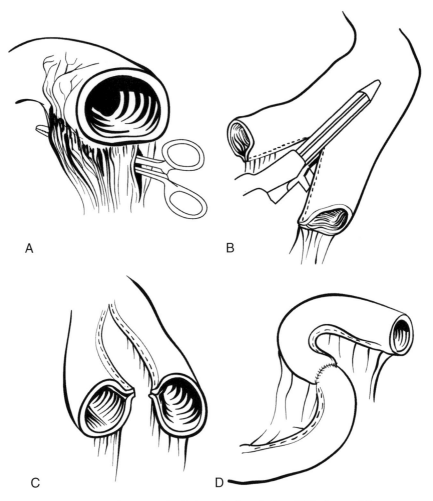

Fig. 30.4 Bianchi procedure—Bianchi longitudinal intestinal lengthening. (A) The leaves of the mesentery are separated, and a tunnel is created to separate the vasculature to alternate sides. (B) and (C) The linear stapler is passed through this tunnel and the bowel is divided longitudinally. (D) A lazy "s" is then formed to bring the open ends together and hand-sewn anastomosis is performed to restore continuity. (From Thompson J, Sudan D. Intestinal lengthening for short bowel syndrome. *Adv Surg.* 2008;42:49–61.)

Case Summary

Complaint/History: A 3-week-old premature infant develops necrotizing enterocolitis, and despite aggressive therapy, he eventually undergoes operative resection of his terminal ileum, ileocecal valve and right colon.

Findings: Watery diarrhea whenever he is fed orally.

Labs/Tests: Metabolic acidosis secondary to gastrointestinal losses.

Diagnosis: Short bowel syndrome.

Treatment: Trophic feeds with a hydrolyzed formula via gastric tube, PN, and ursodeoxycholic acid. Possible bowel lengthening procedure or transplant in the future.

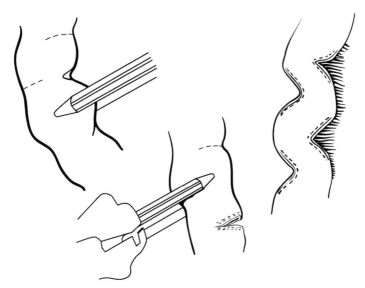

Fig. 30.5 Serial transverse enteroplasty. The bowel lumen is partially transected using a linear stapler, stopping at the point that leaves the normal luminal diameter (generally 1–2 cm) intact. Subsequent staple firings are displaced the same distance as the remnant lumen (usually 1–2 cm), either proximally or distally along the dilated small bowel loop and alternatively placed at 180 degrees from the first firing. This procedure can be performed either by alternating from side-to-side or mesenteric to antimesenteric edge. (From Thompson J, Sudan D. Intestinal lengthening for short bowel syndrome. *Adv Surg.* 2008;42:49–61.)

References

O'Keefe SJ, Buchman AL, Fishbein TM, et al. Short bowel syndrome and intestinal failure: consensus definitions and overview. *Clin Gastroenterol Hepatol.* 2006;4(1):6–10.

Siebert JR. Small intestine length in infants and children. *Am J Dis Child.* 1980;134(6):593–595.

Squires RH, Duggan C, Teitelbaum DH, et al. Natural history of pediatric intestinal failure: initial report from the pediatric intestinal failure consortium. *J Pediatr.* 2012;161(4):723–728.e2.

Thompson J, Sudan D. Intestinal lengthening for short bowel syndrome. *Adv Surg.* 2008;42(9):49–67.

Weaver LT, Austin S, Cole TJ. Small intestinal length: a factor essential to gut adaptation. *Gut.* 1991;32(11):1321–1323.

3-Year-Old Female With Buccal Swelling

Patricia F. Villegas ▦ Mikhaela Cielo

A 3-year-old previously healthy female living in Ethiopia presents with bilateral buccal swelling for 3 weeks. Her mother reports that 3 weeks prior to presenting, she had a febrile illness, with a sore throat and fatigue. At that time, her mother noticed that her right cheek had become swollen. Her mother took her to a physician in Ethiopia and she was prescribed an unknown oral antibiotic that she took for 7 days with minimal effect. She has associated pain with mastication.

What is the differential diagnosis for buccal swelling?

The differential diagnosis for buccal swelling primarily includes parotitis, inflammation of the parotid gland. Causes of parotitis include viral, bacterial (suppurative), and noninfectious causes. Viral pathogens of parotitis include mumps virus, influenza virus, parainfluenza virus, adenovirus, coxsackievirus, Epstein-Barr virus, cytomegalovirus, herpes simplex virus, human immunodeficiency virus (HIV), and lymphocytic choriomeningitis virus. Viral parotitis typically presents with a prodromal illness, followed by acute swelling of the parotid gland, which may progress bilaterally. HIV and *Bartonella henselae* can cause a chronic low-grade infection of the parotid gland.

Bacterial parotitis is an uncommon infection in infants and children. It is usually unilateral and often polymicrobial, with *Staphylococcus aureus* being the most commonly isolated pathogen, as well as streptococci and anaerobes. Gram-negative bacilli can be an important cause in the neonate. Bacterial parotitis manifests as acute-onset swelling, with a firm, tender, erythematous mass. There can be purulent discharge from the parotid gland (Stenson duct) and systemic findings, such as fever and chills. The infection can result from hematogenous spread or direct invasion of oral flora through the Stenson duct.

CLINICAL PEARL	**STEP 2/3**

Suppurative parotitis in the neonate can mimic the appearance of group B *Streptococcus* spp. facial cellulitis.

Recurrent acute parotitis can occur in some cases, from once every few years to several times per year. The pathogenesis is not known. Some bacteria isolated include *Streptococcus pneumoniae*, nontypeable *Haemophilus influenzae,* and oral *Streptococcus* spp. In patients with HIV, cytomegalovirus has also been associated. The condition usually resolves in adolescence.

Noninfectious causes of parotid swelling include Sjögren syndrome, salivary gland stones (sialolithiasis), and salivary gland tumors. Sialolithiasis is diagnosed by radiography. Salivary gland tumors can be identified on imaging, but definitive diagnosis requires biopsy. The diagnosis of Sjögren syndrome is based on clinical criteria, including ocular and oral dryness, inadequate tear production, and impaired salivary gland function, with the presence of autoantibodies and systemic autoimmune disease.

CLINICAL PEARL   STEP 2/3

Given the proximity of the parotid gland to the mandible and lymphatic structures, one must also consider odontogenic infections, trauma, osteomyelitis of the mandible, and malignancy.

Case Point 31.1

The patient is a previously healthy child who is developmentally appropriate for age. She has only received vaccinations up to 9 months of age. She arrived in the United States 4 days prior for a family vacation.

Her temperature is 36.4°C, pulse rate is 80/min, respiratory rate is 20/min, blood pressure is 95/59 mm Hg, and oxygen saturation is 100% on room air. She is well-appearing and cooperative on examination. She has buccal swelling in the region of the bilateral parotid glands, extending posteriorly (right greater than left; Fig. 31.1); the cheek is mildly tender to palpation. There is no increased warmth, erythema, or fluctuance. There is no discharge or exudate from the parotid (Stenson) ducts. The oropharynx is clear, with no tonsillar swelling or exudates and the uvula is midline. There are palpable 1- to 2-cm submandibular and posterior cervical lymph nodes, which are nontender. The remainder of her examination is normal.

What is the most likely diagnosis based on the additional history and physical examination?
In an incompletely vaccinated child presenting with a prodromal illness followed by unilateral buccal swelling, the most likely diagnosis is mumps virus infection. The virus is acquired via respiratory droplets, direct contact, or fomites. The typical incubation period lasts 14 to 18 days. Humans are the only natural host. It is highly infectious, especially in close quarters. Outbreaks in the past have been noted in the military and, more recently, in college dormitories.

BASIC SCIENCE PEARL   STEP 1

Mumps virus is a single-stranded RNA virus with a helical capsule and surface envelope. It is in the Paramyxoviridae family of viruses.

BASIC SCIENCE PEARL   STEP 1

The mumps virus is stable at refrigerator temperature for days but is destroyed by 20 minutes of moderate heat (56°C).

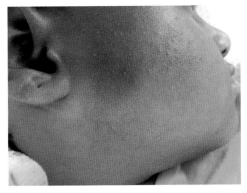

Fig. 31.1 Buccal swelling in the region of the parotid gland.

What steps are necessary to make a diagnosis of mumps?

Before the introduction of the mumps virus vaccine, the prevalence of mumps was high worldwide, and a diagnosis of mumps could be made based on the history of exposure and clinical findings. Typical laboratory findings of parotitis include elevated serum amylase levels (not specific to mumps). Other laboratory findings of mumps infection include leukopenia, with relative lymphocytosis.

Today, in an area with low incidence due to high vaccination rates, a specific diagnosis of mumps should be confirmed or ruled out in patients with parotitis of unknown cause. Potential infections should be reported to the local public health department because it monitors for outbreaks and can assist in the guidance of appropriate testing and precautions.

Although the virus can be isolated, and/or viral antigen can be detected from respiratory secretions, cerebrospinal fluid, and/or urine, serologic testing is more commonly used due to its broader availability and higher ease of collection. An elevated serum mumps immunoglobulin (Ig) M antibody level suggests recent infection. A significant rise of mumps IgG antibody level between acute and convalescent specimens is diagnostic. Reverse transcriptase polymerase chain reaction (RT-PCR) is also used for diagnosis.

Case Point 31.2

> Laboratory testing reveals a normal blood count and metabolic panel. The serum amylase level is elevated, at 1159 U/L (normal, 40–140 U/L). Mumps virus is detected by RT-PCR, and serologic testing of mumps confirms an antibody response.

> Diagnosis: Viral parotitis due to mumps virus infection.

What is the most common syndrome associated with mumps virus infection?

The clinical manifestation of mumps includes a nonspecific prodrome consisting of low-grade fever, malaise, headache, myalgia, and anorexia, followed by parotitis. Parotid swelling is present in 95% of symptomatic cases and is due to direct infection of the ductal epithelium, with resultant local inflammation. Parotid tenderness and occasionally earache precedes the onset of parotid swelling.

CLINICAL PEARL   **STEP 2/3**

Purulent drainage is not seen in mumps. Consider bacterial sialadenitis instead.

On examination of the buccal mucosa, there may be erythema and edema at the opening of the Stensen duct. Enlargement of the contralateral parotid gland occurs in 70% of patients but may be delayed by several days. Parotid swelling can last up to 10 days. Viral shedding precedes the onset of symptomatic illness and can last up to 2 weeks.

BASIC SCIENCE/CLINICAL PEARL   **STEP 1/2/3**

Mumps parotitis is bilateral in over 70% of cases.

What complications are associated with mumps virus infection?

The most common complications associated with mumps include meningoencephalitis and orchitis. Meningitis with or without encephalitis occurs when the mumps virus enters the central nervous system (CNS) via the choroid plexus and infects the choroid epithelium. Symptomatic CNS involvement often manifests 5 days after parotitis; however, it may also occur before or along with the initial presentation. Parotitis is only present in about 50% of cases of mumps meningitis.

Cerebrospinal fluid findings include pleocytosis with lymphocyte predominance, normal glucose level, and normal or elevated protein level. Clinical manifestations of meningitis include fever, vomiting, headache, neck stiffness, lethargy, and seizures. Other rare neurologic complications of mumps virus infection include sensorineural hearing loss, Guillain-Barré syndrome, transverse myelitis, and facial palsy.

BASIC SCIENCE/CLINICAL PEARL	STEP 1/2/3
Approximately 1 in every 60 cases of mumps encephalitis will be fatal.	

Orchitis secondary to mumps can be seen in adolescent and adult males and is rare in prepubescent boys. Males typically report tenderness, with swelling of the testes, which can be unilateral or bilateral. Occasionally, atrophy of the testes may occur, but sterility is rare.

Other organ involvement that has been reported in association with mumps infection include thyroiditis, myocarditis, pancreatitis, interstitial nephritis, and arthritis.

How is mumps treated?

Treatment for mumps is supportive care only—antipyretics for fever, analgesics for pain, and adequate hydration. Acidic or sour foods may be avoided to prevent stimulation of salivation. Hospitalization is indicated if the patient is clinically unstable or is having serious complications (e.g., meningoencephalitis).

CLINICAL PEARL	STEP 2/3
Acidic foods stimulate salivation, which is painful with parotitis.	

CLINICAL PEARL	STEP 2/3
In cases of recurrent (nonmumps) parotitis, the use of sialagogues—in addition to penicillin, parotid massage, and hydration—is a beneficial part of treatment.	

Patients should avoid daycare, school, or work until the risk of transmission is low. Children should be excluded from school for 5 days, starting from the onset of parotid gland swelling. For hospitalized patients, droplet and standard isolation precautions are recommended until 5 days after the onset of parotid swelling. There is no postexposure prophylaxis treatment for nonimmunized persons exposed to infected individuals due to lack of evidence for efficacy.

Case Point 31.3

Lumbar puncture is not performed, given the lack of meningismus and neurologic symptoms. The patient is treated conservatively, with oral hydration and monitoring of her food intake. Her parents are counseled to avoid acidic foods until her parotitis resolves. Ultimately, her disease self-resolves after 2 more weeks.

Her parents ask if this could have been prevented.

How is mumps prevented?

Three years after the mumps virus was first isolated, a vaccine was made available in 1948. Its induced immunity was short-lived, however, and long-lasting immunity was not achievable via immunization until the current vaccine—a live-attenuated virus—was licensed in 1967. Routine use was recommended starting in 1977, leading to a rapid fall in the incidence of mumps infections (Fig. 31.2). A two-dose combined measles-mumps-rubella vaccine (MMR) schedule was introduced in 1989, which led to further decreases in the incidence of mumps infections.

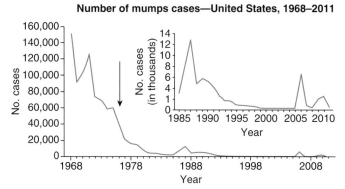

Number of mumps cases—United States, 1968–2011

Fig. 31.2 The effect of routine vaccination *(arrow)* on mumps incidence. *Inset* shows the 2006 outbreak, discussed further below. (From Mason WH. Mumps. In: Kliegman RM, Stanton BF, St. Geme J, Schor N, eds. *Nelson's Textbook of Pediatrics*. 20th ed. Philadelphia: Elsevier/Saunders; 2016:1552–1554; and McLean HQ, Fiebelkorn AP, Temte JL, Wallace GS; Centers for Disease Control and Prevention: Prevention of measles, rubella, congenital rubella syndrome and mumps: summary recommendations of the Advisory Committee on Immunization Practices (ACIP). *MMWR Recomm Rep*. 2013:62(RR-04):1–34.))

BASIC SCIENCE PEARL	STEP 1

The incidence of mumps in the prevaccine era was as high as 50 to 251/100,000 cases. In the postvaccine era, the incidence had significantly declined by 1999, with a reported incidence of <0.1/100,000 cases.

The Centers for Disease Control and Prevention (CDC) has recommended routine universal vaccination as part of the two-dose MMR vaccine series; the first dose is given at 12 to 15 months of age and the second dose is given at 4 to 6 years of age. The efficacy is increased with two doses versus a single dose (88% and 78%, respectively); this led the Advisory Committee on Immunization Practices of the CDC to recommend the two-dose schedule in 1989.

The MMR vaccine contains live attenuated measles (Edmonston-Enders vaccine strain), mumps (Jeryl-Lynn vaccine strain), and rubella (Wistar RA 27/3 vaccine strain) viruses. It is licensed in the United States for routine use in children 12 months of age and older; however, it can be given to infants as young as 6 months of age who are travelling internationally. If a child receives a dose of mumps vaccine before 12 months of age, this dose is not counted toward the required number of doses, and two additional doses are required, beginning at 12 to 15 months of age and separated by at least 28 days. Because it is a live virus vaccine, it should not be given to pregnant women or immunocompromised or immunosuppressed individuals.

Are nonvaccinated and undervaccinated children protected by herd immunity?
In 2006, there was large-scale mumps outbreak in the Midwestern United States (Midwest), with 6584 reported cases. The highest incidence was in the 18- to 24-year-old age group, making up 29% of total cases. Furthermore, in the group of 18- to 24-year-old persons who were infected, 83% of patients had received two doses of the MMR vaccine. In settings of high immunization coverage such as the United States, most mumps cases likely will occur in people who have received two doses. This resurgence among a highly vaccinated population has brought attention to the importance of continued vaccination efforts because the disease is not eradicated, and outbreaks occur as community vaccination rates decrease below the threshold for effective herd immunity. It has also raised questions of waning immunity over time and the possibility of decreased efficacy against current circulating strains.

BASIC SCIENCE PEARL   **STEP 1**

Vaccination rate thresholds to achieve herd immunity are estimated based on the number of susceptible persons, cases of disease, and rates of transmission; the latter is itself dependent on the reproductive rate of the organism and windows of susceptibility. The herd immunity threshold for mumps has been estimated to be a 75% to 86% vaccination rate.

BEYOND THE PEARLS

- The mumps virus genome encodes for only nine proteins.
- Prior to routine vaccination, epidemic outbreaks of mumps virus occurred roughly every 4 years in the United States.
- The serologic presence of anti-mumps IgM develops by the second day of illness and peaks within the first week. It is often undetectable within 3 months of disease onset but may persist for up to 6 months. Anti-mumps virus IgG will be detectable for life.
- Inoculation with mumps virus vaccine will diminish the response to tuberculin skin testing for up to 1 month.
- There are suggested intervals between therapeutic intravenous immune globulin (IVIG) administration and MMR administration, including 11 months following the administration of IVIG for the treatment of Kawasaki disease.
- Epididymo-orchitis is rare in prepubertal patients.
- Mumps infections in the first trimester of pregnancy increases the risk of fetal loss. There are no known fetal malformations associated with intrauterine mumps infection.
- Over 25% of patients with mumps meningoencephalitis will not present with nuchal rigidity. Less than 50% will have parotid swelling.

Case Summary

Complaint/History: A 3-year-old female presents with bilateral buccal swelling, right greater than left.

Findings: She has buccal swelling in the region of the parotid gland extending posteriorly; the cheek is mildly tender to palpation.

Labs/Tests: Mumps virus is detected by the reverse transcriptase polymerase chain reaction assay.

Diagnosis: Viral parotitis due to mumps virus infection.

Treatment: Supportive care.

Bibliography

Anderson LJ, Seward JF. Mumps epidemiology and immunity. *Pediatr Infect Dis J.* 2008;27(suppl):S75–S79.

Centers for Disease Control and Prevention. Mumps. In: Hamborsky J, Kroger A, Wolfe S, eds. *Epidemiology and Prevention of Vaccine-Preventable Diseases.* 13th ed. Washington D.C: Public Health Foundation; 2015.

Cherry JD, Quinn KK. Mumps Virus. In: *Feigin and Cherry's Textbook of Pediatric Infectious Diseases.* 2013:2395–2407.e4.

Dayan GH, Quinlisk MP, Parker AA, et al. Recent resurgence of mumps in the United States. *N Engl J Med.* 2008;358(15):1580–1589.

Fiebelkorn A, Lawler J, Curns AT, et al. Mumps postexposure prophylaxis with a third dose of measles-mumps-rubella vaccine, Orange County, New York, USA. *Emerg Infect Dis.* 2013;19(9):1411–1417.

Fine PE. Herd immunity: history, theory, practice. *Epidemiol Rev.* 1993;15(2):265–302.

Mumps. In: Kimberlin DW, Brady MT, Jackson MA, et al., eds. *Red Book: 2015 Report of the Committee on Infectious Diseases.* Elk Grove Village, IL: American Academy of Pediatrics; 2015:564–567.

Newborn With Hypoglycemia

Priya Shastry ▪ Smeeta Sardesai

A late preterm female infant is delivered via cesarean section to a 24-year-old primigravida mother with type 2 diabetes mellitus. The infant is delivered early for a nonreassuring fetal heart rate tracing. The mother received spotty prenatal care and did not have appropriate monitoring of her diabetes. On the day of delivery, the mother's hemoglobin A1c was high at 8.9% (the normal level is between 4% and 5.6%).

The infant cries spontaneously at birth and has some transient respiratory distress. Her birth weight is 4000 g (>95th percentile) (Fig. 32.1). On examination, she appears large for gestational age. She cries loudly but is consolable. She does not appear lethargic or jittery. The anterior and posterior fontanelles are soft and flat. Her facies are not dysmorphic. She has a good suck reflex. Her tongue is not large. Hard and soft palates are intact. Sclerae are anicteric. There is mild nasal flaring. Her lungs are clear to auscultation without crackles. Her heart rate is regular and there are no murmurs appreciated. Her abdomen is soft, and there is no palpable liver or spleen. Her external genital and rectal examinations are normal. She has good perfusion in her extremities. She does not have any sacral dimples or rashes.

Why are infants of diabetic mothers (IDMs) large for gestational age?

Macrosomia, defined as a birth weight greater than the 90th percentile for gestational age, is the hallmark of a diabetic pregnancy. In this vignette, the infant is macrosomic because her birth weight is greater than the 95th percentile. Fetal hyperinsulinemia is the main cause of fetal over-growth in diabetic pregnancies. Elevated insulin levels in the fetus stimulate glycogen storage in the liver, increasing lipid synthesis and the accumulation of fat. The fetus has normal head growth with an increased growth velocity and fat deposition in the abdominal organs and interscapular areas.

Why did the patient have respiratory distress after she was born?

Respiratory distress is a common complication in IDM. A premature delivery is more likely to occur in IDMs because of a higher rate of preterm labor. There is also an increased rate of iatro-genic prematurity due to early induction of labor to prevent intrauterine fetal death. Respiratory symptoms in IDMs may be due to either respiratory distress syndrome (RDS) due to surfactant deficiency or retained fetal lung fluid causing transient tachypnea of the newborn (TTN) after operative delivery.

BASIC SCIENCE/CLINICAL PEARL   **STEP 1/2/3**

There is an increased risk of surfactant deficiency in IDMs because hyperinsulinemia in the fetus interferes with the induction of lung maturation by glucocorticoids.

What is the next step?

Neonatal hypoglycemia must be ruled out in all IDMs, regardless of symptomatology. In new-borns signs of hypoglycemia include apnea, bradycardia, cyanosis, hypothermia, irritability,

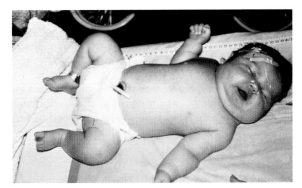

Fig. 32.1 An infant born to a mother with gestational diabetes. She is large for gestational age and has rounded facies. (From Balest AL, Riley M, Bogen D. Neonatology. In: Basil J. Zitelli BJ, McIntire SC, Nowalk AJ, eds. *Atlas of Pediatric Physical Diagnosis.* 7th ed. Philadelphia: Elsevier; 2017:44–70.)

sweating, jitteriness, tremors, poor feeding, weak or high-pitched cry, lethargy, coma, and seizures. Most findings are nonspecific and result from disturbances in central nervous system function.

CLINICAL PEARL   STEP 2/3

Infants with low blood glucose concentrations are frequently asymptomatic. Hypoglycemia in these cases is usually detected by the screening of blood glucose levels in at-risk infants.

Case Point 32.1

Her serum glucose level is 10 mg/dL (abnormal level <30 mg/dL) at 1 hour of life.

What are the causes of hypoglycemia in a newborn?
Infants with excessive insulin production, altered hormone secretion, an inadequate substrate supply, or inadequate amino acid or lipid stores are at risk for transient hypoglycemia. Normal gluconeogenesis and ketogenesis are required to maintain glucose homeostasis. Factors placing neonates at higher risk for developing hypoglycemia are prematurity (limited hepatic glycogen stores), perinatal stress or asphyxia (depleted glycogen stores), small size for gestational age (depleted glycogen stores), and being born to a diabetic mother (excessive insulin production). Other causes include infection, hypothermia, hyperviscosity, and erythroblastosis fetalis. Infants of mothers treated with hypoglycemic agents during pregnancy may also develop neonatal hypoglycemia.

CLINICAL PEARL   STEP 2/3

Infants of mothers receiving intravenous dextrose during delivery may develop neonatal hypoglycemia.

Persistent or recurrent hypoglycemia is far less common and can be separated into four categories: hyperinsulinism, endocrine disorders, inborn errors of metabolism (IEOM), and neuro-hypoglycemia. Hyperinsulinism is seen in congenital hyperinsulinism, such as in Beckwith-Wiedemann syndrome. Endocrine disorders include congenital glucagon deficiency, cortisol deficiency, pituitary insufficiency, and epinephrine deficiency. Neuro-hypoglycemia is due to defective transport of glucose across blood vessels into the brain and cerebrospinal fluid (CSF). IEOM include inherited disorders of carbohydrate, amino acid, or fatty acid metabolism.

Why does this infant have hypoglycemia?

The maternal glucose concentration is higher than the fetal concentration over a broad concentration range, and overall glucose flux follows a maternal-to-fetal concentration gradient. During pregnancy, fetal plasma glucose concentration is 70% to 80% that of the maternal venous plasma glucose concentration. Maternal hyperglycemia thus leads to fetal hyperglycemia.

BASIC SCIENCE/CLINICAL PEARL	STEP 1/2/3

In utero, the fetus is completely dependent on maternal glucose transport across the placenta via facilitated diffusion. Fetal glucose production is minimal.

Pregnancy characterized by maternal/fetal hyperglycemia results in prolonged stimulation of fetal insulin release. This induces hyperplasia of the fetal pancreatic β cells. With the clamping of the umbilical cord, the neonate's maternal supply of glucose suddenly ceases, and the neonate develops hypoglycemia because of insufficient substrate, with continued insulin secretion.

Case Point 32.2

Diagnosis:
Hypoglycemia secondary to hyperinsulinemia is seen in infants of diabetic mothers.

What is the treatment of asymptomatic neonatal hypoglycemia?

Onset of hypoglycemia typically occurs within the first few hours of life. IDMs require close blood glucose monitoring after delivery, and frequently need glucose supplementation. Serum or whole blood glucose levels of less than 47 mg/dL within the first 24 hours after birth is abnormal and requires intervention.

In an asymptomatic term infant, an initial attempt at enteral feeding may be successful in reaching target blood glucose values. Use of a standard infant formula will provide carbohydrate in the form of lactose, and provide protein and fat, which are metabolized more slowly and therefore provide a sustained supply of substrate.

BASIC SCIENCE/CLINICAL PEARL	STEP 1/2/3

Fat intake decreases cellular glucose uptake and stimulates gluconeogenesis, further contributing to the restoration of normal glucose homeostasis.

Infants whose blood glucose concentrations normalize following an enteral feeding should continue to have blood glucose concentrations checked before each feeding for 12 to 24 hours. Infants who fail to achieve targeted glucose values by enteral feeds should be considered for intravenous (IV) glucose therapy.

What is the treatment of symptomatic neonatal hypoglycemia?

Immediate IV therapy with 200 mg/kg of dextrose is required in any symptomatic infant with hypoglycemia. A 10% dextrose solution (D_{10}) provides 100 mg/mL of dextrose, so the starting dose is a 2-mL/kg infusion of D_{10} regardless of the presence of enteral feeds. The initial bolus of dextrose should be followed by a continuous infusion of dextrose at a glucose infusion rate of 6 to 8 mg/kg per minute to avoid rebound hypoglycemia. (Carbohydrate infusion dosing is performed in glucose-equivalent units; 1 mg of dextrose provides the carbohydrate equivalent of 1 mg of glucose.)

CLINICAL PEARL	STEP 2/3

A glucose bolus may result in heightened pancreatic insulin release, leading to rebound hypoglycemia.

The blood glucose concentration should be checked approximately 30 minutes after the bolus, and every 1 to 2 hours until euglycemia is achieved. If a subsequent value falls in the hypoglycemic range, the bolus should be repeated, and the glucose infusion rate increased by 2 mg/kg per minute until euglycemia is achieved. Some infants who have transient or sustained hyperinsulinemia may require as much as 12 to 15 mg/kg per minute of IV glucose to maintain normoglycemia.

Case Point 32.3

She is given 20 mL of formula and transferred to the neonatal intensive care unit (NICU). Her blood glucose level 30 minutes after feeding is 11 mg/dL. In the NICU, she is given a 2 mL/kg bolus of D_{10}, and started on a continuous dextrose infusion. Repeat blood glucose level after the bolus was 44 mg/dL.

The IV dextrose infusion is weaned slowly, as the patient is drinking enough formula and breastmilk to maintain appropriate blood glucose levels. Laboratory tests at 12 hours of life were remarkable for a glucose level of 52 mg/dL, a calcium level of 8.2 mg/dL (normal 8.8–10 g/dL), and a magnesium level of 1.5 mg/dL (normal 1.7–2.2 mg/dL).

What are the metabolic complications noted in infants of diabetic mothers?
The most common metabolic complications seen in IDMs are hypoglycemia, hypocalcemia, and hypomagnesemia.

BASIC SCIENCE/CLINICAL PEARL	STEP 1/2/3

In utero, the fetal parathyroid glands are relatively inactive because of the high transplacental flux of calcium. Abnormalities in calcium metabolism likely represent a delayed transition from fetal to neonatal parathyroid control.

Maternal loss of magnesium, due to diabetes, may decrease available magnesium for placental transport to the fetus, resulting in blunted parathyroid hormone secretion, and causing neonatal hypocalcemia and hypomagnesemia. Hypocalcemia is usually asymptomatic in IDMs and resolves without treatment. Hypomagnesemia is also frequently transient and asymptomatic; thus, it usually is not treated.

CLINICAL PEARL	STEP 2/3

Serum calcium concentration should be measured in infants with jitteriness, lethargy, apnea, tachypnea, or seizures, and in those with prematurity, asphyxia, respiratory distress, or suspected infection. Routine screening is not recommended.

BASIC SCIENCE/CLINICAL PEARL	STEP 1/2/3

Hypomagnesemia can reduce both parathyroid hormone (PTH) secretion and responsiveness. Correction of low magnesium levels is critical to successfully treat hypocalcemia.

Case Point 32.4

On day 3, she is noted to appear mildly jaundiced, and her unconjugated bilirubin is 15 mg/dL (normal <13 mg/dL in a premature baby on day 3 of life). She is diagnosed with hyperbilirubinemia and started on phototherapy.

What is the most likely cause of hyperbilirubinemia in this child, beyond physiologic jaundice?

Polycythemia—a central venous hematocrit of more than 65%—is the most common hematologic complication in an IDM. This is thought to be due to fetal hypoxia, resulting from hyperinsulinemia and fluctuations in fetal glucose concentrations that affect fetal oxygen availability. Chronic fetal hypoxia then triggers erythropoiesis to increase the oxygen carrying capacity in the fetus.

BASIC SCIENCE/CLINICAL PEARL   **STEP 1/2/3**

Infants with polycythemia present with a ruddy appearance, sluggish capillary refill, or respiratory distress. Hyperviscosity resulting from polycythemia may cause renal vein thrombosis, stroke, seizures, and necrotizing enterocolitis. To detect polycythemia, the hematocrit should be measured within 12 hours of birth.

Hyperbilirubinemia, commonly seen in IDMs, is likely secondary to the breakdown of an increased number of circulating red blood cells (RBCs) from polycythemia, along with relative immaturity of hepatic bilirubin conjugation and excretion.

Case Point 32.5

The infant's hyperbilirubinemia stabilizes, and her discharge is prepared. During rounds, your attending asks you about congenital abnormalities associated with IDMs.

What are some of the congenital abnormalities seen in infants of diabetic mothers?

Multiple organ systems are susceptible to the teratogenic effects of diabetes:

- Cardiac anomalies, such as transposition of the great arteries, double outlet right ventricle, ventricular septal defect, truncus arteriosus, tricuspid atresia, and patent ductus arteriosus, are more prevalent in IDMs.
- Spinal agenesis–caudal regression syndrome—a syndrome involving varying degrees of developmental failure in the lower lumbar, sacral, and coccygeal vertebrae—is strongly associated with IDMs.
- Structural abnormalities of the central nervous system in IDMs are related to the failure of neural tube closure, and include meningomyelocele, encephalocele, and anencephaly.
- Renal anomalies such as renal agenesis, ureteral duplication, hydronephrosis, cystic kidneys, and renal vein thrombosis can also occur. Infants affected by renal vein thrombosis present with a flank mass due to renal enlargement.
- The most common intestinal anomalies include atresias of the duodenum and rectum. Neonatal small left colon syndrome, also known as neonatal microcolon or lazy colon syndrome, is a transient anomaly unique to IDMs. This condition presents as intestinal obstruction, with affected infants ultimately developing normal function.

Why are infants of diabetic mothers at risk for cardiomyopathy?

Transient hypertrophic cardiomyopathy, noted in 30% of IDMs, is believed to be caused by fetal hyperinsulinemia. Fetal hyperinsulinemia increases the synthesis and deposition of fat and glycogen in myocardial cells. The most prominent change is asymmetric septal hypertrophy, resulting in a reduction of ventricular chamber size and in left ventricular outflow obstruction.

CLINICAL PEARL   STEP 2/3

Respiratory symptoms may be the first sign of cardiomyopathy if not already detected on prenatal ultrasound.

This cardiomyopathy is transient and resolves as plasma insulin concentrations normalize. Symptomatic infants typically recover after 2 to 3 weeks of supportive care, and echocardiographic findings resolve within 6 to 12 months. Supportive care for symptomatic infants includes increased IV fluid administration and β-blockers, such as propranolol. Inotropic agents are contraindicated because they may decrease ventricular size and further obstruct cardiac outflow.

Are infants of diabetic mothers predisposed to congenital malformations?

IDMs have three times the incidence of congenital anomalies than infants of mothers without diabetes. This risk can be reduced by strict glycemic control during the pre- and periconceptual periods (the first 8 weeks of pregnancy). The risk of isolated and multiple congenital anomalies is highest in infants of mothers with uncontrolled pre-gestational diabetes, as noted by an elevated hemoglobin A1c level.

CLINICAL PEARL   STEP 2/3

Preconceptional euglycemia is critical to reduce perinatal complications such as macrosomia and congenital anomalies.

BEYOND THE PEARLS

- Although the fetus has the potential for gluconeogenesis, the actual formation of glucose from pyruvate is not apparent until after birth because the rate-limiting enzyme, phosphoenolpyruvate carboxykinase, appears only after birth in the immediate newborn period.
- A small subgroup of IDMs, usually delivered to mothers who have advanced diabetes with significant vascular disease, may be affected by growth restriction because of compromised nutrient and oxygen delivery to the fetus.
- IDMs with significant macrosomia should be considered for delivery by cesarean section, as they are at increased risk for shoulder dystocia with vaginal delivery. This can lead to brachial plexus injury.
- It is important to examine the IDMs lower back for lumbar, sacral, and coccygeal vertebral anomalies associated with caudal regression syndrome. These can often be associated with lower limb congenital malformations, such as club foot, hypoplastic femur, defects of the tibia and fibula, and knee and hip contractures. Abnormalities of the lower extremities require a thorough neurologic examination and radiographic evaluation.
- Intrauterine exposure to hyperglycemia may result in an increased risk for obesity later in life. Fetal hyperinsulinemia may affect the development of adipose tissue and pancreatic beta cells, leading to an increased body mass index and impaired glucose metabolism. This effect is seen in IDMs as both pregestational and gestational diabetes in adulthood.

Case Summary

Complaint/History: A preterm infant is delivered to a mother with type 2 diabetes mellitus.

Findings: On physical examination, the infant is found to be macrosomic with mild respiratory distress. She does not have any of the other dysmorphic features associated with her mother's condition.

Labs/Tests: She is noted to have a serum glucose level of 10 mg/dL at 1 hour of life. Labs also show hypocalcemia, hypomagnesemia, and an unconjugated hyperbilirubinemia.

Diagnosis: Hypoglycemia secondary to hyperinsulinemia, as seen in infants of diabetic mothers.

Treatment: The infant is given oral formula and an IV dextrose bolus. She is transferred to the NICU, where her serum glucose level is closely monitored. She is gradually weaned off her IV dextrose drip as she is able to achieve euglycemia on oral feeds alone. Her hypocalcemia and hypomagnesemia resolve without intervention. She is placed under phototherapy until her unconjugated bilirubin reaches an acceptable level for discharge.

References

Ashwal E, Hod M. Gestational diabetes mellitus: where are we now? *Clin Chim Acta*. 2015;451:14–20.

Mitanchez D. Foetal and neonatal complications in gestational diabetes: perinatal mortality, congenital malformations, macrosomia, shoulder dystocia, birth injuries, neonatal complications. *Diabetes Metab*. 2010;36:617–627.

Ogata E. Problems of the infant of the diabetic mother. *Neoreviews*. 2010;11:e627–e631.

Teramo K. Diabetic pregnancy and fetal consequences. *Neoreviews*. 2014;15(3):e83–e90.

Weindling MA. Offspring of diabetic pregnancy: short term outcomes. *Semin Fetal Neonatal Med*. 2009;14(2):111–118.

4-Day-Old Male Infant With Yellow Skin Color

Priya Shastry ▧ Monika Alas-Segura ▧ Smeeta Sardesai

A 4-day-old male infant presents with poor feeding and yellow skin color to clinic.

What is the significance of yellow skin in a neonate?

Yellow skin and sclera in a neonate is jaundice, indicating an elevated serum bilirubin level. Neonatal dermal icterus is noticeable at serum bilirubin levels above 4 mg/dL. The yellow color progresses in a cephalocaudal fashion (head to toe), starting at the face at lower bilirubin levels and progressing toward the feet as the serum bilirubin level increases.

What is the mechanism for hyperbilirubinemia?

Bilirubin is a product of heme catabolism from the red blood cells. Heme oxygenase catalyzes the breakdown of heme into carbon monoxide and water-soluble biliverdin. Biliverdin is converted to water-insoluble bilirubin by biliverdin reductase and is subsequently bound to albumin for transport to the liver.

BASIC SCIENCE PEARL	STEP 1

The carbon monoxide produced via heme breakdown is excreted through the lungs and can be measured in the patient's breath to quantify bilirubin production.

In the liver, bilirubin binds to ligandins. Within the hepatocyte, in the endoplasmic reticulum, bilirubin is conjugated with glucuronic acid by the enzyme uridine diphosphate glucuronosyltransferase (UGT1A1). Conjugated bilirubin is then excreted through the bile ducts and stored in the gallbladder. After a meal, bile is excreted into the duodenum.

BASIC SCIENCE PEARL	STEP 1

Conjugated bilirubin is water-soluble, whereas unconjugated bilirubin is not.

When is jaundice normal (physiologic)?

Transient (physiologic) jaundice in the first weeks of life—caused by normal neonatal changes in bilirubin metabolism—is common among healthy neonates. Physiologic jaundice occurs due to a combination of factors, such as a shorter neonatal red blood cell (RBC) life span, less effective binding and transportation of bilirubin (due to lower albumin levels), decreased activity of UGT1A1, and reabsorption of deconjugated bilirubin in the proximal small intestine through the action of β-glucuronidases located in the brush border.

BASIC SCIENCE/CLINICAL PEARL	STEP 1/2/3

60% of term infants and 80% of preterm infants develop jaundice 2 to 4 days after birth. UGT1A1 activity is low at birth but increases to adult values by 4 to 8 weeks of life.

When is jaundice pathologic?

Jaundice is considered to be pathologic when present in the first 24 hours of life, total serum bilirubin (TSB) levels are greater than 95th percentile for age (refer to the nomogram in Fig. 33.1), TSB rises at a rate greater than 0.2 mg/dL per hour, and/or the onset of jaundice is after 2 weeks of age. These scenarios require further workup for alternate causes of hyperbilirubinemia, such as hemolytic disease, sepsis, and genetic mutations (e.g., Crigler-Najjar syndrome and Gilbert syndrome).

BASIC SCIENCE/CLINICAL PEARL	STEP 1/2/3

Jaundice in infants with hepatosplenomegaly, petechiae, and microcephaly require an evaluation for hemolytic anemia, sepsis, and congenital infections.

Case Point 33.1

The infant was born full term, with a birth weight of 2800 g, via normal spontaneous vaginal delivery. There were no complications. His mother's pregnancy was unremarkable. His mother denies any family history of hemolytic disease but remarks that her daughter also required treatment for jaundice as a newborn.

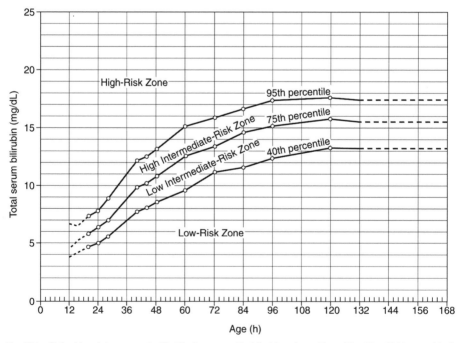

Fig. 33.1 Risk of kernicterus, as stratified by hour-specific bilirubin values. (From Watchko JF. Neonatal indirect hyperbilirubinemia and kernicterus. In: Gleason CA, Juul SE, eds. *Avery's Diseases of the Newborn*. 10th ed. Philadelphia: Elsevier; 2012:1123–1142.)

Case Point 33.2

He was previously breastfeeding every 2 hours, but the frequency has dropped to every 3 to 4 hours. Occasionally, his mother needs to wake him up for feeds. The mother mentions that his suck is not as strong as compared to her prior children. The number of wet diapers per day has decreased as well. He has normal-colored stools daily.

On examination, his sclerae and skin are yellow, he has a mildly sunken fontanelle, is tachycardic, and is sleepy but arousable. There are no subgaleal hematomas, cephalohematomas, or appreciated bruising. His current weight is 2700 g.

What are the risk factors for severe neonatal hyperbilirubinemia?

Hemolytic processes, such as those due to ABO-Rh incompatibility, glucose-6-phosphate dehydrogenase (G6PD) deficiency, and hereditary spherocytosis, increase the risk for hyperbilirubinemia. Infants with congenital infections, polycythemia, cephalohematomas, subgaleal bleeds, bruising, and exclusively breast-fed infants are also at increased risk for developing jaundice. Prematurity of the hepatocytes and slow gastrointestinal motility increase the risk as well. Other risk factors include a history of siblings requiring treatment for jaundice, hypothyroidism, and increased enterohepatic circulation of bilirubin due to delayed meconium passage or bowel obstruction.

The infant in this case has two risk factors for hyperbilirubinemia—suboptimal breastfeeding and a sibling who needed treatment for jaundice.

Which infants need an evaluation for jaundice?

Any infant with history and physical findings suggestive of a pathologic process require a TSB or transcutaneous bilirubinometer (TcB) measurement through the skin. Many centers universally screen all infants with a TSB or TcB prior to discharge from the newborn nursery. The infant in this case warrants evaluation given his history, physical findings of jaundice and dehydration (as evidenced by his tachycardia and sunken fontanelle), and 3.5% weight loss from birth weight.

What is the workup for jaundice?

Once the clinician has a suspicion for jaundice, a TSB, direct bilirubin, complete blood count (CBC) with manual peripheral smear (to evaluate for RBC morphology), reticulocyte count, blood type, Rh determination, direct antiglobulin testing, and serum albumin level should be tested. Bilirubin is bound to albumin in the blood, and low levels of albumin can result in higher levels of unbound bilirubin in the serum, which can lead to toxicity. Measurement of end-tidal carbon monoxide (ETCO) in the breath may assist in identifying infants with increased bilirubin production and thus are at increased risk of developing high bilirubin levels.

BASIC SCIENCE/CLINICAL PEARL   **STEP 1/2/3**

The reticulocyte count provides an indirect insight into accelerated loss and destruction of RBCs when elevated but may be deceptively low in the first few weeks of life due to the physiologic hemoglobin nadir that accompanies the transition from fetal hemoglobin to adult hemoglobin.

Case Point 33.3

A review of his neonatal records indicates that his TSB at 38 hours of life was 9 mg/dL, with a serum conjugated bilirubin level of 1 mg/dL. His newborn screen was normal, and he and his mother have the same blood type, AB+; direct antiglobulin testing was negative. Laboratory tests ordered on admission, at 96 hours of life, demonstrated a TSB of 15 mg/dL and direct bilirubin level of 0.8 mg/dL. His albumin, CBC, and peripheral smear were normal for his age. He did not have jaundice on the first day of life.

What is the cause of jaundice in the infant in this case?

The most likely cause of jaundice in this infant is breastfeeding jaundice. His history and examination are consistent with dehydration and poor caloric intake, and his laboratory test results do not demonstrate immune-mediated hemolysis or a conjugated hyperbilirubinemia. His TSB is less than the 95th percentile at 96 hours (per the nomogram in Fig. 33.1), and the TSB rate of increase is 0.1 mg/dL per hour, suggesting that this is less likely to be pathologic hyperbilirubinemia.

Diagnosis: Breastfeeding jaundice.

What is the relationship between jaundice and breastfeeding in a neonate?

There are two patterns of jaundice noted in breast-fed infants, breastfeeding jaundice and breast milk jaundice. Early-onset breastfeeding jaundice, also known as breastfeeding failure jaundice, is seen in the first week of life. It is believed to be due to decreased volume and frequency of feeds, resulting in relative caloric deprivation, mild dehydration, and delayed passage of meconium in the first few days of life. Early and frequent breastfeeding increases stooling and decreases transit time through the intestine and enterohepatic circulation of bilirubin. The second is breast milk jaundice, seen in the second to sixth weeks of life, and up to 3 months of age in some infants.

This infant's history suggests that he may have breastfeeding failure jaundice.

BASIC SCIENCE PEARL   **STEP 1**

Breast milk jaundice is thought to be due to the presence of β-glucuronidase in breast milk, which enhances intestinal bilirubin reabsorption. In addition, non-esterified fatty acids and lipases in some breast milks may inhibit hepatic UGT1A1, thus disrupting normal bilirubin metabolism

---

What is the treatment for neonatal jaundice?

The primary preferred treatment option for unconjugated hyperbilirubinemia is phototherapy. Phototherapy has three mechanisms of action. The principal mechanism is irreversible structural photoisomerization of bilirubin to the more water-soluble lumirubin. The second mechanism is configurational photoisomerization, which is reversible. The photoisomers of bilirubin are excreted in the bile and, to some extent, in the urine. The third mechanism is a photooxidation reaction that converts bilirubin to a colorless polar compound, which is excreted primarily in the urine.

BASIC SCIENCE PEARL   **STEP 1**

Phototherapy blunts the rate of rise of TSB in almost all cases of hyperbilirubinemia, regardless of the cause of the hyperbilirubinemia. Phototherapy using light in the 460- to 490-nm range (blue light) wavelength is most effective.

A double-volume exchange transfusion, which replaces approximately 85% of the infant's circulating RBCs, is indicated in patients for whom phototherapy is not effective or in infants with signs of bilirubin-induced neurologic dysfunction (BIND). Exchange transfusion is especially useful in cases of isoimmune hemolysis because circulating antibodies and sensitized RBCs also are removed along with the bilirubin.

Should the child be allowed to continue breastfeeding?

Formula supplementation may be necessary in infants who lose more than 10% of their birth weight, but breastfeeding should be continued to maintain breast milk production. Supplemental water or dextrose-water administration should be avoided because it places the newborn at risk for iatrogenic hyponatremia. Other causes of hyperbilirubinemia should be eliminated as contributing factors in breast-fed babies.

Case Point 33.4

This infant's TSB was in the high-intermediate risk zone and he was placed under phototherapy for 24 hours. Lactation specialists worked with the mother and infant to optimize breastfeeding. At 120 hours of life, his TSB had decreased to 10 mg/dL, his feeding improved, and he gained weight. He was discharged home with follow-up in 2 days. His mother asks about potential long-term complications of his hyperbilirubinemia.

What are the long-term neurologic manifestations of hyperbilirubinemia?

The most serious and concerning consequence of severe hyperbilirubinemia is the development of BIND. The fat-soluble nature of unconjugated bilirubin allows it to cross the blood-brain barrier and cause cell death by apoptosis and necrosis. The early manifestations of BIND are referred to as *acute bilirubin encephalopathy* (ABE), and the chronic and permanent sequelae is termed *kernicterus*. In the first few days of life, the infant can present with fever, lethargy, hypotonia, and a high-pitched cry, followed by the development of retrocollis (backward arching of the neck) and opisthotonus (backward arching of the back). Brain regions most commonly involved in BIND include the basal ganglia, oculomotor, and cochlear cranial nerve nuclei. Features of kernicterus include abnormalities in the extrapyramidal, visual, and auditory systems that evolve slowly over the first several years of life in the affected infant. Seizures are not typically associated with acute bilirubin encephalopathy.

Case Point 33.5

Because this infant's bilirubin levels were less than 20 mg/dL, he is assessed to be at a low risk for BIND. His mother is reassured that his poor feeding is likely from poor suck-swallow coordination, not encephalopathy.

BEYOND THE PEARLS

- G6PD deficiency testing should be considered if either parent is of Mediterranean, Nigerian, or East Asian ancestry.
- Drugs that displace bilirubin from albumin and increase the risk of hyperbilirubinemia include ceftriaxone, chloramphenicol, vitamin K, ascorbic acid, antimalaria medications, and sulfa-containing compounds.
- Adverse effects of phototherapy include increased body and environmental temperatures, resulting in increased insensible fluid loss. Although the effect of phototherapy on the eyes of infants is not known, animal studies have indicated that retinal degeneration may occur after 24 hours of continuous exposure, so eye patches are placed during therapy. Phototherapy can cause severe blistering and photosensitivity in patients with porphyria. Phototherapy can produce the bronze baby syndrome in infants with direct hyperbilirubinemia, in which the skin develops a dark, grayish-brown discoloration. When phototherapy is stopped, the cholestasis resolves, and the coloration disappears.
- The bilirubin-to-albumin (B:A) ratio can be used as an additional factor in determining the need for exchange transfusion in conjunction with TSB values. In term neonates, a B:A ratio >7.0 (bilirubin in mg/dL, albumin in g/dL) indicates that all bilirubin-binding sites on albumin are occupied. Any further increase in the bilirubin level would be associated with exponentially increasing levels of free bilirubin.
- The long-term complications of kernicterus include choreoathetoid cerebral palsy, high-frequency sensorineural hearing loss, limitation of upward gaze, and dental enamel hypoplasia.

Case Summary

Complaint/History: A full-term, 4-day-old male presents with yellow skin and poor feeding. He has decreased frequency of breastfeeding and number of wet diapers. He was not noted to be jaundiced at birth. He has pigmented stools.

Findings: His physical examination is significant for skin and scleral icterus, a sunken fontanelle, tachycardia, and no obvious hematoma, bruising, or bleeding.

Labs/Tests: Labs reveal a total serum bilirubin of 15 mg/dL and a conjugated bilirubin level of 0.8 mg/dL at 96 hours of life. His newborn screen was normal, and he had the same blood type as his mother. The serum albumin level, complete blood cell count, and manual peripheral smear were all normal.

Diagnosis: Breastfeeding jaundice.

Treatment: He received phototherapy for 24 hours, and lactation specialists worked with the mother and infant to optimize breastfeeding. At 120 hours of life, his total serum bilirubin had decreased to 10 mg/dL and he had gained adequate weight. He was discharged home, with close follow-up.

Bibliography

Bhutani VK, Johnson L, Sivieri EM. Predictive ability of a predischarge hour-specific serum bilirubin for subsequent significant hyperbilirubinemia in healthy term and near-term newborns. *Pediatrics.* 1999;103(1):6–14.

Dani C, Martelli E, Bertini G, et al. Plasma bilirubin level and oxidative stress in preterm infants. *Arch Dis Child Fetal Neonatal.* 2003;88(2):F119–F123.

Lauer BJ, Spector ND. Hyperbilirubinemia in the newborn. *Pediatr Rev.* 2011;32(8):341–349.

Maheshwari A, Carlo WA, Maheshwari A, et al. Digestive system disorders. In: *Nelson Textbook of Pediatrics.* 20th ed. Philadelphia: Elsevier; 2016:867–880.e1.

16-Year-Old Female With Nausea, Emesis, Icterus, and Abdominal Pain

Alauna K. Hersch ▓ Quin Y. Liu

A 16-year-old female ballerina presents to the emergency room with a 2-day history of yellowing of her eyes, followed by acute onset epigastric abdominal pain, nausea, and nonbloody, nonbilious emesis.

What is your differential diagnosis?

The differential diagnosis for jaundice and abdominal pain includes acute hepatitis (e.g., viral hepatitis), which presents with right upper quadrant abdominal pain and jaundice; gallstone complications (e.g., cholecystitis, choledocholithiasis, gallstone ileus, pancreatitis), often presenting with right upper quadrant abdominal pain with or without jaundice in a patient predisposed to gallstones (due to obesity, chronic total parenteral nutrition use, medications); autoimmune hepatitis, presenting either as acute and severe disease (i.e., acute liver failure), or insidious disease with fatigue, jaundice, abdominal pain, and arthralgias; Wilson disease, with a presentation varying widely from asymptomatic to acute or chronic hepatitis to neurologic abnormalities with or without hepatitis (changes in behavior, micrographia, tremor), or psychiatric abnormalities.

Case Point 34.1

She is otherwise healthy but admits to intentional weight loss of 15 pounds in the 2 months in preparation for an upcoming dance recital. Her previous body mass index (BMI) was 30 kg/m². She denies travel history, sexual activity, and the use of prescribed or illicit drugs. Her mother states her immunizations are up to date.

Why is it important to know a patient's BMI and ask about weight loss or weight gain?

An abnormally high BMI predisposes patients to a variety of gastrointestinal and hepatic medical problems, including cholelithiasis, nonalcoholic steatohepatitis and pancreatitis.

CLINICAL PEARL   **STEP 2/3**

Complications of nonalcoholic fatty liver disease (NAFLD), often asymptomatic, can be seen in patients with obesity. These complications include type 2 diabetes, dyslipidemia, and hypertension.

Weight loss or gain may be intentional or unintentional. Unintentional weight loss can be seen in various types of cancer, inflammatory bowel disease, and rheumatologic diseases.

BASIC SCIENCE/CLINICAL PEARL   **STEP 1/2/3**

Rapid weight loss can cause loss of the fat pad under the superior mesenteric artery, leading to duodenal compression. This condition, known as superior mesenteric artery syndrome, presents with abdominal pain and bilious emesis.

Case Point 34.2

She is ill-appearing, but afebrile. Her pulse rate is 95 beats/min, respiration rate is 13/min, blood pressure is 137/85 mmHg, and oxygen saturation is 99% on room air. On physical examination, she appears thin, with decreased subcutaneous fat stores. She has adequate muscle bulk. She appears well-hydrated. Scleral icterus is prominent, and her abdomen is tender in the epigastric region, with guarding but without rebound. She does not have hepatosplenomegaly or ascites. Neurologically, she is alert and awake and oriented to person, place, and time. She has no skin rashes or abnormal bruising. Her physical examination is otherwise unremarkable.

What is the most likely diagnosis based on the findings thus far?

Given her acute weight loss, emesis, and acute onset pain in the epigastrium, pancreatitis due to gallstones is high in the differential. She is also the right age and gender for the presentation of autoimmune hepatitis. She is also the prime age for hepatitis due to Epstein-Barr virus. Other causes of viral hepatitis seem less likely, given that she denies a travel history (for hepatitis A), her immunizations are up to date (she should have been vaccinated for hepatitis B), and she denies being sexually active or using intravenous drugs (for hepatitis C).

What laboratory tests are indicated in this patient?

Elevations in serum amylase and lipase levels may be diagnostic of acute pancreatitis. The diagnosis is supported by abdominal pain consistent with pancreatitis (mid-epigastrium which may radiate to the back), high serum amylase and lipase, and features of acute pancreatitis on radiographic imaging.

Obtaining a fractionated bilirubin level (to determine if the jaundice is due to unconjugated versus conjugated bilirubin), as well as a liver panel, including aspartate aminotransferase (AST), alanine aminotransferase (ALT), prothrombin time (PT), and gamma-glutamyltransferase (GGT), can help distinguish liver pathology and cholestasis from hemolysis. Hemolysis would result in elevations of unconjugated bilirubin, and AST would be higher than ALT. GGT, which is specific for the biliary system's cholangiocytes, would not be elevated with hemolysis. A prolonged PT may indicate liver failure in the absence of other causes.

A complete blood cell count should be obtained to evaluate for pancytopenia, which can be associated with severe liver dysfunction, or leukocytosis, which can be seen with pancreatitis. The hemoglobin and hematocrit would be low with hemolysis, and the peripheral smear may show schistocytes (fragmented red blood cells). The serum lactate dehydrogenase (LDH) level would be elevated and the serum haptoglobin level would be decreased with hemolysis. A low platelet count may indicate chronic liver disease due to portal hypertension, with splenic sequestration of platelets. In most hemolytic anemias, the platelet count is normal.

A chemistry panel should be obtained to evaluate for the degree of dehydration and electrolyte abnormalities, which can predispose to abdominal pain and nausea (e.g., hypokalemia).

Case Point 34.3

Laboratory tests are remarkable for an amylase level of 1680 U/L (normal 23–85 U/L), lipase level of 2345 U/L (normal 200–300 U/L), total bilirubin of 5.4 mg/dL (normal 0.1–1.2 mg/dL), conjugated bilirubin of 2.4 mg/dL (normal <0.3 mg/dL), AST of 200 U/L (normal 8–48 U/L), and ALT of 234 U/L (normal 7–55 U/L).

Pancreatitis is diagnosed, and gallstone pancreatitis is suspected.

What are the common symptoms of pancreatitis?

The most common presentations of pancreatitis include abdominal pain (seen in 80%–95% of patients), nausea/emesis (seen in 40%–80% of patients), and abdominal distention (seen in 21%–46% of patients). Pancreatitis can be acute (short presentation of onset), chronic (lasting for weeks to months), recurrent (clearance of the disease with relapse), hereditary (seen in cystic fibrosis and mutations in trypsin and trypsin inhibitors), hemorrhagic (bleeding into the gland), and necrotic (death of the gland with a high rate of mortality). Fortunately, most cases of young children with acute-onset pancreatitis resolve quickly without sequelae. The other forms of pancreatitis listed here can result in severe complications, including shock, renal failure, acute respiratory distress syndrome, and chronic malnutrition.

BASIC SCIENCE/CLINICAL PEARL	STEP 1/2/3

The incidence of pancreatitis in the pediatric population is increasing. This has correlated with the obesity epidemic and increased presentations of gallstones in pediatrics.

What are the most common causes of pancreatitis?

The most common cause of pancreatitis in children is cholelithiasis or gallbladder sludge, which account for 10%–30% of cases. Other causes (from most to least common in occurrence) include medications (26%; e.g., valproic acid, prednisone, mesalamine, trimethoprim/sulfamethoxazole, 6-mercaptopurine/azathioprine, tacrolimus), idiopathic (20%; most likely due to an unidentified viral cause), systemic (10%; sepsis/systemic diseases), trauma (9%), identified viral infection (8%), metabolic disease (5%), endoscopic retrograde cholangiopancreatography (4%), cystic fibrosis (2%), and alcohol (1%).

BASIC SCIENCE/CLINICAL PEARL	STEP 1/2/3

In adults, gallstones and alcoholism account for the majority of cases of acute pancreatitis.

What is the next step?

In the setting of elevated serum lipase and conjugated bilirubin levels, the next step is to order an abdominal ultrasound (US). The abdominal US is not to evaluate the pancreas, but rather to evaluate for biliary causes of pancreatitis, such as cholelithiasis (presence of gallstones) and choledocholithiasis (presence of stones in the common bile duct). An US can also be helpful to evaluate underlying anatomic abnormalities, such as choledochal cysts, annular pancreas, and pancreatic divisum, which can also be associated with pancreatitis. The normal developmental embryology of the pancreas is seen in Fig. 34.1.

BASIC SCIENCE/CLINICAL PEARL	STEP 1/2/3

Choledochal cysts are congenital cystic dilations of the intrahepatic and/or extrahepatic biliary tree. They require resection due to the increased risk of contributing to the development of biliary malignancy.

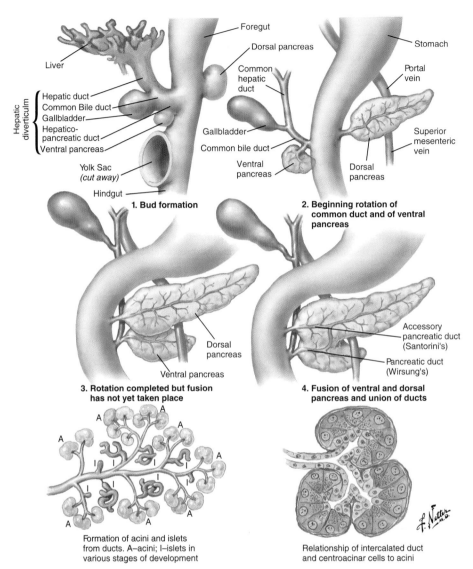

Fig. 34.1 Embryology of the pancreas. 1 Formation of the dorsal and ventral buds from duodenal-level endoderm at 4-weeks' gestation. 2–4 Rotation of the ventral pancreas and common bile duct to fuse with the dorsal pancreas. (Netter medical illustration used with permission of Elsevier. All rights reserved.)

BASIC SCIENCE/CLINICAL PEARL   **STEP 1/2/3**

Annular pancreas is a rare anomaly associated with abnormal embryologic development of the pancreas. This occurs when there is a ring of pancreatic tissue around the second portion of the duodenum. It is associated with low birth weight, feeding problems, and polyhydramnios (a large amount of fluid in the amniotic sac during pregnancy). It is thought to occur in 1 in 12,000–15,000 live births and requires surgical correction if symptomatic.

BASIC SCIENCE / CLINICAL PEARL	STEP 1/2/3

Pancreatic divisum occurs when there is failure of the ventral and dorsal pancreas to fuse. It is estimated that up to 10% of embryos have this abnormality. However, most individuals with this condition will remain asymptomatic, and it can be found incidentally on autopsy. If symptomatic, various surgeries can be attempted to stent, enlarge, or bypass the affected ducts to improve drainage.

Although the likelihood of choledocholithiasis is higher in patients with dilated bile ducts and elevated liver enzymes, an abdominal US can miss a significant portion of patients with stones in the common bile duct. If bilirubin continues to remain elevated, despite the normal appearance of the bile ducts on US, the next best step is to obtain a magnetic resonance cholangiopancreatography (MRCP), which has high sensitivity and specificity in identifying choledocholithiasis as the cause of the pancreatitis.

Case Point 34.4

An abdominal US is obtained which demonstrates normal liver size and echogenicity, and stones visualized in the gallbladder, cystic duct, and common bile duct (Figs. 34.2 and 34.3). The pancreas appears heterogeneous with edema, and no peripancreatic fluid collections are visualized.

Diagnosis: Gallstone pancreatitis.

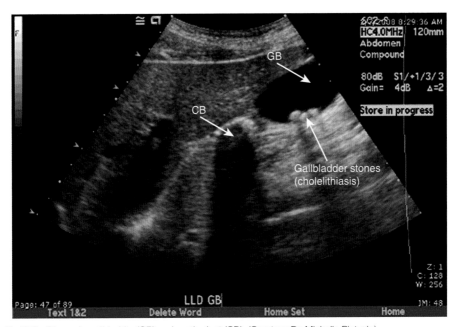

Fig. 34.2 Stones in gallbladder (GB) and cystic duct (CD). (Courtesy Dr. Michelle Pietzak.)

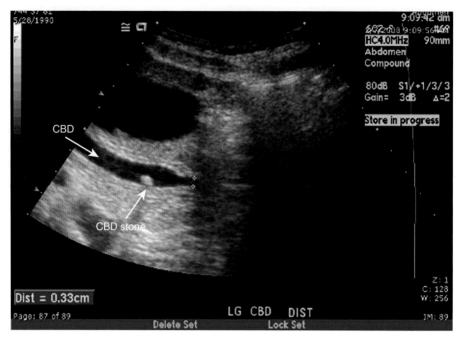

Fig. 34.3   Stone in common bile duct (CBD). (Courtesy Dr. Michelle Pietzak.)

How do gallstones cause pancreatitis?

When gallstones obstruct the bile ducts, the pancreatic enzymes cannot get released into the third portion of the duodenum through the ampulla of Vater. These digestive enzymes then go retrograde into the pancreatic tissue, causing inflammation and edema.

How is pancreatitis treated acutely?

The management of pancreatitis includes initial bowel rest, fluid resuscitation, and pain management. If emesis is persistent due to ileus, a nasogastric (NG) tube can be placed to low intermittent suction. Early initiation of feeds has been shown to decrease morbidity and mortality. Parenteral nutrition should be started via a central line if the patient is expected to be unable to take enteral feeds for more than 3 days. Duodenal acidification can be reduced by giving oral or parenteral histamine-2 receptor antagonists.

Complete pain relief may be difficult, as many opiates have been implicated to worsen pancreatitis symptoms by causing spasm of the sphincter of Oddi. Meperidine has been reported to have the least effect on enterobiliary pressures. Hydromorphone can also be used for pain relief.

If there are clinical signs of sepsis, multiorgan failure or necrosis of the gland, antibiotics should be considered.

CLINICAL PEARL   **STEP 2/3**

Patients may become extremely ill with unstable hemodynamics, such as tachycardia and hypotension, indicative of systemic inflammatory response syndrome (SIRS). These patients require aggressive fluid resuscitation and intensive care monitoring.

Case Point 34.5

The patient is admitted to the hospital and an order is placed to restrict her from all oral intake. She is started on a high-rate intravenous saline infusion. The following morning, her AST has decreased to 100 U/L, ALT to 120 U/L, and total bilirubin to 4 mg/dL.

What is the next best step?

Patients with choledocholithiasis found on imaging studies—as well as any patient with clinical signs of cholangitis (e.g., fever, jaundice, right upper quadrant pain ± elevated white blood cell count and/or clinical signs of sepsis)—require an endoscopic retrograde cholangiopancreatography (ERCP) for duct decompression and stone retrieval.

CLINICAL PEARL   **STEP 2/3**

ERCP is not only a diagnostic procedure for choledocholithiasis, but it can be therapeutic as well, as the operator can remove stones and place stents for drainage. Unfortunately, ERCP can inadvertently result in iatrogenic pancreatitis in about 20% of cases.

Case Point 34.6

The patient undergoes ERCP and choledocholithiasis is found during the procedure. Stones are retrieved from the common bile duct via a basket. A sphincterotomy is performed and a stent is placed to allow further drainage. Over the next 3 days, the patient's pancreatitis resolves, and she is able to be weaned to exclusive oral nutrition. She and her family receive nutritional and weight management counseling from a registered dietician. She is scheduled for a laparoscopic cholecystectomy prior to discharge.

BEYOND THE PEARLS

- In adult studies, abdominal adiposity has been associated with an increased risk of pancreatitis. The cause has yet to be determined, but in animal models it is thought to be due to the increased cytokines associated with adipose tissue.
- Even if choledocholithiasis was not found at the time of pancreatitis, it does not necessarily mean that gallstones were not the cause. A gallstone can still pass through the bile duct and lodge in the papilla, having caused temporary pancreatic duct obstruction leading to pancreatitis, prior to it passing through the papilla and into the intestinal tract.
- People with pancreatic divisum are thought to be protected against gallstone pancreatitis, as the pancreas would drain though the minor papilla via the duct of Santorini. Therefore, if a gallstone were to pass into the papilla, the pancreas would still drain through the minor papilla without obstruction.
- In cases of severe pain due to chronic pancreatitis, an ERCP with sphincterotomy +/− stent placement may be considered to reduce pressure in the gland, even if choledocholithiasis is not present.
- The Puestow procedure can also be considered for patients with chronic, unremitting pain due to pancreatitis. Also called a *longitudinal pancreaticojejunostomy,* this surgery creates a permanent side-to-side anastomosis between the pancreatic duct and jejunum.

Case Summary

Complaint/History: A 16-year-old female presents to the emergency room with acute onset of yellow eyes, epigastric pain, and vomiting. Her history is significant for an intentional weight loss of 15 pounds in 2 months.

Findings: Physical examination reveals an ill-appearing, thin teenage female in moderate pain. She has scleral icterus and moderate epigastric pain with guarding.

Labs/Tests: Labs are significant for an elevated amylase, lipase, total bilirubin, conjugated bilirubin, AST and ALT level. An abdominal ultrasound demonstrates stones in the gallbladder, cystic duct, and common bile duct.

Diagnosis: Gallstone pancreatitis.

Treatment: She is treated with hydration, bowel rest, and intravenous acid-blockage and pain medications. An endoscopic retrograde pancreatography reveals multiple stones in the common bile duct, which were retrieved with a basket. A sphincterotomy and a stent are performed endoscopically. Her diet is advanced, her pain medications are weaned, and she is scheduled for laparoscopic cholecystectomy prior to discharge.

Bibliography

Bai HX, Lowe ME, Husain SZ. What have we learned about acute pancreatitis in children? *J Pediatr Gastroenterol Nutr*. 2011;52(3):262–270.

Hong S, Qiwen B, Ying J, et al. Body mass index and the risk and prognosis of acute pancreatitis: a meta-analysis. *Eur J Gastroenterol Hepatol*. 2011;23(12):1136–1143.

Maple JT, Ben-Menachem T, Anderson MA, et al. The role of endoscopy in the evaluation of suspected choledocholithiasis. *Gastrointest Endosc*. 2010;71(1):1–9.

Sadr-Azodi O, Orsini N, Andrén-Sandberg Å, et al. Abdominal and total adiposity and the risk of acute pancreatitis: a population-based prospective cohort study. *Am J Gastroenterol*. 2013;108(1):133–139.

Şurlin V, Săftoiu A, Dumitrescu D. Imaging tests for accurate diagnosis of acute biliary pancreatitis. *World J Gastroenterol*. 2014;20(44):16544–16549.

Szabo FK, Fei L, Cruz LA, et al. Early enteral nutrition and aggressive fluid resuscitation are associated with improved clinical outcomes in acute pancreatitis. *J Pediatr*. 2015;167(2):397–402.e1.

18-Month-Old Male With Vomiting and Altered Mental Status

Solomon Behar

An 18-month-old male is seen in the pediatric emergency department (ED) for vomiting for 2 hours. The mother noted that after he vomited, he became difficult to arouse. The patient had a rapid return to baseline by the time of arrival to the pediatric ED and now appears well.

What is the differential diagnosis?

Vomiting and altered mental status is a concerning presentation with unique causes in the toddler years. Differential diagnoses include head injury, toxic ingestions, central nervous system (CNS) infections, hydrocephalus, electrolyte and metabolic abnormalities, renal insufficiency, and CNS bleeds from trauma or vascular lesions (e.g., arteriovenous malformation, vasculitis). Additionally, non-accidental head trauma (i.e., child abuse) should always be a consideration in the preverbal or minimally verbal child who is unable to report this injury. Gastrointestinal (GI) illnesses, such as intussusception, appendicitis, and malrotation with volvulus, can present with emesis and altered mental status in a young child.

CLINICAL PEARL	**STEP 2/3**

Determining whether a child in this age group had access to other household members' medications is vital, as unintentional, potentially fatal ingestions commonly occur in this age group.

Case Point 35.1

The mother states that the child has not had fevers, diarrhea, bloody stools, polyuria, polydipsia, weight loss, headaches, or changes in his urine output or quality. The rest of the review of systems is negative.

How does the negative focused review of systems help narrow the differential diagnosis?

An absence of fever helps narrow the differential diagnosis away from infectious processes such as meningitis, urinary tract infection, and viral gastroenteritis. Polyuria (abnormally excessive or frequent passage of urine) and polydipsia (abnormally excessive thirst or drinking) are worrisome for hyperglycemia, most likely due to type I diabetes in this age group. Urinary tract infections can present with vomiting, dehydration, and altered mental status.

CLINICAL PEARL	**STEP 2/3**

Be wary of giving the diagnosis of viral gastroenteritis to patients who experience vomiting without diarrhea, as there are many serious, potentially life-threatening diagnoses that may be missed.

CLINICAL PEARL   **STEP 2/3**

In any patient presenting with vomiting, obtain a surgical history. Patients with prior history of abdominal surgery can have adhesions leading to small bowel obstruction. This can present with vomiting (often bilious), abdominal distention, and altered mental status due to dehydration and/or electrolyte abnormalities.

Case Point 35.2

His vital signs show a temperature of 37°C, pulse rate of 116/min, respiratory rate of 28/min, blood pressure of 97/58 mm Hg, and an oxygen saturation of 100% on room air. The physical examination reveals a well-appearing toddler. His abdomen is soft, without mass, and has active bowel sounds. He has a normal neurologic examination. There is no evidence of trauma or macrocephaly.

What physical examination findings can assist in narrowing the differential diagnosis?
In a toddler with mental status changes, accurate vital signs looking for Cushing triad and performing the Glasgow Coma Scale (GCS) are essential to evaluate whether the patient's altered mental status is due to a CNS disturbance requiring emergent intervention (e.g., intracranial hemorrhage) (Fig. 35.1). The GCS may need to be modified for younger or developmentally delayed pediatric patients.

CLINICAL PEARL   **STEP 2/3**

Cushing's triad consists of vital sign abnormalities that suggest elevated intracranial pressure with herniation. It includes high blood pressure, bradycardia, and irregular Cheyne-Stokes respirations. This pattern of breathing, also called *agonal breathing* is a repetitive pattern of hyperpnea (deep and rapid breaths), followed by shallower respirations and eventually apnea (complete cessation of breathing).

It is also important to note the toddler's anthropometrics—weight, length, weight for length, and head circumference. Macrocephaly (a large head in proportion to weight and length) can be an ominous sign of hydrocephalus (excessive cerebrospinal fluid within the brain) or a space-occupying lesion (such as a brain tumor). Physical examination findings suggestive of skull fracture include blood behind the tympanic membrane (hemotympanum), bruising in the area posterior to the ear (Battle's sign), step-offs in the surface continuity of the skull, and scalp hematomas (especially in non-frontal areas).

In this patient, who appears well with a normal neurologic examination a CNS cause becomes less likely. The GI causes should be considered more thoroughly, particularly those that can present with intermittent altered mental status (e.g., intussusception).

Case Point 35.3

After an hour of observation in the ED, the patient suddenly starts crying while holding his abdomen. He has a small amount of nonbloody, nonbilious emesis. After vomiting, he becomes immediately somnolent, without any evidence of desaturation or seizure-like activity. A repeat abdominal examination demonstrates a sausage-like fullness in the right upper quadrant of the abdomen. There are no focal neurologic deficits beyond him being sleepy. On rectal examination, a stool guaiac test is positive.

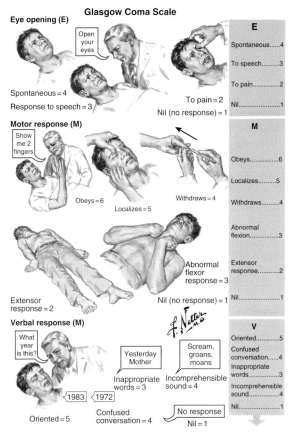

Fig. 35.1 Glasgow Coma Scale. (Netter medical illustration used with permission of Elsevier. All rights reserved.)

CLINICAL PEARL	**STEP 2/3**

Observation and reassessment of patients who look well, but have a concerning history, is a good strategy to help clarify the clinical picture. In this case, a new physical finding helped guide testing and led to the correct diagnosis.

BASIC SCIENCE/CLINICAL PEARL	**STEP 1/2/3**

The stool guaiac test detects occult (hidden) blood from a stool sample. This is useful if the stool is not grossly bloody. A thin layer of stool is smeared on a test card coated with guaiac, a substance from a plant. Drops of indicator fluid change the color.

What is the most probable diagnosis at this point in time?

Leading the list of probable diagnoses at this point in time is intussusception, due to the presence of emesis, mass in the right upper quadrant, positive stool guaiac, and the patient's age. Other considerations for this age group would include a toxic ingestion of a medication, intracranial pathology such as an intracranial bleed (due to accidental or nonaccidental trauma), or a space-occupying mass, such as a brain tumor. Other causes of intestinal obstruction (e.g., malrotation with volvulus), gastroenteritis, new-onset diabetes with ketoacidosis, appendicitis, renal failure, and urinary tract infection are still on the differential but are less likely.

What is the next step?

When intussusception is suspected, radiographic evidence should be sought. Classic findings on plain abdominal films (popularly known as a *KUB—kidney, ureter, bladder—*radiograph) include the paucity of air in the right lower quadrant, and a target or a crescent sign outlining the tip of the apex of the intussusception. However, sensitivity of the KUB for intussusception is poor at around 25% to 45%. Ultrasound is much more sensitive (98%–100%), and specific (88%–100%) for intussusception. A doughnut or target sign is seen on cross section of the bowel. Longitudinal views of the intussusceptum may show a double-walled bowel, representing the small bowel within the large bowel.

Case Point 35.4

A radiograph of the abdomen demonstrates a paucity of gas in the right lower quadrant and proximal dilation of small bowel (Fig. 35.2). Abdominal ultrasound demonstrates an ileoileocolic intussusception (Fig. 35.3).

Diagnosis: Idiopathic ileoileocolic intussusception.

What is intussusception? Why does it occur?

Intussusception occurs when one portion of the bowel telescopes into the adjoining bowel. It is one of the most common surgical emergencies in the toddler age-range. The most common types of intussusception are ileoileocolic (ileum into the cecum) and ileoileal (ileum into ileum), as illustrated in Fig. 35.4. This is due to the presence of Peyer's patches in the distal ileum.

What are the most common causes of intussusception?

Idiopathic intussusception accounts for 90% of cases, and is often associated with preceding viral infections, most notably adenovirus. The peak age for this condition is between 6 months and 3 years of age, with 80% of cases occurring prior to 2 years of age. Some speculate that hypertrophied Peyer's patches in the ileocolic region act as a lead point, allowing the terminal ileum to telescope and get stuck in the proximal colon. About 5% of cases occur outside of the typical age range. These cases are often not idiopathic; a "lead point" such as bowel wall edema from vasculitis (e.g., Henoch-Schönlein purpura), or mass (e.g., Meckel's diverticulum, polyps, lymphoma, mesenteric cysts, or intestinal duplications) can often be identified.

How does intussusception present?

The classic symptoms of intussusception are colicky intermittent abdominal pain, vomiting, and/ or currant jelly stools (a late finding indicative of bowel necrosis). All three symptoms are present in 10% to 82% of cases. Other signs and symptoms may include loud crying or grunting with the pain, pulling the knees up to the chest with relief of pain, and a period of somnolence when the pain resolves.

BASIC SCIENCE/CLINICAL PEARL   **STEP 1/2/3**

In about 17% of cases, lethargy or hypotonia may be the only presenting finding of intussusception, so do not forget to include it in your differential diagnosis of the altered infant or toddler.

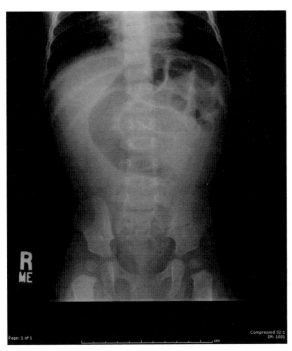

Fig. 35.2 Plain film KUB demonstrating a paucity of air in the right lower quadrant and dilation of the small bowel. (Courtesy Dr. Solomon Behar.)

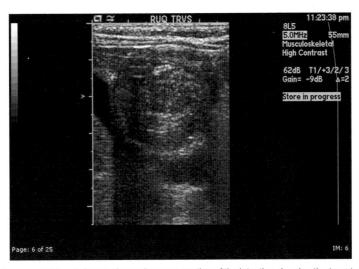

Fig. 35.3 Ultrasound of the abdomen shows the cross section of the intestine showing the target or doughnut sign consistent with intussusception. The terminal ileum is telescoping into the proximal cecum, leading to intestinal obstruction. (Courtesy Dr. Solomon Behar.)

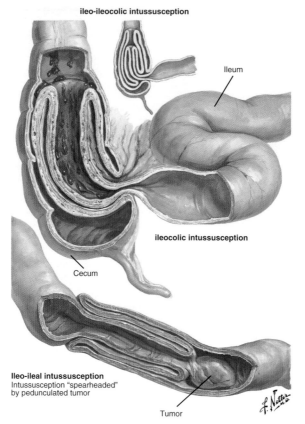

Fig. 35.4   Ileoileocolic and ileoileal intussusception. (Netter medical illustration used with permission of Elsevier. All rights reserved.)

How should this patient be managed?

The initial treatment of intussusception is with either an air or barium enema. The pressure from the air or barium is able to reduce the intussusception by forcing the telescoping ileum back out of the cecum and/or ascending colon. Reduction rates for air enemas range from 60% to 90%, and for barium/aqueous contrast, 60% to 80%. When an enema successfully reduces the intussusception, these children are usually admitted for observation, as up to 10% can recur.

If an initial attempt at nonoperative reduction fails, surgical reduction is necessary. Additionally, bowel perforation during reduction would be an indication for immediate surgery. It is ideal to have an experienced pediatric surgeon in the radiographic suite at the time of reduction of the intussusception.

What complications can occur from intussusception?

Delays in diagnosis of intussusception result in increased rates of requiring surgery and complications. The longer the intussusceptum is present, the more likely the small and large intestine are to undergo obstruction, perforation, or ischemia. This can result in bowel resection, and the patient is at higher risk for the development of sepsis.

CLINICAL PEARL	STEP 2/3

Sepsis is a systemic inflammatory response syndrome (SIRS) in the setting of an identified infection. Symptoms of SIRS include fever (or hypothermia), tachycardia (fast heart rate), tachypnea (rapid breathing), and elevated peripheral white blood cell count. SIRS/sepsis in the setting of ileocolic intussusception is rare but ominous.

Importantly, treatment with an air or barium enema should be performed at an experienced center, and a surgical team with an available operative room should be available on standby. Bowel perforation occurs in approximately 1% of nonoperative reduction procedures and is a medical emergency. Tension pneumoperitoneum resulting from bowel perforation and leading to hypoventilation is rare but may be deadly if not rapidly reversed.

Case Point 35.5

Intravenous fluids and antibiotics are started in the ED. Pediatric surgery is consulted, and the patient is shuttled back to the radiology suite for an air enema. The air enema successfully reduces the intussusception on the first attempt.

The patient was admitted for observation and discharged on hospital day 2 without complications.

BEYOND THE PEARLS

- Intussusception is the most common cause of small intestinal obstruction in infancy.
- Intestinal volvulus is another pediatric surgical emergency that can result in bowel necrosis and death if not treated urgently. This most commonly occurs in children born with malrotation.
- The stool guaiac test is the most common fecal occult blood test (FOBT) performed to screen for colon cancer. Other causes of a positive FOBT include esophagitis, esophageal varices, gastritis, peptic ulcer disease, GI polyps and tumors, and inflammatory bowel disease (Crohn disease and ulcerative colitis). Non–GI causes for FOBT include nosebleeds or hemoptysis (coughing up blood) with subsequent swallowing of the blood into the GI tract. Additionally, some foods can cause a false-positive stool guaiac test result (e.g., cantaloupe, red meat, uncooked broccoli, turnip, and radish, including horseradish), and some medicines may interfere with the stool guaiac test reaction (e.g., aspirin, vitamin C and nonsteroidal antiinflammatory drugs [NSAIDs], such as ibuprofen). Medications containing iron and bismuth can also turn the stool visibly black.
- Some academic centers are moving to discharge patients who undergo successful nonoperative reduction after a short observation period and successful oral trial. This should only be attempted if the reduction was uncomplicated and if the family is reliable, with good access to transportation to come back immediately to the ED should complications arise.

Case Summary

Complaint/History: An 18-month-old male comes to the emergency department with a 2-hour history of vomiting and somnolence.

Findings: On arrival, he appears well without any physical findings. While under observation, he has emesis followed by sleepiness. Repeat physical examination reveals a sausage-shaped mass in his right upper quadrant.

Labs/Tests: A plain abdominal radiograph demonstrates paucity of air in the right-lower quadrant and dilation of the small bowel. Ultrasound of the abdomen shows the cross section of the intestine with a target sign, consistent the terminal ileum telescoping into the proximal cecum, leading to an intestinal obstruction.

Diagnosis: Ileoileocolic intussusception.

Treatment: The patient has a successful air enema reduction and is discharged home after 48 hours of further observation. He does not require surgical intervention.

Bibliography

Comstedt P, Storgaard M, Lassen AT. The systemic inflammatory response syndrome (SIRS) in acutely hospitalized medical patients: a cohort study. *Scan J Trauma Resusc Emerg Med.* 2009;17:67–72.

Henderson AA, Anupindi SA, Servaes S, et al. Comparison of 2-view abdominal radiographs with ultrasound in children with suspected intussusception. *Pediatr Emerg Care.* 2013;29(2):145–150.

Kleizen KJ, Hunck A, Wijnen MH, et al. Neurological symptoms in children with intussusception. *Acta Paediatr.* 2009;98(11):1822–1824.

Lehnert T, Sorge I, Till H, et al. Intussusception in children–clinical presentation, diagnosis and management. *Int J Colorectal Dis.* 2009;24(10):1187–1192.

Okimoto S, Hyodo S, Yamamoto M, et al. Association of viral isolates from stool samples with intussusception in children. *Int J Infect Dis.* 2011;15(9):e641–e645.

16-Month-Old Female With Refusal to Walk

Spencer Liebman ▪ James Homans

A 16-month-old female presents with refusal to walk. One week ago, her grandmother noticed a new limp. This progressed rapidly to refusal to bear weight on her right leg. She was also extremely fussy with diaper changes, and any passive movement of her right hip would cause her to cry out. She has intermittently felt warm to the touch.

What is the differential diagnosis for pain and tenderness in an extremity?

Rheumatic, postinfectious/reactive, neoplastic, hematologic, traumatic, orthopedic, and mechanical causes should be considered. The duration of symptoms, recent exposures, travel history, clinical appearance, age, and other pertinent medical history can help narrow the differential diagnosis and guide further workup.

Common causes of pain and a limp in the infant and toddler include trauma and infection. Trauma may be due to falls—for example, a spiral fracture of the tibia from twisting during a fall (toddler's fracture) is fairly common. Fractures prior to ambulation should raise suspicion for nonaccidental trauma (i.e., child abuse).

Infections to consider include those of the joint (septic arthritis) and bone (osteomyelitis).

BASIC SCIENCE/CLINICAL PEARL	STEP 1/2/3

Developmental hip dysplasia may be the cause of limp in a toddler, but pain would not be a prominent feature.

Case Point 36.1

Her temperature is 37.8°C, pulse is 125/min, respiratory rate is 28/min, and blood pressure is 110/60 mm Hg. Her right hip is tender to both palpation and passive range of motion.

What is the next step?

Septic arthritis is a medical emergency. It must be excluded in a child with fever, articular swelling, erythema, tenderness, or pseudoparalysis. Plain film radiography may help differentiate septic arthritis from bone pathology (e.g., osteomyelitis, Legg-Calvé-Perthes disease, malignancy, trauma). Ultrasound can identify and quantify joint effusions and help guide aspiration. Magnetic resonance imaging (MRI) can provide a more detailed view of bone and soft tissue. However, if septic arthritis is suspected, prompt diagnostic arthrocentesis and rapid initiation of empiric antibacterial therapy are crucial to help prevent further deterioration.

CLINICAL PEARL   **STEP 2/3**

Septic arthritis is a medical emergency, and early initiation of antibiotics is essential to preserve joint function.

Case Point 36.2

Due to the concern for septic arthritis, orthopedic consultation is obtained, and a bedside arthrocentesis is performed. Bloody fluid is drained from the right hip joint, resulting in pain relief. Synovial fluid analysis reveals inflammation but does not meet the criteria for septic arthritis (Table 36.1).

A plain radiograph of the hip reveals a lytic lesion in the proximal epiphysis of the right femur (Fig. 36.1; anatomic diagram in Fig. 36.2).

TABLE 36.1 ■ **Synovial Fluid Analysis**

Test	Findings
Visual appearance	Pink to red
Nucleated cell count	1.065×10^9/L (1065 cells/mm^3)
Cell count differential	87% neutrophils, 4% lymphocytes, 9% monocytes-histiocytes
Gram staining and cultures	No organisms seen or isolated

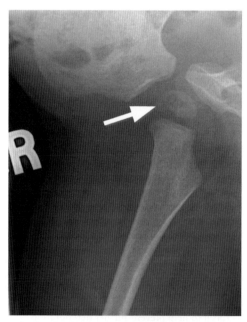

Fig. 36.1 A lucency is seen in the right lateral proximal femoral epiphysis *(arrow)*. The epiphysis normally appears separate from the metaphysis and diaphysis in young children due to the lucency of the growth plate.

What is the most likely diagnosis?

Based on the lytic lesion in the epiphysis and the inflammatory synovial fluid, acute epiphyseal osteomyelitis is the most likely diagnosis. Acute epiphyseal osteomyelitis may present with joint swelling and purulent fluid in the joint space because the epiphyseal-metaphyseal junction is often still within the joint capsule in young children. This may result in a misdiagnosis of septic arthritis.

BASIC SCIENCE PEARL   **STEP 1**

Most cases of hematogenous osteomyelitis occur in the metaphysis, but infants and young toddlers may present with epiphyseal involvement due to transphyseal vessels that involute by 18 months of age.

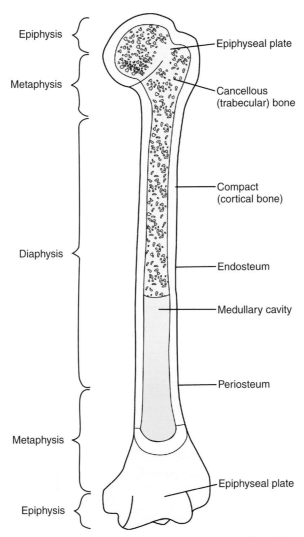

Fig. 36.2 Locations of the epiphysis, metaphysis, and diaphysis in the femur. (From Silverstein JA, Moeller JL, Hutchinson MR. Common issues in orthopedics. In: Rakel RE, Rakel A, eds. *Textbook of Family Medicine.* 9th ed. Philadelphia: Elsevier; 2016:648–683.)

Case Point 36.3

The patient is diagnosed with osteomyelitis and started on the empiric broad-spectrum antibiotics vancomycin and ceftriaxone to cover for suspected organisms, including *Staphylococcus aureus* and *Streptococcus* spp.

What is the pathophysiology of osteomyelitis?

Osteomyelitis occurs because of hematogenous seeding or direct inoculation/adjacent spread of infection. Acute hematogenous osteomyelitis occurs due to seeding of bacteria into the metaphysis, adjacent to the epiphyseal growth plate, via the nutrient arteries feeding the epiphyseal growth plate. Capillaries feeding off these arteries drain into a sinusoidal plexus that ultimately joins the large sinusoidal veins in the bone marrow. Trauma, emboli, or hematogenous spread of bacteria occlude a sinusoidal vessel, causing stasis and conditions favorable for infection.

Inoculum (puncture wound) osteomyelitis occurs when a trauma leads to inoculation of infection into the bone. This is more common with metatarsals and the patella because these areas are more likely to suffer penetrating injuries. The microbiology also includes *Pseudomonas aeruginosa* (often found in the sponge material in shoes), *S. aureus*, and *Streptococcus* spp., as well as *Stenotrophomonas maltophilia* and *Serratia marcescens*.

Osteomyelitis can also be caused by spread from a contiguous focus of infection. This is especially relevant in patients with severe burn injuries, sacral ulcers, or a recent surgical procedure.

Which bones are most commonly affected in osteomyelitis?

Long bones or long bone equivalents—calcaneal apophysis or inferior pubic ramus—are the most common areas for acute hematogenous osteomyelitis (Table 36.2). The combination of rich metaphyseal blood flow and tortuous blood flow in the physis, where capillaries make a sharp turn from the metaphysis, allows bacteria to aggregate and subsequently spread into intraosseous, subperiosteal, or extraperiosteal spaces.

BASIC SCIENCE PEARL   **STEP 1**

More than 80% of osteomyelitis cases involve tubular bones.

What are the clinical manifestations of osteomyelitis?

The initial bacteremic phase may range from asymptomatic to nonspecific symptoms, including low-grade fever and malaise, to high-spiking fevers and chills. In neonates, there is a much higher risk of early spread into the epiphysis, surrounding soft tissue, and joint space, given the poor barriers to spread of infection. This can lead to a swollen, tender, sausage-shaped appearance of the affected limb. The cortex is thicker and periosteum more adherent in older infants, so there is generally less risk of the infection spreading into the joint space and surrounding soft tissue. They are still at high risk of developing subperiosteal abscesses and contiguous edema, however.

CLINICAL PEARL   **STEP 2/3**

Neonates with osteomyelitis present with irritability, pain with movement, and pseudoparalysis of the extremity.

CLINICAL PEARL   **STEP 2/3**

In neonates, hematogenous osteomyelitis may lead directly to septic arthritis due to the decreased integrity of anatomic barriers.

TABLE 36.2 ■ Site of Involvement in Acute Hematogenous Osteomyelitis

Site	%
Tubular bone	
Femur	25
Tibia	24
Humerus	13
Phalanges	5
Fibula	4
Radius	4
Ulna	2
Metatarsal	2
Clavicle	0.5
Metacarpal	0.5
Cuboidal bone	
Calcaneus	5
Talus	0.8
Carpals	0.5
Cuneiform	0.5
Cuboid	0.3
Irregular bone	
Ischium	4
Ilium	2
Vertebra	2
Pubis	0.8
Sacrum	0.8
Flat bone	
Skull	1
Rib	0.5
Sternum	0.5
Scapula	0.5
Maxilla	0.3
Mandible	0.3

From Nelson JD. Acute osteomyelitis in children. Infect Dis Clin North Am. 1990;4:513–522.

In children and adolescents, the thickened metaphyseal cortex and fibrous adherent perios-teum results in less spread and thus more focal signs and symptoms. These children often have point tenderness and a limp (or other restriction of use of the involved bone). Percussion of the bone distal to the site of infection will often lead to pain at the infected site.

What are the most common organisms involved in osteomyelitis?
Common organisms and appropriate empiric antibiotics are summarized in Table 36.3. The causative organism greatly affects the clinical presentation. Osteomyelitis due to *S. aureus* is often a more severe,

TABLE 36.3 ■ Causative Agents of Osteomyelitis by Age Group and Method of Acquisition

Patient Characteristics	Causative Organisms	Empiric Antibiotics
Nosocomial infection	*Staphylococcus aureus*, streptococcal spp., Enterobacteriaceae, *Candida* spp.	Nafcillin or oxacillin + gentamicin or cefotaxime (or ceftriaxone) + gentamicin
Community-acquired infection	*S. aureus*, group B streptococcus, *Escherichia coli*, *Klebsiella* spp.	Nafcillin or oxacillin + gentamicin or cefotaxime (or ceftriaxone) + gentamicin
Infant (2–18 mo)	*S. aureus*, *Kingella kingae*, *Streptococcus pneumoniae*, *Neisseria meningitidis*, *Haemophilus influenzae* type b (nonimmunized)	Immunized—nafcillin, oxacillin, or cefazolin Nonimmunized—nafcillin, oxacillin + cefotaxime, or cefuroxime
Young child (18 mo–3 yr)	*S. aureus*, *K. kingae*, *Streptococcus pneumoniae*, *N. meningitidis*, *H. influenzae* type b (nonimmunized)	Immunized: nafcillin, oxacillin, or cefazolin Nonimmunized: nafcillin, oxacillin + cefotaxime, or cefuroxime
Child (3–12 yr)	*S. aureus*, group A β-hemolytic streptococcus	Nafcillin, oxacillin, or cefazolin
Adolescent (12–18 yr)	*S. aureus*, group A β-hemolytic streptococcus, *Neisseria gonorrhoeae*	Nafcillin, oxacillin, or cefazolin; ceftriaxone and doxycycline for disseminated gonococcal infection

Adapted from Funk SS, Copley LAB. Acute hematogenous osteomyelitis in children: pathogenesis, diagnosis, and treatment. *Orthop Clin North Am.* 2017;48:199–208.

rapidly progressing infection and may be complicated by associated myositis, pyomyositis, intraosseous and subperiosteal abscesses, and septic thrombophlebitis. In younger children, infections with *Kingella kingae* can occur; such infections often present with more than 1 week of symptoms and less specific signs of infection. Nonimmunized infants are at higher risk for infections due to *Haemophilus influenzae* type B and *Streptococcus pneumoniae*. Culture-negative osteomyelitis generally presents with a more indolent course and more nonspecific symptoms than culture-positive osteomyelitis.

What is the next step?

All pediatric patients with suspected osteomyelitis or septic arthritis warrant orthopedic consultation. Blood cultures should be taken at the time of presentation, but their yield is limited. They may only be positive in about 45% of cases, much lower in cases involving fastidious bacteria (e.g., *K. kingae*), fungus, or mycobacteria. Whenever possible, bone biopsy should be obtained for Gram staining, bacterial cultures (aerobic and anaerobic), pathology, and fungal and mycobacterial cultures (if suspected). Microbiology should be alerted if fastidious organisms are suspected. Open fractures warrant early irrigation and debridement.

CLINICAL PEARL   **STEP 2/3**

Culture yield is higher if obtained prior to the administration of antibiotics, but appropriate cultures and studies should be obtained whenever an invasive procedure is performed. In patients with systemic toxicity, empiric antibacterial therapy should not be delayed while waiting for surgery.

Percutaneous needle aspiration may be the only diagnostic modality required in infants and young children with soft tissue and periosteal involvement or subperiosteal fluid collections. Percutaneous techniques are more limited in older children and adolescents because infection limited

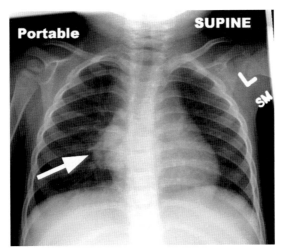

Fig. 36.3 A chest radiograph reveals right hilar adenopathy *(arrow)*.

to the metaphysis requires biopsy for a specimen. The risk of damaging the growth plate must be weighed against that of not identifying a causative organism.

Is there a role for surgery in hematogenous osteomyelitis?

Acute osteomyelitis is characterized by purulent inflammation that may include abscess formation and/or necrosis of bone. Surgery is frequently necessary for diagnosis, drainage of purulent material, and/or debridement of necrotic nonviable bone to allow healing.

If the inflammation extends into the subperiosteal space, it may fully entrap a necrotic piece of bone (sequestrum) away from the primary bone. The resulting periosteal reaction above the sequestrum is termed the *involucrum*. Formation of a sequestrum results in a chronic osteomyelitis that is resistant to antibiotic therapy and must be surgically debrided to allow healing.

Case Point 36.4

The patient does not improve, despite empiric antibacterial treatment. Both blood cultures and synovial fluid cultures are negative by Gram staining and culture. MRI does not reveal sequestrum.

On further questioning, the patient's grandmother states that the patient's mother was diagnosed and treated for tuberculosis *(Mycobacterium tuberculosis)* infection. The patient was also prescribed tuberculosis therapy in early life to eradicate any latent infection but it was not administered.

A tuberculin skin test is positive. A chest radiograph reveals hilar adenopathy consistent with tuberculosis (Fig. 36.3). Acid-fast stain of the patient's gastric aspirate fluid is unrevealing but a polymerase chain reaction assay and culture are positive for *M. tuberculosis*.

Diagnosis: Hematogenous epiphyseal osteomyelitis due to *Mycobacterium tuberculosis*.

What features help distinguish tuberculous osteomyelitis from bacterial osteomyelitis? What bones are usually involved in tuberculous osteomyelitis?

Nearly 20% of tuberculous infections among children are classified as extrapulmonary tuberculosis (EPTB). During initial infection, bacilli can spread widely to organs, bones, and synovial tissue. Local immune responses then usually control local infection, leading to subclinical (latent) infection associated with granuloma formation. Reactivation then occurs if local immune defenses fail.

CLINICAL PEARL   **STEP 2/3**

In young children and neonates, EPTB can occur during initial infection due to immature local defenses, unlike immunocompetent adults, in whom EPTB generally occurs with reactivation.

Although any bone can be infected by *M. tuberculosis*, the most commonly affected areas include vertebral (Pott disease) and long bones of the upper and lower extremities. Unifocal infections are most common, but multifocal tuberculous osteomyelitis occurs in 10% to 15% of cases. The onset of symptoms occurs over weeks to months and includes low-grade fever, chills, mild erythema, pain, and little to no warmth of the affected bone. An associated abscess may not have intense inflammatory signs (i.e., a cold abscess).

BASIC SCIENCE/CLINICAL PEARL   **STEP 1/2/3**

Skeletal tuberculosis usually affects the vertebrae (spondylitis); this is known as Pott disease.

How is tuberculous osteomyelitis treated?

The approach to treatment of tuberculous osteomyelitis is similar to that of pulmonary tuberculosis. It varies with concomitant HIV infection and/or drug resistance. Neurosurgical evaluation is recommended for all patients with Pott disease. Surgery may be needed if there are advanced neurologic deficits, worsening deficits while on appropriate therapy, or severe kyphosis (>40 degrees) at the time of presentation. Those with cold abscesses—especially chest wall abscesses—may also warrant surgical intervention.

Initial treatment should include a 2-month intensive phase consisting of four-drug treatment (e.g., isoniazid, rifampin, pyrazinamide, and ethambutol). Those with fully sensitive *M. tuberculosis* can then begin a continuation phase for 6 to 10 months with two drugs, including rifampin (e.g., isoniazid and rifampin). The drugs used and treatment duration are modified for any drug resistance.

Patients should be monitored for toxicity due to antituberculous drugs. In particular, isoniazid can cause hepatic toxicity (rare in children) and neurotoxicity, rifampin and pyrazinamide can cause hepatic toxicity, and ethambutol can cause optic neuropathy leading to blindness. Isoniazid toxicity is responsive to vitamin B_6 (pyridoxine).

CLINICAL PEARL   **STEP 2/3**

Due to the contagious nature of tuberculosis, patients with active pulmonary tuberculosis are often treated with directly observed therapy (DOT), usually administered by a staff member in a local department of public health.

CLINICAL PEARL   **STEP 2/3**

The common four-drug empiric regimen for *M. tuberculosis*—isoniazid, rifampin, pyrazinamide and ethambutol—is often remembered by the acronym RIPE.

Case Point 36.5

The patient is started on multidrug therapy against *M. tuberculosis* with isoniazid, rifampin, pyrazinamide, and ethambutol. Coverage is reduced to isoniazid and rifampin once the absence of drug resistance is proven. The patient ultimately completes 1 year of directly observed therapy.

BEYOND THE PEARLS

- Subacute osteomyelitis can sometimes cause an intraosseous abscess, known as a *Brodie abscess*. This is more common in adolescents and presents with a target sign on MRI that represents a lytic lesion with sclerotic margins.
- Fracture superinfection should be considered with increasing pain 1 to 6 weeks after initial reduction and casting. Unlike fracture pain, the pain associated with osteomyelitis does not improve with immobilization.
- Neonates, patients with sickle cell disease, and patients on chronic hemodialysis are all at higher risk for developing osteomyelitis. Immunodeficiencies such as chronic granulomatous disease and acquired immunodeficiency syndrome also predispose to osteomyelitis.
- *Actinomyces* is an unusual cause of osteomyelitis and favors the bones of the jaw and cervical spine. Diffuse honeycombing lesions may be seen on radiographs.
- Debridement with antimicrobial therapy is the treatment of choice for chronic osteomyelitis. However, in some cases, the limb cannot be salvaged, and partial or total amputation is warranted.

Case Summary

Complaint/History: A 16-month-old female presents with refusal to walk.

Findings: Her right hip is tender to both palpation and passive range of motion.

Labs/Tests: Synovial fluid analysis reveals inflammation but does not meet the criteria for septic arthritis; a plain radiograph of the hip reveals a lytic lesion in the proximal epiphysis of the right femur. Polymerase chain reaction testing reveals *Mycobacterium tuberculosis*.

Diagnosis: Epiphyseal osteomyelitis due to *M. tuberculosis*.

Treatment: Rifampin, isoniazid, pyrazinamide, and ethambutol.

Bibliography

Conrad DA. Acute hematogenous osteomyelitis. *Pediatr Rev.* 2010;31(11):464.

Cruz AT, Starke JR. Tuberculosis. In: *Feigin and Cherry's Textbook of Pediatric Infectious Diseases.* 2013:1335–1380.

Funk SS, Copley LA. Acute hematogenous osteomyelitis in children: pathogenesis, diagnosis, and treatment. *Orthop Clin North Am.* 2017;48(2):199–208.

Krogstad P. Osteomyelitis. In: *Feigin and Cherry's Textbook of Pediatric Infectious Diseases.* 2013:711–727.

Nahid P, et al. Official American Thoracic Society/Centers for Disease Control and Prevention/Infectious Diseases Society of America clinical practice guidelines: treatment of drug-susceptible tuberculosis. *Clin Infect Dis.* 2016;63(7):e147–e195.

Pigrau-Serrallach C, Rodríguez-Pardo D. Bone and joint tuberculosis. *Eur Spine J.* 2013;22(4):556–566.

Teo HE, Peh WC. Skeletal tuberculosis in children. *Pediatr Radiol.* 2004;34(11):853–860.

Ware JK, et al. Chronic osteomyelitis. In: *Skeletal Trauma: Basic Science, Management, and Reconstruction.* 2014:609–635.

16-Year-Old Female With Cola-Colored Urine

Sunniya Basravi ▪ Richard Fine ▪ Lawrence Opas

A 16-year-old female presents with 2 days of cough, runny nose, body aches, and 1 day of bloody urine.

What is hematuria?

Hematuria is defined as five or more red blood cells (RBCs) per high power field (HPF) (>40×) on three consecutive fresh, centrifuged specimens of urine (Fig. 37.1).

Why is confirmation of hematuria important?

A urine dipstick positive for blood may not always be due to actual blood present in the urine sample. For example, a positive urine dipstick may result from myoglobinuria or hemoglobinuria, in which the urine may appear pink or red but no RBCs are present on the microscopic evaluation of the specimen. To confirm that there is in fact true hematuria, there must be at least five or more RBCs seen on the microscopic evaluation of the urine specimen.

How do you approach hematuria in a child?

Once it has been confirmed that there are RBCs in the urine specimen, the source of hematuria must be determined. Hematuria can be from glomerular or extraglomerular causes. Glomerular causes of hematuria are most often described as smoky and tea or cola-colored red and does not present with clots (Table 37.1), and urinalysis is usually positive for dysmorphic RBCs, proteinuria, and RBC and white blood cell (WBC) casts. Extraglomerular causes of hematuria often have pink or red urine, with blood clots. Urinalysis shows normal RBCs and no casts and mild to no proteinuria. Both glomerular and extraglomerular causes of hematuria may occasionally present as microscopic hematuria, in which the urine is clear in color but five or more RBCs/HPF present in the microscopic study of the urine, which makes the workup more challenging.

What is the differential diagnosis of hematuria?

It is easier to divide the urinary tract into sections and then think of the differential in the two different parts (Box 37.1).

Case Point 37.1

The patient states that her urine is uniformly dark reddish brown in color, similar to cola, and without any blood clots. Her urinalysis shows amber-colored urine with a specific gravity of 1.016. It is significant for urine protein more than 300 mg/dL, large blood, and small leukocytes. Microscopy shows more than 50 RBCs/HPF, 31 to 50 WBCs/HPF, positive RBC casts, no crystals, and no bacteria.

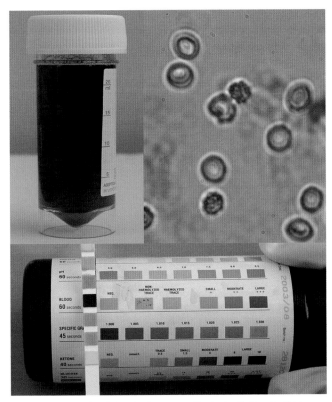

Fig. 37.1 Hematuria detection by dipstick and microscopy. Contact with the dipstick's reagent strip causes the hemolysis of urine RBCs. The released hemoglobin causes oxidation of the strip's chromogen indicator, causing a change in color. Oxidation can also be caused by myoglobin or other oxidizing agents, resulting in the reagent strip's low specificity. A positive dipstick test for hematuria requires confirmation by microscopy of the centrifuged urine specimen. The presence of 5+ RBCs/ HPF is considered abnormal. (From Bryant R, Catto J. Haematuria. *Surgery.* 2008:26(4):150–153.)

TABLE 37.1 ■ **Characteristics of Hematuria**

	Gross Hematuria		Microscopic Hematuria
Glomerular	**Extraglomerular**		**Glomerular or Extraglomerular**
Tea or cola-colored urine	Pink or red urine		Clear or yellow urine
No blood clots	Blood clots present		No blood clots
Red blood cells (RBCs) present, ± casts	RBCs present		RBCs present

What is the likely source of this patient's hematuria?
Because her urine is uniformly dark red in color, without clots, and confirmed RBCs and RBC casts on the microscopic study, the hematuria likely has a glomerular cause.

BOX 37.1 ■ Differential Diagnosis of Hematuria[a]

Upper Urinary Tract (Renal Parenchyma)

Poststreptococcal glomerulonephritis
IgA nephropathy
IgA vasculitis (formerly known as Henoch-Schönlein purpura)
Alport syndrome
Thin basement membrane disease
Systemic lupus erythematosus
Nephrotic syndrome
Hemolytic-uremic syndrome
Renal vein thrombosis
Renal calculi
Wilms' tumor
Renal cell carcinoma
Cystic kidney disease
Urinary tract infection
Trauma
Sickle cell disease
Bleeding diathesis

Lower Urinary Tract (Ureters, Bladder, Urethra)

Hemorrhagic cystitis
Urinary tract infection
Trauma
Transitional cell carcinoma
Bladder polyp
Urinary tract obstruction

---

[a]Based on location along the urinary tract.

Case Point 37.2

The patient states that she has a current illness consisting of cough and runny nose. She denies any other symptoms and denies prior hematuria. There is no family history of autoimmune or renal disease. On physical examination, her blood pressure is slightly elevated, with systolic and diastolic pressures in the 90th to 95th percentiles for age, and she has edema (1+) of her bilateral lower extremities. She is awake, alert, and in no distress. The remainder of the examination is otherwise unremarkable.

What is the next step in the workup?

Urinalysis results were already discussed (see earlier), which indicated a likely glomerular cause of hematuria. The next step is to rule out postinfectious glomerulonephritis, particularly poststreptococcal glomerulonephritis (PSGN). Specific laboratory tests include anti–streptolysin O (ASO) titers and complement components 3 (C3) and 4 (C4). PSGN would show low C3, normal C4, and elevated ASO titer. If laboratory test results support PSGN as the diagnosis, the patient can be observed over time and, if renal disease improves, there is no need for biopsy. However, if history, examination, and laboratory results do not support the diagnosis of the PSGN, a renal biopsy will be necessary to make the diagnosis.

CLINICAL PEARL	STEPS 1/2/3

Poststreptococcal glomerulonephritis (PSGN) usually presents with nephritis symptoms (e.g., hematuria, proteinuria, hypertension, edema) about 2 weeks after an acute streptococcal pharyngitis and about 4 to 6 weeks after a streptococcal skin infection.

CLINICAL PEARL	STEPS 1/2/3

In PSGN, laboratory tests should show elevated ASO titer, low C3, and normal C4 levels.

CLINICAL PEARL	STEPS 2/3

ASO titer may peak at about 2 to 4 weeks after a streptococcal pharyngitis and remain elevated for several months. The ASO titer does not typically increase secondary to pyodermal skin infections.

CLINICAL PEARL	STEPS 2/3

C3 can remain low for up to 8 weeks following a streptococcal pharyngitis or pyodermal infection.

Serum albumin level and urine protein-to-creatinine ratio would also be helpful in that they could indicate to what extent protein is being lost in the urine. If proteinuria is in the nephrotic range, a diagnosis other than PSGN should also be considered.

CLINICAL PEARL	STEPS 1/2/3

Nephrotic-range protein is urine protein >3 g in 24 hours or urine protein-to-creatinine ratio >2. Nephritic-range proteinuria is when there is protein present in the urine but less than 3 g in 24 hours. Also, a urine calcium-to-creatinine ratio would be another noninvasive test to rule out hypercalciuria as a possible cause of the hematuria.

Case Point 37.3

The patient's serum creatinine level is 1.0 mg/dL (normal, 0.8–1.3 mg/dL). The urine protein-to-creatinine ratio is 1.74 (normal, <0.2) and urine calcium-to-creatinine ratio is 0.003 (normal, <0.2). A rapid streptococcal antigen test and ASO titer are negative. C3 is 180 mg/dL (normal, 90–180 mg/dL), and C4 is 39 mg/dL (normal, 10–40 mg/dL). Urine culture is negative.

These results rule out PSGN, hypercalciuria, and urinary tract infection (UTI) as possible causes for the patient's hematuria.

What is the next step in the workup?

The next step is to rule out autoimmune or rheumatologic disease as a cause for this patient's hematuria.

CLINICAL PEARL	STEP 1

Positive results for both antinuclear antibody (ANA) and anti–double-stranded DNA (anti-dsDNA) is indicative of possible nephritis due to systemic lupus erythematosus (SLE).

CLINICAL PEARL   **STEP 1**

A positive cytoplasmic antineutrophil cytoplasmic antibody screen (c-ANCA) is suggestive of granulomatous polyangiitis.

CLINICAL PEARL   **STEP 1**

Positive perinuclear antineutrophil cytoplasmic antibody screen (p-ANCA) is more commonly seen in microscopic polyangiitis.

Case Point 37.4

Antinuclear antibody (ANA), anti–double-stranded DNA (dsDNA) antibody, and antineutrophilic cytoplasmic antibody (ANCA) screen are negative. Renal ultrasound is normal.

These rheumatologic laboratory results can only help indicate the possible diagnosis. Because PSGN is unlikely for our patient, and she continues to have hematuria and nephritic-range proteinuria, a kidney biopsy is still required to make a definitive diagnosis.

Case Point 37.5

The patient undergoes a renal biopsy that shows mesangial deposition of immunoglobulin A (IgA) and C3 on immunofluorescence microscopy.

Diagnosis: Immunoglobulin A nephropathy.

What is immunoglobulin A nephropathy?

IgA nephropathy is characterized by mesangial deposition of the IgA1 subclass of IgA. Deposition of IgG and C3 may also be seen in IgA nephropathy. Unlike in other diseases, in which you may also see IgA deposits in the glomeruli (e.g., IgA vasculitis), in IgA nephropathy, the disease is localized to the kidneys and does not involve other systems. IgA nephropathy is one of the most common causes of progressive renal failure worldwide. When IgA nephropathy presents in childhood, the disease is usually fairly benign. About 20% of children with IgA nephropathy may have a slowly progressive disease, eventually leading to end-stage renal disease in adulthood.

How does immunoglobulin A nephropathy typically present?

Usually, IgA nephropathy presents as hematuria during or immediately after an upper respiratory tract illness. Most commonly, the disease presents with gross hematuria, with or without mild proteinuria. Less commonly, IgA nephropathy may present as an asymptomatic microscopic hematuria, with nephritic-range proteinuria and mild hypertension. Additionally, IgA nephropathy may rarely present with nephrotic-range proteinuria or a mixed nephritic-nephrotic picture.

The cause of IgA nephropathy is still largely unclear; although it seems to follow an infection, there has been no specific organism linked to the disease. Because the disease seems to be rarely clustered in families and varies in presentation in different parts of the world, the hypothesis is that there are likely genetic and environmental factors that play a role in the pathogenesis of IgA nephropathy. Additionally, abnormally glycosylated IgA1 has been found in the urine of patients with IgA nephropathy which further supports the theory that a person may be genetically predisposed to the disease. Abnormal glycosylation of the O-linked hinge region of IgA1 leads to the production of autoantibodies, which increases the likelihood that immune complexes will deposit in the mesangium of the glomerulus.

Can immunoglobulin A nephropathy be confirmed with laboratory tests alone?

IgA nephropathy cannot be confirmed by laboratory tests alone. Although C3 and C4 levels can be ordered, which help distinguish IgA nephropathy from other common causes of hematuria, such as postinfectious (e.g., poststreptococcal) glomerulonephritis, IgA nephropathy can only be definitively diagnosed by a renal biopsy. IgA nephropathy can be confirmed by the presence of IgA and C3 deposits seen in the mesangium on immunofluorescence microscopy (Fig. 37.2). Normally, C3 is equal to or less than the amount of IgA deposits present. IgG deposits may also be seen in the mesangium. Additional histologic findings include mesangial hyperexpansion and hypercellularity seen using periodic acid–Schiff stain (PAS; Fig. 37.3 shows normal glomerulus; Fig. 37.4 illustrates IgA nephropathy). Mesangial widening and deposition can be seen with electron microscopy (EM; Fig. 37.5, normal glomerulus; Fig. 37.6, IgA nephropathy).

How is immunoglobulin A nephropathy treated?

There is no definitive treatment for IgA nephropathy. The initial management of the disease involves the control of high blood pressure and proteinuria if these are present. Angiotensin-converting enzyme (ACE) inhibitors are first-line therapy for reducing proteinuria and thus slowing progression of the disease. Angiotensin-II receptor antagonists (ARBs) can also be used for this purpose and are equally as effective. If proteinuria is refractory to ACE inhibitors or ARBs, the next choice is the administration of glucocorticoids; however, the significant side effect profile makes this a much less favorable option.

CLINICAL PEARL	STEP 1

ACE inhibitors prevent the conversion of angiotensin-I to angiotensin-II, preventing vasoconstriction.

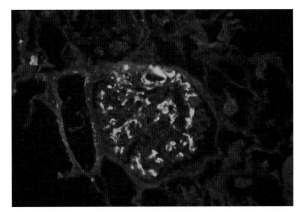

Fig. 37.2 Immunofluorescence microscopy showing IgA and C3 deposits in the mesangium, consistent with IgA nephropathy. (From Fogo AB, Lusco MA, Najafian B, Alpers CE. AJKD Atlas of Renal Pathology: IgA nephropathy. *Am J Kidney Dis.* 2015:66(5):e33–e34.)

CLINICAL PEARL   STEP 1

The angiotensin converting enzyme (ACE) normally inactivates bradykinin. Bradykinin stimulates the release of nitric oxide and prostacyclin, which causes vasodilation. ACE inhibitors result in higher levels of bradykinin, leading to vasodilation.

Case Point 37.6

The patient is started on an ACE inhibitor (enalapril, 5 mg/day) for her hypertension and proteinuria. She will require lifelong nephrology follow up to monitor her renal function and hypertension.

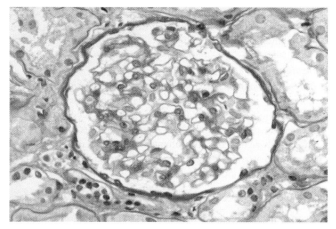

Fig. 37.3 Normal glomerulus seen with periodic acid–Schiff staining. Shown is the glomerulus with normal cellularity and mesangium with a thin capillary wall. (From Weidner N, Cote R, Suster S, et al. *Modern Surgical Pathology*. 2nd ed. Philadelphia: Saunders/Elsevier; 2009.)

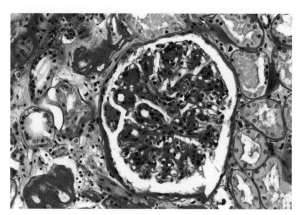

Fig. 37.4 Periodic acid–Schiff staining showing mesangial proliferation and hypercellularity in IgA nephropathy. (From Fogo AB, Lusco MA, Najafian B, Alpers CE. AJKD Atlas of Renal Pathology: IgA nephropathy. *Am J Kidney Dis*. 2015:66(5):e33–e34.)

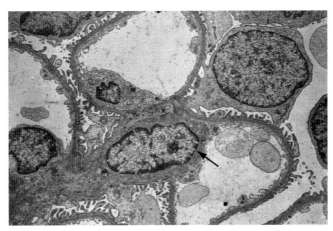

Fig. 37.5 Normal glomerulus seen on electron microscopy showing the mesangium with mesangial cell *(arrow)*, basement membrane, and visceral epithelial cells, with foot processes and endothelial cells. (From Weidner N, Cote R, Suster S, et al. *Modern Surgical Pathology*. 2nd ed. Philadelphia: Saunders/Elsevier; 2009.)

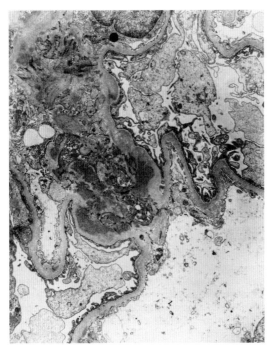

Fig. 37.6 Electron microscopy in IgA nephropathy showing mesangial widening with deposits. (From Weidner N, Cote R, Suster S, et al. *Modern Surgical Pathology*. 2nd ed. Philadelphia: Saunders/Elsevier; 2009.)

What is the long-term outcome for patients with immunoglobulin A nephropathy?

Although most people with IgA nephropathy do not develop end-stage renal disease during childhood, long-term follow up is important because about 20% of these patients will go on to develop signs of significant renal disease after reaching adulthood. IgA nephropathy patients with little or no proteinuria (<500–1000 mg/day) usually have a low risk of progression of renal disease.

Among those who develop overt proteinuria and/or elevated serum creatinine levels, progression to end-stage renal disease is about 15% to 25% in 10 years and 20% to 30 % in 20 years.

Case Summary

Complaint/History: 16-year-old female with cola-colored urine preceded by upper respiratory tract infection symptoms.

Findings: Physical examination shows blood pressure in the 90th to 95th percentile for age and bilateral lower extremity edema.

Labs/Tests: Microscopic urinalysis shows more than 50 RBCs/HPF and an elevated urine protein-to-creatinine ratio (1.74). Renal biopsy and immunofluorescence microscopy show mesangial deposition of IgA and complement C3.

Diagnosis: IgA nephropathy.

Treatment: ACE inhibitor with long-term pediatric nephrology follow-up to monitor for progression of renal disease.

BEYOND THE PEARLS

- Poststreptococcal glomerulonephritis (PSNG) and IgA nephropathy present with similar findings (hematuria, proteinuria, hypertension, edema). However, in PSGN, the hematuria presents a few weeks after the infection, whereas in IgA nephropathy, the hematuria presents concurrently with the acute infection.

- Elevated serum levels of IgA alone does not guarantee the development of IgA nephropathy. Mesangial deposition of IgA is associated with a high proportion of abnormal glycosylation of the IgA1 subclass.

- Mesangial deposition can be seen in 3% to16% of healthy individuals. In these patients, the renal biopsy indicates IgA nephropathy while there may be no clinical signs of nephritis.

- Familial IgA nephropathy affects 10% to 15% of all cases, with transmission as an autosomal dominant trait with incomplete penetrance.

- Most cases of IgA nephropathy are clinically restricted to the kidneys, however, the disease has been associated with other conditions, such as celiac disease, HIV infection, cirrhosis, and granulomatosis with polyangiitis. Less frequently, IgA nephropathy may also be associated with ankylosing spondyloarthritis, lymphoma, disseminated tuberculosis, inflammatory bowel disease, bronchiolitis obliterans, and small cell carcinoma.

- There is a subset of IgA nephropathy patients who present with acute-onset nephrotic syndrome, little or no hematuria, preserved renal function, and histologic findings similar to those of minimal change disease (diffuse fusion of the foot processes of glomerular epithelium on electron microscopy). These patients benefit from glucocorticoid treatment alone.

- At the time of initial presentation of IgA nephropathy, hematuria is almost always present, whereas proteinuria may or may not be there. However, over time, persistence of proteinuria is the strongest indicator of likely progression to end-stage renal disease.

- ACE inhibitors also block the renin-angiotensin system (RAS), which normally stimulates proinflammatory cytokine release, resulting in an antiinflammatory effect.

- Omega-3 fatty acid in fish oil supplementation in adults with IgA nephropathy may decrease proteinuria and stabilize renal function. However, randomized controlled trials among pediatric IgA nephropathy patients have not shown any benefit.

Bibliography

Fogo AB, Lusco MA, Najafian B, et al. AJKD atlas of renal pathology: IgA nephropathy. *Am J Kidney Dis.* 2015;66(5):e33–e34.

Hogg R. Idiopathic immunoglobulin A nephropathy in children and adolescents. *Pediatr Nephrol.* 2010;25:823–829.

Pan C, Avner E. IgA nephropathy (Berger nephropathy). In: *Nelson Textbook of Pediatrics.* 20th ed. Philadelphia: Elsevier; 2016.

15-Month-Old Male With Renal Calculi

Sunniya Basravi ■ Richard Fine ■ Shoji Yano

A 15-month-old male is seen for well-child care. The mother reports that since his last well-child check, the patient was admitted for treatment of a urinary tract infection with sepsis. She reports that an ultrasound of the kidneys was performed, and renal calculi were seen in the left kidney, with associated obstructive pelviectasis (Fig. 38.1). The patient was treated successfully with antibiotics.

What are the most common causes of renal calculi in children?

The most common types of renal stones are calcium oxalate and calcium phosphate stones. The most common cause is idiopathic hypercalciuria. However, dependent and independent hyperparathyroidism are other common causes of hypercalcemia.

The second most common types of renal stones are ammonium and magnesium phosphate stones. These are usually due to infections from urease-positive organisms (e.g., *Proteus vulgaris*, *Klebsiella* spp.). Clinically, these types of stones are associated with staghorn calculi in the renal calices, which can act as a nidus for infection.

Uric acid stones are the third most common type of renal stones. These are usually seen in the setting of hyperuricemia.

Case Point 38.1

A plan is made to test the patient's urine prior to the next well-child visit at 18 months of age. During a routine discussion of the patient's development, the patient's mother reports that the child has not learned to crawl. Furthermore, the mother reports seeing flinging motions from the patient's arms and legs, as well as other nonpurposeful movements.

On physical examination, dystonia is noted throughout. Truncal spasms are occasionally noted.

What is the differential diagnosis for generalized dystonia in childhood?

Dystonia, a movement disorder with involuntary muscle contractions, is described as primary or secondary in nature. Primary, or early-onset, dystonia is usually due to an underlying genetic disorder or is idiopathic in nature. Secondary dystonia—the more common type of dystonia in children—is secondary to another disease process, such as cerebral palsy following a hypoxic brain injury, metabolic disorders, exposure to different drugs or toxins, basal ganglia infarction, neoplasm, or stroke.

Case Point 38.2

Microscopic examination of the urine reveals crystals (Fig. 38.2). Urinalysis reveals markedly increased excretion of uric acid (i.e., hyperuricosuria), with a urine uric acid-to-creatinine ratio of 5 (normal, <2). The patient does not have hypercalciuria, hyperoxaluria ,or hypocitraturia.

A serum uric acid level is obtained and found to be elevated at 15 mg/dL (normal, <4 mg/dL).

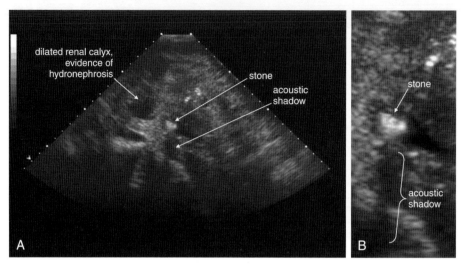

Fig. 38.1 (A) A renal calculus (stone) is seen in the renal pelvis, with associated hydronephrosis. (B) Close-up of panel A. (From Broder JS: *Diagnostic Imaging for the Emergency Physician*. Philadelphia: Saunders; 2011.)

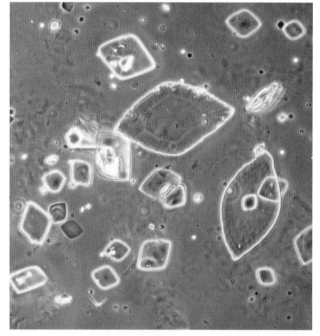

Fig. 38.2 Rhomboid-shaped uric acid crystals seen under phase contrast microscopy. (From Fogazzi GB, Garigali G. Urinalysis. In: Johnson R, Feehally J, Floege J, eds. *Comprehensive Clinical Nephrology*. 5th ed. London: Saunders/Elsevier; 2014:39–52.)

What can cause hyperuricemia and hyperuricosuria? What is the most likely diagnosis, given the constellation of findings?

Hyperuricemia can occur secondary to excess uric acid production, a purine-rich diet, impaired uric acid excretion, and disorders of purine metabolism. Disorders that can cause increased production of uric acid include malignancy, Reye syndrome, Down syndrome, psoriasis, sickle cell anemia, obesity, hypothyroidism, cyanotic congenital heart disease, glycogen storage disease types I, III, IV, and V, hereditary fructose intolerance, and acyl-coenzyme A dehydrogenase deficiency.

Increased purine ingestion is seen with excess alcohol ingestion, ingestion of liver, game meat, anchovies, sardines, gravy, dried beans, peas, and/or mushrooms, diuretic use (e.g., furosemide or hydrochlorothiazide), and/or immunosuppressive medications.

Renal insufficiency from any cause can lead to hyperuricemia due to low uric acid excretion— hyperuricosuria would not be seen in this scenario.

Some genetic conditions associated with disorders in purine metabolism, and thus with hyperuricemia and hyperuricosuria include hypoxanthine-guanine phosphoribosyltransferase (HPRT or HGPRT) deficiency, adenylosuccinate lyase deficiency, adenosine deaminase deficiency, phosphoribosyl pyrophosphate synthetase superactivity syndrome, and purine nucleoside phosphorylase deficiency.

Most of these listed causes for hyperuricemia were ruled out by initial history and physical examination in this patient. However, given the developmental delay, dystonia, and hyperuricemia, HPRT deficiency—eponymously known as Lesch-Nyhan disease (LND)—is the most likely diagnosis.

How do you make the diagnosis of Lesch-Nyhan disease?

Diagnosis is based on clinical and laboratory evidence. Some helpful laboratory test results include elevated serum uric acid levels and an elevated urine urate-to-creatinine ratio more than 2. However, disease confirmation requires demonstration of low HPRT enzyme activity (in blood or cultured fibroblasts) or a mutation in the *HPRT1* gene.

An HPRT enzyme activity level lower than 1.5% is consistent with classic LND. There are milder variants of the disease that have residual enzyme activity between 1.5% and 8%. These include HPRT-related hyperuricemia (HRH), which is the mild form, and HPRT-related dysfunction (HND), which is the moderate form. Compared to classic LND, HRH and HND have milder neurocognitive symptoms.

The *HPRT1* gene is located on the long arm of the X chromosome. The various mutations documented in LND are dispersed through the gene, with some locations more commonly associated with a disease-causing mutation. Specific disease features have not been associated with any specific mutation location, but the less severe clinical manifestations typically have mutations that allow some degree of enzyme activity.

BASIC SCIENCE PEARL   **STEP 1**

The *HPRT1* gene is located on the long arm of the X chromosome (Xq26-q27). This disorder can be due to a wide variety of mutations in the *HPRT1* gene, which codes for the HPRT protein.

BASIC SCIENCE/CLINICAL PEARL   **STEP 1/2/3**

Although more common in males, Lesch-Nyhan disease can be seen in females. Females have only one functioning copy of the *HPRT1* gene because the other is silenced by CpG cluster methylation.

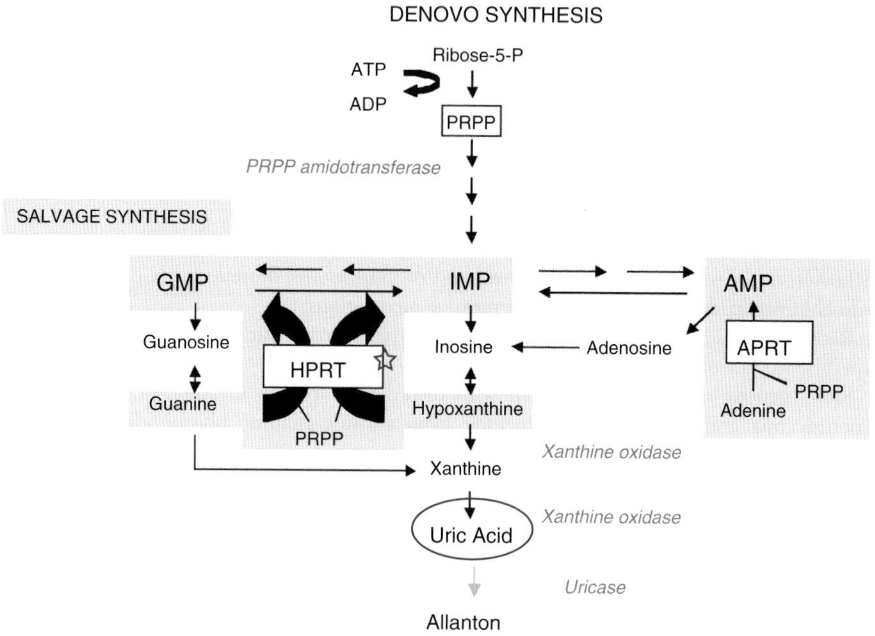

DENOVO SYNTHESIS

Fig. 38.3 Schematic of purine metabolism. Deficiency in hypoxanthine-guanine phosphoribosyl trans-ferase *(star)* in the salvage pathway results in overproduction of xanthine and ultimately uric acid *(circle).* *ADP,* Adenosine diphosphate; *AMP,* adenosine monophosphate; *APRT,* adenine phospho-ribosyltransferase; *ATP,* adenosine triphosphate; *GMP,* guanosine monophosphate; *HPRT,* hypo-xanthine-guanine phosphoribosyltransferase; *IMP,* inosine monophosphate; *PRPP,* phosphoribosyl pyrophosphate; *Ribose-5-P,* ribose 5-phosphate. (From Roche A, Pérez-Dueñas B, Camacho JA, et al. Efficacy of rasburicase in hyperuricemia secondary to Lesch-Nyhan syndrome. *Am J Kidney Dis.* 2009;53(4):677–680.)

Case Point 38.3

Gene sequencing identifies a hemizygous frameshift mutation in the *HPRT1* gene.

Diagnosis: Lesch-Nyhan disease (hypoxanthine-guanine phosphoribosyltransferase deficiency).

What is the pathophysiology of Lesch-Nyhan disease?

LND is a rare neurodevelopmental and metabolic disorder that occurs because of a genetic mu-tation in *HPRT1* that encodes for HPRT, an enzyme acting in the purine metabolite salvage pathway. Purines form the basis of nucleotides in deoxyribonucleic acid (DNA) and provide the primary source of cellular energy through adenosine triphosphate (ATP). An inability to salvage the metabolic products leads to shunting into the catabolic pathway and thus leads to increased production of uric acid (Fig. 38.3).

Uric acid is poorly soluble and must be continuously excreted to avoid toxic accumulation in the body. Uric acid is mostly eliminated by the kidneys; however, a small portion is also excreted by the gastrointestinal tract in biliary and intestinal secretions.

BASIC SCIENCE PEARL	STEP 1

Normal serum uric acid concentration is already near saturation. Hyperuricemia thus leads to precipitation.

BASIC SCIENCE/CLINICAL PEARL	STEP 1/2/3

Despite marked overproduction of uric acid, hyperuricemia may be mild or nonexistent due to rapid renal clearance.

The biologic basis for neurobehavioral abnormalities in LND is less well understood. It is thought to be due to the HPRT deficiency in developing neurons, rather than the effects of hyperuricemia. Allopurinol—a drug that treats hyperuricemia (see later)—does not prevent the cognitive impairment, dystonia, or behavioral symptoms of the disease.

How does Lesch-Nyhan disease present?
In classic LND, the hallmark of behavior problems includes typical self-injurious behavior, such as biting of the lips, fingers, hands, or cheeks, and banging of the head and limbs. Self-injurious behavior usually manifests between 2 and 4 years of age and is compulsive in nature—that is, patients do not wish to inflict self-harm but are unable to resist the behavior.

A severe motor disorder similar to dyskinetic cerebral palsy is seen; most patients never walk. Severe generalized dystonia is common. Dysarthria is severe, and most patients can only be understood by caregivers and close friends and family members. Choreoathetosis, ballismus, and corticospinal dysfunction—manifesting with findings such as spasticity and clonus—are also seen in a substantial minority of patients. Feeding may be impaired enough to render patients dependent on gastrostomy tube feeds.

Cognitive impairment is essentially universal but generally overestimated due to comorbid dysarthria and behavioral issues. Formal testing reveals only mild to moderate impairment.

Uric acid overproduction leads to a number of symptoms, which include gouty arthritis and nephrolithiasis. Nephrolithiasis may result in hematuria, dysuria, obstructive nephropathy and uropathy, repeated urinary tract infections, and ultimately renal failure if not treated appropriately at the time of diagnosis.

CLINICAL PEARL	STEP 2/3

If gouty arthritis is not treated, permanent articular deformities and dysfunction will result.

Less severe mutations of the *HPRT1* gene may result in milder disease (Fig. 38.4). Self-injurious behavior is generally seen only in classic (severe) disease.

How is Lesch-Nyhan treated?
There is no cure for the syndrome. Currently, treatment efforts are focused on reducing serum uric acid levels and thus minimizing the symptoms of hyperuricemia. Allopurinol is the most common drug of choice for this purpose. This is a xanthine oxidase inhibitor that helps inhibit the progression of the pathway from the hypoxanthine to xanthine to uric acid, thus slowing down or reducing the overall production of uric acid.

CLINICAL PEARL	STEP 2/3

Conditions that predispose hypovolemia, such as fever or diarrhea, increase the risk for nephrolithiasis and gout. Ensuring adequate hydration is essential.

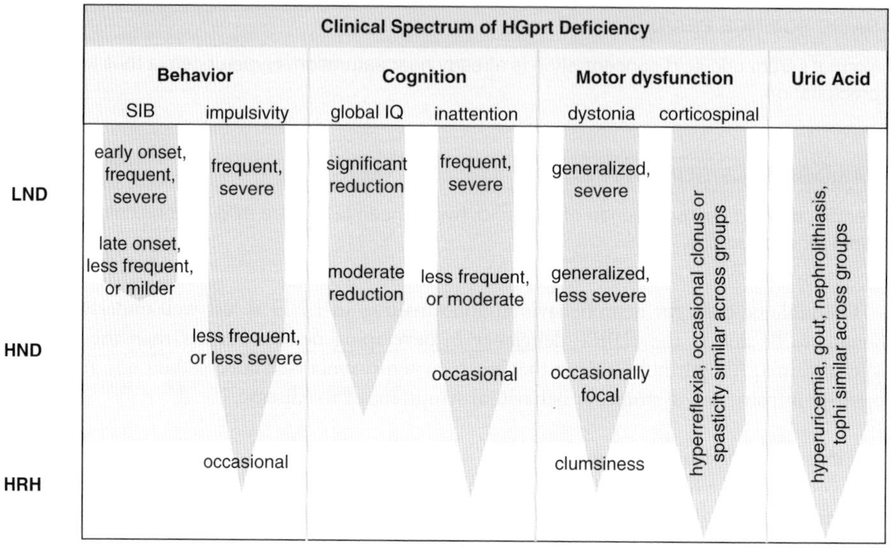

Clinical Spectrum of HGprt Deficiency						
Behavior		Cognition		Motor dysfunction		Uric Acid
SIB	impulsivity	global IQ	inattention	dystonia	corticospinal	
LND early onset, frequent, severe	frequent, severe	significant reduction	frequent, severe	generalized, severe	hyperreflexia, occasional clonus or spasticity similar across groups	hyperuricemia, gout, nephrolithiasis, tophi similar across groups
late onset, less frequent, or milder		moderate reduction	less frequent, or moderate	generalized, less severe		
HND	less frequent, or less severe		occasional	occasionally focal		
HRH	occasional			clumsiness		

Fig. 38.4 Clinical spectrum of hypoxanthine-guanine phosphoribosyltransferase deficiency. *HGprt,* Hypoxanthine-guanine phosphoribosyltransferase; *HND,* hypoxanthine-guanine phosphoribosyltransferase-related dysfunction; *HRH,* hypoxanthine-guanine phosphoribosyltransferase-related hyperuricemia; *LND,* Lesch-Nyhan disease; *SIB,* self-injurious behavior. (From Kamatani N, Jinnah HA, Hennekam RCM, van Kuilenburg ABP. Purine and pyrimidine metabolism. In: Rimoin DL, Pyeritz RE, Korf BR, eds. *Emery and Rimoin's Principles and Practice of Medical Genetics.* 6th ed. San Diego, CA: Academic Press; 2013:1–38.)

CLINICAL PEARL   **STEP 2/3**

Allopurinol reduces uric acid formation by inhibiting the conversion of xanthine to uric acid. As a result, xanthine oxide calculi may occur.

Other supportive treatments include the use of restraints, removal of teeth, and use of mouth guards to reduce self-injury. The time needed to be in restraints may vary from patient to patient, depending on the severity of impulsive behavior. Simply being aware of the patient's needs plays an important role in reducing self-injurious behavior.

CLINICAL PEARL   **STEP 2/3**

Using punishments for self-injurious behavior often has the paradoxic effect of increasing these behaviors.

Case Point 38.4

Allopurinol is prescribed, and the dose is titrated up to suppress hyperuricosuria. After several months of therapy, repeat renal ultrasound shows resolution of his nephrolithiasis.

Care is established with several subspecialists, including a pediatric nephrologist to monitor renal function, pediatric neurologist to manage his dystonia, developmental-behavioral pediatric specialist for early intervention services, and clinical geneticist to follow the overall progression of his disease. Additionally, physical and occupational therapy is prescribed. His parents are given anticipatory guidance regarding self-injurious behavior that has not yet begun to manifest.

BEYOND THE PEARLS

- More than 400 mutations in *HPRT* have been documented in Lesch-Nyhan disease and its variants.
- Loss of HPRT function in Lesch-Nyhan disease increases the production of uric acid by three- to fivefold.
- Analogous to gallbladder disease, hyperuricosuria can cause not only nephrolithiasis but also uric acid sludging. The sludgelike material—described as sandy—can cause the same obstructive symptoms as stones.
- Physically aggressive behaviors (e.g., hitting others) and the inappropriate use of foul and sexual language are common in addition in self-injurious behavior. Patients report the behavior to be impulsive and compulsive and afterward often feel embarrassed and/or remorseful.
- Motor dysfunction is often confused with cerebral palsy. Like cerebral palsy, it is static in nature, rather than progressive.
- Genetic testing is available for prenatal diagnosis as well. Identification of a specific mutation in the mother—who is either affected or is a carrier—is performed first, so that targeted sequencing can be carried out on the fetus.
- Although currently there is no standard therapy to treat or reduce the self-injurious behavior, there have been several case reports on deep brain stimulation of the internal globus pallidus, leading to the improvement of dystonia and disappearance of self-injurious behavior.

Case Summary

Complaint/History: A 15-month-old male presents after a recent admission for renal calculi.

Findings: Dystonia.

Labs/Tests: Serum and urine studies reveal hyperuricemia and hyperuricosuria, respectively.

Diagnosis: Hypoxanthine-guanine phosphoribosyltransferase deficiency (Lesch-Nyhan disease).

Treatment: Allopurinol and anticipatory guidance for his predicted neurologic disease.

Bibliography

Fu R. Clinical severity in Lesch-Nyhan disease: the role of residual enzyme and compensatory pathways. *Mol Genet Metab*. 2015;114:55–61.

Harris JC. Disorders of purine and pyrimidine metabolism. In: *Nelson Textbook of Pediatrics*. Philadelphia: Elsevier; 744–752.

Jinnah HA, Sabina RL, Van Den Berghe G. Metabolic disorders of purine metabolism affecting the nervous system. *Handb Clin Neurol*. 2013;113:1827–1836.

Kamatani N, et al. Purine and pyrimidine metabolism. In: Rimoin D, Pyeritz R, Korf B, eds. *Emery and Rimoin's Principles and Practice of Medical Genetics*. Philadelphia: Elsevier; 2013:1–38.

McRea N. Childhood dystonia. *Paediatr Neurol*. 2013;13(5):18–20.

Piedimonte F, Andreani J. Remarkable clinical improvement with bilateral globus pallidus internus deep brain stimulation in a case of Lesch–Nyhan disease: five-year follow-up. *Neuromodulation*. 2015;18:118–122.

17-Year-Old Female With Fatigue and Yellow Eyes

Franklyn Fenton   ■   Michelle Pietzak

A 17-year-old previously healthy female presents to your clinic with 1 week of fatigue, malaise, and diffuse body aches, in addition to her eyes turning yellow. She has had nausea and a 5-pound unintentional weight loss. Her urine appears to her to be a darker yellow. Her skin is also more yellow in appearance.

What is the differential diagnosis?

The yellowing of the eyes and skin indicate jaundice, which in turn is caused by an elevation of the serum bilirubin level. Causes of hyperbilirubinemia can be divided into prehepatic (indirect, unconjugated hyperbilirubinemia), hepatic (mixed hyperbilirubinemia), and posthepatic (direct, conjugated hyperbilirubinemia). Prehepatic jaundice is caused by the overproduction of bilirubin, indicating a hemolytic anemia. Hepatic jaundice is caused by inadequate processing of bilirubin in the liver, which is seen in disorders that result in hepatocellular injury and/or liver failure. Posthepatic jaundice is caused by problems with excretion of bilirubin from the biliary system (cholestasis).

BASIC SCIENCE PEARL   **STEP 1**

Acute liver failure is defined as the triad of abnormal liver test results, encephalopathy, and coagulopathy, whereas acute liver injury (without failure) is defined by abnormal liver test results without encephalopathy or coagulopathy.

Case Point 39.1

Her mother has systemic lupus erythematosus (SLE). There is no family history of jaundice, liver disease, other autoimmune diseases, or hemolytic anemias.

She is afebrile, and all other vital signs are within normal limits. On physical examination, she has scleral icterus and jaundice. Her liver edge is palpated 3 cm below the right costal margin at the midclavicular line; it is nontender and soft. Her abdomen is otherwise soft, not tender and not distended, and there is no splenomegaly or ascites. The remainder of her physical examination is normal.

What is your differential diagnosis at this point?

The enlarged liver suggests a hepatic cause of hyperbilirubinemia, although cholestasis should also be considered. Given the acute onset of the patient's illness, infections and drug-induced liver disease should be high on the list.

Viral infections to consider include hepatitis A virus (HAV), hepatitis B virus (HBV), hepatitis C virus (HCV), hepatitis E virus (HEV), Epstein-Barr virus (EBV), cytomegalovirus (CMV), and human immunodeficiency virus (HIV). HAV and HEV are transmitted through water or food contaminated by the feces of someone who has these viruses. Blood transfusion as a neonate could have put her at some risk for HBV, HCV, and HIV, although contaminated blood products would be extremely rare in the United States due to routine screening; additionally, HBV vaccination is nearly universal in children in the United States. Cholestatic hepatitis can uncommonly occur with EBV and CMV infections; the lack of complaints of fever, rash and sore throat, and the absence of adenopathy and splenomegaly on physical examination make these viral infections less likely in our patient.

BASIC SCIENCE/CLINICAL PEARL	STEP 1/2/3

HAV usually causes mild disease in children. In adults, it can present with fulminant liver failure. HAV infection should spontaneously resolve in an immunocompetent host.

CLINICAL PEARL	STEP 2/3

HEV can cause epidemics of infection, usually in developing countries. Like HAV, it usually resolves with only supportive care. However, in pregnant women in certain geographic areas, it is associated with miscarriage, fulminant hepatic failure, and death.

Given the acuity of her symptoms, drug-induced liver injury (DILI) is also high on the differential. Acetaminophen is the most common drug of choice used in suicide attempts in teenage females. Measuring a blood level of this drug is a simple and rapid test, and early treatment with N-acetylcysteine can potentially prevent a patient from going into fulminant liver failure. Alcoholic hepatitis is another consideration in a teenage patient with acute symptoms; however, this is more common with chronic alcohol abuse in the setting of preexisting liver disease.

CLINICAL PEARL	STEP 2/3

If acetaminophen overdose is left untreated for 3 to 4 days, weakness, hematuria, blurred vision, tachycardia, confusion, coma, and/or death can occur.

Although hepatomegaly suggests a hepatic cause of jaundice, cholestasis should still be considered due to its high prevalence. Gallstones with impaction in the common bile duct commonly cause a cholestatic jaundice but would be associated with severe pain in the right upper quadrant; gallstones are usually seen in those with obesity, pregnancy, rapid weight loss, and hemolytic disease. Cholestasis of pregnancy can present with jaundice and pruritus (itching) but usually occurs in late pregnancy.

What other liver diseases should be considered in a teenage girl?
After infections, DILI, and cholestasis, less common diseases that should be considered include Wilson disease, alpha-1 antitrypsin deficiency, and autoimmune disease. Wilson disease is a rare inherited disorder of abnormal copper storage in the liver and other organs; along with jaundice, it can present with neurologic and psychiatric symptoms due to the deposition of copper into the basal ganglia. The total bilirubin in Wilson disease can be extremely high due to a combination of liver disease and hemolysis seen with copper overload. Alpha-1 antitrypsin deficiency results from a mutation in *SERPINA1*, which encodes alpha-1 antitrypsin, a serine protease inhibitor secreted from hepatocytes; the mutation results in the accumulation of an abnormal alpha-1 antitrypsin protein that hepatocytes cannot secrete. Hepatocyte inflammation (hepatitis) and eventually scarring (cirrhosis) result. Both diseases can present in the teenage years with a wide clinical spectrum, from asymptomatic elevated transaminase levels all the way to fulminant liver failure.

BASIC SCIENCE PEARL	STEP 1

Alpha-1 antitrypsin deficiency also results in early adult-onset chronic obstructive pulmonary disease (COPD).

Also high on the differential would be autoimmune diseases, particularly given a family history of SLE. Autoimmune diseases to consider include autoimmune hepatitis (AIH), primary sclerosing cholangitis (PSC), and SLE or inflammatory bowel disease with liver involvement. PSC is more common in males, and about 80% will also have ulcerative colitis.

What laboratory tests are indicated?

Serum chemistries should be ordered to characterize the hyperbilirubinemia. Both unconjugated (indirect) and conjugated (direct) serum bilirubin levels should be measured. If the indirect fraction is greater than 80% of the total, hyperbilirubinemia is most likely resultant from hemolysis, whereas if it is less than 80%, the cause is most likely hepatic or cholestatic jaundice. Additionally, a complete blood cell count and reticulocyte count can help rule out hemolytic anemia.

BASIC SCIENCE PEARL	STEP 1

The one liver disease that violates the 80% rule is Wilson disease because both direct and indirect bilirubin levels are elevated due to the hemolysis induced by copper overload.

Other serum chemistries are helpful to evaluate the liver and biliary system. Elevated serum aspartate aminotransferase (AST) and/or alanine aminotransferase (ALT) levels suggest liver inflammation and hepatocellular injury but are nonspecific. An elevated serum alkaline phosphatase (AP) level suggests cholestasis, whereas a decreased serum albumin level and/or prolonged prothrombin time (PT) suggests diminished liver synthetic function and thus hepatocellular injury and/or liver failure.

BASIC SCIENCE/CLINICAL PEARL	STEP 1/2/3

AST and ALT are often referred to as *liver function tests;* however, they are neither specific to the liver nor its function. These enzymes are also found in red blood cells and muscle cells. Also, when the liver is cirrhotic, transaminase levels are often normal or low due to low hepatocyte volume.

CLINICAL PEARL	STEP 2/3

Hepatocellular liver injury usually has greater elevations in AST and ALT levels, usually more than 500 U/L. Cholestatic liver injury has a more severe elevation in bilirubin and AP levels, with lesser elevations of aminotransferase levels.

Case Point 39.2

The patient's serum chemistry panel reveals the following: AST, 1381 U/L (normal 10–40 U/L); ALT, 1752 U/L (normal 7–56 U/L); total protein, 9.0 g/dL (normal, 6–8.3 g/dL); albumin, 3.0 g/dL (normal, 3.5–5.5 g/dL); total bilirubin, 6.0 mg/dL (normal < 1.2 mg/dL); and direct bilirubin, 4.0 mg/dL (normal < 0.3mg/dL). AP is normal, and PT is normal. Viral serologies are negative. The serum acetaminophen level is undetectable. A urine pregnancy test is negative.

What radiographic would you do at this point?

An abdominal ultrasound would be helpful to examine liver and spleen anatomy and to look for gallstones and ascites. A Doppler investigation should be done to look at flow through the hepatic, portal, and splenic veins.

Case Point 39.3

Her abdominal ultrasound demonstrates a slightly enlarged liver and spleen, without gallstones, ascites, or abnormal portal venous flow.

What further workup would you do at this point?

Given that common infections, acetaminophen overdose, gallstones, and pregnancy have been ruled out, workup for AIH, Wilson disease, and alpha-1 antitrypsin deficiency should be started. Her age, gender, family history of SLE, and elevated globulin fraction put AIH at the top of the differential.

BASIC SCIENCE/CLINICAL PEARL	STEP 1/2/3

The globulin fraction is calculated by subtracting the albumin from the total protein. A high globulin fraction suggests increased amounts of circulating antibodies, suggestive of an auto-immune disease or paraproteinemia. Paraproteinemia is the elevation of a single monoclonal gamma globulin in the blood due to an underlying hematologic malignancy. It is extremely rare in the pediatric population.

Case Point 39.4

Further laboratory investigation reveals a ceruloplasmin level of 40 g/L (usually <20 g/L in Wilson disease) and no mutation in her *SERPINA1* gene. Antibody screening detects antinuclear antibodies (ANAs) at 1:80 titer and anti–smooth muscle antibody (SMA). Anti–liver-kidney microsomal antibody (LKM-1) is not detected.

BASIC SCIENCE/CLINICAL PEARL	STEP 1/2/3

ANA can be positive in many autoimmune diseases, such as SLE, scleroderma, polymyositis-dermatomyositis, rheumatoid arthritis, Sjögren syndrome, and mixed connective tissue diseases. Smooth muscle Ab can also be seen in some cancers and in primary biliary cirrhosis (PBC).

What is your next step?

The patient's laboratory test results are highly suggestive of AIH. Liver biopsy is required for confirmation.

Case Point 39.5

The patient has a percutaneous liver biopsy done under ultrasound guidance. It demonstrates an interface hepatitis, with lymphocytic infiltration and hepatocyte necrosis (Fig. 39.1).

Diagnosis: Autoimmune hepatitis (AIH).

What is autoimmune hepatitis?

AIH is a chronic inflammatory disorder of the liver thought to be caused by an environmental trigger in a genetically susceptible individual. It is more common in females and is diagnosed by typical clinical presentation, liver histology, and positive autoantibodies: ANA, SMA, LKM-1, and anti–liver cytosol type 1 Ab (LC-1).

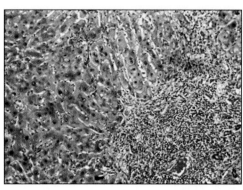

Fig. 39.1 Liver biopsy showing interface hepatitis with lymphocytic infiltration and hepatocyte necrosis consistent with AIH. (Netter medical illustration used with permission of Elsevier. All rights reserved.)

There are two main types of AIH, associated with specific ages, autoantibodies, and human leukocyte antigen (HLA) types. Both types overwhelmingly occur in females. Type I AIH has bimodal peaks between ages 10 to 20 and 45 to 70 years, has positive ANA and SMA, and is associated with HLA-B8, DR3, and DR4. Type 2 AIH peaks at age 2 to 14 years, has positive LKM-1, and is associated with HLA-B14 and DR3. Our patient's laboratory test results are more consistent with type 1 AIH, which has a better prognosis.

How does autoimmune hepatitis present?

The true incidence and prevalence of AIH in the United States is not known. Type I AIH, which represents 80% of cases, may present anywhere from asymptomatic elevations of the transaminase levels (in 25%, found on routine chemistries) all the way to cirrhosis, with portal hypertension and/or liver failure. Type 2 AIH usually presents with fulminant liver failure in children and has a worse prognosis. If symptoms are present, the most common are generalized malaise and fatigue, vague abdominal pain, joint pain, and occasionally jaundice. Patients in liver failure may present with a first variceal hemorrhage, ascites and peripheral edema, and hepatic encephalopathy.

How is autoimmune hepatitis diagnosed?

Criteria for the diagnosis of AIH are shown in Table 39.1. Diseases that should be ruled out before a diagnosis of AIH is considered include HAV, HBV, HCV, HIV, EBV, and CMV infection, Wilson disease, and alpha-1 antitrypsin deficiency. In adults, hemochromatosis should be ruled out. An obese female should be checked for gallstones and nonalcoholic fatty liver disease (NAFLD) by abdominal ultrasound. Serum acetaminophen levels and a urine pregnancy test should also be routine. A thorough history of prescription medication use, illicit drug use, blood transfusions, and alcohol ingestion is also important.

An algorithm for the diagnosis of AIH is presented in Fig. 39.2.

How is autoimmune hepatitis treated?

Once diagnosis is confirmed, treatment should be considered in all patients, including those who are asymptomatic. There are two phases of treatment, induction and maintenance, which may use different medications. The goal of induction therapy is to induce clinical remission. Maintenance therapy is used to preserve remission. The gold standard of treatment

TABLE 39.1 ■ **Diagnostic Criteria for Autoimmune Hepatitis (AIH)**

	Diagnostic Criteria	
Requisites	**Definite**	**Probable**
No genetic liver disease	Normal alpha-1 antitrypsin phenotype Normal serum ceruloplasmin, iron, and ferritin levels	Partial alpha-1 antitrypsin deficiency Nonspecific serum copper, ceruloplasmin, iron, and/or ferritin abnormalities
No active viral infection	No markers of current infection with hepatitis A, B, and C viruses	No markers of current infection with hepatitis A, B, and C viruses
No toxic or alcohol injury	Daily alcohol < 25 g/day and no recent use of hepatotoxic drugs	Daily alcohol < 50 g/day and no recent use of hepatotoxic drugs
Laboratory features	Predominant serum aminotransferase abnormality Globulin, gamma globulin, or immunoglobulin G level ≥ 1.5× normal	Predominant serum aminotransferase abnormality Hypergammaglobulinemia of any degree
Autoantibodies	ANA, SMA, or anti-LKM1 ≥ 1:80 in adults and ≥ 1:20 in children; no AMA	ANA, SMA, or anti-LKM1 ≥ 1:40 in adults, or other autoantibodies[a]
Histologic findings	Interface hepatitis No biliary lesions, granulomas, or prominent changes suggestive of another disease	Interface hepatitis No biliary lesions, granulomas, or prominent changes suggestive of another disease

[a]Includes perinuclear antineutrophil cytoplasmic antibodies and the not generally available antibodies to soluble liver antigen–liver pancreas, actin, liver cytosol type 1, and asialoglycoprotein receptor.
AMA, Antimitochondrial antibodies.
From Alvarez F, Berg PA, Bianchi FB, et al. International AIH Group Report: review of criteria for diagnosis of AIH. *J Hepatol.* 1999;31:929–938.

in pediatrics is induction therapy with a glucocorticoid (e.g., prednisolone) and concomitant maintenance therapy with azathioprine. This combination achieves remission in 80% of patients. Second-line therapies include mycophenolate mofetil and/or tacrolimus with prednisolone. Remission is defined as a normalization of serum aminotransferase levels, a normal level of IgG, and an inactive liver histology. After 3 years of remission, treatment withdrawal can be attempted. However, reinduction therapy may be more difficult than with the first induction therapy.

CLINICAL PEARL **STEP 2/3**

Pediatric patients (e.g., young adults) are more likely to fail conventional therapy for AIH than older adults.

Case Point 39.6

The patient is started on oral prednisone and azathioprine. Her symptoms of fatigue and general malaise improve within the first 3 days of treatment. Her transaminase levels normalize within 1 month, and her bilirubin normalizes in 3 months.

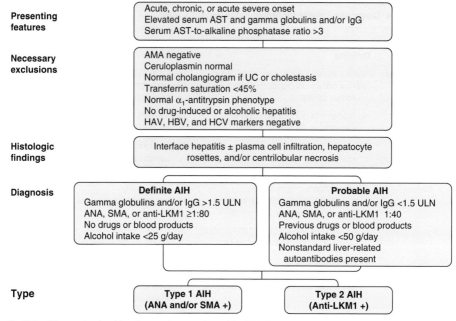

Presenting features

Acute, chronic, or acute severe onset
Elevated serum AST and gamma globulins and/or IgG
Serum AST-to-alkaline phosphatase ratio >3

Necessary exclusions

AMA negative
Ceruloplasmin normal
Normal cholangiogram if UC or cholestasis
Transferrin saturation <45%
Normal α_1-antitrypsin phenotype
No drug-induced or alcoholic hepatitis
HAV, HBV, and HCV markers negative

Histologic findings

Interface hepatitis ± plasma cell infiltration, hepatocyte rosettes, and/or centrilobular necrosis

Diagnosis

Definite AIH
Gamma globulins and/or IgG >1.5 ULN
ANA, SMA, or anti-LKM1 ≥1:80
No drugs or blood products
Alcohol intake <25 g/day

Probable AIH
Gamma globulins and/or IgG <1.5 ULN
ANA, SMA, or anti-LKM1 1:40
Previous drugs or blood products
Alcohol intake <50 g/day
Nonstandard liver-related autoantibodies present

Type

Type 1 AIH (ANA and/or SMA +)

Type 2 AIH (Anti-LKM1 +)

Fig. 39.2 Diagnostic algorithm for autoimmune hepatitis. AIH, Autoimmune hepatitis; ANA, anti-nuclear antibodies; AST, aspartate aminotransferase; HAV, hepatitis A virus; HBV, hepatitis B virus; HCV, hepatitis C virus; IgG, immunoglobulin G; LKM1, liver-kidney microsome type 1; SMA, smooth muscle antibodies. (From Czaja AJ. Autoimmune hepatitis. In: Sleisenger MH, Fordtran JS, Feldman M, et al, eds. *Sleisenger and Fordtran's Gastrointestinal and Liver Disease.* Philadelphia: Elsevier; 2015:1493–1511.)

BEYOND THE PEARLS

- AIH is more likely to present with cirrhosis in persons of African descent or Hispanic ethnicity in comparison to (white) European descent. They are also more likely to have liver failure and/or a need for liver transplantation at diagnosis.
- Patients can satisfy criteria for AIH, but lack detectable autoantibodies. Such patients are labeled with cryptogenic disease but may still respond to immunosuppressive therapies.
- AIH can be associated with other autoimmune diseases, such as autoimmune thyroid disease (Grave disease, Hashimoto thyroiditis), ulcerative colitis, idiopathic thrombocytopenia, hemolytic anemia, type 1 diabetes, celiac disease, and autoimmune polyendocrinopathy–candidiasis–ectodermal dystrophy (APCED).
- Drug-induced AIH may result from exposure to certain drugs such as nitrofurantoin, minocycline, isoniazid, propylthiouracil, and infliximab. Although drug withdrawal ultimately treats the disease, glucocorticoids should still be used in initial therapy.
- Overlapping autoimmune disease of the liver can occur in pediatrics, such as PSC-AIH overlap syndrome. In these cases, all the criteria for both AIH and PSC are met. Diagnostic criteria for this biliary tract disease includes AP or gamma-glutamyl transpeptidase (GGT) five times the upper limit of normal and histologic or radiographic evidence (via magnetic resonance cholangiopancreatography or endoscopic retrograde cholangiopancreatography) of large bile duct disease. PBC-AIH overlap can be seen in adult patients.
- Patients with evidence of end-stage liver disease due to AIH are less likely to respond to conventional glucocorticoid therapy.

BEYOND THE PEARLS—cont'd

- Prior to the initiation of azathioprine for AIH, patients should be checked with a blood test for polymorphisms in the *TPMT* gene. *TPMT* encodes thiopurine methyltransferase, an enzyme that metabolizes thiopurines. Loss of thiopurine methyltransferase results in excessive bone marrow toxicity, leading to cytopenias, sepsis, and even death. In patients with homozygous *TPMT* mutations, resulting in negligible concentrations of this enzyme, azathioprine should be avoided.

Case Summary

Complaint/History: A 17-year-old previously healthy female presents with 1 week of fatigue, malaise and diffuse body aches, and yellow eyes.

Findings: Scleral icterus and jaundice.; hepatomegaly, with a liver edge 3 cm below the right costal margin; it is nontender and soft.

Labs/Tests: Serum antinuclear antibodies and anti–smooth muscle antibodies are detected. Percutaneous liver biopsy demonstrates an interface hepatitis with lymphocytic infiltration and hepatocyte necrosis.

Diagnosis: Autoimmune hepatitis.

Treatment: Oral prednisone and azathioprine.

Bibliography

Alvarez F, Berg PA, Bianchi FB, et al. International autoimmune hepatitis group report: review of criteria for diagnosis of autoimmune hepatitis. *J Hepatol.* 1999;31:929–938.

Floreani A, Rodrigo L, Vergani D, et al. Autoimmune hepatitis: contrasts and comparisons in children and adults – a comprehensive review. *J Autoimmun.* 2013;46:7–16.

Heneghan MA, Yeoman AD, Verma S, et al. Autoimmune hepatitis. *Lancet.* 2013;382(9902):1433–1444.

Invernizzi P. Autoimmune liver diseases. *World J Gastroenterol.* 2008;14(21):3290–3291.

Lohse AW, Giorgina MV. Autoimmune hepatitis. *J Hepatol.* 2011;55(1):171–182.

Maggiore G. Juvenile autoimmune hepatitis: spectrum of the disease. *World J Hepatol.* 2014;6(7):464–476.

18-Month-Old Female With Acute-Onset Refusal to Walk

Tracey Samko ■ Cynthia H. Ho

An 18-month-old female presents with refusal to walk for 2 days. Her parents also report tactile fevers and fussiness.

What are the causes of refusal to walk in children?

Musculoskeletal causes include diskitis, septic arthritis, toxic (transient) synovitis, and pyomyositis. Meningitis, appendicitis, trauma, malignancy, and intussusception can also present as refusal to walk in young children.

CLINICAL PEARL **STEP 2/3**

Make sure to perform a thorough physical examination because young children may not be able to localize their pain and cannot clearly communicate their symptoms. Lower extremity conditions, spinal pathology, acute abdomen, and child abuse can all present with refusal to walk.

Case Point 40.1

Her temperature is 103°F, pulse rate is 180/min, and respiratory rate is 25/min. On physical examination, she appears tired but responsive. She is lying supine in bed, with her right hip rotated externally (Fig. 40.1). She cries when her right thigh is compressed into her hip. The abdomen and spine are nontender to palpation. The remainder of her physical examination is normal.

What is concerning about her physical examination?

Observation is a critical part of the pediatric physical examination. Pay particular attention to the child's mental status and position of comfort because certain diagnoses are suggested by the ways in which children reduce their pain. For example, a child with acute abdomen (e.g., due to acute appendicitis or peritonitis) will lie supine and avoid movement because movement causes peritoneal irritation. On the other hand, irritability and lethargy in a febrile child with tachycardia should raise concern for sepsis and represents decreased cerebral perfusion.

In this particular patient, the patient's positioning is concerning for septic arthritis of the left hip. Children with hip arthritis maintain their hip flexed with slight abduction and in external rotation to alleviate arthralgia because this position minimizes intraarticular pressure.

CLINICAL PEARL **STEP 2/3**

The position of comfort in hip arthritis—flexion, **ab**duction and external rotation—can be remembered by the FABER acronym.

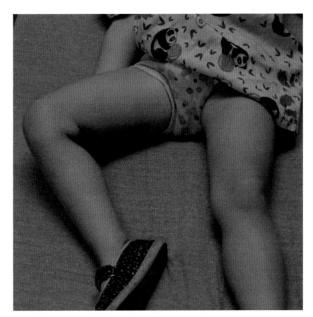

Fig. 40.1 This child's right thigh is held in flexion and external rotation, which relieves hip joint pressure. (From Neville DNW, Zuckerbraun N. Pediatric nontraumatic hip pathology. *Clin Pediatr Emerg Med.* 2016;17:13–28.)

What is the difference between arthralgia and arthritis?

Arthralgia means joint pain; arthritis means joint inflammation. Although arthritis will generally result in arthralgia, not all causes of arthralgia result in arthritis. Arthritis can often be identified by the cardinal signs of inflammation—rubor (erythema), calor (warmth), tumor (edema), and dolor (pain).

CLINICAL PEARL	STEP 2/3

Arthritis involving the knee and ankle are usually readily apparent. However, because the hip is a deeper joint, it may be challenging to detect erythema, warmth, and swelling.

What are the causes of arthritis in children?

The most common causes of arthritis in children include toxic (transient) synovitis, juvenile idiopathic arthritis (JIA), septic arthritis, hemarthrosis due to trauma and, rarely, pseudogout. Although the differential diagnosis is broad, benign and emergent causes can usually be distinguished by whether the child will bear weight. Patients with septic arthritis will not typically bear weight, whereas patients with noninfectious causes of arthritis bear weight but walk with a limp.

CLINICAL PEARL	STEP 2/3

In nonambulatory children, lifting the child—or asking the parents to lift the child—to a standing position with support and trying to see if she or he will bear weight on the affected extremity may help differentiate infectious from noninfectious causes of arthritis.

In a young child with acute monoarticular arthritis with fever, the most common causes are septic arthritis and toxic (transient) synovitis. Septic arthritis is due to infection of the synovial fluid, usually by bacteria. Transient synovitis, a nonpyogenic arthritis (frequently of the hip), may

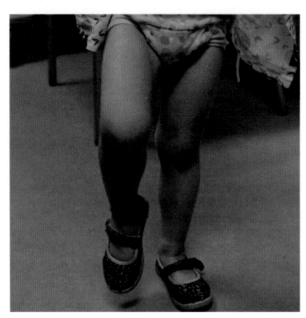

Fig. 40.2 The patient refuses to bear weight on her right leg. (From Neville DNW, Zuckerbraun N. Pediatric nontraumatic hip pathology. *Clin Pediatr Emerg Med.* 2016;17:13–28.)

be confused with septic arthritis but is benign and self-limited. The incidence of transient synovitis peaks in children 3 to 10 years old. In contrast to transient synovitis, children with septic arthritis appear more systemically ill—often with a high fever, tachycardia, and irritability—and avoid weight bearing on the affected extremity. The white blood cell count and serum C-reactive protein (CRP) level may be elevated.

BASIC SCIENCE/CLINICAL PEARL	STEP 1/2/3

The presence of three or more of the following—fever, erythrocyte sedimentation rate >40 mm/hr, white blood cell count > 12 × 10^9/L, and inability to bear weight, collectively known as the Kocher criteria—is predictive of septic arthritis over toxic synovitis.

Case Point 40.2

An attempt is made to have the child stand, but she refuses to bear weight on her right leg (Fig. 40.2).

What is the next step in determining the cause of her hip pain?

In a patient with suspected septic arthritis, immediate arthrocentesis (needle aspiration of synovial fluid) performed by an experienced health care provider is the next step (Fig. 40.3). Synovial fluid appears cloudy in septic arthritis. Synovial fluid should be sent for cell count, glucose, Gram staining, and culture.

Other laboratory studies. such as an elevated white blood cell count (leukocytosis), increased erythrocyte sedimentation rate (ESR), and elevated serum CRP level may be suggestive, but not diagnostic, of septic arthritis.

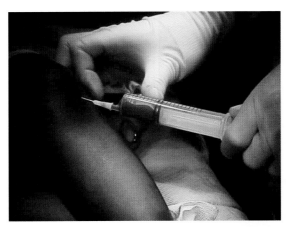

Fig. 40.3 Arthrocentesis (from the knee). Note the bloody and purulent appearance of the fluid. (From Paterson M, Joseph B. Musculoskeletal infection. In: Luqmani R, Robb J, Porter D, Joseph B, eds. *Textbook of Orthopaedics, Trauma and Rheumatology*. 2nd ed. Edinburgh: Elsevier; 2013:93–100.)

Plain radiographs of the hip may show increased joint space of the hip, suggesting an effusion. In addition, they may help identify tumors or fractures if other causes are suspected. However, hip radiographs are not sensitive in detecting hip arthritis.

Ultrasound is a more sensitive modality than pain radiography in detecting a hip effusion and can help guide the needle during arthrocentesis. Ultrasound is generally preferred over fluoroscopy in young children because the latter modality does not show cartilage.

CLINICAL PEARL   **STEP 2/3**

Needle aspiration of a hip effusion should almost always be performed under imaging guidance.

Magnetic resonance imaging (MRI) of the hip is very sensitive in identifying effusions and joint pathology; however, it is an expensive study and requires patient cooperation to lie still for more than 30 minutes to obtain images. In a young child, procedural sedation is often used for MRI. Therefore, the risks of potential diagnostic delay and procedural sedation when obtaining an MRI scan should be weighed against the potential benefits of the study.

Case Point 40.3

Radiographs of the hip are obtained, and findings suggest a hip effusion (Fig. 40.4). Ultrasound confirms the hip effusion (Fig. 40.5), and arthrocentesis is performed under ultrasound guidance at the same time. Empiric antibiotics are initiated while waiting for laboratory test results to return.

How are synovial fluid cell counts and chemistries interpreted?
A synovial fluid white blood cell count more than 50,000/µL, with more than 90% polymorphonuclear leukocytes (PMNs) and synovial fluid glucose less than 30% of serum glucose, are highly suggestive of septic arthritis. A summary of synovial fluid findings is presented in Table 40.1.

Isolation of a causative organism in synovial fluid culture is the gold standard for diagnosis of septic arthritis. However, synovial fluid culture is only 60% to 70% sensitive for septic arthritis.

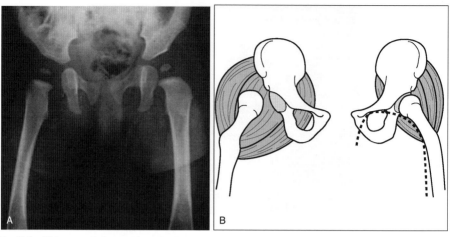

Fig. 40.4 (A) Increased distance from the femoral head to the acetabulum is suggestive of right hip effusion. (B) Joint effusion results in disruption of the Shenton line *(dashed line)*. (From Krogstad P. Septic arthritis. In: Cherry J, Demmler-Harrison G, Kaplan S, et al., eds. *Feigin and Cherry's Textbook of Pediatric Infectious Diseases.* Philadelphia: Elsevier/Saunders; 2013:727–734.)

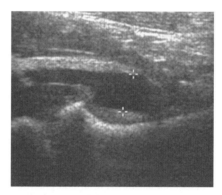

Fig. 40.5 Increased fluid is seen in the joint space of the left hip *(space between cross markers)*. (From Schwartz-Doria A, Babyn P. Imaging investigation of arthritis in children. In: Weissman BN, ed. *Imaging of Arthritis and Metabolic Bone Disease.* Philadelphia: Saunders/Elsevier; 2009:428–456.)

Therefore, a clinical diagnosis is often determined based on the examination, imaging studies, and laboratory studies when cultures are negative.

Case Point 40.4

The synovial fluid cell count finds 100,000/μL mononuclear cells that are 92% PMNs. Gram staining of the synovial fluid reveals gram-positive cocci in clusters.

What organisms are responsible for septic arthritis?

Staphylococcus aureus is the most common cause of septic arthritis in all age groups, with community-acquired methicillin resistant *S. aureus* (CA-MRSA) accounting for more than

TABLE 40.1 ■ **Findings in Synovial Fluid**

Condition	Feature	WBC Count (cells/µL)	PMNs (%)	Other
Normal	Clear; yellow	<200	<10	—
Juvenile rheumatoid arthritis	Turbid	25–50,000	50–70	50% with decreased complement
Reactive arthritis	Cloudy to turbid; may be clear	1000–150,000	50–70	Increased complement
Lyme arthritis	Turbid	500–100,000	>50	—
Septic arthritis	Turbid; white-gray	10,000–250,000	>75	Low glucose, high lactate levels

PMNs, Polymorphonuclear leukocytes (neutrophils); *WBC,* white blood cell.
From McQuillen KK. Musculoskeletal disorders. In: Walls RM, Hockberger RS, Gausche-Hill M, eds. *Rosen's Emergency Medicine: Concepts and Clinical Practice.* Philadelphia: Saunders/Elsevier, 2018. 2201–2217.

25% of isolates. Group A *Streptococcus* spp. (e.g., *Streptococcus pyogenes*) and *Streptococcus pneumoniae* account for 10% to 20% of cases. In the prevaccination era, *Haemophilus influenzae* type b (Hib) comprised about 50% of the cases of septic arthritis in children; now septic arthritis due to Hib is rare.

Other organisms to consider depend on the child's age, comorbid conditions, and geographic location. In neonates, group B *Streptococcus* spp. and gram-negative organisms are often isolated. *Kingella kingae* has been described in patients younger than 3 years. In sexually active adolescents, *Neisseria gonorrhoeae* infection should be considered. In patients with sickle cell disease, *Salmonella* spp. must be considered. In endemic areas, Lyme disease should be considered because it may cause septic arthritis, generally affecting the knee. Tuberculosis should be considered in those with a history of exposure or in endemic areas.

What antibiotics would you start?

Empiric antibiotic choice should take into account the most commonly isolated organisms and local resistance patterns. In an 18-month-old child, *S. aureus*, *S. pyogenes*, and *K. kingae* should be considered. Cephalexin or nafcillin would be appropriate choices for *S. aureus* and *S. pyogenes.* In areas where the incidence of CA-MRSA is 10% or higher, clindamycin or vancomycin should be used instead. A third-generation cephalosporin should be initiated when there is concern for *K. kingae.*

The duration of antibiotic therapy should be tailored to the organism and the patient's clinical status. Historically, intravenous antibiotics were recommended for 4 to 6 weeks; recent studies have supported a shorter duration of therapy, with transition to oral antibiotics when clinical signs and inflammatory markers improve. Two weeks is sufficient for streptococcal spp. or *K. kingae,* whereas longer courses are indicated for *S. aureus* and gram-negative infections.

What are complications of septic arthritis?

Complications can be seen in the immediate or long-term period following diagnosis. The initial course can be complicated by osteomyelitis of the adjacent bone. Failure of early joint decompression can result in avascular necrosis and impaired bone growth. Damage to the growth plate may not be noticed immediately and may present months to years following treatment. Additionally, decreased range of motion or chronic joint dislocation may occur. Recurrence or chronic infection may complicate the treatment course.

BASIC SCIENCE/CLINICAL PEARL   **STEP 1/2/3**

Delay in the initiation of therapy for septic arthritis increases the risks of long-term complication such as permanent hip dislocation. Infections with *S. aureus* also increase the risk of
long-term complications in comparison to other bacteria, such as *Haemophilus influenzae*.

What is the treatment of septic arthritis?

The treatment of septic arthritis is dependent on the clinical course. Fluid resuscitation is often
indicated to achieve euvolemia in patients presenting with sepsis. Antibiotics should be promptly
initiated. Pain control may require opioids. Joint decompression can be achieved through serial
arthrocentesis or open surgical arthrotomy. Patients who present earlier in the course tend to have
better outcomes without surgery compared with those presenting after 5 days.

CLINICAL PEARL   **STEP 2/3**

The presence of fibrin, loculations, and/or other tissue debris in the synovial fluid may preclude the use of arthrocentesis for joint decompression.

Case Point 40.5

The patient undergoes surgical irrigation and debridement (I&D) of the hip. Two days later, the
wound culture grows methicillin-sensitive *S. aureus* (MSSA). The patient successfully completes
a prolonged course of oxacillin.

BEYOND THE PEARLS

- Septic arthritis in the neonate is a very challenging diagnosis to make because of the
  frequent lack of fever, leukocytosis, and sepsis. Neonatal septic arthritis of the hip generally presents with a swollen thigh and flexed hip but may present as an abdominal mass
  after the hip effusion spontaneously drains up into the pelvis, along the obturator internus
  muscle.
- Indolent septic arthritis should prompt suspicion for fungus, particularly in areas that are
  endemic for species such as *Coccidioides immitis*, *Blastomyces dermatitidis*, and *Histoplasma capsulatum*. Additionally, species such as *Candida* spp. should be considered in
  the immunocompromised patient.
- When synovial fluid cultures from repeated arthrocentesis procedures are persistently positive, open drainage of the joint is indicated.
- When an organism is isolated and identified, antibiotics should be narrowed to the narrow-
  est spectrum that is effective against the causative organism. This enhances patient health
  outcomes, reduces the development of antibiotic resistance, and decreases costs.
- Intraarticular antibiotic administration is not indicated in pediatric septic arthritis because
  it causes joint irritation, and adequate synovial penetration is achieved with systemic
  antibiotics. Antibiotics rapidly penetrate joint fluid from the systemic circulation, whereas
  diffusion back into the systemic circulation is very slow.
- The use of dexamethasone in addition to standard of care to reduce long-term sequelae
  has been studied in several randomized trials. The results have been mixed.

Case Summary

Complaint/History: An 18-month-old female presents with fever, fussiness and refusal to walk.

Findings: She is lying supine in bed, with her right hip rotated externally, and she cries when
her right thigh is compressed into her hip.

Labs/Tests: Plain radiographs reveal a hip effusion. Needle arthrocentesis reveals a pyogenic infection.

Diagnosis: Septic arthritis.

Treatment: Antibiotics and surgical debridement.

Bibliography

Basmaci R, Lorrot M, Bidet P, et al. Comparison of clinical and biologic features of kingella kingae and staphylococcus aurea arthritis at initial evaluation. *Pediatr Infect Dis J*. 2011;30(10):902–903.

Fordham L, Gunderman R, Blatt ER, et al. Limping child–ages 0-5 years. *Am Coll Radiol (ACR)*. 2007:5.

Kocher MS, Zurakowski D, Kasser JR. Differentiating between septic arthritis and transient synovitis of the hip in children: an evidence-based clinical prediction algorithm. *J Bone Joint Surg Am*. 1999;81(12):1662–1670.

Krogstad P. Septic Arthritis. In: *Feigin and Cherry's Textbook of Pediatric Infectious Diseases*. Published December 31, 2013:727–734.e2. © 2014.

Pääkkönen M, Kallio MJ, Peltola H, Kallio PE. Pediatric septic hip with or without arthrotomy: retrospective analysis of 62 consecutive nonneonatal culture-positive cases. *J Pediatr Orthop B*. 2010;19(3):264–269.

Shmerling RH. Synovial fluid analysis: a critical reappraisal. *Rheum Dis Clin North Am*. 1994;20:503.

6-Year-Old Male With Cough and Fever

Vidhi Doshi ▥ Mikhaela Cielo

A 6-year-old male presents in January with 2 days of low-grade fevers. The fevers have been daily, with a maximum temperature of 39°C. He has had associated headache, cough, rhinorrhea, and generalized malaise. On first impression, he is well-appearing.

What is the most likely diagnosis based on the symptoms and time of year?
The most likely diagnosis based on the cough and runny nose in an otherwise well-appearing child is the common cold. The common cold has high prevalence during fall and winter months; however, it can occur year-round. In North America, rhinovirus starts with a small wave in March and April and then has a larger peak in September. Parainfluenza viruses follow in October and November. In winter, influenza viruses, coronaviruses, and respiratory syncytial virus are the most prevalent. Enteroviruses are mostly seen in the summer months but occur year-round. Adenoviruses are seen continuously at low rates, but epidemics occur primarily in the winter, spring, and summer.

BASIC SCIENCE PEARL	STEP 1

The most common viruses implicated in the common cold—in order of most to least common—include rhinovirus, coronavirus, influenza virus, parainfluenza virus, respiratory syncytial virus, adenovirus, and enterovirus.

Case Point 41.1

He has no past medical history and has otherwise been well, although during review of systems his mother reports that his appetite is markedly decreased. He has received all his vaccines, except for his annual flu shot. He is enrolled in first grade, and a number of children have been ill with cold symptoms. His mother states that his best friend was diagnosed with influenza virus infection yesterday.

His temperature is 38.7°C, pulse rate is 110/min, and respiratory rate is 18/min. On physical examination, he appears tired but is interactive. He has clear rhinorrhea and is coughing intermittently on examination. The rest of his physical examination is normal, including auscultation of the chest.

What is the most likely diagnosis?
Although any of the seasonal respiratory viruses listed should be considered, the recent exposure history should raise the suspicion for influenza virus infection. Clinical diagnosis of influenza virus infection can be difficult, given that other viruses cause similar symptoms, but it should be considered in the influenza season regardless of immunization status and during any outbreaks.

Laboratory testing is not required unless it will change the clinical care of the patient or others (e.g., cohorting infected patients in the hospital or giving prophylaxis to family members) because generally treatment will be supportive.

CLINICAL PEARL   **STEP 2/3**

Testing for influenza virus should be performed in patients who have a high risk of complications (or who reside with a household member in a high-risk category), children younger than 2 years, and all children who are hospitalized with an acute respiratory illness or may have neurologic complications of influenza virus, such as meningitis. Other children may be treated presumptively.

If testing is to be pursued, reverse transcriptase-polymerase chain reaction (RT-PCR), viral culture, or rapid influenza molecular assays are recommended as the tests of choice. An RT-PCR assay and viral culture are considered gold standards; however, rapid influenza molecular assays can yield results within 20 minutes and have a sensitivity of 50% to 70% and specificity of 90% to 95%.

CLINICAL PEARL   **STEP 2/3**

If providers do not obtain a true nasopharyngeal swab specimen when testing for influenza (e.g., the swab is not inserted far enough into the nare), results may be inaccurate.

CLINICAL PEARL   **STEP 2/3**

In immunocompetent older children and adults, there is little viral shedding after 5 days of illness, and negative tests during this period do not reliably exclude influenza. In infants, young children, and immunocompromised hosts, the duration of viral shedding may exceed 1 week.

Case Point 41.2

A rapid influenza nasopharyngeal molecular assay swab is positive for influenza A virus.

Diagnosis: Upper respiratory tract infection due to influenza virus.

What is influenza virus?

Influenza virus is a single-stranded RNA of three types—A, B, and C (Fig. 41.1). Influenza A and B viruses are the primary human pathogens that cause seasonal epidemics, whereas influenza virus type C is a sporadic cause of mild upper respiratory tract illness. Influenza A viruses are divided into subtypes based on surface proteins called hemagglutinin (HA) and neuraminidase (NA).

Small changes in the HA gene occur through point mutations during viral replication and result in new influenza strains of the same HA type, a phenomenon known as *antigen drift*. This antigenic drift occurs yearly resulting in annual epidemics (Fig. 41.2). Major changes in subtypes are not as common but can occur through reassortment of viral gene segments when more than one strain of influenza simultaneously infects a single host, a phenomenon known as *antigen shift*. This can occur in humans or animal hosts, resulting in the emergence of novel subtypes.

BASIC SCIENCE PEARL   **STEP 1**

Worldwide epidemics, known as pandemics, occur every few decades. Both antigenic drifts and antigenic shifts can result in a pandemic.

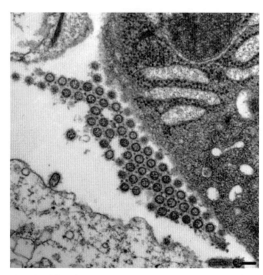

Fig. 41.1 The influenza virus, budding from an infected cell in tissue culture. (Courtesy Cynthia Goldsmith, Centers for Disease Control and Prevention.)

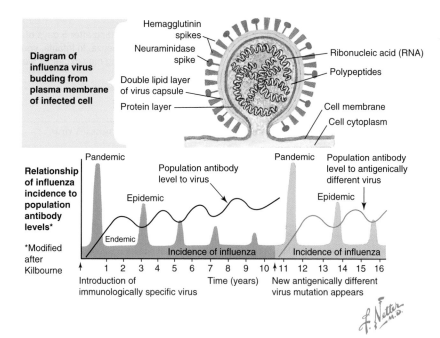

Fig. 41.2 The influenza virus and its epidemiology. (From Yeh SH. Influenza. In: Jong EC, Stevens DL, eds. *Netter's Infectious Diseases*. Philadelphia: Elsevier/Saunders; 2012:34–38.)

BASIC SCIENCE PEARL	STEP 1

Although influenza A and B viruses both express HA and NA, only influenza A undergoes significant antigen drift and shift. Only two distinct lineages of influenza B have been observed in circulation since 1983.

What is the transmission modality and epidemiology of influenza virus?
Influenza virus is spread primarily by respiratory tract droplets that are released by coughing and sneezing. Secondarily, when the droplets land on surfaces, autoinoculation can occur with someone touching the object and then touching respiratory mucosa.

BASIC SCIENCE/CLINICAL PEARL   **STEP 1/2/3**

Handwashing is one of the most effective methods to prevent the spread of the virus. Children should also be taught to sneeze into their sleeves and to wash their hands or use alcohol sanitizer after coughing and sneezing.

Incidence of influenza in healthy children ranges from 10% to 40%/year. The highest incidence of community outbreaks occurs with school-age children who then spread the virus to the adults in the family. The incidence varies based on rates of immunity in the community from having had the disease or having had the influenza vaccine with the circulating strain or a related strain.

How do patients with influenza virus infection present?
Presenting symptoms and complications vary by age (Table 41.1). Influenza in healthy children is most often an acute, self-limited, and uncomplicated disease. Typically, symptoms include fever, malaise, headaches, myalgia, cough, sore throat, and rhinitis. Younger children tend to have higher fevers, less prominent respiratory findings, and more gastrointestinal complaints. Patients with uncomplicated influenza usually improve in 1 week; however, cough and weakness can persist for

---

TABLE 41.1 ■ Clinical Manifestations of Influenza Virus Infection by Age

Age	Manifestation	Frequency
Infant, toddler < 5 yr	Afebrile URI	+
	Febrile URI	+++
	Acute otitis media	++
	Pneumonia	+
	Laryngotracheobronchitis	+
	Bronchiolitis	+
	Sepsis syndrome	+
Child ≥ 5 yr	Afebrile URI	+
	Flulike syndrome[a]	+++
	Acute otitis media	++
	Pneumonia	+
	Myositis	+
	Myocarditis	Rare
	Encephalopathy	Rare

[a]Fever, cough, headache, myalgia, and malaise.
URI, Upper respiratory tract infection; +++, most common manifestation; ++, common manifestation; +, infrequent manifestation.
From Dawood FS, Bresee J. Influenza viruses. In: Long S, Prober C, and Fischer M, eds. *Principles and Practice of Pediatric Infectious Diseases.* 5th ed. Philadelphia: Elsevier; 2018:1181–1190.

several weeks. Infection with influenza virus does not preclude further infection with a different influenza type or subtype later in the season.

Children younger than 24 months are at a higher risk of hospitalization and mortality related to influenza virus. Risk factors for increased morbidity and mortality from influenza virus are summarized in Box 41.1. However, 40% of pediatric deaths from influenza virus are not associated with any high-risk conditions. There were at least 148 deaths from influenza in the United States in children younger than 18 years old in the 2014 to 2015 season.

What treatments are available for influenza virus?

There are two classes of antiviral medications for treatment or prophylaxis of influenza infections, NA inhibitors (e.g., oseltamivir, zanamivir) and adamantanes. NA inhibitors are the recommended influenza antiviral drugs, given the widespread resistance to adamantanes.

Antiviral treatment is recommended as soon as possible for patients with suspected or confirmed influenza requiring hospitalization, those who have severe or complicated illness regardless of previous health or vaccination status, and those who are at high risk for influenza complications. Diagnostic confirmation of influenza virus is not required, and the start of therapy should not be delayed for testing results. Treatment is associated with reduced morbidity and mortality.

Case Point 41.3

The patient is given treatment for influenza with oseltamivir for 5 days and given strict return precautions.

The patient initially improves after finishing oseltamivir, but he then develops a worsening cough, with fevers 1 week afterward. On examination, he has tachypnea and crackles in his right lower lung fields.

BOX 41.1 ■ Children and Adolescents at High Risk for Influenza Complications[a]

- Children < 5 years; highest risk for children < 2 years
- Persons with chronic pulmonary (including asthma), cardiovascular (except hypertension alone), renal, hepatic, hematologic (including sickle cell disease), or metabolic disorders (including diabetes mellitus), or neurologic and neurodevelopmental conditions (including disorders of the brain, spinal cord, peripheral nerve, and muscle, e.g., cerebral palsy, epilepsy [seizure disorders], stroke, intellectual disability [mental retardation], moderate to severe developmental delay, muscular dystrophy, or spinal cord injury)
- Persons with immunosuppression, including that caused by medications or by HIV infection
- Adolescents who are pregnant or postpartum (within 2 weeks after delivery)
- Persons < 19 years who are receiving long-term aspirin therapy
- Native Americans, Alaska Natives
- Persons who are morbidly obese
- Residents of long-term care facilities

---

[a]As identified by the Centers for Disease Control and Prevention.
Adapted from Havers FP, Campbell AJP. Influenza viruses. In: Kliegman RM, Stanton B, St Geme J, Schor NF, EDS. *Nelson Textbook of Pediatrics.* Philadelphia: Elsevier; 2015:1598–1603.

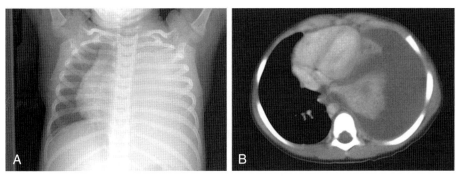

Fig. 41.3 (A) A complicated pneumonia with left hemithorax opacification. (B) Computed tomography scan reveals lung collapse and pleural effusion. (From Harper MB. Pneumonia. In: Bergelson J, Zaoutis T, Shah SS, eds. *Pediatric Infectious Diseases: The Requisites in Pediatrics.* Philadelphia: Mosby/Elsevier; 2008:117–124.)

What are the common complications of influenza?

The most common complication of influenza is otitis media because it can complicate the course of 10% to 50% of children with influenza. Respiratory complications include viral pneumonia, laryngotracheitis, tracheobronchitis, bronchitis, respiratory failure, and exacerbations of underlying chronic lung diseases, such as asthma. Pneumonia due to a co-infection with influenza virus and either *Streptococcus pneumoniae* or *Staphylococcus aureus* is synergistic, often leading to severe and possibly even fatal disease (Fig. 41.3).

Neurologic complications are less common and include febrile seizures, encephalitis, aseptic meningitis, acute cerebellar ataxia, transverse myelitis, Guillain-Barré syndrome, acute postinfectious encephalitis, encephalopathy, and acute mental status changes. Acute myositis can occur but is frequently mild. Cardiac complications such as myocarditis and pericarditis are rare.

Case Point 41.4

> The chest radiograph reveals pneumonia. The patient is given amoxicillin and clindamycin to treat a bacterial pneumonia complicating his influenza virus infection. During a follow-up phone call, his mother reports that he has had resolution of all his symptoms except for a dry cough, which is improving.
>
> His mother inquires about whether he should be receiving a yearly influenza vaccination.

What are the indications and contraindications for the different influenza vaccines?

Each year, the seasonal vaccine changes in anticipation of the predominant influenza strains that are expected to circulate. There are two forms of the vaccine, the inactivated influenza vaccine (IIV) that is given intramuscularly and the live-attenuated influenza vaccine (LAIV) that is given intranasally. The LAIV is not recommend in children younger than 2 years, children with asthma or recurrent wheezing, children with a history of anaphylaxis to gentamycin, arginine, or gelatin, children with medical conditions that increase risk of complications (see Table 41.1), pregnant patients, or children who are in close contact with severely immunocompromised individuals. The IIV is licensed for use in children as young as 6 months, and the only contraindication is a history of severe allergic reaction to the influenza vaccine.

CLINICAL PEARL	STEP 2/3

In children younger than 9 years who are receiving the IIV for the first time, two doses separated by 4 weeks are recommended. In subsequent years, only one dose is necessary.

CLINICAL PEARL	STEP 2/3

Annual immunization is necessary, even if the previous season's vaccine contained one or more of the antigens to be administered in the current season because immunity declines during the year following vaccination.

BEYOND THE PEARLS

- The most recent influenza pandemic, due to a novel H1N1 influenza A virus appearing in 2009, led to more than 60 million cases of influenza virus infection and more than 12,500 deaths in the United States alone.
- Neuraminidase inhibitor treatment in children with influenza only reduces the duration of illness by 1 day but decreases the incidence of otitis media by 50%.
- Postexposure chemoprophylaxis can be used to prevent infection in high-risk children who are not fully immunized but is not a substitution for vaccination. Postexposure prophylaxis should be given within 48 hours of the most recent exposure.
- Children with a mild egg allergy (e.g., hives) can receive the influenza virus vaccine with observation in clinic for 30 minutes after vaccine administration, as long as trained personnel and appropriate resuscitative equipment are available. If the patient has a history of anaphylaxis or a severe allergy to egg, however, he or she should be referred for consultation with an allergist prior to any vaccination being administered.
- Children who receive the nasal live attenuated influenza vaccine have detectable vaccine virus shedding for up to 3 weeks.
- The use of aspirin during influenza virus infection is associated with Reye syndrome, a rapidly progressive and often fatal encephalopathy with liver involvement. Parents should be instructed to avoid giving aspirin to young children unless prescribed, and chronic aspirin therapy should be temporarily stopped for confirmed or suspected influenza virus infections in young children.

Case Summary

Complaint/History: A 6-year-old male presents in winter with low-grade fevers, cough, and rhinorrhea.

Findings: He is coughing through his examination, but his pulmonary examination is normal.

Labs/Tests: A rapid influenza nasopharyngeal molecular assay swab is positive for influenza A virus.

Diagnosis: Upper respiratory tract infection due to influenza virus.

Treatment: Oseltamivir.

Bibliography

American Academy of Pediatrics. Influenza. In: Kimberlin DW, Brady MT, Jackson MA, Long SS, eds. *Red Book®: 2015 Report of the Committee on the Infectious Diseases.* American Academy of Pediatrics; 2015:476–493.

Centers for Disease Control and Prevention. Influenza. In: Hamborsky J, Kroger A, Wolfe S, eds. *Epidemiology and Prevention of Vaccine-Preventable Diseases.* 13th ed. Washington D.C: Public Health Foundation; 2015.

Fry AM, Goswami D, Nahar K, et al. Efficacy of oseltamivir treatment started within 5 days of symptom onset to reduce influenza illness duration and virus shedding in an urban setting in Bangladesh: a randomised placebo-controlled trial. *Lancet Infect Dis.* 2014;14(2):109.

Hendley JO. Epidemiology, pathogenesis, and treatment of the common cold. *Semin Pediatr Infect Dis.* 1998;9:50.

Robert M, Kliegman RM, Stanton BF, Geme JW, Schor NF. Influenza. *Nelson Textbook of Pediatrics.* 20th ed. 2016. Chapter 258.

Sung RY, Murray HG, Chan RC, et al. Seasonal patterns of respiratory syncytial virus infection in Hong Kong: a preliminary report. *J Infect Dis.* 1987;156:527.

Wong KK, Jain S, Blanton L, Dhara R, Brammer L, Fry AM, et al. Influenza-associated pediatric deaths in the United States, 2004-2012. *Pediatrics.* 2013;132(5):796.

10-Year-Old Male With Dysphagia

Vrinda Bhardwaj ■ Michelle Pietzak

A 10-year-old Caucasian male presents with a chief complaint of an acidic feeling in his throat and a dull burning sensation in his chest during meals for the last 6 months. He has associated nausea without frank vomiting.

What is the most likely diagnosis?

The symptoms are suggestive of esophagitis, which is most commonly due to gastroesophageal reflux disease (GERD). GERD is characterized by the passage of acidic gastric contents backward into the esophagus. It is diagnosed clinically by eliciting symptoms consistent with heartburn and then treating empirically with acid suppression. Radiologic tests, such as upper gastrointestinal (GI) contrast studies, may also show GERD but are more helpful in looking for anatomic abnormalities. If there is no response to acid suppression after 2 to 3 months, other causes of the GI symptomatology must be explored.

BASIC SCIENCE/CLINICAL PEARL	STEP 1/2/3

Gastroesophageal reflux is a normal physiologic event in everyone and consists simply of the passage of gastric contents into the esophagus. GERD, with a "D," is a disease that develops when there are complications of the reflux, such as esophagitis, erosions, or strictures. In contrast, vomiting is defined as an expulsion of refluxed gastric contents from the mouth. It can be a component of GERD. Rumination, on the other hand, is the deliberate regurgitation of food into the mouth, which is often then reswallowed. Patients with rumination often have underlying psychiatric or neurologic conditions.

Case Point 42.1

He is prescribed omeprazole, a proton pump inhibitor (PPI).

BASIC SCIENCE	STEP 1

The proton pump exchanges hydrogen (to make hydrochloric acid) for potassium (which goes intracellularly). PPIs selectively inactivate this proton pump in the parietal cell, the final step in acid production. Once inhibited by the PPI, the pump becomes unresponsive to stimulation by histamine, gastrin, and acetylcholine. Histamine-2 receptor antagonists (H2RAs) only block stimulation of the parietal cell by histamine. Thus, upregulation of gastrin or acetylcholine can overcome the effect of these drugs. This is why PPIs are more effective than H2RAs in healing erosive esophagitis due to GERD.

He returns to clinic 3 months later. His mother reports that the PPI has not had any significant effect on his symptoms. Furthermore, he has begun to have dysphagia (difficulty swallowing) in the last 2 months, worsening over the last month with globus pharyngis (sensation of a lump in the throat) and water brash (regurgitation of saliva back into the mouth with acid).

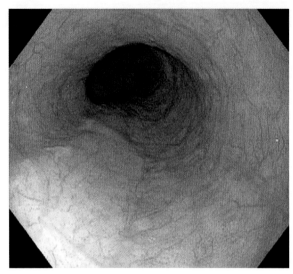

Fig. 42.1   Normal-caliber esophagus seen by endoscopy. (Courtesy Dr. Vrinda Bhardwaj.)

What is the differential diagnosis at this point?

Eosinophilic esophagitis (EoE), resistant or refractory GERD, esophageal stricture, and congenital vascular rings or slings should be considered in a patient with symptoms of dysphagia and gastroesophageal reflux. EoE, an atopic inflammatory disease sometimes referred to as *asthma of the esophagus,* should be considered if the patient has symptoms of GERD that do not respond to acid suppression therapy. Esophageal strictures in the pediatric population are often congenital rather than acquired, and should present with more prolonged symptoms, likely since birth. Acquired esophageal strictures should be suspected in patients with a history of caustic ingestion or chronic GERD. Vascular rings or slings should be suspected in a newborn with feeding intolerance and breathing difficulties. In a toddler with these complaints, an accidental or deliberately ingested foreign body must be in the differential.

BASIC SCIENCE/CLINICAL PEARL	STEP 1/2/3

Both GERD and EoE, left untreated, can cause esophageal stricture formation. An esophageal stricture is a narrowing in the esophagus caused by chronic inflammation leading to circumferential scar tissue formation (Figs. 42.1 and 42.2). Esophageal strictures can be treated by endoscopic balloon dilation (Figs. 42.3 and 42.4).

What is the next step?

Resistant or refractory GERD and EoE are the most likely diagnoses at this time, and a detailed dietary history can help differentiate between the two. GERD is often exacerbated by alcohol, caffeinated and carbonated beverages, and acidic foods (e.g., tomato sauce, fruit juices). Patients with EoE often are not able to identify specific trigger foods; rather, they have functional problems with eating. Younger patients with EoE tend to present with feeding dysfunction, vomiting, and fussiness; adolescents with EoE tend to have complaints of dysphagia and food impaction. A need to consume water with meals and taking "wet swallows" suggest EoE. Patients with dysphagia due to EoE also tend to cut up solid foods into small pieces and often take a long time to finish their meals.

It is also useful to obtain a personal and family history of atopy (e.g., eczema, allergic rhinitis, asthma, food allergies) because EoE is often seen with concurrent allergic diathesis.

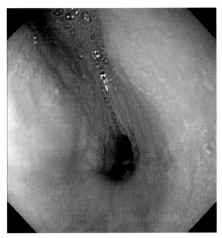

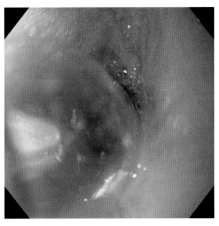

Fig. 42.3 Placement and expansion of balloon dilator. (Courtesy Dr. Vrinda Bhardwaj.)

Fig. 42.2 Esophageal stricture. (Courtesy Dr. Vrinda Bhardwaj.)

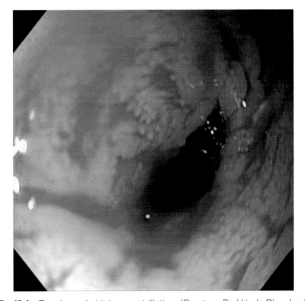

Fig. 42.4 Esophageal stricture postdilation. (Courtesy Dr. Vrinda Bhardwaj.)

Case Point 42.2

He has a history of food allergies, allergic rhinitis, and eczema. His family history is significant for maternal food allergies.

On physical examination, he is afebrile. His pulse rate is 85 beats/min, respiration rate is 18/min, blood pressure is 118/70 mm Hg, and oxygen saturation is 97% on room air. His weight is 28 kg (fifth percentile for age) and his height is 138 cm (50th percentile for age). He has nasal creases, pharyngeal cobblestoning, and a dry scaly rash (eczema) on the flexor surfaces of his arms bilaterally. The rest of the physical examination, including an abdominal examination, is normal.

CLINICAL PEARL	STEP 2/3

Although EoE is often seen in the setting of atopy, GERD is also often seen in patients with atopy; the latter occurs simply due to the high prevalence of GERD. (GERD itself is not associated with atopy.) Therefore, atopy is not a specific discriminator for EoE.

What is the next step?

The physical examination is useful to identify abnormal growth patterns that suggest severe and/or uncontrolled disease but would not be expected to differentiate between GERD and EoE. Stigmata of atopy (e.g., nasal congestion, allergic shiners, pharyngeal cobblestoning) can be seen if comorbid allergic diseases exist; however, no features on physical examination are specific in making the diagnosis of EoE. Laboratory testing may reveal peripheral eosinophilia on complete blood count (CBC), but this finding is neither sensitive nor specific for EoE.

BASIC SCIENCE/CLINICAL PEARL	STEP 1/2/3

Cobblestoning refers to the presence of small, round, uniform nodules on a mucosal surface, resembling a cobblestone street. Oropharyngeal cobblestoning is thought to be due to inflamed lymphoid tissue and can be seen in viral infections, Crohn disease, and allergic rhinitis due to postnasal drip into the posterior pharynx.

Because the physical examination and laboratory workup are nonspecific for EoE or complications of GERD, the next step would be direct endoscopic visualization of the esophageal lumen with biopsy. This procedure is known as *esophagogastroduodenoscopy* (scoping the upper GI tract—esophagus, stomach, and duodenum; EGD). EGD is able to identify and remove foreign bodies and identify erosions and ulcers in the esophagus and stomach seen in GERD and peptic ulcer disease, EoE-associated erosions, ulcers, and exudates, and esophageal narrowing or strictures seen in chronic GERD or EoE. EGD allows for esophageal biopsy, which remains the only reliable diagnostic test for EoE.

BASIC SCIENCE/CLINICAL PEARL	STEP 1/2/3

Eosinophil count in the CBC differential can be elevated in many different circumstances, including parasitic infections, food allergies, environmental allergies, malignancy, and systemic illnesses (e.g., inflammatory bowel disease).

Case Point 42.3

The patient undergoes EGD. Visually, his esophagus shows furrows, rings, and white plaques (Fig. 42.5). He does not have a stricture. Multiple biopsies are taken. Pathology shows a high eosinophil count and basal cell hyperplasia in his esophageal biopsies, consistent with EoE (Figs. 42.6–42.8).

Diagnosis: Eosinophilic esophagitis.

How is eosinophilic esophagitis treated?

EoE can be treated with medical or dietary approaches. Medical therapies for EoE include PPIs, corticosteroids, leukotriene modifiers, and biologic agents. Topical corticosteroids delivered to the esophagus (swallowed and not inhaled) have become the mainstay of pharmacotherapy for patients with EoE, given their substantially better safety profile.

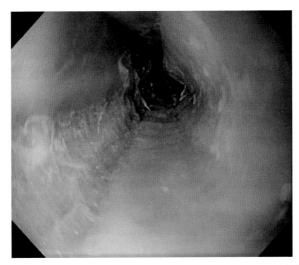

Fig. 42.5 Direct visual examination of the esophageal lumen showing furrows, rings and white plaques. (Courtesy Dr. Vrinda Bhardwaj.)

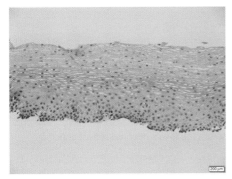

Fig. 42.6 Normal esophageal biopsy. (Courtesy Dr. Vrinda Bhardwaj.)

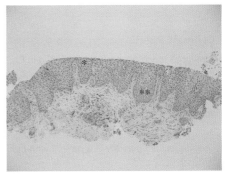

Fig. 42.7 Esophageal biopsy with increased eosinophils *(*)* and basal cell hyperplasia *(**)*. The basal cell hyperplasia is the lower part of the top cells (bottom of the epithelial layer). (Courtesy Dr. Vrinda Bhardwaj.)

Dietary therapies can be targeted or empiric. In targeted dietary therapy, food allergy testing via skin prick or determination of serum IgE levels is performed, and allergenic foods are eliminated from the patient's diet. In empiric dietary therapy, the six most commonly considered allergenic foods are excluded from the diet—milk, soy, eggs, wheat, nuts, and fish. Patients may react to one or multiple foods.

CLINICAL PEARL   **STEP 2/3**

In young children with vomiting, chest radiographs should also be considered to evaluate for a radiopaque foreign body, such as coins or magnets.

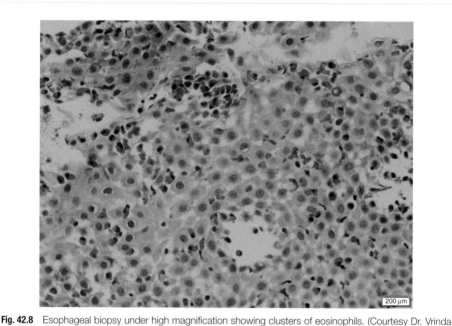

Fig. 42.8 Esophageal biopsy under high magnification showing clusters of eosinophils. (Courtesy Dr. Vrinda Bhardwaj.)

CLINICAL PEARL	STEP 2/3

Almost all foods have been implicated in EoE, but the most common are milk, egg, nuts, tree nuts, beef, wheat, fish, shellfish, corn, and soy.

BASIC SCIENCE/CLINICAL PEARL	STEP 1/2/3

Allergy testing via skin prick or determination of serum IgE levels may not reflect specific esophageal antigenicity in a patient with EoE.

If strict elimination diets and medications do not work, an elemental diet can be tried. An elemental allergen-free liquid formula (with predigested protein) is exclusively ingested for a minimum of 1 to 3 months to induce healing. Over time, various foods are introduced. Multiple EGDs with biopsies are often needed to assess clinical response and dilate strictures, if present.

CLINICAL PEARL	STEP 2/3

Unfortunately, once medications or specific food elimination diets are stopped, EoE generally relapses.

Case Point 42.4

Milk, soy, eggs, wheat, nuts, and fish are eliminated from the patient's diet for 3 months and his symptoms resolve. The foods are reintroduced—one new food per week—and his symptoms return with the reintroduction of fish. He is successfully able to treat his EoE with dietary restriction alone.

BEYOND THE PEARLS

- Of reported EoE cases, 75% are white males.
- The incidence of EoE is thought to be 1/10,000 people. However, it is likely underreported and underdiagnosed. The incidence is thought to be increasing, along with other allergic diseases.
- The most common clinical manifestations of EoE reported in pediatric studies are as follows: dysphagia (16%–100%), emesis (8%–100%), GERD (5%–82%), abdominal pain (5%–68%), food impaction (10%–50%), chest pain (17%–20%), diarrhea (1%–24%) and failure to thrive (5%–19%).
- The esophageal biopsy should demonstrate more than 15 eosinophils/high power field to confirm the diagnosis of EoE. Smaller numbers of eosinophils, which are usually located more superficially, are more suggestive of GERD.
- Inflammation should be restricted to the esophagus alone in EoE. If inflammation is present further down the GI tract, eosinophilic gastroenteritis (esophagus and stomach) should be diagnosed. This condition is often associated with abdominal pain, emesis, and diarrhea. Eosinophilia of the GI tract can also involve the small bowel and colon.
- GERD symptoms that respond to PPIs do not rule out EoE. PPI-responsive EoE has been described. Such a diagnosis must be made on repeat esophageal biopsy after several months of therapy.
- Humanized monoclonal antibodies against interleukin-5 (IL-5) and IgE (omalizumab) may be therapeutic options for disease that does not respond to dietary therapy or routine medications. Results from a small case series using the IL-5 antibodies reslizumab and mepolizumab have suggested that these biologics are well tolerated and may improve clinical symptoms, histology, and quality of life in patients with EoE.

Case Summary

Complaint/History: A 10-year-old Caucasian male presents with an acidic feeling in his throat, a burning sensation in his chest during meals, and nausea without frank vomiting for the past 6 months. His past medical history is significant for eczema, allergic rhinitis, and food allergies. He is prescribed a proton pump inhibitor for 3 months, without improvement. He has now developed dysphagia, globus pharyngis, and water brash.

Findings: The physical examination is significant for being underweight, with normal height for age. He has nasal creases, pharyngeal cobblestoning, and eczema on the flexor surfaces of his arms bilaterally. The rest of the physical examination, including an abdominal examination, is normal.

Labs/Tests: During esophagogastroduodenoscopy, his esophagus shows furrows, rings, and white plaques. Esophageal biopsies show high eosinophil counts.

Diagnosis: Eosinophilic esophagitis.

Treatment: The top food allergens are eliminated from the patient's diet for 3 months, and his symptoms resolve. The foods are reintroduced as one new food per week, and his symptoms return with the reintroduction of fish. He is successfully able to treat his eosinophilic esophagitis with dietary restriction alone.

Bibliography

Arora AS, Yamazaki K. Eosinophilic esophagitis: asthma of the esophagus? *Clin Gastroenterol Hepatol.* 2004;2(7):523–530.

Bhardwaj V, Harb R, Naon H. Eosinophilic esophagitis: a clinicopathological review. *Ann Pediatr Child Health.* 2015;3(2):1040–1045.

Carr S, Watson W. Eosinophilic esophagitis. *Allergy Asthma Clin Immunol.* 2011;7(Suppl 1):S8–S15.

Furuta GT, Liacouras CA, Collins MH, et al. Eosinophilic esophagitis in children and adults: a systematic review and consensus recommendations for diagnosis and treatment. *Gastroenterology.* 2007;133(4): 1342.63.

Liacouras CA, Furuta GT, Hirano I, et al. Eosinophilic esophagitis: updated consensus recommendations for children and adults. *J Allergy Clin Immunol.* 2011;128(1):3–20.e6.

Moawad FJ, Veerapan GR, Wong RK. Eosinophilic esophagitis. *Dig Dis Sci.* 2009;54(9):1818–1828.

10-Year-Old Male With Fast Breathing

Anne Zepeda-Tiscareno ▦ Monika Alas-Segura ▦ Keith Lewis

A 10-year-old male presents for evaluation after 1 week of cough and rhinorrhea, nasal congestion, and low-grade fever. In the past 2 days, he has developed a productive cough and fever to 103°F. He says that there are other children who are sick at school with "colds," but his parents note that he is more tired, eating and drinking less, and breathing faster. His parents state that he is otherwise healthy and does not have any chronic illnesses. He has occasional headaches, stomach aches, and emesis. The parents have given him antipyretics and cough medicine over the course of the illness. They are concerned and bring the patient to the emergency department (ED).

What are the pertinent positives and negatives from the history, and how do they help in identifying the problem in this patient?

The pertinent positives for this patient include the symptoms of an upper respiratory infection that has developed over the course of a week and is now worsening. The patient has had a decrease in appetite and fluid intake and in energy, as well as tachypnea, which have made the parents decide to take him to the ED. Pertinent negatives include the absence of diarrhea, making acute viral gastroenteritis less likely.

Why is the patient breathing faster?

The neurologic, respiratory, musculoskeletal, cardiovascular, and hematologic systems can affect a patient's respiratory rate. Stimuli that affect respiratory rate is obtained from chemoreceptors, lung stretch receptors, irritant receptors, juxtacapillary (J) receptors, and joint muscle receptors. In our patient's situation, because his illness may now be a lower respiratory tract infection—fevers, tachypnea, and worsening of an upper respiratory infection—tachypnea is a way for the body's attempt to match the metabolic demand for oxygenation. In our patient's case, the central and peripheral chemoreceptors play more of a role due to the hypoxemia.

CLINICAL PEARL   **STEP 1**

Hypoxemia can be caused by dysfunctions in oxygen uptake, delivery, and utilization. Pulmonary mechanisms for impaired oxygen uptake include hypoventilation, diffusion impairment, pulmonary shunting, and ventilation/perfusion (V/Q) mismatch (Table 43.1). Impairment in oxygen transport to tissues includes causes such as anemia and carbon monoxide poisoning. Cyanide poisoning interferes with oxygen utilization in the tissue's mitochondrial cytochrome c oxidase, thereby preventing the formation of adenosine triphosphate (ATP).

How do the central and peripheral chemoreceptors function?

Central chemoreceptors in the medulla respond to the change in pH of the cerebrospinal fluid (CSF). If the central chemoreceptors detect a decrease in pH, a prompt increase in respiratory rate is triggered. Carbon dioxide (CO_2) readily crosses the blood-brain barrier due to its lipid solubility. When CO_2 combines with water in the CSF, the resulting hydrogen ions act directly on the

TABLE 43.1 ■ Pulmonary Mechanisms of Hypoxemia

Mechanism	Description	Causes
Ventilation/perfusion (V/Q) mismatch	Low V/Q causes decreased alveolar oxygen (PAo$_2$) and concomitant decreased arterial oxygen (Pao$_2$) Corrects with supplemental oxygen Wide A-a gradient	Asthma COPD Bronchiectasis Cystic fibrosis ILD Pulmonary hypertension
Shunt	Extreme degree of V/Q mismatch—no ventilation with normal perfusion No response to supplemental oxygen Normal Paco$_2$	Pneumonia Pulmonary edema ARDS Pulmonary AVM
Diffusion impairment	Impaired oxygen transport across alveolar-capillary membrane Corrects with supplemental oxygen Worsened by exercise Widened A-a gradient Normal Paco$_2$	Bronchopulmonary dysplasia Emphysema Pulmonary fibrosis Shortened capillary transit time (exercise)
Hypoventilation	Corrects with supplemental oxygen Normal A-a gradient Elevated Paco$_2$ Pao$_2$ and Paco$_2$ deviate in opposite directions to some extent	Impaired respiratory drive (sedation, brainstem injury, infarction, primary alveolar hypoventilation) Weakness (Guillain-Barré syndrome, myasthenia gravis, Eaton-Lambert syndrome) Chest wall defects (kyphoscoliosis)

A-a, Alveolar-arterial; *ARDS,* acute respiratory distress syndrome; *AVM,* arteriovenous malformation; *COPD,* chronic obstructive pulmonary disease; *ILD,* interstitial lung disease.

central chemoreceptors in the medulla. This means that an increase in partial pressure of CO_2 (pco$_2$) leads to hyperventilation, which then leads to returning the arterial pco$_2$ to within normal range. Peripheral chemoreceptors located in the carotids and aortic bodies detect changes in the partial partial pressure of oxygen (po$_2$), pco$_2$, and hydrogen ion (H$^+$) concentration. Although the chemoreceptors in the aortic bodies respond to a decrease in po$_2$ or an increase in pco$_2$, the carotid chemoreceptors respond directly to an increase in H$^+$.

CLINICAL PEARL	STEP 1/2/3

The bicarbonate buffer system is a balance of ions that maintains pH so that there is appropriate metabolic function. The enzyme carbonic anhydrase catalyzes the reactions for the conversion of CO_2 and H_2O to carbonic acid (H_2CO_3) in human tissues in which there is a high concentration of CO_2. Carbonic acid readily dissociates to hydrogen (H$^+$) and bicarbonate (HCO$_3^-$) ions. In organs with low carbon dioxide, such as the lungs and kidneys, the reaction is reversed.
CO_2 + H_2O {ReversReact} H_2CO_3 {ReversReact} H$^+$ + HCO$_3^-$

CLINICAL PEARL	STEP 1

The Henderson-Hasselbalch equation describes the relationship between arterial pH and the bicarbonate buffer system: pH = pK + log [HCO$_3^-$]/(0.03 × pco$_2$), where pK refers to the characteristic equilibrium constant for bicarbonate buffering system ions. The solubility constant for CO_2 in the blood, 0.03 mmol/L/mm Hg, is used to express the partial pressure of CO_2. The equation indicates how hypoventilation and increased pco$_2$ lead to acidemia (decreased pH).

Case Point 43.1

In the ED, the patient has normal blood pressure for age, pulse rate is 125 beats/min, respiration rate is 35 breaths/min, and oxygen saturation 88% on room air. His temperature is 102.6°F.

What are concerning/worrisome signs to look for in this patient?
The general inspection of our patient would need to include an assessment of his level of alertness. A depressed mental status suggests severe hypoxia and may be a harbinger for acute respiratory failure. Other concerning signs would include increased work of breathing, cyanosis, and poor perfusion.

What does the respiratory examination consist of?
After the general inspection, if the patient were stable, you would want to inspect, palpate, percuss, and auscultate the torso. During inspection, look at the patient's posture, use of accessory muscles, and expansion of the chest wall, and note if there are any abnormalities of the chest surface. By inspecting, you can also assess the depth and inspiratory-to-expiratory ratio of each breathing cycle (normal, 1:2). A normal lung would have a resonant percussion note (low pitch). Auscultation allows you to hear adventitious noises, such as wheezing, rhonchi, or crackles.

CLINICAL PEARL	STEP 2/3

Other percussion notes include a hyperresonant percussion note (lower than normal pitch is heard, like in those with emphysema), dull percussion note (higher than normal pitch, similar to percussing the liver), and flat percussion note (higher than normal pitch heard in those with an effusion).

CLINICAL PEARL	STEP 1

The air movements responsible for the production of breath sounds are dependent on the size of the airway. There are three types of movement that may take place along the tracheobronchial tree: (1) laminal airflow, which is characteristic of a small peripheral airway—it is slow and referred to as silent movement; (2) vorticose airflow is faster and thought of as a mixed type of flow because it may resemble both laminal and turbulent airflows; and (3) turbulent airflow, which is very rapid, noisy, and complex and more typical of larger airways.

What findings/information would help you differentiate an upper airway disease from a lower airway disease?
The upper airway (extrathoracic) consists of the nasal passages through the pharynx to the vocal cords, whereas the lower airway (intrathoracic) is composed of the lung parenchyma, bronchi, and alveoli. Stridor would imply an upper airway process. Signs of a lower airway infection include tachypnea, decreased breath sounds, crackles, rhonchi over the area of consolidation, which can sound dull during percussion.

CLINICAL PEARL	STEP 1

Stridor is a loud, long, high-pitched, inspiratory sound that always indicates upper airway obstruction, best heard at the neck region. The extrathoracic region is exposed to atmospheric pressure. When there is edema, air travels through a smaller area, thereby increasing the velocity. According to the Bernoulli principle (Fig. 43.1), the increase in air velocity occurs simultaneously with a decrease in pressure, allowing the external atmospheric pressure to collapse the upper airway further with inspiration, leading to stridor.

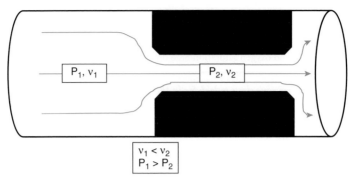

Fig. 43.1   Bernoulli principle. The velocity of airflow increases as it enters an area of constriction. The conservation of total energy results in a decrease in potential energy, manifesting in a lower pressure. P_1, P_2, Pressure; v_1, v_2, velocity.

What would make a pulmonary source likely in this patient?

The history of a productive cough, rhinorrhea, and contact with someone with a cold, indicates that this patient had an upper respiratory infection initially. By the time the patient is brought in to be evaluated, tachypnea and desaturation on pulse oximetry shows that his initial infection has proceeded to a lower airway disease. After narrowing the source to a pulmonary cause, you would want to differentiate whether it is an obstructive or restrictive disease process.

What findings would help you differentiate an obstructive versus a restrictive disease process?

With both inspection and auscultation, you would be able to differentiate between an obstructive and restrictive disease process. An obstructive disease process can be thought of as a disease of the airways or parenchyma that affects the amount of air that is exhaled. During the physical examination, an obstructive disease process would be noted to have expiratory wheezing or increased expiratory time. In severe and progressive obstructive airway disease, wheezing may be heard during both the inspiratory and expiratory limbs of the respiratory cycle. In a restrictive lung disease, inspiration is limited by reduced compliance of the lung parenchyma, abnormality of the chest wall, or weakness of the inspiratory muscles. During the physical examination, you can inspect the chest wall for skeletal conditions such as scoliosis or kyphosis. During auscultation, you can listen for decreased breath sounds in a particular lobe—noted in those with pneumonia—indicating a decrease in lung volume.

CLINICAL PEARL   **STEP 2/3**

A forced expiratory test can help distinguish between an obstructive and restrictive disease process. Forced expiratory volume (FEV) is lower than forced vital capacity (FVC), producing a low FEV/FVC ratio. In a restrictive disease process, both the FEV and FVC are low, so the FEV/FVC ratio is normal or increased. Normally, the FEV is about 80% of the FVC.

CLINICAL PEARL   **STEP 1**

Lung compliance is equal to the change in volume divided by the change in pleural pressure. Of note, alveolar size and number continue to increase during childhood. Lung compliance also increases with age.

CLINICAL PEARL	**STEPS 1/2/3**

The thorax in an infant and young child is more cartilaginous, making it more compliant. When an infant has respiratory distress, the chest readily retracts inward, making the increase in negative intrathoracic pressure ineffective in causing an increase in the tidal volume, which then prompts an increase in the work of breathing.

Why is it important to know about the pattern of breathing—depth, muscle use, retractions, inspiration-to-expiration ratio—and the rate of breathing in this patient?
Knowing the pattern of breathing allows us to determine if the patient is able to maintain adequate minute ventilation and oxygenation when there is pulmonary compromise. If the patient has increased work of breathing and is still able to meet the demand of oxygenation, then the patient may be experiencing respiratory distress. If the demand of oxygenation is not met, there is the concern for respiratory failure. On examination, signs of increased work of breathing, including nasal flaring, tachypnea, and retractions, are seen with respiratory distress. Retractions include the use of the subcostal, intercostal, and suprasternal muscles. Because of the limitation in inhalation experienced by those with restrictive lung disease, the depth of the breath will be more limited, and the inspiratory phase will be longer compared to someone with an obstructive disease process. Severe increases in the work of breathing portend risk for fatigue and respiratory failure.

CLINICAL PEARL	**STEP 1**

Smaller anatomic conducting airways in children may produce high resistance if they become narrower due to inflammation, edema, mucus or bronchospasm. Higher peripheral airway resistance may alter exhalation and cause dynamic closure of the airways.

CLINICAL PEARL	**STEP 1**

Other anatomic differences of infants and small children that may contribute to a quick progression to respiratory failure due to the reduced thoracic volume include soft tissue retractions, rib alignment, position of the diaphragm, and immature intercostal muscles. The rib alignment of infants is on a more horizontal plane, and the position of the diaphragm is also more horizontal, which means that the lower thorax may be drawn inward during inspiration, contributing to a reduced inspiratory volume. The immature intercostal muscles are not able to assist in active ventilation, meaning that infants depend more on diaphragmatic function.

Case Point 43.2

On physical examination, the patient is noted to have nasal flaring, grunting, and difficulty in answering questions in full sentences. He is tachypneic, with subcostal and subdiaphragmatic retractions. Auscultation demonstrates decreased breath sounds in the left lower lobe, with crackles. He complains of abdominal pain in the left upper quadrant (LUQ).

What is the significance of your physical examination findings?
The patient's presentation further suggests that this is a lower respiratory tract infection. He not only appears ill overall, but he is also manifesting increased work of breathing. The auscultation examination reveals that there is decreased airflow and a possibly of a consolidation in the left lower lobe. The patient's abdominal pain may be due to referred pain because the lung and abdomen share the T9 dermatome.

CLINICAL PEARL	STEPS 2/3

Parietal pain is localized, sharp, and intense and travels through myelinated afferent fibers. This information is transmitted to a specific dorsal root ganglia of a dermatome level. This is different from visceral pain, which is usually dull and poorly localized. This type of information travels via unmyelinated fibers that can be transmitted to different dorsal root ganglia.

What are your management priorities?

Supportive care is very important initially. Providing the patient with oxygen is a priority to increase oxygenation and maintain saturation above 92% to 95%. If the patient is not able to maintain appropriate fluid intake, intravenous (IV) fluids may be indicated.

After physically assessing the patient, what laboratory tests would you consider?

Laboratory tests may be needed in those who are hypoxic or in severe respiratory distress, unlike those who are stable and can be treated in an outpatient setting. This patient is hypoxic, appears ill, is in respiratory distress, and requires treatment in the inpatient setting. Laboratory tests include a complete blood count with differential (CBC with diff), peripheral smear, and C-reactive protein (CRP) level, which would help monitor response to treatment, complete metabolic panel to detect electrolyte abnormalities, and blood cultures to detect concomitant bacteremia. Microbiologic diagnostic testing for suspicion of a lower respiratory tract infection includes blood cultures, Gram staining and culture of sputum (typically for older children who can produce a sputum sample), and pleural fluid, if present. Rapid diagnostic testing such as immunofluorescence and a polymerase chain reaction (PCR) assay is recommended for hospitalized patients for treatment and cohorting decision making. Rapid testing is required for certain microbes, including respiratory syncytial virus (RSV), influenza, parainfluenza, adenovirus, human metapneumovirus, and *Chlamydia* and *Mycoplasma* spp. The results of these rapid tests should be used with caution because differentiation among colonization and acute, mixed, or secondary infections may not be possible.

CLINICAL PEARL	STEP 2/3

Indications for inpatient admission include oxygen saturation < 90%, tachypnea for age (>50 breaths/min), physical examination findings, such as respiratory distress (apnea, grunting, and difficulty breathing), signs of dehydration, inability to maintain hydration or oral intake, and a toxic appearance. Such a patient is suspected or confirmed to have infection with a virulent organism.

CLINICAL PEARL	STEPS 2/3

You can usually have an expectation of laboratory results but be aware that it may be variable. You can expect an elevated white blood cell count (leukocytosis) with a left shift (neutrophil predominance) with bandemia on a CBC with differential. The CRP may also be elevated because it is an inflammatory marker. Positive blood cultures may be present if the patient is very ill.

What imaging modality would you order, and what results would you expect?

A chest radiograph would be helpful in this case. The presence of infiltrates, along with fever and respiratory stress, confirms the diagnosis of pneumonia. However, if you still suspect pneumonia, and there is no infiltrate on the chest radiograph, this does not necessarily rule out pneumonia because you have to consider that the findings on imaging may be delayed from the patient's clinical status. It is not uncommon for radiographic abnormalities to appear after IV fluid resuscitation in severely ill patients. Radiographs may also reveal nonpulmonary findings that may be helpful, including signs of cardiomegaly, presence of foreign bodies, and airway abnormalities.

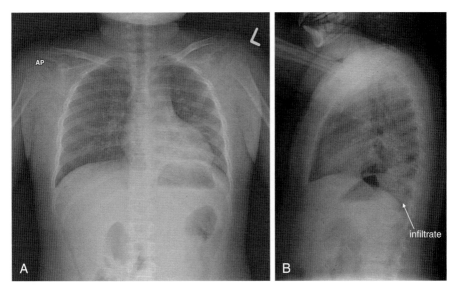

Fig. 43.2 Pneumonia, left lower lobe. (A) Anterior-posterior (AP) chest x-ray shows increased subtle hyperdensity in the left lower lobe. (B) Lateral chest x-ray shows definite increased density overlying the lower thoracic spine, a left lower lobe pneumonia. (From Broder J. Imaging the chest: the chest radiograph. In: Broder J, ed. *Diagnostic Imaging for the Emergency Physician*. Philadelphia: Elsevier/Saunders; 2011:185–296.)

Case Point 43.3

Laboratory testing showed leukocytosis, with a left shift and elevated bands. Blood cultures were drawn and sent to the laboratory. The chest x-ray showed a left lower lobe infiltrate (Fig. 43.2). The constellation of findings from the physical examination, laboratory tests, and x-ray confirms suspicion for community-acquired pneumonia in our patient. He is admitted to the hospital for hypoxia requiring oxygen supplementation.

What causative organisms would you consider for this patient?
Infectious causes for pneumonia may classified by age group (Table 43.2). Because our patient is 10 years old, you would consider *Staphylococcus aureus* and *Streptococcus pneumoniae* as the most likely bacterial organisms, given the findings on chest x-ray. Keep in mind, however, that atypical organisms such as *Mycoplasma pneumoniae* are more common in school-age children. Other organisms include *Chlamydia pneumoniae* and *Mycobacterium tuberculosis*. Vaccines have played an important role in decreasing infections from *Haemophilus influenzae type B*. With the rise in antibiotic resistance, a presentation of a patient with a complicated pneumonia (e.g., a patient with an empyema) may have a methicillin-resistant *S. aureus* (MRSA) infection.

What are some of the risk factors for developing pneumonia?
Certain factors need to be considered when a child develops pneumonia. These include underlying medical conditions and socioeconomic and environmental factors. Some underlying medical conditions include asthma, neuromuscular disorders, immunodeficiency disorders, diabetes mellitus, and chronic lung disease. Examples of socioeconomic and environmental factors include poor access to health care, air pollution, and exposure to cigarette smoke.

TABLE 43.2 ■ Causative Agents Grouped by Age of Patient

Age Group	Frequent Pathogens (in order of frequency)
Neonates <3 wk	Group B streptococci, *Escherichia coli*, gram-negative bacilli, *Streptococcus pneumoniae*, *Haemophilus influenzae* (type b,[a] nontypeable)
3 wk–3 mo	Respiratory syncytial virus, other viruses (e.g., rhinovirus, parainfluenza, influenza, adenovirus), *S. pneumoniae*, *H. influenzae* (type b,[a] nontypeable), *Chlamydia trachomatis* (consider in afebrile infants)
4 mo–4 yr	Respiratory syncytial virus, other viruses (e.g., rhinovirus, parainfluenza, influenza, adenovirus), *S. pneumoniae*, *H. influenzae* (type b,[a] nontypeable), *Mycoplasma pneumoniae*, group A streptococci
≥5 yr	*M. pneumoniae, S. pneumoniae, Chlamydophila pneumoniae, H. influenzae* (type b,[a] nontypeable), influenza, adenovirus, other respiratory viruses, *Legionella pneumophila*

[a]*H. influenzae* type b is uncommon with routine *H. influenzae* type b immunization.
Adapted from Kliegman RM, Marcdante KJ, Jenson HJ, et al., eds. *Nelson Essentials of Pediatrics.* 5th ed. Philadelphia: Elsevier; 2006:504.

How would you proceed with treatment?

IV ampicillin was chosen for this patient. Third-generation cephalosporins are alternatives in nonvaccinated patients and those at high risk for organisms with resistance to penicillin. Azithromycin treats atypical pneumonia; vancomycin or clindamycin (based on regional susceptibility data) should be provided in addition to β-lactam therapy if there is concern for *S. aureus* infection.

What other treatment adjuncts would you consider?

Aside from supplemental oxygen, IV fluids, and antibiotics in a patient who is febrile or in pain, consideration can be given to an antipyretic such as acetaminophen that is weight-appropriate, which may be 10 to 15 mg/kg.

What are possible complications?

Parapneumonic effusions can complicate 2% to 12% of pediatric pneumonia cases, as high as 28% for those requiring hospitalization. A minimally sized effusion can be treated without aspiration, whereas a larger one requires thoracentesis for microbiologic identification and/or chest tube drainage, with or without fibrinolytic agents. Effusions unresponsive to medical treatment or causing respiratory compromise may require video-assisted thoracoscopic surgery (VATS). Empyemas may also occur, and there are three phases—exudative, fibrinopurulent, and organizing phases. Pneumatoceles, necrotizing pneumonia (associated with prolonged fever), lung abscess, fistulas, and pneumothorax may occur in protracted cases.

CLINICAL PEARL	STEPS 2/3

The lateral radiograph can be used, along with the measurement of the rim of the fluid being less or more than 10 mm. The occupation of the effusion is also looked at—for example, whether the fluid occupies less than 25% or 50% of the hemithorax. A small effusion has less than a 10-mm rim of fluid, with less than 25% of the hemithorax affected, meaning that there would be no need for chest tube drainage in this case.

CLINICAL PEARL	STEPS 2/3

Complications of a lung abscess includes intracavitary hemorrhage, septicemia, cerebral abscess, and inappropriate secretion of antidiuretic hormone.

Case Point 43.4

After receiving oxygen, IV fluids, and IV antibiotics for 2 days, the patient's work of breathing decreased, his fever curve decreased, and he was able to answer questions comfortably. His pulse oximetry values were greater than 92%, and his supplemental oxygen requirement was titrated down to room air. He was started on a regular diet, which he tolerated with no bouts of emesis.

What are the discharge criteria for a patient hospitalized with pneumonia?
The patient must be able to have an increase in activity and appetite. Fever curves may decrease but usually a child who is afebrile and on room air for at least 24 hours demonstrates stability. Improving vital signs, with particular attention to the respiratory rate, as well as examination findings that include no nasal flaring, no retractions, and an improved inspiratory-to-expiratory ratio, are helpful signs. The ability to tolerate oral antibiotics is also important, as well as fluids and feeds. It is important to have appropriate hospital discharge follow-up with a primary care physician to ensure that the patient finished the course of antibiotics and has an improved physical examination. Microbiologic diagnosis in this case of uncomplicated community-acquired pneumonia was not obtained.

Case Point 43.5

The patient was transitioned from IV antibiotics to oral antibiotics and was able to ambulate and maintain appropriate oxygen saturation levels on room air. The blood culture sent initially was negative. Because the oral medications were effective, and the patient was afebrile for 48 hours, with an improved physical examination, he was discharged home, with follow-up in 1 week with his pediatrician.

BEYOND THE PEARLS

- Children with tachypnea, as defined by World Health Organization (WHO) respiratory rate thresholds, are more likely to have pneumonia than children without pneumonia. The WHO thresholds are as follows: Children aged 2 to 11 months—50 breaths/min or more; children aged 12 months to 5 years—40 breaths/min or more.
- The information from the receptors travels via the vagus and glossopharyngeal nerves to the medullary respiratory center—in particular, the dorsal respiratory group. This center is in the reticular formation where there are two groups, dorsal and ventral. The information out of the dorsal respiratory group travels via the phrenic nerve to the diaphragm, leading to contraction.
- The incidence of bacteremia with uncomplicated community-acquired pneumonia is 7%. The incidence of bacteremia in cases complicated by parapneumonic effusion is 21%.
- If the patient appears to be in respiratory distress, you may also consider determining an arterial blood gas value to know the pH (acidemia vs. alkalemia), partial pressure of CO_2 (hypercapnia vs. hypocapnia), and O_2 (hypoxemia). If the patient appears to have increased work of breathing, but the pH and $Paco_2$ are within normal limits, it may actually indicate that the patient is fatigued and at risk for impending respiratory failure.

Case Summary

Complaint/History: A 10-year-old male with 2 days of cough and high fevers.
Findings: Examination findings include tachypnea, tachycardia, 88% O_2 saturation on room air, increased work of breathing, decreased breath sounds, and crackles on the left lower lobe (LLL).
Labs/Tests: Leukocytosis with neutrophil predominance and bandemia; chest x-ray with LLL infiltrate.

Diagnosis: Community-acquired pneumonia.

Treatment: IV ampicillin during hospitalization and oral penicillin for continued outpatient treatment.

Bibliography

Bradley John S, et al. The management of community-acquired pneumonia in infants and children older than 3 months of age: clinical practice guidelines by the Pediatric Infectious Diseases Society and the Infectious Diseases Society of America. *Clin Infect Dis.* 2011. cir531.

Costanzo L. *Physiology.* Philadelphia: Saunders Elsevier; 2006.

Gereige RS, Laufer PM. Pneumonia. *Pediatr Rev.* 2013;34(10):438–455.

Leung AK, Sigalet DL. Acute abdominal pain in children. *Am Fam Physician.* 2003;67(11): 2321–2328.

Mangione S. *Physical Diagnosis Secrets: With Student Consult Online Access.* St. Louis: Elsevier Health Sciences; 2012.

Myers A, Hall M, et al. Prevalence of bacteremia in hospitalized pediatric patients with community acquired pneumonia. *Pediatr Infect Dis J.* 2013;32(7):736–740.

Society of Critical Care Medicine. *Pediatric Fundamental Critical Care Support.* Second Printing. 2011.

West JB. *Respiratory Physiology: The Essentials.* Philadelphia: Lippincott Williams & Wilkins; 2012.

12-Month-Old Male With Stridor

Brittany Middleton

A 12-month-old male presents to the emergency department with worsening stridor for 3 days. The male's mother also reports tactile fever and decreased oral intake.

What is stridor, and what causes it?

Stridor is a high-pitched noise with breathing that indicates air passing through a narrow upper airway. Stridor is best heard over the anterior neck using the diaphragm of the stethoscope. It may be louder during inspiration or expiration, depending on the location of the airway narrowing. The upper airway can be divided into the extrathoracic and intrathoracic structures. The extrathoracic airway includes the nasopharynx, epiglottis, larynx, aryepiglottic folds, vocal folds, and proximal trachea. The intrathoracic upper airway is composed of the distal trachea and mainstem bronchi. Normally, during inspiration, the extrathoracic pressure (atmospheric pressure) exceeds the pressure in the trachea. With obstruction or narrowing of the extrathoracic airway, the pressure in the airway falls below atmospheric pressure during inspiration, causing worsening of the obstruction and stridor (think about sucking through a partially clogged straw and the walls of the straw collapsing inward). With narrowing of the intrathoracic airway, the intrathoracic pressure falls below the pressure in the airway during inspiration, causing the narrowed portion to open. With expiration, the opposite occurs, and the pressure in the airway drops below intrathoracic pressure; therefore, stridor is more audible during expiration with an intrathoracic airway obstruction (Fig. 44.1).

BASIC SCIENCE PEARL	STEP 1

The bell of the stethoscope is used to listen to low-pitched sounds; the diaphragm is better for hearing medium- or high-pitched sounds.

What are causes of stridor in children?

Extrathoracic causes of stridor include croup, retropharyngeal abscess, pharyngitis (Fig. 44.2), epiglottitis, subglottic stenosis, and laryngomalacia. In a patient with suspected laryngomalacia, ask the caregiver if the stridor improves with prone positioning. Prone positioning moves the redundant and floppy tissue of laryngomalacia out of the airway and alleviates stridor. Intrathoracic causes of stridor include congenital malformations such as tracheal webs, esophageal foreign body, vascular rings, and vascular slings. Tracheomalacia, bacterial tracheitis, anaphylaxis, airway compression from a tumor, and foreign body aspiration may occur in the extrathoracic and/or intrathoracic upper airway.

BASIC SCIENCE PEARL	STEP 1

If a child presents in significant distress, avoid performing unnecessary examinations and evaluations. The degree of airway obstruction is dynamic and dependent on relative pressures in the airway and outside the airway; therefore, causing more stress and anxiety worsens the obstruction.

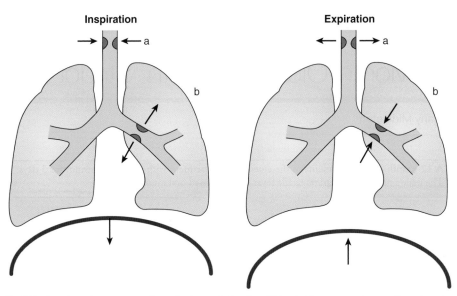

Fig. 44.1 Intrathoracic versus extrathoracic airway obstruction. (A) Inspiration causes airway collapse in extrathoracic obstruction and airway opening in intrathoracic obstruction. (B) Exhalation causes airway opening in extrathoracic obstruction and airway collapse in intrathoracic obstruction. (From Bersten A, Soni N. *Oh's Intensive Care Manual.* 7th ed. London: Elsevier, 2014.)

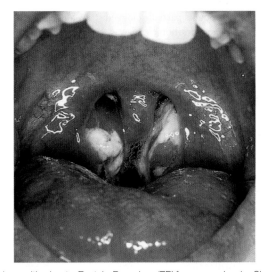

Fig. 44.2 Exudative pharyngitis due to Epstein-Barr virus (EBV) mononucleosis. Shown is severe pharyngotonsillitis, with enlarged tonsils covered with exudate. (From Michaels M, Williams J. Infectious diseases. In: Zitelli BJ, McIntire SC, Nowalk AN, eds. *Zitelli and Davis' Atlas of Pediatric Physical Diagnosis.* 7th ed. Philadelphia: Elsevier; 2018:455–509.)

CLINICAL PEARL	STEPS 2/3

Ask the child's caregiver about changes in the child's voice or cry. A hoarse voice or cry may help localize the disease process to the vocal folds.

Case Point 44.1

The male's mother denies choking or gagging episodes. He has no previous history of stridor or hospitalizations. Examination reveals a tired-appearing male, with decreased capillary refill at 3 seconds, neck stiffness, a muffled cry, and excessive drooling. Stridor is worse with inspiration.

What is a capillary refill test? How do you perform and interpret the test?
The capillary refill test is measured by holding the child's hand higher than heart level and pressing the fingernail until it blanches. If there is good perfusion to the nail bed, color should return in less than 2 seconds. Prolonged capillary refill may be a sign of dehydration.

BASIC SCIENCE PEARL	STEP 1

Capillary refill can be affected by ambient temperature because peripheral vessels vasoconstrict in cold temperatures and vasodilate with heat. The capillary refill test is an important component in evaluating hydration status but should be interpreted with caution.

How would you proceed with your evaluation to make a diagnosis?
A lateral neck film may be helpful in patients with suspected retropharyngeal abscess and may show increased prevertebral soft tissue. A computed tomography (CT) scan is helpful for presurgical evaluation of a retropharyngeal abscess and for patients with suspected vascular rings and slings. Chest radiographs are not necessary but should be considered in case of suspected foreign body ingestion or aspiration (Figs. 44.3–44.6).

CLINICAL PEARL	STEPS 2/3

A pseudo–steeple sign, which is a normal variant, may be seen in children without airway obstruction.

What organisms should be considered in retropharyngeal abscess?
Most retropharyngeal abscesses are polymicrobial infections. Cultures of the drained fluid often reveal both aerobes and anaerobes. The most common causative organisms are group A β-hemolytic *Streptococcus* (e.g., *Streptococcus pyogenes)*, *Staphylococcus aureus,* and anaerobes. α-Hemolytic *Streptococcus* (e.g., *Streptococcus viridans*) and *Haemophilus influenzae* are less commonly isolated (Table 44.1).

BASIC SCIENCE PEARL	STEP 1

α-Hemolysis refers to the ability of bacteria to hemolyze hemoglobin partially to methemoglobin via hydrogen peroxide production. Bacteria with β-hemolytic activity induce complete red blood cell lysis via streptolysin activity. γ-Hemolysis actually refers to the absence of any bacterial hemolytic activity.

What antibiotics should be initiated for this patient?
Initial intravenous (IV) antibiotic treatment should be broad to cover gram-positive and gram-negative aerobes, anaerobes, and β-lactamase–producing bacteria. Appropriate choices include an aminopenicillin (e.g., ampicillin) with a β-lactamase inhibitor (e.g., sulbactam), clindamycin, or a carbapenem. Antibiotic coverage should be narrowed when fluid cultures result. IV antibiotics

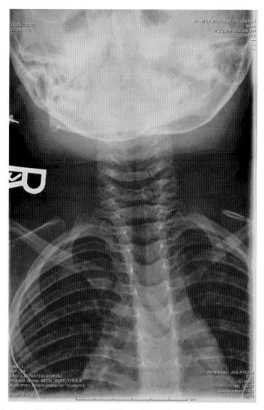

Fig. 44.3 Steeple sign (wine bottle sign) in croup. This radiograph of the neck shows narrowing of the subglottic area of the trachea.

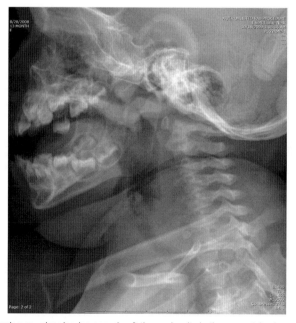

Fig. 44.4 Lateral neck x-ray showing increased soft tissue density in the prevertebral space, suggestive of a retropharyngeal abscess.

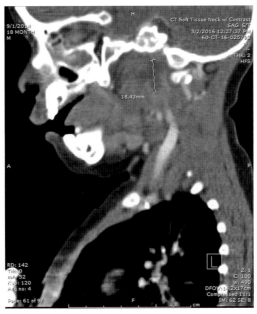

Fig. 44.5 CT scan of neck confirming a retropharyngeal abscess.

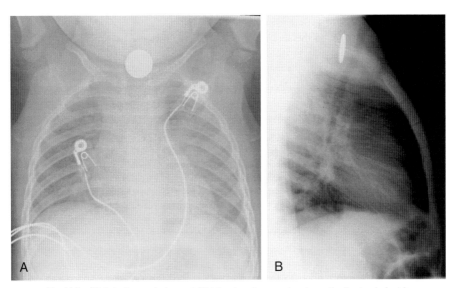

Fig. 44.6 (A) Anterior-posterior and (B) lateral neck x-ray showing a foreign body (coin).

TABLE 44.1 ■ **Bacterial Causes of Retropharyngeal Abscess**

Type of Bacteria	Cause
Aerobic	Gram-positive—group A β-hemolytic *Streptococcus, Staphylococcus aureus*, α-hemolytic *Streptococcus* Gram-negative—*Haemophilus influenzae* type B
Anaerobic	*Bacteroides, Fusobacterium, Prevotella, Porphyromonas, Peptostreptococcus* spp.

should be continued until there is clinical improvement, usually characterized by fever and symptom resolution. Total duration depends on the clinical course, but 10 to 14 days is generally accepted.

CLINICAL PEARL   **STEPS 2/3**

Penicillins with β-lactamase inhibitors are bactericidal with a broad spectrum of activity but do not cover methicillin-resistant *Staphylococcus aureus* (MRSA). Carbapenems are bactericidal agents with a very broad spectrum of activity but are susceptible to β-lactamases and do not cover MRSA. Clindamycin has excellent gram-positive and anaerobic activity, including MRSA coverage, but is bacteriostatic, with limited gram-negative coverage. Local and institutional antibiograms should be used to assist in antibiotic selection.

What complications can occur in a patient with a retropharyngeal abscess?
Complications associated with a retropharyngeal abscess are uncommon but should be recognized as serious and potentially fatal. Direct airway compression or abscess rupture, leading to airway compromise, aspiration, and pneumonia, are the most commonly seen complications. Other potential complications include extension of the abscess into the mediastinum (mediastinitis), jugular suppurative thrombophlebitis (Lemierre syndrome), and sepsis.

What is the treatment of a retropharyngeal abscess?
Systemic antibiotics are always indicated. Surgical drainage, usually via the intraoral route, is often required in the presence of a discrete pus collection. Medical management alone is reserved for cases of small abscesses or in the absence of an organized abscess. The patient may initially be trialed on intravenous antibiotics without surgical drainage and monitored for improvement over a period of 24 to 48 hours. Steroids may be added in cases of very large abscesses and/or marked inflammation, with concern for airway compromise.

Case Point 44.2

A lateral x-ray of his neck shows a soft tissue density in the prevertebral space, suggestive of a retropharyngeal abscess. The patient is taken to the operating room by an otolaryngologist, where incision and drainage are performed under general anesthesia. The patient receives clindamycin IV postsurgery. His fever defervesce. A culture of abscess fluid obtained during surgery grows *Streptococcus pyogenes*. Three days after surgery, he is tolerating a regular diet and discharged home with sufficient amoxicillin-clavulanate to complete a 10-day course.

BEYOND THE PEARLS

- The term *danger space* refers to an area posterior to the retropharyngeal space through which infection can easily spread to the mediastinum. Its borders are delineated by the skull, the diaphragm, and the prevertebral and alar fascia.
- Patients are usually placed supine when performing a computed tomography scan of the chest. Be aware that airway obstruction from mass effect anterior to the airway may worsen when patients are placed in a supine position.
- Foreign body aspiration or an esophageal foreign body should be suspected in any child who is developmentally able to grasp and release objects (≈5–6 months of age), especially if they are independently mobile (≈8–9 months of age).

Case Summary

Complaint/History: A 12-month-old male with fever and noisy breathing for 3 days.

Findings: The examination reveals a fatigued male with stridor, delayed capillary refill, drooling, neck stiffness, and a muffled cry.

Labs/Tests: An x-ray of the lateral neck shows hyperdensity in the prevertebral space.

Diagnosis: Retropharyngeal abscess; culture of abscess fluid positive for *Streptococcus pyogenes*.

Treatment: Incision and drainage of abscess under general anesthesia; an IV antibiotic (clindamycin) is given during hospitalization. Amoxicillin-clavulanate is prescribed to complete a 10-day course at the time of discharge.

Bibliography

Brook I. Microbiology and management of peritonsillar, retropharyngeal, and parapharyngeal abscesses. *J Oral Maxillofac Surg*. 2004;62:1545–1550.

Brook I. Microbiology of retropharyngeal abscesses in children. *Am J Dis Child*. 1987;141:202–204.

Page C, Biet A, Zaatar R, Strunski V. Parapharyngeal abscess: diagnosis and treatment. *Eur Arch Otorhinolaryngol*. 2008;265:681–686.

16-Year-Old Female With Right Knee Pain

Cecilia Weaver ▪ Adler Salazar

A 16-year-old female presents to the emergency department with 3 months of right knee pain. The pain was initially mild but has slowly worsened and has limited her ambulation due to her inability to extend the knee due to pain.

How can you identify the cause of this child's knee pain?

The differential diagnosis for a child with knee pain can be extensive due to the variety of injuries or diseases that may be involved (Table 45.1). Information obtained during the history and physical examination can effectively narrow the workup and initial management for most cases. Important information to obtain includes the duration of onset, constitutional or systemic symptoms, history of travel, insect bites, sexual activity (as appropriate), and current or past infection. The priority would be to determine the presence of limb- or life-threatening conditions requiring immediate medical and surgical intervention.

BASIC SCIENCE PEARL	**STEP 1**

Acute septic arthritis is a limb- or life-threatening cause of knee pain that requires immediate diagnosis and treatment. Most cases are caused by hematogenous spread of the bacteria with *Staphylococcus aureus* being the most common cause among pediatric cases. Up to 65% of these *S. aureus* cases are caused by a community-acquired, methicillin-resistant variant (MRSA).

Case Point 45.1

The patient reports that her knee pain is at its worst in the mornings, decreases in intensity throughout the day, and is not relieved by over-the-counter pain relievers. She reports that her left knee and bilateral ankles have also developed similar pain in recent weeks. On review of symptoms, she reports fatigue and weight loss for the past month, coughing with blood-tinged sputum for 2 weeks, and intermittent, dark, tea-colored urine for 1 week. On the day of admission, she developed fever and abdominal pain (left lower quadrant), prompting for her to be brought to the emergency room. Her family history is significant for maternal aunts with type 1 diabetes mellitus (DM), systemic lupus erythematosus (SLE), or rheumatoid arthritis (RA) and cousins with thyroid disease.

CLINICAL PEARL	**STEPS 2/3**

The combination of the presence of constitutive symptoms, chronicity of the symptoms, multisystemic involvement, and familial predisposition for autoimmune conditions suggest a systemic disease rather than an isolated musculoskeletal injury. The differential diagnosis can be narrowed to rheumatologic, oncologic, and chronic infective causes.

TABLE 45.1 ■ **Differential Diagnosis for Knee Pain in a Child**

Type of Condition	Diagnosis
Limb- or life-threatening condition	**Infection** Septic arthritis, osteomyelitis **Malignancy** Osteosarcoma, Ewing sarcoma, lymphoma, leukemia
Stress injury	Patellofemoral syndrome, quadriceps or patellar tendinopathy, pre-patellar bursitis, Baker cyst, collateral ligament sprain (medial, lateral, anterior), osteochondritis dissecans
Benign bone tumor	Osteochondroma, osteoid osteoma, aneurysmal bone cyst, nonos-sifying fibroma
Inflammatory, rheumatologic	Systemic lupus erythematosus, juvenile idiopathic arthritides, rheu-matoid arthritis, vasculitides, inflammatory bowel disease
Infectious	**Bacterial** Lyme disease, *Neisseria gonorrhoeae* **Viral** Parvovirus, rubella virus, hepatitis virus, Ebstein-Barr virus
Hematologic	Sickle cell disease, hemophilia A, thrombophilic conditions,
Other	Growing pains, Osgood-Schlatter disease, slipped capital femoral epiphysis, acute traumatic injury

Case Point 45.2

In the emergency room (ER), her vital signs are temperature 37.6°C, heart rate, 118 beats/min, respira-tions, 25 breaths/min, blood pressure, 101/61 mm Hg, and 96% O_2 saturation on room air. She has right conjunctival infection. Her abdomen is soft but tender to deep palpation in the left lower quadrant, without rebound or guarding. She has mild swelling of her right knee without warmth or erythema, with limited flexion and extension due to pain. The chest x-ray is abnormal, with nodular hyperdensities in the right lower lobe (Fig. 45.1). Initial labs sent from the ER show the white blood cell count (WBC) to be 16,000/mL. The patient is determined to have systemic inflammatory response syndrome (SIRS). Additional laboratory tests, including a blood culture, are ordered. She is given a normal saline (NS) bolus for fluid resuscitation and a dose of ceftriaxone and is transferred to the pediatric ward.

CLINICAL PEARL   **STEP 2/3**

The definition of systemic inflammatory response syndrome (SIRS) in pediatrics is the pres-ence of two of the following: (1) core temperature < 36°C or > 38.5°C; (2) leukocyte count el-evated or decreased for age or > 10% immature neutrophils; (3) respiratory rate > 2 standard deviations (SD) above normal for age or mechanical ventilation requirements; (4) tachycardia > 2 SD above normal for age; and (5) for infants younger than 1 year, bradycardia below the 10th percentile for age. In pediatric SIRS, one of the findings must include an abnormal tem-perature or leukocyte count, a requirement not defined for SIRS in adults.

Case Point 45.3

In the pediatric ward, the patient continues to have tachycardia, despite pain control, antipyretics, and multiple NS boluses. She is transferred to the pediatric intensive care unit (PICU) for closer monitoring and further evaluation of her persistent tachycardia to rule out septic shock, myocarditis, and arrhythmia. The electrocardiogram (ECG) shows findings of myocardial inflammation (myocarditis; Fig. 45.2).

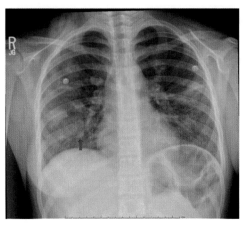

Fig. 45.1 The patient's chest x-ray shows shows nodular densities in the right lower lobe, including one measuring up to 2.9 cm *(red arrow)*.

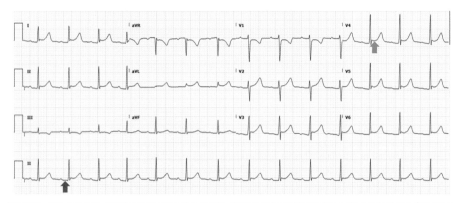

Fig. 45.2 The patient's electrocardiogram shows first-degree atrioventricular block *(red arrow)* and S-T elevation in leads V3, V4, V5, and V6 *(green arrow)*.

BASIC SCIENCE PEARL	STEP 1

ECG findings in myocarditis can be variable; these include sinus tachycardia, QRS/QT prolongation, diffuse T wave inversion, ventricular arrhythmias, and AV conduction defects. The most common abnormality seen in myocarditis is sinus tachycardia, with nonspecific ST-segment and T wave changes.

Case Point 45.4

A complete blood count (CBC) with peripheral smear evaluation is positive for leukocytosis and normocytic anemia, but there is an absence of any abnormal cells. The metabolic panel shows elevated liver enzyme levels but normal hepatic and renal function. The urinalysis (UA) shows pyuria, hematuria, and proteinuria, with an elevated protein-to-creatinine ratio. An elevated erythrocyte sedimentation rate (ESR) and C-reactive protein (CRP) level confirm suspicion of an inflammatory process (Table 45.2). Radiography and ultrasound of the right knee show an absence of bony abnormalities or a discrete fluid collection. The workup for indolent infections is negative.

TABLE 45.2 ■ Patient's Laboratory Test Results

Substance Analyzed	Finding
Leukocytes	16,000/μL
Hemoglobin	10.5 g/dL
Hematocrit	37%
Mean corpuscular volume (MCV)	87.2%
Aspartate transaminase (AST)	146 U/L
Alanine transaminase (ALT)	81 U/L
Urine protein-to-creatinine ratio	0.95
Urine white blood cell count	11–30/hpf
Urine red blood cell count	>50/hpf
Erythrocyte sedimentation rate (ESR)	102 mm/h
C-reactive protein (CRP)	144.8 mg/L
Cytoplasmic antineutrophil cytoplasmic antibody (cANCA)	Positive
Proteinase-3 antibody	228.6 U
Myeloperoxidase antibody	Negative
Antineutrophilic antibody (ANA)	Negative
Anti–glomerular basement membrane antibody (AGBM)	Negative
Lupus anticoagulant	Negative

What is the differential diagnosis?

The multisystem complaints suggest a likely mixed connective tissue disorder or small vessel vasculitis, such as granulomatosis with polyangiitis (GPA, formerly Wegener granulomatosis), anti–glomerular basement membrane (AGBM) disease (formerly Goodpasture syndrome), microscopic polyangiitis, juvenile idiopathic arthritis (JIA), or SLE. Given the history of blood-tinged sputum and renal involvement, GPA and AGBM disease are highest on the differential because they can result in alveolar hemorrhage.

GPA is a small vessel vasculitis causing granulomatous inflammation, usually affecting the lungs and kidneys (Fig. 45.3). Respiratory manifestations are most common, occurring in around 90% of patients, and can occur anywhere along the respiratory tract. Upper airway and respiratory tract manifestations include sinus disease, subglottic stenosis, and nasal septum perforations. Lower respiratory tract disease can cause nodular infiltrates, cavitary lesions, or ground glass infiltrates. Glomerulonephritis is present in 20% of patients on presentation but eventually 80% of patients with GPA will develop it. Ocular and cutaneous findings can be present in approximately 50% of patients, but these findings are variable and nonspecific to GPA compared with other rheumatologic diseases. Cardiac manifestations such as pericarditis and myocarditis are also seen but are less common.

AGBM disease also presents with concurrent pulmonary and renal manifestations. Its course is more rapid than GPA and can result in fatal pulmonary hemorrhages. Even with treatment, patients often progress to end-stage renal failure. Polyarticular JIA has a more chronic presentation, with arthritis in four joints over 6 months. In systemic JIA, fever must last a minimum of 2 weeks, and arthritis lasts longer than 6 weeks.

Oncologic and infectious causes are less likely at this point, given the absence of any abnormal findings in the radiographic studies and peripheral smear evaluation. Tuberculosis (TB) can also

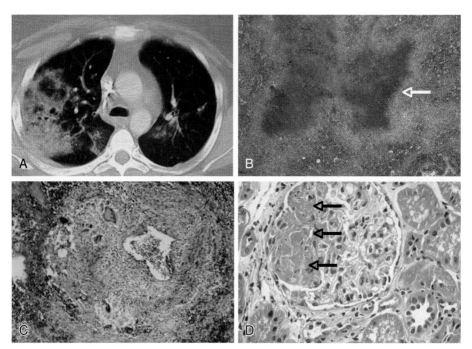

Fig. 45.3 Granulomatosis with polyangiitis. (A) Chest computed tomography (CT) scan shows cavitated nodular lung infiltrate. (B) Low-power view of biopsy of a lung granuloma showing inflammation and necrosis *(arrow)*. (C) Granulomatous vasculitis of small pulmonary artery—thickened vessel wall with infiltration and multinucleated giant cells. (D) Glomeruli showing necrosis and early crescent formation *(arrows)*. (From Adkinson NF, Bochner BS, Burks AW, et al, eds. *Middleton's Allergy: Principles and Practice.* 8th ed. Philadelphia: Elsevier/Saunders; 2014.)

cause chronic infection, hemoptysis, and constitutive symptoms. Specific TB testing should be performed with this patient to determine its presence or absence.

Case Point 45.5

Rheumatologic laboratory tests show a positive cytoplasmic antineutrophil cytoplasmic antibody (c-ANCA) screen and elevated serine protease proteinase-3 (PPR3) antibody levels. Antinuclear and AGBM antibody tests are negative. A high-resolution chest CT scan shows peribronchial pulmonary nodules, with cavitary and wedge-shaped lesions (Fig. 45.4).

Diagnosis: Granulomatosis with polyangiitis.

BASIC SCIENCE PEARL   **STEP 1**

There are two types of antineutrophil cytoplasmic antibodies (ANCAs). One is directed against neutrophil serine protease proteinase-3 (PPR3), which is located in the cytoplasm. On immunofluorescence, the cytoplasm lights up—hence, the name *cytoplasmic ANCA* (cANCA). The other targets the neutrophil enzyme myeloperoxidase (MPO), which causes a perinuclear immunofluorescence pattern termed *perinuclear ANCA* (pANCA; Fig. 45.5).

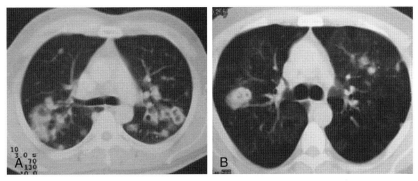

Fig. 45.4 CT scan showing pulmonary nodules. (A) Consolidation, noncavitated and cavitated nodules. (B) Mosaic pattern, cavitated nodules, and centrilobular micronodules on the periphery of the anterior segment of the left upper lobe. (From Gomez-Gomez A, Martinez-Martinez U, Cuevas-Orta E, et al. Pulmonary manifestations of granulomatosis with polyangiitis. *Reumatol Clin.* 2013;10(5):288–293.)

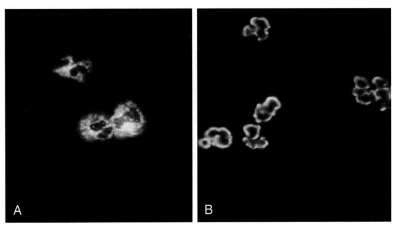

Fig. 45.5 Immunofluorescence staining for antineutrophilic cytoplasmic antibodies. (A) Diffuse cytoplasmic staining in c-ANCA. (B) Perinuclear staining in p-ANCA. (From Kelly A, Jane-Tizar E. Vasculitis in children. *Paediatr Child Health.* 2010;20(2):6–72.)

CLINICAL PEARL   **STEPS 2/3**

If you suspect GPA, chest imaging must be performed because one-third of patients will be asymptomatic but will have abnormal radiographic findings on a chest x-ray.

The diagnosis of GPA can be made based on clinical features, histologic findings, and laboratory values. Biopsy can be done on affected tissues to show compatible histology for diagnosis. Even when specimens are obtained from affected tissue, usually lung parenchyma, they may not be diagnostic and so are not routinely done.

How would you proceed with treatment?

For respiratory and renal manifestations, initial treatment includes intravenous (IV) corticosteroids and oral cyclophosphamide. Once in remission, therapy is transitioned to a less toxic regimen, such as methotrexate, azathioprine, or mycophenolate mofetil. Disease relapse occurs in up to 60% of patients.

BASIC SCIENCE PEARL   **STEP 1**

The studies needed to determine the diagnosis take days to obtain results but the patient
needs to be treated. The initial treatment for our top diagnoses on our differential is the same,
so treatment should not be delayed by your diagnostic workup. Anti–glomerular basement
membrane disease is also treated with IV corticosteroids and cyclophosphamide, plus plasmapheresis. The decision to carry out plasmapheresis can be made based on the patient's
initial response to medications.

Case Point 45.6

The patient is treated with IV methylprednisolone, 1 g daily for 3 days (pulse steroid therapy),
followed by rituximab, 1 g IV. Her heart rate decreases to normal range during the course of antiinflammatory treatment. She is discharged home to continue a maintenance dose of prednisone,
2 mg/kg per day. She will be followed by the pediatric rheumatologist as an outpatient.

Case Summary

Complaint/History: A 16-year-old female has a 3-month history of right knee pain and
the development of systemic symptoms, including fatigue, weight loss, fever, multiple joint
pains, cough with blood-tinged sputum, and dark-colored urine.

Findings: Mildly swollen right knee, pallor, persistent tachycardia, and tachypnea.

Labs/Tests: Chest x-ray with nodular hyperdensities; laboratory tests show leukocytosis, normocytic anemia, elevated liver enzyme levels, hematuria, proteinuria, and pyuria. Her ECG
shows myocarditis. A chest CT scan shows pulmonary nodules with cavitary lesions. The
c-ANCA and PPR3 tests are positive.

Diagnosis: Granulomatosis with polyangiitis (GPA).

Treatment: Pulse steroid (methylprednisolone, 1 g IV for 3 days) and rituximab, 1 g IV for
acute management, followed by a maintenance prednisone regimen.

BEYOND THE PEARLS

- Granulomatous disease may be found in granulomatosis with polyangiitis (GPA), microscopic angiitis, anti-GBM disease, and Henoch-Schönlein purpura (HSP). GPA can be
  differentiated from these other conditions by the presence of upper airway disease (nasal,
  sinus), lower airway disease with necrosis, granulomas on lung biopsy with vasculitis, and
  glomerulonephritis.
- Major causes of hemoptysis, pulmonary infiltrates, and renal involvement, as seen in our
  patient, include GPA and anti-GBM disease.
- Anti-GBM disease causes rapidly progressive pulmonary hemorrhage and renal failure,
  which may be acutely life threatening.
- Autoantibodies against the cytoplasmic granules of neutrophils (ANCAs) are found in 90%
  of GPA cases. A small number of patients can still develop the clinical findings of GPA in
  the absence of detectable ANCA.
- Perinuclear ANCA (pANCA) and cytoplasmic ANCA (cANCA) are named for the part of the
  cell that lights up with immunofluorescence.
- A chest x-ray must be obtained if there is a suspicion for GPA because it may still be positive, even if the patient does not have pulmonary symptoms.
- The identification of an active or latent tuberculosis infection is crucial in patients with a
  potential autoimmune condition, not only for adequate treatment, but for the risk of TB
  reactivation once immunosuppressive treatment is initiated.

Bibliography

Ardoin SP, Fels E. Vasculitis syndromes. *Nelson Textbook of Pediatrics*, Philadelphia: Elsevier; 1215–1224.e2

Bohm M, et al. Clinical features of childhood granulomatosis with polyangiitis (Wegener's granulomatosis) Bohm, et al. *Pediatr Rheumatol.* 2014;12:18.

Cooper A, et al. A 14-year-old boy with sore throat and tea-colored urine. *Pediatrics.* 2014; 133:e1377–1380. Number 5.

Langford C. Clinical features and diagnosis of small-vessel vasculitis. *Cleve Clin J Med.* 2012; 79(suppl 3).

Saxena R, et al. Antiglomerular basement membrane disease. *Medscape.* 2015. 3 Feb 2016.

Specks U. Controversies in ANCA testing. *Cleve Clin J Med.* 2012; 79(suppl 3).

Van Why SK, Avner ED. Goodpasture disease. *Nelson Textbook of Pediatrics,* Philadelphia: Elsevier; 2507–2507.e2

6-Week-Old Female Infant With Persistent Jaundice

Christine Kassissa-Mourad

A 6-week-old ex–preterm female infant presents for outpatient evaluation for persistent jaundice. Today, her father states that she is doing well at home. She is taking 2 ounces of formula every 3 hours. She has adequate urine output and two to three yellow-colored stools per day. Otherwise, her father states that she is acting like her normal self and his only concern is that her skin and eyes remain yellow.

What is the significance of the stool color provided in the patient's history?

One of the most concerning causes of persistent neonatal jaundice that must be ruled out quickly is biliary atresia, because there is a small window of time for intervention. Biliary atresia is a disease of the extrahepatic biliary tree that presents with biliary obstruction resulting in conjugated hyperbilirubinemia. Early surgical intervention, generally within 2 months of life, is associated with a better outcome. An infant will generally present within the first 8 weeks of life with jaundice, acholic stools, and a firm liver, with an enlarged spleen. Although we have not yet heard about the physical examination for this patient, it is reassuring to know that her stools are pigmented, making biliary atresia less likely.

Case Point 46.1

She was born at 34 weeks via cesarean section due to maternal preeclampsia. Her mother was adequately treated with glucocorticoids. Both maternal and baby blood types are O+. Her Apgar scores were 7 and 9, and she was noted to be small for gestational age. Maternal screening laboratory tests were negative (rapid plasma reagin [RPR], hepatitis B, rubella, HIV). She was admitted to the neonatal intensive care unit (NICU) for prematurity. Her hospital course was complicated by thrombocytopenia of unknown cause, requiring platelet transfusion. She required total parenteral nutrition (TPN) for 1 week. She was noted to have unconjugated hyperbilirubinemia and required phototherapy for 2 days, with an adequate response. She was discharged from the NICU after 4 weeks. She did not pass her hearing screen on the first attempt.

What is the clinical significance of her birth history?

There are clues in both the maternal history and birth history that can aid in your diagnosis. The ability to obtain important information, such as the infant being jaundiced, having thrombocytopenia, and being small for gestational age, are characteristics of many TORCH infections (*t*oxoplasmosis, *o*ther agents, *r*ubella, *c*ytomegalovirus, and *h*erpes simplex). She was also on TPN, which can cause cholestasis and jaundice. Although many infants do not pass the hearing screen on the first attempt, this fact should not be overlooked in this patient because it may be relevant to the case. Her history of prematurity is important in that it makes her vulnerable to chronic illnesses inherent in this patient population.

Case Point 46.2

On physical examination, she is afebrile, alert, and responsive. She is microcephalic. Her anterior fontanelle is open, soft, and flat. She has normal facies. The respiratory and cardiovascular examinations are unremarkable. Her abdomen is soft. Both the liver edge and spleen tip are palpable 2 cm below the costal margin. Her skin is notable for jaundice to the lower trunk and petechiae; otherwise, she is warm and well-perfused.

Would you order any imaging at this point?

The physical examination suggests that the infant has hepatosplenomegaly. This is a very subjective finding, so it would be beneficial to order an abdominal ultrasound to evaluate both the liver and spleen. This will aid in providing accurate measurements and showing any gross structural abnormalities. Now that you have a physical examination with evidence of jaundice and hepatosplenomegaly, a cholescintigraphy or hepatobiliary iminodiacetic acid (HIDA) scan should be done because there is still concern for biliary atresia.

CLINICAL PEARL   **STEPS 2/3**

In a HIDA scan, a radioactive tracer (usually Tc^{99m} iminodiacetic acid analogues) is injected and travels to the liver, where it is taken up by the bile-producing cells. It then travels through the bile ducts. Biliary atresia is diagnosed when there is failure of tracer excretion into the bowel.

Case Point 46.3

Abdominal ultrasound is significant for a liver of 9 cm and spleen of 8 cm, which are both greater than the 97th percentile for age. The HIDA scan shows tracer excretion into the bowel, effectively ruling out biliary atresia.

CLINICAL PEARL   **STEP 1**

In patients presenting with multisystem complaints, it is beneficial to create a problem list to organize your thoughts and ensure that you do not miss any problems. It will also allow you to combine the problems to formulate one most likely diagnosis.

What is the differential diagnosis?

In summary, the patient is a 6-week-old female infant with the following problem list: jaundice, thrombocytopenia, hepatosplenomegaly, small for gestational age, microcephaly, and failed hearing screen. As already mentioned, it is important to rule out biliary atresia because this diagnosis requires prompt intervention. A normal HIDA scan in a neonate that has pigmented stools excludes biliary atresia. The constellation of symptoms and signs that the patient has makes a TORCH infection the most likely diagnosis. The three TORCH infections that may present in this fashion include rubella, toxoplasmosis, and cytomegalovirus (CMV). Rubella is associated with sensorineural deafness, cataracts, cardiac malformations, growth retardation, radiolucent bone disease, hepatosplenomegaly, thrombocytopenia, hyperbilirubinemia, and purpuric skin lesions, typically known as *blueberry muffin spots* (Fig. 46.1).

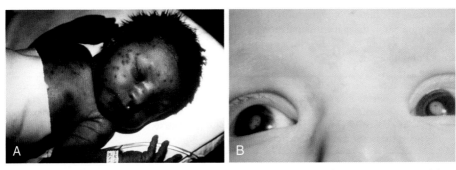

Fig. 46.1 Congenital Rubella infection. (A) Purpuric blueberry muffin rash. (B) Cataracts in a newborn infant. (From Neu N, Duchon J, Zachariah P. TORCH infections. *Clin Perinatol*. 2015;42(1):77–103.)

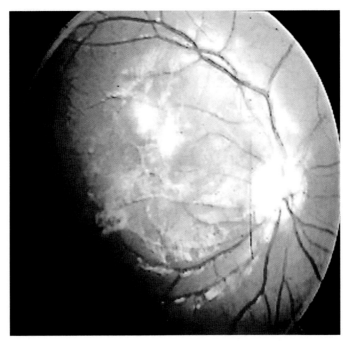

Fig. 46.2 Toxoplasmosis chorioretinitis. Shown is active chorioretinitis from reactivation of a congenital toxoplasmosis infection. (From Amaya L. Congenital infections of the eye. In: Lambert SR, Lyons CJ, eds. *Taylor and Hoyt's Pediatric Ophthalmology and Strabismus*. 5th ed. Philadelphia, Elsevier;2017:101–108.)

Maternal laboratory tests indicate that the mother is immune to rubella, making this infection less likely. Toxoplasmosis presents with fever, maculopapular rash, hepatosplenomegaly, microcephaly, seizures, jaundice, and thrombocytopenia. Active chorioretinitis occurs with the reactivation of a congenital toxoplasmosis infection (Fig. 46.2). There are no maternal risk factors such as feline exposure, making this diagnosis less likely. CMV is associated with petechiae, jaundice, hepatosplenomegaly, thrombocytopenia, small for gestational age, microcephaly, intracranial calcifications (Fig. 46.3), sensorineural hearing loss, chorioretinitis, and seizures. She has most of the listed symptoms, making this the most likely diagnosis. Also on the differential is Alagille

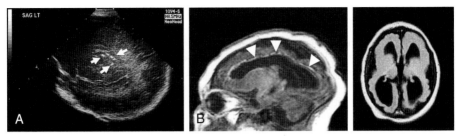

Fig. 46.3 Congenital CMV infection. (A) Head ultrasound showing intracranial and periventricular calcifications *(arrows)*. (B) Brain MRI scan with T1-weighted, 1.5-T images demonstrating ventriculomegaly, periventricular calcifications *(arrowheads)*, and marked loss of brain volume. This sagittal view demonstrates the calcifications. (From Swanson E, Schleiss M. Congenital cytomegalovirus infection. *Pediatr Clin North Am.* 2013;60(2):335–349.)

syndrome, although this is unlikely in an infant with normal facies and no cardiac anomalies. Although administering TPN may have contributed to the jaundice, it does not explain the other findings in this patient, making TPN cholestasis unlikely. Neonatal sepsis can have a variable presentation, so this should always be on the differential diagnosis. It is reassuring to hear that the infant is at baseline mental status, afebrile, and otherwise clinically well appearing, making sepsis less likely.

CLINICAL PEARL   **STEPS 2/3**

Many of the TORCH infections have variable and nonspecific manifestations, and infants may present with one, many, or most of the clinical signs and symptoms, so you must always have a high index of suspicion.

Case Point 46.4

Laboratory testing reveals a complete blood count (CBC) with thrombocytopenia, comprehensive metabolic panel (CMP) with elevated liver function tests (LFTs), and elevated direct and indirect bilirubin levels. The blood culture and urine culture are negative. The C-reactive protein (CRP) level is normal. The hepatitis panel is negative. The TORCH panel is negative for rubella, toxoplasma, herpes virus, and parvovirus. The CMV IgM antibody is found to be positive. A CMV DNA polymerase chain reaction (PCR) assay result is elevated, at 25,000 copies/mL. A lumbar puncture shows elevated protein.

Diagnosis: Neonatal CMV infection.

CLINICAL PEARL   **STEPS 2/3**

The method of diagnosing CMV is age-dependent. From birth to 3 weeks of age, the diagnosis can be made by analyzing urine or saliva for the presence of the virus. However, when older than 3 weeks of age, as in this case, a positive urine or saliva test cannot differentiate between congenital and postnatal CMV. CMV IgM antibodies are suggestive of infection, but there can be false-positives, so confirmatory testing with a PCR assay is recommended.

What additional testing would you order?

When an infant has hepatosplenomegaly and elevated LFTs, you want to evaluate for liver synthetic function. The liver is responsible for making many of the clotting factors; thus the most sensitive tests for the liver synthetic function are the prothrombin time (PT) and international normalized ratio (INR). The serum albumin level can also tell you about liver synthetic function.

Case Point 46.5

The PT and INR are prolonged, and the serum albumin level is within normal range.

Would you order any additional imaging now that you have confirmed the diagnosis of CMV?

In neonates with CMV, you should order cranial ultrasound imaging because they can have the following findings: periventricular intracranial calcifications, white matter disease, ventriculomegaly, periventricular leukomalacia, and cystic abnormalities.

Case Point 46.6

The cranial ultrasound is normal.

When is treatment indicated?

Treatment with intravenous ganciclovir or oral valganciclovir should be initiated in infants with symptomatic congenital CMV infection because it is shown to improve long-term audiologic and neurodevelopmental disabilities, such as cerebral palsy, intellectual disability, and seizures. Some physicians also recommend treating asymptomatic infants who have failed the hearing screen to prevent the progression of hearing loss. Another indication to treat is infants with primary immunodeficiency. Treatment is not recommended for infants who are asymptomatic and have passed their newborn hearing screen.

Case Point 46.7

She was treated with valganciclovir for 6 months.

CLINICAL PEARL	STEPS 1/2/3

Infants who are being treated with valganciclovir or ganciclovir should be monitored carefully for the following medications side effects: neutropenia, thrombocytopenia, hepatotoxicity, and nephrotoxicity.

What follow-up interventions are needed for infants with CMV?

Treatment response is followed by measuring the level of viremia with a CMV DNA PCR assay. Infants need hearing evaluations every 3 to 6 months during the first 3 years of life, and annually thereafter until they are at least 18 years old. They should also be seen by an ophthalmologist for eye examinations annually. Regular dental visits are also recommended because CMV is associated with hypoplasia and hypocalcification of tooth enamel.

Case Point 46.8

She has improved clinically, with improvement in her viral load, as well as normalization of her LFTs, PT, INR, and bilirubin level.

CLINICAL PEARL   **STEPS 2/3**

Chorioretinitis is the most common eye finding in infants with CMV, but infants can also have retinopathy, optic atrophy, and strabismus.

BEYOND THE PEARLS

- CMV infection is asymptomatic in most infants but can cause severe infection when congenital and is more severe in preterm infants.
- There is no routine maternal screening for CMV infection in the United States.
- Congenital CMV is the most common cause of sensorineural hearing loss.
- The most common findings in symptomatic infants include jaundice, hepatosplenomegaly, hearing loss, microcephaly, petechiae, and brain calcifications.
- Common laboratory findings include anemia, thrombocytopenia, elevated liver enzyme levels, hyperbilirubinemia, and increased CSF protein.
- All infants should undergo an ophthalmic examination to evaluate for chorioretinitis.
- All infants should undergo an audiology examination to evaluate for hearing loss.

Case Summary

Complaint/History: A 6-week-old female infant presents with jaundice.

Findings: Neonatal history significant for 34-week prematurity and thrombocytopenia. Examination findings include jaundice, microcephaly, and hepatosplenomegaly.

Labs/Tests: Laboratory tests indicate thrombocytopenia, hyperbilirubinemia, CMV IgM antibody-positive, CMV DNA PCR positive; abdominal ultrasound shows liver and spleen size greater than 95th percentile, confirming hepatosplenomegaly.

Diagnosis: Congenital cytomegalovirus infection.

Treatment: Valganciclovir for 6 weeks.

Bibliography

Banatvala JE, Brown DW. Rubella. *Lancet.* 2004;363:1127.

Boppana SB, Pass RF, Britt WJ, et al. Symptomatic congenital cytomegalovirus infection: neonatal morbidity and mortality. *Pediatr Infect Dis J.* 1992;11:93.

Capretti MG, Lanari M, Tani G, et al. Role of cerebral ultrasound and magnetic resonance imaging in newborns with congenital cytomegalovirus infection. *Brain Dev.* 2014;36:203.

Dreher AM, Arora N, Fowler KB, et al. Spectrum of disease and outcome in children with symptomatic congenital cytomegalovirus infection. *J Pediatr.* 2014;164:855.

Fink KR, Thapa MM, Ishak GE, Pruthi S. Neuroimaging of pediatric central nervous system cytomegalovirus infection. *Radiographics.* 2010;30:1779.

Ghekiere S, Allegaert K, Cossey V, et al. Ophthalmological findings in congenital cytomegalovirus infection: when to screen, when to treat? *J Pediatr Ophthalmol Strabismus.* 2012;49(274):899.

Gottesman LE, Del Vecchio MT, Aronoff SC. Etiologies of conjugated hyperbilirubinemia in infancy: a systematic review of 1692 subjects. *BMC Pediatr.* 2015;15:192.

Gwee A, Curtis N, Connell TG, et al. Ganciclovir for the treatment of congenital cytomegalovirus: what are the side effects? *Pediatr Infect Dis J.* 2014;33:115.

Haber BA, Russo P. Biliary atresia. *Gastroenterol Clin North Am.* 2003;32:891.

Kimberlin DW, Lin CY, Sánchez PJ, et al. Effect of ganciclovir therapy on hearing in symptomatic congenital cytomegalovirus disease involving the central nervous system: a randomized, controlled trial. *J Pediatr.* 2003;143:16.

Lombardi G, Garofoli F, Villani P, et al. Oral valganciclovir treatment in newborns with symptomatic congenital cytomegalovirus infection. *Eur J Clin Microbiol Infect Dis.* 2009;28:1465.

Oh M, Hobeldin M, Chen T, et al. The Kasai procedure in the treatment of biliary atresia. *J Pediatr Surg.* 1995;30:1077.

Pinninti SG, Ross SA, Shimamura M, et al. Comparison of saliva PCR assay versus rapid culture for detection of congenital cytomegalovirus infection. *Pediatr Infect Dis J.* 2015;34:536.

Stagno S, Pass RF, Thomas JP, et al. Defects of tooth structure in congenital cytomegalovirus infection. *Pediatrics.* 1982;69:646.

Tamma P. Toxoplasmosis. *Pediatr Rev.* 2007;28:470.

20-Month-Old Female With Fever and Convulsions

Colette Vassilian ▦ Arthur Partikian

A 20-month-old female is brought into the emergency department via ambulance. Her mother had called 911 after the child became unresponsive and exhibited convulsions of her arms and legs. The patient's convulsions stopped after approximately 5 minutes and had ended prior to the arrival of the paramedics. She had developed fever, rhinorrhea, and cough and has been less playful than normal that day. The patient's mother states that her temperature was 103.3°F 1 hour prior to the event.

What is this mother describing?

The female's mother is describing what is called a *febrile seizure*. Febrile seizures are defined as convulsive episodes occurring in childhood after 1 month of age, associated with febrile illness but not caused by infection of the central nervous system (CNS), unassociated with metabolic derangements and previous neonatal seizures or unprovoked seizures, and not meeting criteria for other acute symptomatic seizures. A simple febrile seizure is a generalized seizure that lasts less than 15 minutes and does not recur within 24 hours. Febrile seizures affect 2% to 5% of children and most commonly occur between the ages of 6 to 60 months. Epidemiologically, they represent the most common convulsive event that occurs in children younger than 5 years of age.

CLINICAL PEARL   **STEP 2/3**

A complex febrile seizure is focal, lasts 15 minutes or longer and/or recurs within 24 hours. A febrile seizure is also considered complex if it occurs in an atypically developing child or in a child who has had an abnormal neurologic examination. Febrile status epilepticus is a febrile seizure lasting more than 30 minutes.

What are other important elements of the history?

Obtaining a history of present illness (HPI) from an individual who witnessed the event is of highest yield. Be sure to ask about the duration of the convulsive episode and what it looked like. Questions should focus on how the seizure begins and evolves:

- Prior to any convulsions, did the child experience unresponsive staring?
- Did it involve both arms and legs versus one limb or one side of the body?

In addition, it is critical to obtain an immunization history and a developmental assessment of the child from the parents' perspective. This will lead you to obtain a comprehensive medical history to determine whether the child has other risk factors that predispose her or him to seizures. If the child is not developing normally, he or she cannot truly be described as having a simple febrile seizure.

Case Point 47.1

The child has no significant past medical history. She was born full term via normal vaginal delivery and is meeting all of her developmental milestones. The mother states that she has received all of her vaccines thus far.

What are the main predisposing factors to simple febrile seizures?

The main factors are as follows:

1. The peak temperature of a fever is a child's main risk factor.
2. Viral infections (as opposed to bacterial) are usually associated with febrile seizures. Patients with viral infections associated with very high fevers (e.g., human herpes virus 6, influenza) are at greatest risk of febrile seizures, although several other viral infections have been implicated (e.g., respiratory syncytial virus, adenovirus, herpes simplex virus, cytomegalovirus). Febrile seizures have also occurred in the setting of otitis media and shigellosis.
3. A genetic predisposition is a well-known risk factor for febrile seizures. Approximately 10% to 20% of patients will have a first-degree relative that has had or will have a febrile seizure.

CLINICAL PEARL	STEP 2/3

Fever with seizure has also been shown to occur following administration of measles-mumps-rubella (MMR), diphtheria, tetanus, acellular pertussis (DTap), and influenza vaccines.

BASIC SCIENCE/CLINICAL PEARL	STEP 1/2/3

A predisposition to febrile seizures is inherited as an autosomal dominant trait, and numerous single genes that can predispose to the disorder have been identified. A gene associated with febrile seizures whose function is best understood is the *SCN1A* gene located on chromosome 2q24. This gene encodes for a sodium channel and is also implicated in the following epilepsy syndromes: generalized epilepsy with febrile seizure plus (GEFS+) and severe myoclonic epilepsy of infancy (SMEI), which is also known as Dravet syndrome. These syndromes are often preceded by multiple and/or prolonged febrile seizures.

Case Point 47.2

As the child is wheeled into the emergency room, she is noted to be sleepy but opening her eyes in response to her name being called. Her vital signs are notable for a temperature of 39°C and heart rate of 112 beats/min. She is breathing comfortably, and her examination is only remarkable for a clear discharge at her bilateral nares. Her neurologic examination is nonfocal and within normal limits.

When is a lumbar puncture indicated?

Providers will have a low threshold for lumbar puncture in children with meningeal signs, including neck stiffness, a positive Kernig or Brudzinski sign (Fig. 47.1), or other signs and symptoms suggestive of a CNS infection, including a bulging fontanel, notable lethargy or irritability, and focal findings on a neurologic examination. Otherwise, it is generally recommended that a lumbar puncture be performed in children younger than 12 months of age if their immunization status—specifically for *Haemophilus influenzae* type B and *Streptococcus pneumoniae*—is either incomplete or unknown or if a patient is on antibiotics, given concern for partially treated meningitis.

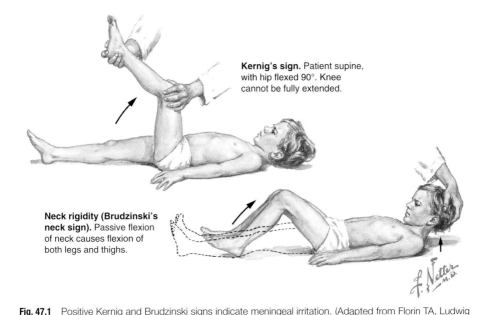

Kernig's sign. Patient supine, with hip flexed 90°. Knee cannot be fully extended.

Neck rigidity (Brudzinski's neck sign). Passive flexion of neck causes flexion of both legs and thighs.

Fig. 47.1   Positive Kernig and Brudzinski signs indicate meningeal irritation. (Adapted from Florin TA, Ludwig S. *Netter's Pediatrics.* Philadelphia: Elsevier/Saunders; 2011.)

CLINICAL PEARL	STEP 2/3

In terms of other laboratory studies, blood tests, including a complete blood count (CBC) and determination of serum electrolyte, calcium, magnesium, and phosphorus levels are not routinely recommended for a child with a first simple febrile seizure. Blood glucose testing should be considered for children with a prolonged postictal period (altered level of consciousness following an epileptic episode) or those with a history of poor oral intake. These tests should only be performed if they are deemed to be clinically indicated.

Case Point 47.3

The patient is given a dose of oral acetaminophen and a respiratory swab is sent. Over the next 2 hours, her fever diminishes and she becomes progressively more interactive. The mother notes that her child is back to her normal self as she feeds her daughter. You then receive a call from the laboratory that her respiratory swab is positive for influenza.

Should this child undergo brain imaging?
The American Academy of Pediatrics (AAP) has recommended against neuroimaging in children with simple febrile seizures based on the risks of radiation associated with computed tomography (CT) scans, and high cost, as well as the need for sedation with magnetic resonance imaging (MRI). Although parents may request imaging, it is important to reassure them that it likely would not change the medical management of their child.

CLINICAL PEARL	STEP 2/3

Similar to neuroimaging, there is little utility in obtaining an electroencephalogram (EEG) in patients with simple febrile seizures who have no neurologic or developmental abnormalities.

Case Point 47.4

Given this child's return to baseline, the medical team prepares to send her home. Prior to her discharge, the patient's mother is counseled regarding seizure management and appropriate treatment.

What other treatment is necessary?

For patients with one or more simple febrile seizures, neither intermittent nor continuous antiepileptic therapy is recommended. However, parents should be counseled regarding acute therapies for prolonged seizures (seizures lasting > 5 minutes). Rectal diazepam is often prescribed for recurrence of a febrile seizure lasting more than 5 minutes. Although antipyretics have the ability to decrease a child's discomfort, they do not decrease the risk of the incidence of febrile seizures because these seizures often occur as the child's temperature is rising or falling.

What are the long-term consequences of simple febrile seizures?

In general, simple febrile seizures are not associated with long-term adverse effects. After experiencing one febrile seizure, approximately 30% of patients will experience another. Following two or more episodes, the recurrence rate increases to about 50%. The risk of developing epilepsy after a simple febrile seizure is about 1%.

BEYOND THE PEARLS

- For seizures lasting longer than 5 minutes and/or for status epilepticus, benzodiazepines are first-line therapy to abort seizure activity. Lorazepam (0.1 mg/kg), administered intravenously, is typically used as initial pharmacotherapy by medical personnel. Rectal diazepam can be prescribed to be administered by nonmedical personnel, including parents, for prolonged seizures or seizure clustering.
- Major risk factors for the recurrence of febrile seizures include age younger than 1 year, less than a 24-hour duration of fever, low peak temperature of 38°C to 39°C, and having a family history of febrile seizures
- Complex febrile seizures confer a twofold increased risk of mortality as compared to the general population over the 2 years following the episode.
- Risk factors for the development of epilepsy after a febrile seizure include neurodevelopmental abnormalities, a family history of epilepsy, multiple febrile seizures, and complex febrile seizures.

Case Summary

Complaint/History: 20-month-old female with fevers and convulsions.

Findings: Otherwise healthy female infant with febrile illness and generalized tonic-clonic seizure of 5 minutes duration.

Labs/Tests: Influenza positive.

Diagnosis: Febrile seizure.

Treatment: Conservative management.

Bibliography

American Academy of Pediatrics. Subcommittee on febrile seizures. Febrile seizures: guideline for the neurodiagnostic evaluation of the child with a simple febrile seizure. *Pediatrics.* 2011;127(2):389–394.

Berg AT, Shinnar S, Hauser WA, et al. A prospective study of recurrent febrile seizures. *N Engl J Med.* 1992;327(16):1122–1127.

Hesdorffer DC, Benn EK, Bagiella E, et al. FEBSTAT Study team. Distribution of febrile seizure duration and associations with development. *Ann Neurol.* 2011;70(1):93–100.

Kimia A, Ben-Joseph E, Prabhu S, et al. Yield of emergent neuroimaging among children presenting with a first complex febrile seizure. *Pediatr Emerg Care.* 2012;28(4):316–321.

Mikati MA. Febrile seizures. In: Kliegman RM, Stanton B, St. Geme J, et al., eds. *Nelson Textbook of Pediatrics.* 19th ed. Philadelphia: Elsevier; 2011:2017–2018.

Sidhu R, Velayudam K, Barnes G. Pediatric seizures. *Pediatr Rev.* 2013;34(8):333–341.

7-Week-Old Male Infant With Apnea

Iris A. Perez

A 7-week-old term male infant is brought in by his mother to the emergency department (ED) for the second time, with the chief complaint of episodes of pauses in breathing during sleep. These episodes are associated with perioral cyanosis lasting about 15 to 20 seconds, which resolves with gentle stimulation, such as tickling of his feet. Sometimes, these episodes are associated with pallor. His past medical history is significant for low Apgar scores requiring observation in the neonatal infant care unit (NICU), where he was noted to have periodic breathing. He was first seen at the ED at 1 month of age for short apnea and pallor, where he was observed overnight and diagnosed with a brief, resolved, unexplained event (BRUE). On physical examination, temperature is 36.9°C, heart rate is 130 beats/min, blood pressure is 87/50 mm Hg, respiratory rate is 32 breaths/min, and oxygen saturation is 97% on room air. He is well nourished, well developed, and not in respiratory distress. The breath sounds are clear. The rest of the physical examination is normal.

What is a brief, resolved, unexplained event?

A BRUE refers to a sudden, brief, and now resolved event characterized by one or more of the following characteristics: (1) cyanosis or pallor; (2) absent, decreased or irregular breathing; (3) marked change in tone (hypo- or hypertonia); and (4) altered level of responsiveness occurring in an infant younger than 1 year. It was previously called an *apparent life-threatening event* (ALTE). It is a diagnosis of exclusion that is made only when there is no explanation after an appropriate history and physical examination are performed.

CLINICAL PEARL	**STEPS 2/3**

A diagnosis of BRUE is given only when there is no explanation of the event. BRUE is a diagnosis of exclusion, and its presentation may be a clue to an underlying medical condition. Therefore, a meticulous medical, environmental, and social history and thorough physical examination are required to identify the cause and predisposing factors, as well as to determine the risk of recurrence.

What is the workup for an infant who experiences a brief, resolved, unexplained event?

When an infant experiences a BRUE, it is essential to perform a thorough history and physical examination to characterize the event, assess the risk of recurrence, and identify an underlying disorder. Infants without identifiable risk factors are considered low risk and will not require extensive investigation. Factors associated with a higher risk of a BRUE are noted in Box 48.1. Using these criteria, this infant is younger than 2 months old and is presenting with a history of apneas for the second time ; the previous history of low Apgar scores and periodic breathing is concerning and thus warrants further investigation. There is an array of conditions that can present as a BRUE (Table 48.1), and the evaluation should focus on the area of concern.

BOX 48.1 ■ Characteristics of a Higher Risk, Brief, Resolved, Unexplained Event (BRUE)

Age < 60 days
Prematurity ≤ 32-wk gestation
>One event, events in clusters
≥1-min duration
Cardiopulmonary resuscitation (CPR) by trained provider

TABLE 48.1 ■ **Differential Diagnosis of a Brief Resolved Unexplained Event**

System	Causes
Respiratory	Upper and lower respiratory tract infections, obstructive sleep apnea (OSA), airway anomalies, congenital central hypoventilation syndrome (CCHS)
Cardiac	Congenital heart disease, cardiomyopathy, Wolff-Parkinson-White syndrome;, arrhythmias
Gastrointestinal	Gastroesophageal reflux disease (GERD), feeding dysfunction, intussusception
Infectious disease	Sepsis, respiratory syncytial virus, pertussis
Central nervous	Seizure, intracranial hemorrhage, anatomic abnormalities
Metabolic	Fatty acid oxidation disorders, mitochondrial disorders, electrolyte abnormalities
Other	
Exposure	Adverse reaction to medication, toxin, drugs of abuse, sedatives
Social	Child abuse

CLINICAL PEARL   **STEPS 2/3**

An infant meeting the criteria for low-risk BRUE—age > 2 months; gestational age ≥ 32 weeks; postconceptional age ≥ 45 weeks; first BRUE lasting <1 minute and not in clusters; no CPR by trained medical provider, and without concerning history and physical examination findings—will not benefit from unnecessary testing. Only when an infant has normal vital signs, physical examination, and oximetry can the event be categorized as low-risk BRUE. Infants with recurrent BRUE and presenting at younger than 2 months of age warrant an investigation because they are more likely to have an infectious or congenital cause that confers an adverse outcome.

Case Point 48.1

At the ED, this infant has several episodes of brief apneic spells and occasional emesis with feeding. He is admitted for evaluation and management. His routine laboratory test results are unremarkable. The respiratory viral panel is negative for adenovirus, human metapneumovirus, influenzas A and B, parainfluenza types 1, 2, and 3, respiratory syncytial virus (RSV), rhinovirus, and enterovirus. The urinalysis was not suggestive of a urinary tract infection. His chest X-ray is unremarkable (Fig. 48.1). Blood gas results, when the patient is awake, show respiratory alkalosis. In contrast, results obtained when the patient is asleep show respiratory acidosis (Table 48.2). An overnight polysomnography reveals central sleep apneas (CSAs), periodic breathing, hypercapnia, and hypoxemia (Fig. 48.2). A diagnosis of congenital central hypoventilation syndrome (CCHS) is suspected.

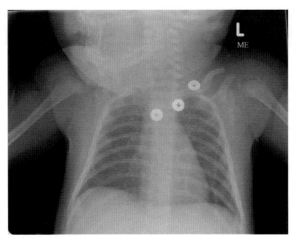

Fig. 48.1   Normal chest x-ray.

TABLE 48.2 ■ **Capillary Blood Gas (CBG) Values**

Parameter	Awake	Sleeping
pH	7.46	7.27
pco_2	33 mm Hg	78 mm Hg
po_2	75 mm Hg	56 mm Hg
HCO_3	23 mEq/L	28 mEq/L

When is congenital central hypoventilation syndrome suspected?

CCHS is suspected when an infant presents with apneas, cyanosis, hypercapnia, and hypoxemia that cannot be explained by other conditions or disorders. Severe hypoventilation is present and is worse during sleep, but my also extend into wakefulness. These events may result in respiratory failure requiring intubation and assisted mechanical ventilation.

Most CCHS patients present in the neonatal period with apnea and cyanosis, as seen in this infant. There is significant hypoventilation and hypoxemia, without the expected increase in respiratory rate or tidal volume. When intubated, these infants cannot be weaned off mechanical ventilation. This patient presents with apneas and cyanosis. The awake partial pressure of carbon dioxide (Pco_2) was normal but was noted to be elevated significantly during sleep.

Beyond the neonatal period, CCHS patients may present with recurrent apnea, cyanosis, or apparent life-threatening events, or a BRUE. They lack objective responses to hypoxemia and hypercapnia and therefore will not present with respiratory distress or tachypnea, in spite of significant hypoventilation or hypoxemia. Older children or adults can present with diaphoresis during sleep and pulmonary hypertension from prolonged hypoventilation and hypoxemia. They may have significant hypoventilation or apneas following exposure to general anesthesia or lower respiratory tract infection. When a patient cannot be extubated or weaned from assisted ventilation following sedation or general anesthesia for a procedure or lower respiratory tract infection, one must suspect CCHS.

CCHS is an autonomic nervous system disorder. About 20% of CCHS patients have Hirschsprung disease, and 6% have neural crest tumors (neuroblastoma and ganglioneuroma). Other

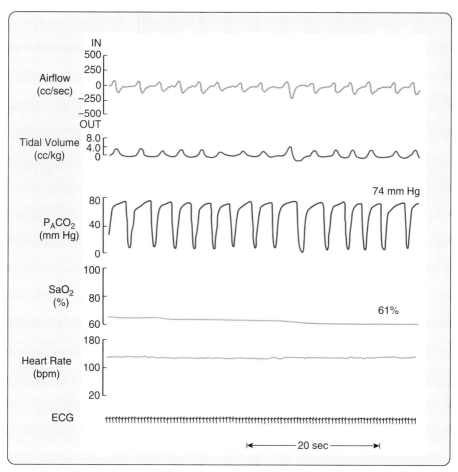

Fig. 48.2 Polysomnography in congenital central hypoventilation syndrome (CCHS)—inappropriate regular breathing (20 breaths/min), shallow breathing (tidal volume averaging 3.5 mL/kg). Progressive hypercarbia and hypoxemia did not stimulate ventilation, arousal, or beat-to-beat heart rate variability. (From Weese-Mayer DE, Silvestri JM, Menzies LJ, et al: Congenital central hypoventilation syndrome: diagnosis, management, and long-term outcome in thirty-two children. *J Pediatr.* 1992;120:38–387.)

associated conditions include postural hypotension, bradyarrhythmia, ocular abnormalities (strabismus, slow pupillary reaction), esophageal dysmotility, hyperinsulinism, temperature dysregulation, and abnormal sweating. Therefore, CCHS should be suspected in a patient with autonomic nervous system dysfunction and evidence of respiratory control abnormalities (apneas, hypoventilation, and hypoxemia).

BASIC SCIENCE/CLINICAL PEARL	STEPS 1/2/3

Suspect CCHS in an infant with unexplained and recurrent apneas, cyanosis, and ALTE or BRUE who cannot be weaned off assisted ventilation. Patients with CCHS generally do not increase their minute ventilation, in spite of significant hypercapnia. The hypoventilation is worse during sleep, so the awake P_{CO_2} may be normal but the sleeping P_{CO_2} is markedly elevated.

How is congenital central hypoventilation syndrome diagnosed?
The diagnosis of CCHS is established by the clinical presentation and confirmed by the presence of mutation in the *PHOX2B* gene that codes for transcription factor, which is essential in the development of the autonomic nervous system and chemosensory drive to respiration.

Case Point 48.2

> In this patient, blood is sent for *PHOX2B* gene mutation testing and is positive for the *PHOX2B–20/25* polyalanine repeat mutation (PARM). Genetic counseling is provided to the family.

BASIC SCIENCE PEARL	STEP 1

Genetic testing showing the presence of PHOX2B gene mutation confirms the diagnosis of CCHS. Of CCHS patients, 90% are heterozygous for PARM in the PHOXB gene and 10% are heterozygous for nonsense, missense, and frameshift mutations (NPARM). All PARMS are located within the second polyalanine repeat of exon 3, and almost all NPARMS are located at the 3′ end of exon 2 and in exon3. CCHS is inherited in an autosomal dominant pattern, but most parents do not carry the genetic mutation, indicating high de novo mutations in the affected patients.

What is congenital central hypoventilation syndrome?
CCHS is a rare genetic disorder characterized by severe alveolar hypoventilation and autonomic nervous system dysfunction. The reported prevalence is 1 in 148,000 live births (Japan) and 1 in 200,000 live births (France). It is due to a mutation in the *PHOX2B* gene that codes for transcription factor, which is essential in the development of the autonomic nervous system and chemosensory drive for respiration. Most CCHS cases are due to an increased polyalanine repeat mutation (PARM) in exon 3 of the *PHOX2B* gene (24–33 repeats; normal, 20; Fig. 48.3). The remainder is due to a nonpolyalanine repeat mutation (NPARM). The longer PARMs (20/27–20/33) and NPARMS are generally associated with more severe respiratory and autonomic nervous system dysfunction. On the other hand, fewer PARMs (20/25 or 20/26) are generally associated with a milder disease. Patients with this genotype usually breathe adequately during wakefulness and require ventilatory support only during sleep. They do not usually have Hirschsprung disease, neural crest tumors, or life-threatening bradyarrhythmia.

Patients with an NPARM, in general, have a more severe clinical phenotype, with severe alveolar hypoventilation and the need for ventilatory support for 24 hours a day, as well as Hirschsprung disease, cardiac arrhythmias, and neural crest tumors. However, recent case reports of mildly symptomatic individuals with NPARM and CCHS patients with longer PARMS who require ventilator support only during sleep have highlighted the clinical variability of this rare disorder.

BASIC SCIENCE/CLINICAL PEARL	STEPS 1/2/3

In general, the genotype can predict the presentation with patients having longer PARMS or NPARMS requiring 24-hour ventilator dependence, having associated arrhythmias (sinus pauses), Hirschsprung disease, or neural crest tumors; however, newer reports suggest clinical variability.

How is a patient with congenital central hypoventilation syndrome managed?
CCHS is a lifelong disorder. It does not resolve spontaneously and does not respond to pharmacologic stimulants. In general, oxygen administration alone is inadequate because, although it improves the Pao$_2$ and relieves cyanosis, hypoventilation persists. Because patients usually do not have significant lung disease, they have a variety of options for chronic ventilatory support in

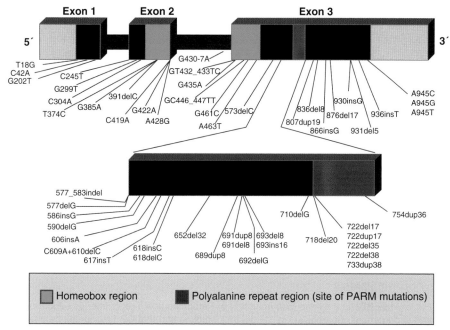

Fig. 48.3 *PHOX2B* gene mutations, with location of all CCHS-associated mutations identified. All polyalanine repeat expansion mutations (PARMs) are located within the second polyalanine expansion region of exon 3 *(shown in red).* (From Rand C, Carroll M, Weese-Mayer D. Congenital central hypoventilation syndrome. *Clin Chest Med.* 2014;35(3):535–545.)

the form of positive-pressure ventilation (PPV) via tracheostomy, noninvasive positive-pressure ventilation (NPPV), or diaphragm pacing. PPV via tracheostomy is the most common form of ventilatory support and is recommended for infants and young children. NPPV delivered via nasal mask or face mask can be considered for older children.

For those ventilated by NPPV, craniofacial development monitoring is recommended, because midface hypoplasia and dental malocclusion have been reported. Diaphragm pacing is an attractive option because it improves the quality of life in ideal candidates. In diaphragm pacing, breathing is generated using the patient's own diaphragm by surgically implanted bilateral phrenic nerve electrodes. The phrenic nerves are electrically stimulated by an external transmitter placed over surgically implanted receivers, resulting in diaphragm contractions. Diaphragm pacing has the advantage of being easily portable, allowing full-time, ventilator- dependent patients to be free of the home mechanical ventilator, and for decannulation in those who are ventilator-dependent only during sleep.

Case Point 48.3

Once the diagnosis of CCHS is established, the infant undergoes a tracheostomy and receives mechanical ventilation. After 6 weeks of family education and training, the patient is discharged with a home mechanical ventilator via the tracheostomy. He is able to breathe spontaneously while awake and uses the ventilator at night and during naps.

What is involved in the follow-up of congenital central hypoventilation syndrome patients after hospital discharge?

Key components of the long-term management of CCHS patients include the following: (1) yearly polysomnography (sleep study) to assess oxygenation and ventilation and adjust ventilator settings as the child grows; (2) periodic echocardiography to assess for pulmonary hypertension; (3) comprehensive eye examinations to assess for ophthalmologic abnormalities; (4) updated vaccinations; and (5) depending on the genotype, periodic Holter monitoring to assess for life-threatening sinus pauses and monitoring for neural crest tumors. Because upper respiratory infections could cause ventilatory control to deteriorate temporarily, the need for increased respiratory support on these occasions is essential.

Case Summary

Complaint/History: A 7-week-old infant is brought to the ED for pauses in breathing during sleep.

Findings: Normal physical examination; capillary blood gas results show respiratory alkalosis when awake and respiratory acidosis when asleep.

Lab/Tests: Overnight polysomnography shows central sleep apneas, periodic breathing, hypercapnia, and hypoxemia. *PHOX2B* gene mutation testing is positive (*PHOX2B* 20/25 polyalanine repeat mutation [+]).

Diagnosis: Congenital central hypoventilation syndrome (CCHS).

Treatment: Mechanical ventilation via tracheostomy during sleep is initiated. The patient breathes unassisted while awake.

BEYOND THE PEARLS

- For low-risk BRUE, the American Academy of Pediatrics (AAP) recommends education and engagement of caregivers in the decision making and that CPR resources be offered to caregivers. Pertussis testing may be performed because pertussis can cause ALTE, and infants may be afebrile and not have lower respiratory symptoms right away. An electrocardiogram may also have to be obtained to identify channelopathies, preexcitation, cardiomyopathy, and other cardiac diseases that pose a risk for sudden cardiac death.
- Infants with low-risk BRUE do not need to be admitted for cardiorespiratory monitoring. However, they may be observed for up to 4 hours with serial examination and continuous pulse oximetry. When discharged, it is essential that they have a follow-up within 24 hours.
- The 2016 AAP guidelines addresses the management for low-risk BRUE but do not provide recommendations for those with higher risk BRUE
- High-risk BRUE, as seen in infants < 2 months, born < 32-wk gestation, event > 1 minute in duration, or recurrent events, require further evaluation because they are more likely to have a serious underlying cause and outcome.
- BRUE, formerly referred to as ALTE, can be a presenting symptom of CCHS.
- CCHS is a lifelong disorder of severe hypoventilation and autonomic dysfunction.
- The presence of the *PHOX2B* gene mutation is essential in establishing the diagnosis. When the *PHOX2B* mutation is absent, consider other causes of hypoventilation and/or autonomic dysfunction.
- Hirschsprung disease is present in 20% of cases, particularly in those with NPARM and 20/27 PARM. When constipation is present, CCHS patients should be evaluated with a barium enema, manometry, or even a full-thickness rectal biopsy.
- CCHS patients with NPARM and 20/29 and longer PARMs are at risk for neural crest tumors (e.g., neuroblastoma, ganglioneuroblastoma); thus, serial chest and abdominal imaging would be beneficial.
- CCHS patients are at risk for life-threating sinus pauses that are 3 seconds or longer, indicating the need for yearly Holter monitoring in these patients.
- Recent reports have indicated that preschool CCHS patients have neurodevelopmental impairment shown by lower Bayley mental and motor scores, particularly those with prolonged breath-holding spells, sinus pauses, and 24-hour ventilator dependence. Thus, these patients need neurodevelopmental monitoring and intervention.

Bibliography

Chen ML, Keens TG. Congenital central hypoventilation syndrome: not just another rare disorder. *Paediatr Respir Rev.* 2004;5(3):182–189.

Diep B, Wang A, Kun S, et al. Diaphragm pacing without tracheostomy in congenital central hypoventilation syndrome patients. *Respiration.* 2015;89(6):534–538.

Kasi A, Perez I, Kun S, Keens T. Congenital central hypoventilation syndrome: diagnostic and management challenges. *Pediatr Heal Med Ther.* 2016;7:99–107.

Kasi AS, Jurgensen TJ, Yen S, et al. Three-generation family with congenital central hypoventilation syndrome and novel PHOX2B gene non-polyalanine repeat mutation. *J Clin Sleep Med.* 2017;13(7):925–927.

Tieder JS, Bonkowsky JL, Etzel RA, et al. Brief resolved unexplained events (formerly apparent life-threatening events) and evaluation of lower-risk infants. *Pediatrics.* 2016;137(5):e20160590–e20160590.

Weese-Mayer DE, Berry-Kravis EM, Ceccherini I, et al. An official ATS clinical policy statement: congenital central hypoventilation syndrome: genetic basis, diagnosis, and management. *Am J Respir Crit Care Med.* 2010;181(6):626–644.

3-Year-Old Male With Worsening Rash for 5 Days

Mariya Zakiuddin ▦ Justin Greenberg ▦ Jeffrey Johnson

The patient is a 3-year-old Caucasian male with a significant past medical history of myoclonic epilepsy who was referred to our emergency department by an outside dermatologist for further evaluation of a rash. Prior to presentation, his neurologist initiated a taper of valproic acid while starting him on lamotrigine. Five days prior to presentation, his mother noticed a rash that appeared first on his thighs and then spread upward to his face. The rash continued to worsen, spreading to other body parts, and was noticed to blister in areas that had previously been red. The patient has had decreased oral intake and could only drink liquids through a straw; however, he is still able to speak in full sentences. The parents deny any recent illness or sick contacts, recent travel, bug bites, chills, shortness of breath, chest pain, headache, easy bleeding or bruising, nausea, vomiting, diarrhea, and constipation, and upper respiratory infection symptoms.

CLINICAL PEARL   **STEPS 2/3**

Rashes associated with the use of medications, including antiepileptics, may indicate serious illness and should be promptly evaluated.

What is the best approach to a patient with a skin rash?

The general practitioner is commonly asked to see a patient who has a skin rash. It is first important to assess the ABCs as in any situation, especially if the rash involves mucosal surfaces such as the mouth, because the airway may become compromised. The physician should be able to elicit an adequate history regarding the morphology, duration, and distribution of the rash. The history should also include the child's age, gender, family history, past and current medications, and known allergies and exposures (e.g., infection, travel, insect or animal exposure). It is also important to be able to differentiate rashes that may be associated with life-threatening conditions from those that are more benign. Rashes that progress rapidly or accompany physical symptoms such as fever or other signs that suggest compromise of the respiratory, cardiovascular, or central nervous system require immediate evaluation. Examples of this may be diffuse oral mucosal involvement that affects oral intake or breathing, changes in capillary refill, skin temperature, and/or changes in mental status or behavior, even if subtle.

CLINICAL PEARL   **STEPS 2/3**

The presence of mucosal involvement is always a serious finding that warrants rapid and expert evaluation.

What is the differential diagnosis for the rash and this patient's presentation?

The broad differential for a rash can be focused by the history and physical examination. The key points in this patient's history include that he is on a chronic and new medication, has the rash described as blistering, and is not eating normally, potentially suggesting systemic illness.

The medication history will bring to mind drug reactions as a trigger, some of which, such as Stevens-Johnson syndrome (SJS), toxic epidermal necrolysis (TEN), drug reaction with eosinophilia and systemic symptoms (DRESS), or anaphylaxis, can be serious. The description of the rash as blistering is also important and suggests some other possibilities, which could include infections such as staphylococcal scalded skin syndrome (SSSS) and disseminated herpes virus infections, in addition to the drug reactions mentioned earlier. The prudent physician should always consider other potentially life-threatening infections in an acutely ill child that can have associated rashes (e.g., meningococcal disease, Rocky Mountain spotted fever, toxic shock syndrome). In this case, the antiepileptic drug (AED) history and description of a potentially vesicular rash affecting mucosal surfaces should push SJS/TEN to the top of the diagnostic considerations. Occasionally, the early presentation of life-threatening illnesses such as SJS/TEN or meningococcemia may also mimic urticaria, other drug eruptions, erythema multiforme, numerous viral exanthems, and Kawasaki disease. It is essential to maintain a high index of suspicion for these serious conditions.

CLINICAL PEARL   **STEPS 2/3**

The medication history and the presence of a spreading vesicular rash affecting mucosal surfaces is strongly indicative of SJS/TEN.

Case Point 49.1

On examination, patient is afebrile, with heart rate, 106 beats/min, blood pressure, 12/33 mm Hg, respiratory rate, 20 breaths/min, and 98% O_2 saturation on room air. He is uncomfortable but nontoxic and in no respiratory distress. The eye examination shows bilateral palpebral and bulbar conjunctival erythema, periorbital edema, and copious mucoid secretions, with limited ability to open his eyelids. There is blistering and erythema of the lips. Skin findings include crusting vesicles on the face, lips, ears, and nose, with confluent irregular erythematous, raised, blanching, patches to the cheeks, forehead, face, and ears. Multiple discrete, erythematous, raised, blanching, circular lesions with darker centers, coalescing in some areas, are noted on the chest, abdomen, back, extremities, groin, penile tip, rectum, and palms and soles of the hands and feet. There are vesicles and bullae noted on the chest and back, most unroofed, some filled with clear fluid. Body surface area (BSA) involvement of the rash is estimated to be 30% at presentation.

The physical examination indicates that the patient is able to maintain his airway and is not currently in cardiorespiratory failure. His vitals, except for his elevated blood pressure, are within normal limits for age. It is very important to note the mental status and general behavior of the child. Young children can be difficult to assess when ill, but appropriate responses to painful or stressful parts of an examination, followed by an assessment of the consolability of the child by parents, can be very helpful in distinguishing a child who is merely irritated by the examination from one who is truly encephalopathic.

A clear description of the rash is also critical to making a correct diagnosis. The rash described is clearly disseminated over much of the body, but the presence of vesicles and bullae with involvement of multiple mucosal surfaces—eyes, mouth, and genitalia—is especially important. The 30% BSA involvement is also relevant and concerning. An accurate description of a rash is a special skill that a physician should be able to acquire because it is useful and important when tracking its progression and relaying it to specialists. The physical examination of this patient affirms the concerning features of the history and is consistent with SJS/TEN. This type of rash is one that needs immediate evaluation in a facility capable of resuscitating critically ill children, ideally one with support of multiple pediatric specialists (dermatologists, ophthalmologists, burn and critical care medicine personnel). If this multispecialty care is not available, transfer to an appropriate referral center will be necessary.

CLINICAL PEARL   **STEPS 2/3**

SJS and TEN are currently considered by many experts to be a spectrum of the same pathophysiologic process. Successful management of this disease requires multispecialty support.

Case Point 49.2

In the emergency department, the child is recognized to have a potentially life-threatening complication of antiseizure medication use, SJS/TEN. SSSS and DRESS are considered as possibilities, but the significant erosive mucosal changes on multiple surfaces make them less likely. The patient is given a fluid bolus intravenously. The pediatric intensive care unit (PICU), dermatology, and ophthalmology services are consulted. Laboratory tests are ordered, including venous blood gas (VBG), complete blood count (CBC) with differential, and a full chemistry panel, including hepatic function and C-reactive protein (CRP) and prealbumin levels. All results are within normal limits except for elevation of the aspartate aminotransaminase (AST) and alanine aminotransaminase (ALT) levels to 450 U/L and 495 U/L, respectively. The dermatology team performs a frozen biopsy for a pathologic specimen. Electron microscopy shows necrosis and separation between the epidermis and the dermis with lymphocytic infiltration (Fig. 49.1).

Diagnosis: Stevens-Johnson syndrome/toxic epidermal necrolysis.

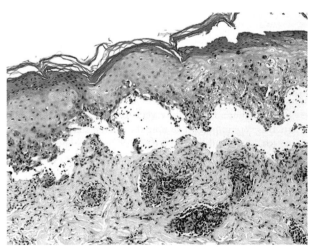

Fig. 49.1 Histopathology of Stevens-Johnson syndrome/toxic epidermal necrolysis. There are multiple apoptotic keratinocytes throughout the full thickness of the epidermis, and a subepidermal split is forming a bulla. There is perivascular lymphocytic infiltrate within the epidermis. (From Creamer D, Walsh S, Dziewulski P, et al. UK guidelines for the management of Stevens Johnson syndrome/toxic epidermal necrolysis in adults 2016. *J Plast Reconstr Aesthet Surg.* 2016;69(6):e119–e153.)

Although not pathognomonic, full-thickness skin sloughing on frozen biopsy can help confirm the clinical suspicion of SJS/TEN (see Fig. 49.2).

The diagnosis SJS/TEN is made clinically and can be confirmed with skin biopsy showing full-thickness epidermal necrosis and changes consistent with the constellation of findings seen in the spectrum of erythema multiforme (EM) and SJS/TEN. To gauge the clinical severity of a presentation, a scoring system has been developed that predicts outcome in adult patients with SJS/TEN based on the presence or absence of known risk factors. Called the SCORTEN (severity of illness score for toxic epidermal necrolysis), it assigns points for the presence of any of the following: age older than 40 years, presence of malignancy, heart rate more than 120 beats/min, more than 10% epidermal detachment at presentation, serum urea level more than 10 mmol/L, serum glucose level more than 14 mmol/L, serum bicarbonate level more than 20 mmol/L. One point is assigned to each criterion, with a score of 5 or more conferring greater than 90% mortality in adults. The mortality of pediatric patients with SJS/TEN appears to be lower than adult counterparts with similar scores, but SCORTEN on day 1 of hospitalization can be used like other measures of predicted pediatric mortality (e.g., pediatric risk of mortality [PRISM]-III or pediatric index of mortality [PIM]-2) as markers of severity of illness overall.

Case Point 49.3

The patient is transferred to the PICU. All unnecessary medications, including AEDs, are stopped. The burns team is consulted for wound care regarding the extent of skin involvement and desquamation. A nasogastric feeding tube is placed to ensure that the patient receives adequate nutrition in anticipation of the increased caloric requirements expected for wound healing. Within several hours of admission to the PICU, the patient develops worsening respiratory distress and oropharyngeal swelling and is subsequently intubated and mechanically ventilated. Over the next day, erythematous areas of the body progress to vesicles on the trunk, legs, arms, and face. The burns team debride the skin lesions and apply silver-based dressings and mupirocin to the face. Ophthalmology and applied ocular amniotic membrane rings help protect against the complications of ocular synechiae and corneal scarring. The patient's lesions progress to cover his entire face and about 40% of his body (Fig. 49.2). Wound checks and dressing changes are performed every 3 to 4 days.

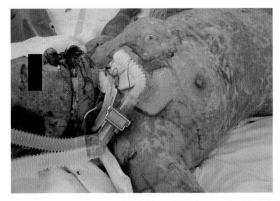

Fig. 49.2 Patient with toxic epidermal necrolysis (TEN). There is widespread epithelial detachment over more than 30% of the body surface area, with mucous membrane involvement. (From Downey A, Jackson C, Harun N, et al. TEN: review of pathogenesis and management. *J Am Acad Dermatol.* 2012;66:995–1003.)

> **BOX 49.1 ■ Associated Triggers for Stevens-Johnson Syndrome and Toxic Epidermal Necrolysis**
>
> ■ Antibiotics: sulfonamides, amoxicillin, co-trimoxazole
> ■ Nonsteroidal antiinflammatory drugs (NSAIDs)
> ■ Anticonvulsants: lamotrigine, phenytoin, hydantoin, phenobarbital, and carbamazepine
> ■ Allopurinol
> ■ Nevirapine
> ■ Sulfasalazine
> ■ Infections: *Mycoplasma pneumoniae,* human immunodeficiency virus (HIV), Ebstein-Barr virus (EBV)
> ■ Systemic lupus erythematous (SLE)

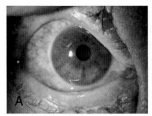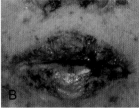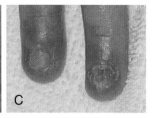

Fig. 49.3 (A) Conjunctivitis in Stevens-Johnson syndrome. There is extensive loss of the bulbar conjunctival epithelium. (B) Swollen and crusted mucous membranes. (C) Fingernail loss and deformation with paronychia. (From Sotozono C, Uetz M, Koizumi N, et al. Diagnosis and treatment of Stevens-Johnson syndrome and toxic epidermal necrolysis with ocular complications. *Ophthalmology.* 2009;116(4):685–690.)

A multidisciplinary care team consisting of the PICU and neurology, burns, dermatology, and ophthalmology providers care for the patient throughout his hospitalization. Over the next 2 weeks, the patient's wounds heal appropriately. He is successfully extubated and receives ongoing occupational and physical therapy. A tapering protocol was initiated for his opiate and benzodiazepine withdrawal. He did not have any seizure activity, despite removal of his antiepileptic medications. He is then transferred to an inpatient physical rehabilitation center for children.

CLINICAL PEARL   **STEPS 2,3**

It is essential that all potentially offending medications be stopped immediately, including any similar medications in the same class. Often, benzodiazepines can be used if patients on AEDs have breakthrough seizures while being treated.

What are Stevens-Johnson syndrome and toxic epidermal necrolysis?
SJS and TEN are immune complex–mediated hypersensitivity reactions. Prior medication exposure and other triggers are implicated in 50% and 95% of SJS and TEN cases, respectively (Box 49.1). SJS and TEN are characterized by multisystem disease, with skin and mucous membrane necrosis (Fig. 49.3). The two conditions are differentiated based on the total body surface area involved and likely represent a spectrum of severity for the same illness. SJS is defined as an affected BSA less than 10%, and TEN is defined as an affected BSA of more than 30%, with an SJS/TEN overlap used to describe patients with between 10% and 30% affected BSA. TEN is the most severe disorder in the spectrum. It is histologically recognized and differentiated from other conditions such as SSSS by findings of full-thickness epidermal necrosis and a minimal to absent dermal infiltrate.

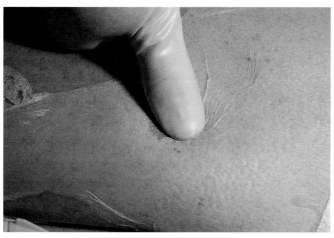

Fig. 49.4 Nikolsky sign. With slight thumb pressure, the skin wrinkles, slides laterally, and separates from the dermis. (Adapted from Kliegman R, Stanton B, St Geme J, et al., eds. *Nelson Textbook of Pediatrics.* 20th ed. Philadelphia: Elsevier; 2016.)

The incidence of SJS/TEN is approximately two to seven cases per million people per year, with SJS being more common than TEN. When comparing mortality rate in adults, SJS has a mortality rate of around 10%, whereas TEN has a higher mortality rate of around 30%. As mentioned previously, reported mortality rates in children are less than adults (0%–7.5% respectively), but this has not been well studied.

The pathogenesis of SJS/TEN is not completely characterized but the epidermal necrosis is believed to be due to the generation of drug-specific CD8+ cytotoxic T cells. This leads to extensive keratinocyte apoptosis through the production of granulysin, a cytolytic protein found in activated T cells and natural killer (NK) cells.

What are the clinical features of Stevens-Johnson syndrome and toxic epidermal necrolysis?
Both SJS and TEN have cutaneous and mucosal involvement. The cutaneous lesions are usually erythematous macules that will later quickly develop central necrosis to form vesicles, bullae, and other areas of denudation. There are usually two or more mucosal areas involved, which may include the eyes, oral cavity, upper airway or esophagus, gastrointestinal (GI) tract, and anogenital mucosa. Some patients will exhibit a flulike prodrome prior to this, and some patients may have no preceding signs. The timing of symptoms and the onset of rash is important to clarify when evaluating for possible triggering candidate drugs. Skin tenderness is commonly reported, and the mucosal lesions can be especially painful, with more severe presentations seen with TEN. In TEN, it is common to see full-thickness epidermis lost in large sheets due to the flaccid bullae that develop. There may be a positive Nikolsky sign, which is denudation of the skin with gentle tangential pressure (Fig. 49.4). A Nikolsky sign is the manifestation of the cleavage of the epidermal layer from the dermis. SJS and TEN can cause multisystem disease that may be life threatening without appropriate treatment (Table 49.1).

What studies or tests should be considered?
It is important to get a biopsy of one of the cutaneous sites and send it for histology evaluation and interpretation from the dermatologist. There are many nonspecific laboratory abnormalities that might be seen with SJS/TEN such as leukocytosis and elevated erythrocyte sedimentation rate (ESR) and CRP levels. Anemia and lymphopenia are common, and the more severely affected

TABLE 49.1 ■ **Multisystemic Manifestations of Stevens-Johnson Syndrome and Toxic Epidermal Necrolysis**

System	Clinical Manifestation
Dermatologic	Macular rash, vesicles, bullae, skin denudation, dehydration
Respiratory	Bronchitis, pneumonitis, bronchial stricture
Cardiac	Myocarditis
Gastrointestinal	Electrolyte imbalances, esophagitis, hepatitis, enterocolitis, esophageal stricture
Renal	Acute tubular necrosis, hematuria
Ophthalmologic	Corneal scarring and/or ulceration, anterior uveitis, panophthalmitis
Infectious disease	Superimposed bacterial infection (e.g., *Staphylococcus aureus*, *Pseudomonas aeruginosa*)
Musculoskeletal	Polyarthritis

patient will often show low serum albumin and elevated transaminase levels. Typically, the need for ongoing monitoring of the CBC, electrolyte levels, and blood gas levels is especially important early in the patient's course and will follow patterns typical for other similarly critically ill children.

What is the treatment of Stevens-Johnson syndrome and toxic epidermal necrolysis?
The mainstay of treatment for patients with SJS/TEN is to discontinue the offending agent and avoid any agents that may have similarities to the drug in question, if one has been identified. Failure to remove a culprit drug is associated with worse prognosis for the patient and extreme medicolegal risk to the physician. The second mainstay of treatment is supportive care—intubation if acute respiratory failure is imminent; IV fluid rehydration (treating SJS/TEN as an often large but superficial burn); meticulous attention to nutritional status and early enteral feeding as soon as tolerated; prevention of secondary infection; and wound management with expert consultation with dermatology, burn and wound care, and ophthalmology (the specifics may vary from center to center). There are no specific therapies that have been shown to change the outcome in pediatric patients. Although intravenous immunoglobulin (IVIG) (1 g/kg × 3 days) is commonly used by many centers, current evidence does not support its efficacy. Similarly, the use of systemic corticosteroids is not currently supported by evidence; these have little effect on the disease course and may mask symptoms of sepsis. Recent studies in adult populations have indicated that early treatment with tumor necrosis factor alpha inhibitors (e.g., infliximab, etanercept) may halt the progression of skin denudation and shorten the disease course. Their efficacy in pediatric populations has not been established.

Case Summary
   Complaint/History: A 3-year-old male with a rash.
   Findings: The skin examination is significant for crusting vesicles of the face, lips, ears, and nose, with irregular erythematous raised, blanching patches to the cheeks, forehead, and face. The patient has discrete scattered erythematous raised, blanching, circular lesions with darker centers, coalescing in some areas, diffusely throughout his body, with some vesicles and bullae on the back, with multisystem complications present.
   Labs/Tests: Elevated AST and ALT levels. Biopsy of skin lesions confirms the diagnosis of TEN (full-thickness epidermal necrosis).
   Diagnosis: Toxic epidermal necrolysis.
   Treatment: The patient was intubated for respiratory failure, all antiepileptic medications were discontinued, and he was treated with supportive care.

BEYOND THE PEARLS

- Stevens-Johnson syndrome/toxic epidermal necrolysis (SJS/TEN) has been a reported adverse outcome to over 200 medications, most commonly sulfonamide antibiotics, anti-convulsants, allopurinol, and NSAIDs.
- SJS/TEN can also be triggered by infections such as *Mycoplasma pneumoniae.*
- A prodrome of a flulike illness is common.
- The Asboe-Hansen sign describes the special features of the blisters in SJS/TEN. They break easily and can be extended sideways by slight pressure of the thumb as more necrotic epidermis is laterally displaced.
- Mucosal involvement is a requirement for the diagnosis of SJS/TEN.
- SJS/TEN and staphylococcal scalded skin syndrome (SSSS) can be differentiated from one another by electron microscopy of biopsy samples. SSSS displays a subcorneal cleavage, with intact epidermis. SJS/TEN shows cleavage between the epidermal and derma layer.
- Recent studies on adult patients have suggested that biologic agents such as the TNF-alpha inhibitors, infliximab or etanercept, may halt progression of skin denudement and improve outcomes. Their role in children has yet to be elucidated.

Bibliography

Bastuji-Garin S, et al. SCORTEN: a severity-of-illness score for toxic epidermal necrolysis. *J Invest Dermatol.* 2000;115(2):149–153.

Nizamoglu M, et al. Improving mortality outcomes of Stevens Johnson syndrome/toxic epidermal necrolysis: a regional burns centre experience. *Burns.* 2017.

Pereira F, et al. Toxic epidermal necrolysis. *J Am Acad Dermatol.* 2007;56(2):181–200.

Sorrell J, et al. Score of toxic epidermal necrosis predicts the outcomes of pediatric epidermal necrolysis. *Pediatr Dermatol.* 2017;34(4):433–437.

16-Year-Old Female With Down Syndrome With Abdominal Pain and Epistaxis

Neha Mahajan ■ Shoji Yano

A 16-year-old female with Down syndrome (DS) presents to the emergency department (ED) for a 1-day history of abdominal pain and epistaxis. Due to moderate intellectual disability and anxiety, she can only respond to "yes" or "no" questions and is unable to characterize the pain fully.

CLINICAL PEARL   STEP 2/3

When working with patients who have an intellectually disability, they should be approached based on their developmental (rather than chronologic) age. History may be limited, and therefore the parental report and physical examination become the main source of information.

What is Down syndrome, and how is it inherited?

DS is a genetic disorder in which patients have three copies of the genes on chromosome 21, leading to a typical phenotype, such as hypotonia, flat facies, epicanthal folds with upward-slanting palpebral fissures, short neck, and a single palmar crease (Fig. 50.1) and a spectrum of physical and intellectual capabilities (Table 50.1). Most cases (95%) are not inherited and occur via meiotic nondisjunction of chromosome 21, leading to trisomy 21 (Fig. 50.2). About 2% to 4% of the cases are caused by a Robertsonian translocation, in which the longer arm of chromosome 21 breaks at the centromere and joins another, leading to multiple copies of affected genes. This translocation may be a *de novo* mutation or may be inherited from a parent carrying the abnormal chromosome 21. In 1% to 2% of the cases, the mosaic form of DS is present, in which some cells carry the trisomy 21 mutation and the rest contain the normal number of chromosomes. Although the risk of DS increases with maternal age, most cases still occur in women younger than 35 years, given the higher birth rate among this group.

BASIC SCIENCE PEARL   STEP 1/2/3

Given the variety of inheritance patterns, it is important for a geneticist to be involved in family discussions of recurrence risks after appropriate genetic testing is completed.

What other autosomal trisomies can lead to live births?

Patau syndrome is caused by trisomy 13 and presents with polydactyly, cleft lip and palate, and holoprosencephaly. Edwards syndrome is caused by trisomy 18 and is characterized by clenched fists with overlapping fingers, micrognathia, and horseshoe kidney. Both have intellectual disability, rocker bottom feet, and congenital heart disease and lead to death prior to the age of 1 year.

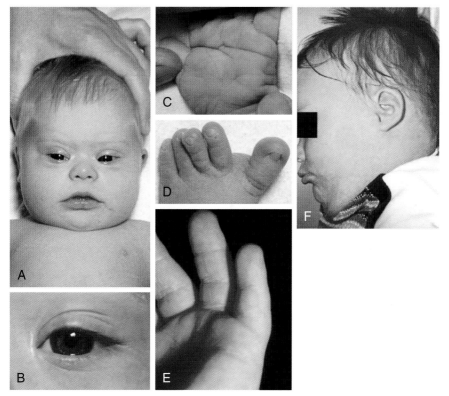

Fig. 50.1 Physical examination findings in Down syndrome. (A) Upward slanting of palpebral fissures, epicanthal folds, flat nasal bridge. (B) Brushfield spots. (C) Bridged palmar crease (two palmar creases connected by a line). (D) Widened toe space. (E) Short fifth finger. (F) Small ears, flat occiput. (From Zitelli BJ, Davis HW: *Atlas of Pediatric Physical Diagnosis*. 4th ed. St. Louis: Mosby; 2002.)

TABLE 50.1 ▓ **Clinical Features of Down Syndrome in the Neonatal Period**

System	Features
Central nervous	Poor Moro reflex, developmental delay, hypotonia
Craniofacial	Brachycephaly with flat occiput, flat face, upward slanting palpebral fissure, epicanthal folds, speckled irises (Brushfield spots), three fontanels, delayed fontanel closure, frontal sinus and midfacial hypoplasia, mild microcephaly, short hard palate, small nose, flat nasal bridge, protruding tongue, open mouth, small dysplastic ear
Cardiovascular	Endocardial Cushing defects, ventricular septal defects, atrial septal defects, patent ductus arteriosus, aberrant subclavian artery, pulmonary hypertension
Musculoskeletal	Joint hyperflexibility, short neck with redundant skin, short metacarpals and phalanges, short fifth digit with clinodactyly, single transverse palmar crease, wide gap between first and second toes, pelvic dysplasia, short sternum, two sternal manubrium ossification centers
Gastrointestinal	Duodenal atresia, annular pancreas, tracheoesophageal fistula, Hirschsprung disease, imperforate anus, neonatal cholestasis
Cutaneous	Cutis marmorata (skin mottling in cold temperatures)

Adapted from Kliegman R, Stanton B, St Geme J, et al, eds. *Nelson Textbook of Pediatrics*. 20th ed. Philadelphia: Elsevier; 2016.

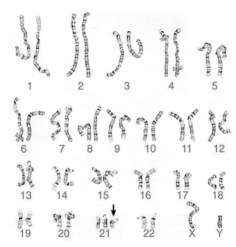

Fig. 50.2 Trisomy 21 karyotype (47XX, +21). Note three copies of chromosome 21 *(arrow)*. (From Bacino CA, Lee B. Cytogenetics. In: Kliegman R, Stanton B, St Geme J, et al, eds. *Nelson Textbook of Pediatrics.* 20th ed. Philadelphia: Elsevier; 2016:604–626.)

TABLE 50.2 ■ **Prenatal Screening Laboratory Tests for Down Syndrome**

Trimester	Screening Test Results
First	↑ Nuchal translucency ↑ Human chorionic gonadotropin (hCG) ↓ Pregnancy-associated plasma protein A (PAPP-A)
Second (quad screen)	↑ hCG ↑ Inhibin A ↓ Alpha-fetoprotein (AFP) ↓ Estriol (uE3)

How do we screen for Down syndrome prenatally?

Screening can begin in the first trimester and includes imaging and blood tests, whereas the second-trimester quad screen consists only of blood tests (Table 50.2). Noninvasive screening via cell-free fetal DNA taken from the maternal blood is also becoming more common. Abnormal results in these screening tests should trigger a discussion with the family regarding whether diagnostic testing is desired (e.g., chorionic villus sampling [CVS] between 10 and 13 weeks of gestation or amniocentesis between 15 and 20 weeks of gestation).

Case Point 50.1

The patient was born with a congenital heart defect (patent ductus arteriosus) and imperforate anus, both requiring surgical correction in the neonatal period. Since then, she has not had any major medical problems. She communicates with simple phrases, ambulates independently but slowly, and requires assistance with all activities of daily living.

What are common complications associated with Down syndrome?

Patients with DS have increased risk of complications in almost every major organ system. At birth, they should be immediately evaluated for life-threatening issues related to hypotonia, congenital heart disease (mainly atrioventricular septal defect), gastrointestinal (GI) tract abnormalities (e.g., small bowel obstruction from an annular pancreas, imperforate anus, Hirschsprung disease). Over time, the physician and parents should continue to monitor for other complications, including delayed milestones, atlantoaxial instability, seizures, hearing and visual impairments (including cataracts and otitis media), short stature, obesity, GI disorders (e.g., celiac disease), oncologic disorders (e.g., acute lymphocytic leukemia, testicular cancer), autoimmune disorders (e.g., hypothyroidism, type 1 diabetes), sleep apnea, and dermatologic conditions (e.g., eczema, tinea). As they approach adulthood, they have an increased risk and earlier presentation of dementia. Life expectancy has improved drastically in the last several decades due to decreased institutionalization and better management of the major causes of mortality (e.g., congenital heart disease, infections). The median age of survival has been approaching 60 years, with higher survival among whites and males.

BASIC SCIENCE PEARL	STEP 2/3

When presenting patients with specific syndromes, be sure to look up the complications associated with those disease processes and the routine screenings required for these populations. For example, young adults with DS should have annual screening for thyroid disease and biennial ophthalmology examinations.

Are psychiatric disorders more common in children with Down syndrome?
Although there are several mental illnesses occurring concurrently in children with DS (e.g., depression, autism spectrum disorder), the rates of these conditions are not necessarily increased (and possibly even lower) when compared to children with intellectual disability in general. However, given their intellectual impairments, there is often a delay in the diagnosis of these conditions. The situation is further complicated by difficulties differentiating abnormal behaviors from expected behaviors for their mental age. For example, imaginary friends and self-talk may be misinterpreted as hallucinations. Further research is needed concerning pediatric mental illness in DS patients.

Case Point 50.2

The physical examination reveals normal vital signs. She is anxious but does not appear toxic. Her abdominal examination reveals suprapubic distention but without signs concerning for an acute surgical abdomen. There is no active bleeding or petechial rash. Cranial nerves are intact and equal bilaterally. The strength of the extremities is normal. Her rectal tone is normal. Sensation cannot be assessed due to the patient's intellectual capacity.

Why is it important to do a full neurologic examination on a patient with Down syndrome?
Atlantoaxial instability occurs in 10% to 20% of patients with DS due to diffuse ligamentous laxity (Fig. 50.3). If symptoms of spinal cord compression occur, this is a medical emergency requiring immediate neurosurgical consultation. Patients may present with neck pain, abnormal gait, clumsiness of upper extremities, and/or change in sphincter control. On examination, they will have signs of upper motor neuron lesions (e.g., hyperreflexia). Although routine imaging is not indicated for all individuals with DS, a full neurologic examination should be performed yearly, and parents should be educated on the symptoms of instability. In addition, cervical spine precautions should be maintained during all surgical procedures, regardless of the results of imaging, because radiologic and clinical findings do not always correlate.

Case Point 50.3

The patient's laboratory tests results indicate uremia, elevated creatinine level, and normocytic anemia (Box 50.1).

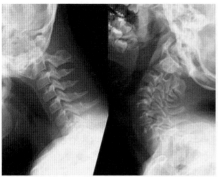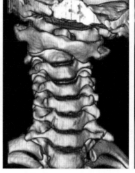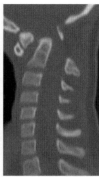

| Flexion view | extension view | 3D-CT frontal view | mid-sagittal view |

Fig. 50.3 Thirteen-year-old male with Down syndrome incidentally found to have C1-C2 instability. (A-D) The anterior dens interval (ADI) measured 11 mm, and the space available for the cord (SAC) was reduced to about 9 mm as seen on the static lateral and dynamic flexion-extension radiographs. (E) MRI shows evidence of chronic spinal cord impingement. (F) Because of the severe atlanto-axial instability (AAI) and concerns about impending catastrophic neurologic injury, decompression of the posterior ring of C1 and in situ fusion from occiput to C2 was performed using transarticular C1-C2 screw fixation and occipitocervical instrumentation. (From Mencio GA, Devin CJ. Fractures of the spine. In Green, Swiontkowski, *Skeletal Trauma in Children,* ed 4. Elsevier, 2009, p 313–354, Fig 11-16.)

BOX 50.1 ■ Patient's Laboratory Test Results

- Creatinine, 5 mg/dL (2 years ago was 1 mg/dL)
- Blood urea nitrogen, 77 mg/dL
- Potassium, 3.8 mmol/L
- Bicarbonate, 23 mmol/L
- Hemoglobin, 8.8 g/dL
- Mean corpuscular volume, 87 fL
- Platelets, 195,000/µL
- Urinalysis with large blood, but negative leukocytes and nitrite; culture negative.

How would you work up the cause of the patient's renal failure?

Renal injury is first classified as acute versus chronic kidney disease (CKD). This is not always apparent on presentation because it requires a prior creatinine value and monitoring for resolution. The cause of the renal failure should further be categorized anatomically—prerenal injury (hypoperfusion), intrinsic renal (vascular, glomerular, tubular, interstitial disease), and postrenal injury (obstruction). Evaluation starts with a thorough history, review of medications, and physical examination. Laboratory tests should include a basic metabolic panel (to estimate the glomerular filtration rate [GFR] and evaluate for alkalosis and hyperkalemia), complete blood count (anemia indicates chronic illness), urinalysis with microscopy (urinary tract infection, signs of nephrolithiasis, proteinuria, nephritic syndrome), and determination of urine electrolyte levels (to calculate the fractional excretion [FE] of sodium [FE_{Na}] or urea [FE_{urea}]). Renal imaging can also suggest causative factors by showing signs of obstruction (e.g., hydronephrosis), and parenchymal disease. If an elevated creatinine level does not normalize over time, CKD can be diagnosed and staging done by GFR (Table 50.3).

Does this patient require emergent dialysis?

Indications for dialysis are easily recalled by using the mnemonic AEIOU—*A*cidosis, *E*lectrolyte disturbance, *I*ntoxication, (fluid), *O*verload, *U*remia. This patient does not meet the criteria for emergent dialysis but should be closely monitored for further signs of uremia, given the presence of epistaxis (sign of platelet dysfunction).

TABLE 50.3 ■ **Staging of Chronic Kidney Disease (CKD)**

CKD Stages	Estimated Glomerular Filtration Rate (eGFR) (mL/min/1.73 m²)
1	≥90
2	60–89
3a, 3b	45–59, 30–44
4	15–29
5	<15

Case Point 50.4

Renal ultrasonograms show severe bilateral hydronephrosis and hydroureter. A urinary (Foley) catheter is placed. The patient's serum creatinine levels decrease and stabilize at CKD stage 3b. Formal urodynamic studies demonstrate detrusor hyperactivity, inability of the patient to void spontaneously, and elevated postvoid residual volume. These findings confirm the diagnosis of nonneurogenic neurogenic bladder. Due to her intellectual disability, she does not tolerate intermittent urinary catheterization. The patient undergoes surgery for suprapubic bladder catheterization.

What is a nonneurogenic neurogenic bladder?
A nonneurogenic neurogenic bladder (or learned voiding dysfunction) presents in childhood or even adulthood with urinary issues (e.g., incontinence, infrequent voiding, urinary tract infections) that are similar to those of a neurogenic bladder. However, the cause is psychological, with the patient voluntarily contracting the external sphincter to avoid enuresis. Over time, this leads to increased intravesicular pressure, without an actual neurologic abnormality. The treatment focuses on addressing the underlying psychological problems and bladder retraining. Additionally, catheterization and antispasmodic medications may be required.

BEYOND THE PEARLS

- Down syndrome is named after the British physician John Langdon Down, who photographed and meticulously described the DS phenotype in the 1860s. He used the commonality of the features across races to support his argument of the unity of mankind.
- Knowing the medical and surgical history of patients with DS is crucial to anticipating future complications.
- Evaluating intellectually delayed patients can be challenging, but this can be done by using a systematic approach, starting with a developmentally appropriate interview of the patient, collaborating history from caregivers, comprehensive physical examination, and appropriate laboratory and radiologic workup—ruling out the most dangerous conditions on your differential diagnoses first.
- Aside from leukemia and testicular cancer, patients with DS have a decreased risk of solid tumors. There may be a protective effect on malignancies from trisomy 21, but research is still underway.

Case Summary
  Complaint/History: A 16-year-old female with DS presents with abdominal pain and epistaxis for 1 day.
  Findings: The physical examination shows suprapubic distention.

Labs/Tests: Laboratory tests indicate uremia, elevated serum creatinine level, and normocytic anemia. Ultrasonography shows hydronephrosis and hydroureter. Urodynamic studies indicate detrusor hyperactivity, inability to void, and elevated postvoid residual volume.

Diagnosis: Chronic kidney disease from nonneurogenic neurogenic bladder.

Treatment: Foley catheter on diagnosis; surgical suprapubic bladder catheterization for long-term management.

Bibliography

Ali FE, et al. Cervical spine abnormalities associated with down syndrome. *Int Orthop*. 2006;30(4):284–289. PMC. Web. 1 Sept. 2017.

Alldred SK, et al. First and second trimester serum tests with and without first trimester ultrasound tests for Down's syndrome screening. *The Cochrane Library*. 2017.

Bratman SV, et al. Solid malignancies in individuals with down syndrome: a case presentation and literature review. *J Natl Compr Canc Netw*. 2014;12(11):1537–1545.

Bull MJ. Health supervision for children with down syndrome. *Pediatrics*. 2011;128(2):393–406.

Dykens EM, et al. Psychiatric disorders in adolescents and young adults with Down syndrome and other intellectual disabilities. *J Neurodevelop Disord*. 2015;7(1):9.

Groutz A, et al. Learned voiding dysfunction (non-neurogenic, neurogenic bladder) among adults. *Neurourol Urodyn*. 2001;20(3):259–268.

Holmes G. Gastrointestinal disorders in down syndrome. *Gastroenterol Hepatol Bed Bench*. 2014;7(1): 6–8.

Kliegman R, Stanton B, St Geme J. *Nelson's Textbook of Pediatrics*. 20th ed. Philadelphia: Elsevier; 2016.

Walker JC, et al. Depression in down syndrome: a review of the literature. *Res Dev Disabil*. 2011;32(5): 1432–1440.

15-Month-Old Female With Left Arm Pain

Nicole Samii ▪ Catherine DeRidder

A 15-month-old female presents for evaluation in the emergency department for a 1-week history of left arm swelling. The father reports that she was jumping on the bed and fell, landing onto her left elbow on the hardwood floor 1 week prior. She cried immediately, with no loss of consciousness, and was consoled by her father. The father appreciated the swelling of the elbow but did not see any other deformities. He noticed that she was not using her left arm and made a sling for her to wear. She was still playful but her arm was not improving, so he decided to bring her to the emergency department. He denies fevers, open breaks in her skin, or other injuries.

What is an important question to ask regarding young children and injuries?
It is important to ask about the child's developmental history. Determining the developmental abilities of the child is imperative when assessing the validity of the story and mechanism of injury. A child's developmental milestones can be categorized into gross motor, fine motor, communication, and social skills (Table 51.1).

Case Point 51.1

The father states that she is learning how to walk, picks up cereal with her thumb and index finger, says five words, and plays well with other children.

CLINICAL PEARL   **STEP 2/3**

Suspicion should be raised when the history given by the caregiver regarding the injuries do not match the child's developmental capabilities. Additionally, if there is a delay in presentation to seek care, it is important to obtain a further history to determine the reasons why. Delayed presentation and vague or inconsistent explanations should always raise concern.

Case Point 51.2

The father states that he did not seek care earlier because she is "clumsy," and her injuries usually resolve on their own. In this case, however, there was no improvement. In terms of her past medical history, she was born full term, with no complications. She has never been hospitalized but has been seen in several emergency departments in the past for different injuries, including a finger fracture and a head injury after falling off a slide. She has not undergone any surgeries, is not taking any medications, and has no known drug allergies. There is no family history of easy fractures, bruising, or bleeding. She eats a regular diet and drinks 12 ounces of milk daily.

TABLE 51.1 ▪ Developmental Milestones in Typically Developing Children[a]

Age (mo)	Gross Motor	Visual, Fine Motor, Social, Language
1	Raises head from prone position	Visually follows to midline, alerts to sound, regards face
2	Lifts chest off table	Smiles socially, recognizes parent, follows object past midline
4	Rolls over	Laughs, orients to voice
6	Sits unsupported	Babbles
9	Pulls to stand, cruises	Says "mama" and "dada" indiscriminately, plays games such as pat-a-cake
12	Walks alone	Two words other than "mama"
15	Creeps upstairs, walks backward	Uses four to six words
18	Runs	Uses seven to ten words, knows five body parts
24	Walks up and down stairs independently	Vocabulary, 50 words, two-word sentences

[a]Up to 2 years old.
Adapted from Engborn B, Flerlage J. *The Harriet Lane Handbook*. 20th ed. Philadelphia: Elsevier/Saunders: 2015.

CLINICAL PEARL   STEP 2/3

Risk factors for child abuse in a home include factors involving the caregiver, such as depression, mental illness, posttraumatic stress disorder, alcoholism, drug use, and history of being abused. Social risk factors include family crisis, domestic violence, single parenting, financial stress, inexperience, and poor parenting skills. Risk factors inherent in the child include chronic illness, mental disability, and age younger than 5 years.

Case Point 51.3

The father states that she lives with him and her older brother, who is 5 years old. The mother is incarcerated for drug abuse. The father has sole custody of the children. He hesitates when asked if there are any drugs or weapons in the home but denies any substance abuse or gun use. On physical examination, she is afebrile, with normal vital signs. Her growth parameters and head circumference are within normal limits. She is happy and interactive and is wearing a make-shift sling out of a belt and T-shirt. Her head is normocephalic and atraumatic, with no scalp lacerations or hematomas. Her conjunctivae are white, with no evidence of subconjunctival hemorrhage. Her nares are patent, with no discharge. Her oropharynx is clear, with a small intact frenulum below her tongue. Her tympanic membranes are pearly bilaterally, with no hemotympanum.

The cardiac and respiratory examinations are unremarkable. The abdominal examination is benign and nontender to palpation. The genital and rectal examinations are unremarkable. Her left arm is noted to have a gross deformity, with significant swelling and tenderness to palpation over the left lateral epicondyle. She is able to wiggle her fingers, perform the "OK" sign, cross her second and third digits, and give the thumbs-up sign. She is unable to move her left upper extremity due to the pain and swelling. There is decreased sensation to light touch. Strength in her hand is 5/5, but you are unable to assess strength in the biceps muscle. Her radial pulse is 2+, and capillary refill is appropriate. On skin examination, there is a 5- × 4-cm ecchymosis over the lateral epicondyle without skin breakdown. Ecchymosis was noted throughout her right external ear (Fig. 51.1). Multiple linear bruises at different stages of healing are seen on the posterior surfaces of her bilateral lower extremities. Once the bruising and marks are noticed, the father is questioned regarding how they occurred. The father states that he did not notice the bruises or marks and is unsure how they happened.

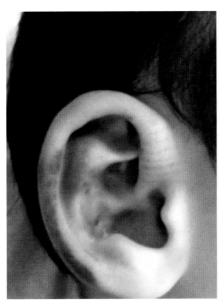

Fig. 51.1 Child's right external ear with multiple areas of ecchymosis. (From Leetch A, Woolridge D. Emergency department evaluation of child abuse. *Emerg Med Clin North Am.* 2013;32(3):853–873.)

What is the most likely diagnosis?

Physical abuse is high on the differential diagnosis, given the history of recurrent emergency department visits for trauma, delayed presentation, bruising on the ear, and patterned bruising on the legs. Accidental bruises are typically found over bony prominences. Bruises from physical abuse are more likely to be located on the cheeks, neck, ears, genitals, buttocks, and back. The TEN-4 bruising rule states that any bruising in a child younger than 4 months or bruising of the Torso, Ears, or Neck in a child younger than 4 years is 97% sensitive for abuse.

The location, shape, and pattern of bruising and marks are also important to note. Common objects used to inflict injury often leave patterned marks, including hands, looped cords, belts, hangers, and cigarettes (Fig. 51.2). Another point to note is that while the patient's arm injury was consistent with the reported mechanism, the findings on the legs and ear were not. Any injury inconsistent with the reported mechanism is cause for concern. Additionally, the father's report of the mother being incarcerated, and his hesitation to describe the safety of the home, should raise suspicion for physical abuse. Vague or inconsistent explanations should also provoke alarm. The patient's arm injury is concerning for neglect due to the delay in seeking care. Neglect is often an overlooked problem but accounts for approximately 75% of maltreatment cases yearly. The characteristic ear bruising is very suspicious for physical abuse. Bleeding disorders, such as hemophilia or coagulopathies, must be ruled out.

Case Point 51.4

Laboratory testing reveals normocytic anemia with a normal prothrombin time (PT), partial thromboplastin time (PTT), international normalized ratio (INR), and von Willebrand panel. An x-ray of her left arm confirms a humeral fracture with dislocation. Orthopedic subspecialists are consulted for surgical management, including closed reduction and immobilization.

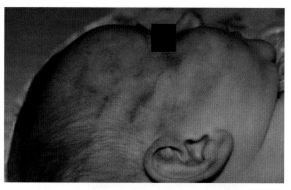

Fig. 51.2 Facial bruising on a nonambulating child. The parallel, linear bruising pattern results when capillaries rupture outward between fingers—a slap mark. (From Lindberg D. Rosen's *Emergency Medicine: Concepts and Clinical Practice,* 9th ed. Philadelphia: Elsevier; 2018.)

BASIC SCIENCE PEARL	STEP 1

Normocytic anemia is defined as anemia with a normal mean corpuscular volume (MCV) for age. Common causes include blood loss, infection, hemolytic anemia, medication, and anemia of chronic disease. A reticulocyte count can help determine the cause for the normocytic anemia. Children with an appropriate (high) reticulocyte response have anemia as a consequence of ongoing hemolysis or chronic bleeding. Children with a low or inappropriate reticulocyte response have decreased red blood cell production, as seen in anemia of chronic disease, malignancy, and acute bleeding.

Case Point 51.5

After discovering that the patient has a normocytic anemia, a reticulocyte count and total and direct bilirubin are ordered. The patient is found to have a high reticulocyte count, with a normal total and direct bilirubin level. The presence of normocytic anemia with an appropriate reticulocyte response is concerning for bleeding or ongoing hemolysis. The normal bilirubin level makes hemolysis unlikely.

What imaging tests would you want to order?

Given the patient's history of prior head trauma in the setting of a normocytic anemia and with no acute neurologic signs, noncontrast magnetic resonance imaging (MRI) of the brain should be performed to evaluate for intracranial bleed. MRI is the preferred imaging modality in asymptomatic patients because it allows for better estimation of the age of intracranial blood products, can detect parenchymal injuries, and can further delineate the location of any intracranial bleeding (e.g., subdural vs. subarachnoid). MRI does not involve radiation, although sedation is often required. However, if a MRI cannot be performed in a timely manner, or the patient is symptomatic (i.e., presents with seizure, altered mental status, or focal neurologic deficits), computed tomography (CT) is indicated. A skeletal radiographic survey should also be performed if there are suspicions for physical abuse in a child younger than 2 years. This includes radiographs of the skull, cervical spine, chest, ribs (including oblique views), pelvis, abdomen, thoracic and lumbar spine, and individual limb segments, hands, and feet. If the skeletal survey is negative, it can be

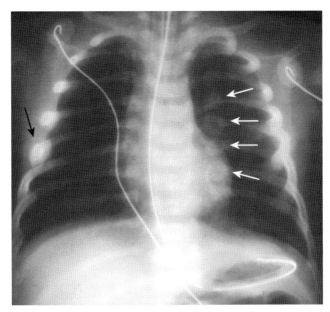

Fig. 51.3 Classic posterior rib fractures with bulbous callus formation at the costovertebral junction at multiple adjacent levels *(white arrows)*. A lateral margin rib fracture, with callus on the right, is also present *(black arrow)*. (From Kriss VM, Carole, J. *Child Abuse and Neglect: Diagnosis, Treatment and Evidence.* St. Louis: Elsevier/Saunders; 2011.)

repeated in 2 weeks to reveal healing fractures that have been missed. Fractures with high specificity for physical abuse include metaphyseal corner lesions, posterior or first rib fracture, scapular fracture, sternal fracture, and spinous process fracture.

Case Point 51.6

Noncontrast MRI scanning of the brain reveals a mixed-density subdural hemorrhage. The skeletal survey shows a fracture of the left humerus, as seen on prior imaging, as well as multiple healing posterior rib fractures (Fig. 51.3).

Diagnosis: Physical abuse.

What are the next steps?

Neurosurgery should be consulted in the setting of an intracranial bleed. However, given that the patient is asymptomatic, there is unlikely to be a surgical intervention. Ophthalmology should also be consulted in the setting of intracranial hemorrhage to evaluate for retinal hemorrhages and other eye injuries. Screening laboratory studies for abdominal trauma should also be ordered, including liver function tests, pancreatic enzyme levels, and urinalysis. If the results are abnormal, there should be consideration for an abdominal CT scan to assess for further injuries.

Most importantly, the Department of Child and Family Services (DCFS) needs to be notified. Physicians are mandated by law to report any concern for child abuse or neglect. They should contact DCFS at the first sign of concern to prevent any future injuries to the child. Once DCFS is aware, they will begin an investigation regarding the accusation and assess the need for any changes in the living situation to protect the child.

Case Point 51.7

To summarize the outcome, DCFS was notified and, given the high index of suspicion for physical abuse, the patient and her brother were removed from the home and placed into foster care. The brother should also have an urgent medical evaluation to assess for physical abuse because he was living in the same home environment.

Case Summary

Complaint/History: 15-month-old female with left arm pain.

Findings: Left humerus fracture, ecchymosis of right external ear, multiple linear, patterned bruising of the posterior surface of the bilateral lower extremities, subdural hemorrhage, multiple healing posterior rib fractures.

Labs/Tests: CBC = normocytic anemia.

Diagnosis: Nonaccidental trauma (child abuse).

Treatment: Humerus fracture—orthopedic closed reduction and immobilization; nonaccidental trauma—referral to Department of Children and Family Services and local law enforcement agency.

BEYOND THE PEARLS

- Physical abuse presents in a variety of ways, including skin injuries, fractures, seizures, altered mental status, and failure to thrive. Often, these clinical signs and symptoms are nonspecific, such as vomiting and decreased level of consciousness.
- Medical mimics for child abuse include the following: pathologic fractures in osteogenesis imperfecta, Caffey disease, leukemia, deficiencies in vitamins C and D, and copper, skin findings in congenital melanocytic nevi (Mongolian spots), hemangiomas, cultural practices including coin rubbing and cupping, and hematologic conditions such as idiopathic thrombocytopenic purpura (ITP), hemophilia, and von Willebrand disease
- Abusive burns, similar to bruising, typically involve the hands, buttocks, legs, and feet. Forced immersion burns present with sharp demarcation, such as the stocking-glove pattern and doughnut sign. The doughnut sign refers to the sparing of thermal injury of the buttocks, as when the buttocks are pressed against the bottom of the bathtub while the surrounding immersed skin is scalded by water.
- Physical abuse is often missed on the first presentation to a health care provider. Always notify the child protection authorities of any concern for child abuse, neglect, or safety concerns to prevent future harm or death to the child.

Bibliography

Glick J. Physical abuse of children. *Pediatr Rev.* 2016;37(4):146–158.

Lerner NB. The anemias. *Nelson Textbook of Pediatrics.* Philadelphia: Elsevier; 2016:2309–2312.e1.

Paul AR, Adamo MA. Non-accidental trauma in pediatric patients: a review of epidemiology, pathophysiology, diagnosis and treatment. *Translat Pediatr.* 2014;3(3):195–207.

4-Month-Old Male Infant With Fever and Difficulty Breathing

Rashmi Tunuguntla   ■   Adler Salazar

A 4-month-old, fully vaccinated, ex–full-term male infant is brought to the emergency department (ED) by his parents due to difficulty breathing. They report that he was in his usual state of health until 2 days prior, when he developed a runny nose and cough. They noticed that other children in his daycare were having similar symptoms, and that 1 day prior he developed a fever and was breast-feeding less frequently than normal. Today, his parents noticed that he is breathing faster and noisier.

What is the initial management for infants presenting in respiratory distress?
It is important for the first responder to have a systematic approach in the evaluation and stabilization of a child in respiratory distress. The priority is to identify life-threatening causes of respiratory distress and intervene promptly. The initial task is to evaluate if the patient's airway is patent or at risk for compromise. Examination of the infant's oropharynx can determine if there is obstruction caused by the tongue, a foreign body, or vomit. The next step involves evaluating the patient's breathing efforts. Depending on the cause, an infant can present with tachypnea, bradypnea or, in severe cases, apnea. The patient may have increased work of breathing, which can manifest as accessory muscle use, abdominal breathing, tracheal tugging, or nasal flaring. Next, the lung fields can be auscultated to assess the quality and symmetry of breath sounds. Abnormal (adventitious) lung sounds include stridor, wheeze, crackles, and rub. The mechanism whereby each adventitious lung sound is made differs and correlates to the pathophysiology of disease. Careful identification of the adventitious sound can help differentiate the cause of the patient's respiratory symptoms (Table 52.1). After evaluating and stabilizing the patient's respiration, proceed to assess his cardiovascular status. Respiratory distress is a sign that the patient is hypoxic. Severe hypoxia can lead to cardiovascular compromise that requires interventions beyond oxygen supplementation.

CLINICAL PEARL   **STEP 2/3**

Tension pneumothorax is an acute, life-threatening condition that can be diagnosed by lung auscultation alone without the need for imaging, which may delay treatment. Decompression can be quickly performed by inserting a large-bore needle into the second intercostal space, which is palpated below the clavicle adjacent to the sternal angle.

Case Point 52.1

The infant's vital signs on presentation include a temperature of 38.7°C, respiratory rate of 48 breaths/min, heart rate of 140 beats/min, blood pressure of 78/53 mm Hg, 88% O_2 saturation on room air. The nurse administers oxygen supplementation by nasal cannula at a rate of 2 L/min, with improvement of O_2 saturation to 96%. Examination shows that the infant is crying and fussy but consolable by his mother. He has clear nasal secretions and occasionally coughs. His anterior fontanelle is flat and his mucous membranes appear dry. He is tachypneic and tachycardic but has good perfusion. Auscultation reveals coarse crackles bilaterally and expiratory wheezing.

TABLE 52.1 ■ Adventitious Respiratory Sounds

Sound	Continuous or Discontinuous	Pitch	Inspiratory or Expiratory	Mechanism	Associated Conditions
Stridor	Continuous	High	Inspiratory	Upper airway obstruction, heard loudest over the neck	Croup, epiglottitis, foreign body, laryngeal edema
Wheeze (rhonchus)	Continuous	High (wheeze); low (rhonchus)	Expiratory; both in severe cases of obstruction	Lower airway obstruction, heard loudest over lung fields	Asthma, bronchiolitis, intrathoracic airway obstruction
Crackles (crepitation, rales)	Discontinuous	High (fine); low (coarse)	Inspiratory	Opening of collapsed distal airway during inspiration; fine crackles—smaller distal airways; coarse crackles—larger, more proximal airways	Pneumonia, pulmonary edema, heart failure, pulmonary fibrosis
Pleural rub	Continuous	Low	Expiratory predominantly, but can be both	Inflamed pleura, decreased lubrication cause grating sounds during sliding of the parietal and visceral pleural membranes	Pleuritis, pneumonia, pleural effusion

Wheezing is a common presenting symptom for obstructive airway disease (OAD) in children. It is a continuous musical sound lasting longer than 250 ms, usually auscultated during exhalation in diseases affecting the airways. Wheezing can originate anywhere along the airways. The different caliber of the affected airway leads to the difference in pitch, where high-frequency wheezing (>400 Hz) occurs in the smaller distal airways and lower frequency wheezing—termed *rhonchi*— in the larger proximal airways. The noise is created when airflow causes oscillation of the airway walls in a section that is narrowed or obstructed. Wheezing can be a sign of different respiratory conditions (Table 52.2). The cause of a child's wheezing can be determined by obtaining a further history, such as the age of onset and acuteness or chronicity and recurrence of the wheezing. For example, congenital anatomic abnormalities such as tracheoesophageal fistula or malacia of the central airway presents in early infancy, whereas asthma presents in older children.

BASIC SCIENCE PEARL | **STEP 1**

In wheezing caused by asthma, the airflow must generate enough pressure and turbulence to overcome airway obstruction and cause the walls to oscillate, respectively. Absence of wheezing in an asthmatic patient (so-called silent chest) is concerning and may signal impending respiratory failure.

TABLE 52.2 ■ **Causes of Wheezing in Infancy**

Cause	Features, Examples
Aspiration syndrome	Gastroesophageal reflux disease, pharyngeal swallow dysfunction
Infection	
• Viral	Respiratory syncytial virus, human metapneumovirus, influenza, parainfluenza adenovirus, bocavirus, rhinovirus, coronavirus, enterovirus
• Other	*Chlamydia trachomatis, Mycobacterium tuberculosis,* histoplasmosis, papillomatosis
Asthma	
• Transient wheezer	• Resolves by 6 years of age; initial risk factor is diminished lung size
• Persistent wheezer	• Persists beyond 6 years of age; risk factors—family asthma history, atopic dermatitis, allergen sensitization, peripheral eosinophilia (<4%) and wheezing unrelated to colds in first year of life; increased risk for asthma
• Late-onset wheezer	• Presents after 3 years of age and persists
Anatomic abnormalities	
• Central airway abnormalities	• Malacia of larynx, trachea, and/or bronchi; laryngeal or tracheal web; tracheoesophageal fistula; laryngeal cleft
• Extrinsic airway anomalies	• Vascular sling or ring; mediastinal lymphadenopathy from infection or tumor; mediastinal mass or tumor; esophageal foreign body
• Intrinsic airway anomalies	• Airway hemangioma; cystic adenomatoid malformation; bronchial or lung cyst; congenital lobar emphysema; aberrant tracheal bronchus; sequestration; congenital heart defect with left-to-right shunt (pulmonary edema); foreign body
Immunodeficiency	Immunoglobulin A deficiency, B cell deficiency, AIDS, bronchiectasis
Mucociliary disorder	Cystic fibrosis, pulmonary ciliary dyskinesia, bronchiectasis
Other	Bronchopulmonary dysplasia, interstitial lung disease (e.g., bronchiolitis obliterans), heart failure, anaphylaxis, inhalational injury (e.g., burns)

Adapted from Kliegman R, Stanton B, St Geme J. *Nelson's Textbook of Pediatrics.* 20th ed. Philadelphia: Elsevier; 2016.

Case Point 52.2

On further questioning, the mother reports that the patient only had one wet diaper today rather than the usual four that he usually has per day. A normal saline (NS) intravenous (IV) bolus of 10 mL/kg is given for fluid resuscitation.

CLINICAL PEARL   **STEP 2/3**

Parental report of symptoms and signs of dehydration (e.g., emesis, diarrhea, poor fluid intake, decreased urine output, weak cry, sunken fontanelle, sunken eyes, decreased tears, dry mouth, cool extremities) have a 73% to 100% sensitivity but poor specificity in predicting moderate to severe dehydration in children. In a systematic literature review, it was found that the most useful signs to predict 5% hypovolemia are delayed capillary refill time, reduced skin turgor, and deep respirations, regardless of respiratory rate.

Case Point 52.3

A chest x-ray is obtained and shows bilateral patchy infiltrates, with signs of left lobe air-trapping (Fig. 52.1). The patient's O_2 saturation, heart rate. and respiratory rate improve after the supplemental oxygenation and NS bolus. He is then transferred to the pediatric ward for further management.

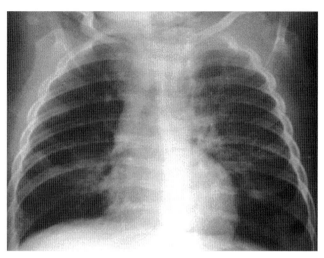

Fig. 52.1 Chest radiograph of patient with bronchiolitis. Seen are patchy, bilateral, perihilar, linear opacities, with slight depression of the left diaphragm, due to left lower lobe air trapping. (Adapted from Broaddus V, Mason R, Ernst J, et al. *Murray and Nadel's Textbook of Respiratory Medicine.* 6th ed. Philadelphia: Elsevier; 2016; courtesy Dr. Michael Gotway.)

What is the differential diagnosis?

Based on the case presented above, one should be able to enumerate a list of possible diagnoses. Possible causes for this case include bronchiolitis, reactive airway disease, pneumonia (bacterial vs. viral vs. atypical), foreign body, croup, and pertussis. The chest x-ray lacks findings associated with bacterial pneumonia. Foreign body ingestion is unlikely given the 3-day course of symptoms and lack of evidence on the chest x-ray. The patient does not seem to have a cough pattern that is consistent with pertussis. The patient was resting and not in a tripod position or drooling and is fully vaccinated, making epiglottitis unlikely. Additionally, the lack of stridor heard during the examination lessens the possibility of croup. At this point, the most likely diagnosis is bronchiolitis.

CLINICAL PEARL	STEP 2/3

It is often difficult to differentiate bronchiolitis from asthma with the patient's first presentation. Asthma usually presents with recurrent wheezing in a child older than 2 years with a personal or family history of atopy, allergic rhinitis, or asthma.

CLINICAL PEARL	STEP 2/3

Bacterial pneumonia in an infant manifests as a toxic appearance, high fevers, and focal findings on the chest x-ray. Bacterial pneumonias usually cause a restrictive lung disease (RLD), with findings of tachypnea and decreased tidal volumes. Wheezing is usually absent.

What is bronchiolitis?

Bronchiolitis is an infection/inflammation of the lower respiratory tract, specifically the terminal bronchioles. Lymphocytic infiltration occurs at these sites (Fig. 52.2) and causes edema, mucous plugging, and necrosis of the bronchiolar epithelium (Fig. 52.3). The cellular debris, mucus, and edema cause obstruction of the bronchiolar lumen and turbulent airflow. This is a dynamic process affected by the intrathoracic pressures during the respiratory cycle. The negative intrathoracic pressure during inspiration causes the bronchioles to open, whereas the positive pressure generated during exhalation causes

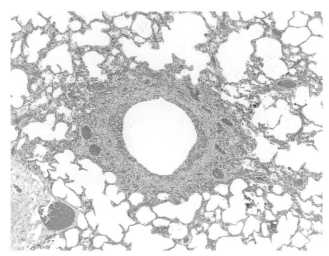

Fig. 52.2 Histologic appearance of RSV bronchiolitis. There is circumferential infiltration of lymphocytes and macrophages in the submucosa of bronchioles (H&E stain, original magnification × 12.5). (From Procop G, Pritt B. *Pathology of Infectious Disease.* Philadelphia: Elsevier/Saunders; 2015.)

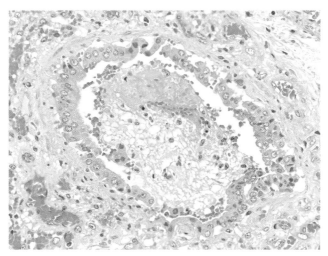

Fig. 52.3 Bronchiole lumen obstructed by granular debris comprised of sloughed epithelium, macrophages, and serum proteins (H&E stain, original magnification × 12.5). (From Procop G, Pritt B. *Pathology of Infectious Disease.* Philadelphia: Elsevier/Saunders; 2015.)

collapse of the airway, leading to progressive hyperinflation of the lung due to the air-trapping phenomenon (known as *auto-PEEP*—auto–positive end-expiratory pressure), notably in the upper lobes of the lung. On the other hand, the effects of gravity on the bases of the lung predisposes these lung tissue segments to collapse (atelectasis). Bronchiolitis typically causes symptoms in children 24 months of age or younger, with a peak incidence in the fall and winter seasons. This is one of the leading causes of hospitalization in children and affects males more frequently than females.

What are the clinical manifestations of bronchiolitis?
The first sign of bronchiolitis is often rhinorrhea. Approximately 1 to 3 days later, coughing develops, followed by fevers and wheezing. As the disease process progresses, signs of respiratory

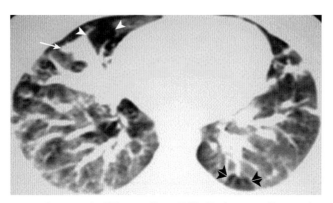

Fig. 52.4 Chest computed tomography (CT) scan of bronchiolitis. Patchy areas of increased attenuation are due to atelectasis *(arrow,)* and areas of decreased attenuation are due to air trapping *(single arrowheads)* in some areas with lobular configuration *(double arrowheads)*. (Adapted from Broaddus V, Mason R, Ernst J, et al. *Murray and Nadel's Textbook of Respiratory Medicine.* 6th ed. Philadelphia: Elsevier; 2016; courtesy Dr. Michael Gotway.)

distress can manifest as tachypnea, intercostal and subcostal retractions, hyperexpansion of the chest, restlessness, peripheral cyanosis, and even apneic spells. Symptoms typically peak around days 5 to 6 of the illness. In healthy infants older than 6 months, the average length of hospitalization, if required, is 3 to 4 days. However, in infants younger than 6 months or those with comorbid conditions, hospitalization can last longer and may require added respiratory/ventilatory support.

How is bronchiolitis diagnosed?

Bronchiolitis is diagnosed based on the classic history and clinical findings. Laboratory and radiograph tests are not required to make the diagnosis for uncomplicated cases. Identifying the viral cause is useful in hospitalized cases for the purpose of patient cohort during the winter season, when the incidence is at its peak. A chest x-ray may be needed for bronchiolitic patients who are immunocompromised or who have high-risk comorbid pulmonary and cardiac diseases or a history of prematurity. Chest imaging for respiratory syncytial virus (RSV) is nonspecific and can show hyperinflation, peribronchial thickening, or patchy atelectasis, with volume loss due to airway narrowing and mucous plugging (Fig. 52.4; see also Fig. 52.1).

CLINICAL PEARL   **STEP 2/3**

Normal chest x-ray results are seen in as much as 87.7% of uncomplicated bronchiolitis cases among infants younger than 12 months.

Case Point 52.4

Conservative management, including nasal suctioning, IV fluids, antipyretics, and supplemental oxygen, is continued. During the course of the next few hours, the patient's work of breathing increases. His respiratory rate is 62 breaths/min, heart rate is 160 beats/min, and O_2 saturation is 91% on 2 L/min nasal cannula oxygen (NCO_2). He is grunting while breathing, with nasal flaring and subcostal retractions. He appears sleepier but is arousable during the examination. High-flow, nasal cannula oxygen ($HFNCO_2$) is started at 8 L/min. He is placed on NPO. He is observed closely to determine whether intubation and invasive mechanical ventilation would be required. After 1 hour of initiating $HFNCO_2$, the patient's O_2 saturation improves to 98%. His heart rate and respiratory rate decrease, and he appears more comfortable. Conservative management is continued.

Pathogenesis of respiratory
failure in bronchiolitis

Possible mechanisms of
CPAP/HFNC

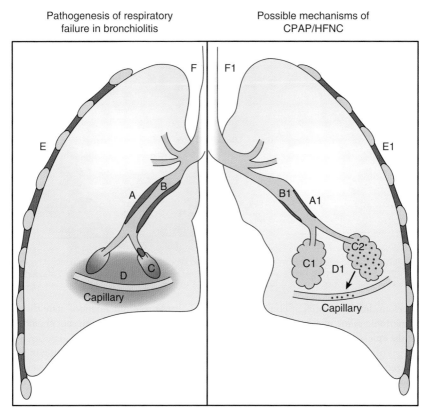

Fig. 52.5 Mechanisms of respiratory failure in bronchiolitis and actions of high-flow, nasal cannula oxygen (HFNCO$_2$) and continuous positive airway pressure (CPAP). Intraluminal mucus and debris cause airway obstruction and resistance, resulting in atelectasis. Interstitial edema limits oxygen transport, contributing to hypoxemia. Warm humidified oxygen may reduce intraluminal mucus and positive end-expiratory pressure (PEEP) from CPAP, and HFNCO$_2$ may overcome resistance, preventing atelectasis and increase oxygen transport. The result may be a reduction in respiratory muscle fatigue. (From Sinha I, McBride A, Smith R, et al. CPAP and high-flow nasal cannula oxygen in bronchiolitis. *Chest.* 2015;148(13):810–823.)

How is bronchiolitis treated?

Treatment of uncomplicated cases that do not require hospitalization is supportive care. For patients who are hospitalized, respiratory support is likely needed. Initially, nasal suctioning is recommended to relieve nasal obstruction. Supplemental oxygen should be provided via nasal cannula or face mask to maintain an oxygen saturation greater than 90% to 92%. Noninvasive respiratory support includes continuous positive airway pressure (CPAP) and heated, humidified, HFNCO$_2$; this can be used for cases unresponsive to conventional oxygen supplementation (Fig. 52.5). HFNCO$_2$ has been shown to decrease the need for invasive mechanical ventilation, length of hospital stay, and medical complications in bronchiolitic infants younger than 12 months.

Inhaled bronchodilators, glucocorticoids, leukotriene inhibitors, heliox, and chest physiotherapy are not routinely used in the management and treatment of bronchiolitis. Managing a patient with bronchiolitis using nebulized hypertonic saline remains controversial; there are several conflicting studies. Physiologic evidence has suggested that nebulized hypertonic saline increases mucociliary clearance. Because mucous plugs are a major factor involved in the development of respiratory distress in patients with bronchiolitis, nebulized hypertonic saline should, theoretically,

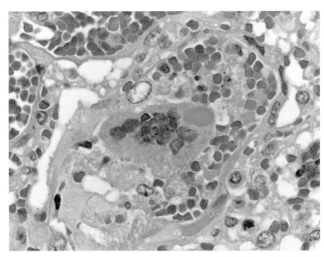

Fig. 52.6 RSV infection causing the formation of multinucleated syncytial cell in the alveoli (H&E stain, original magnification × 25). (From Procop G, Pritt B. *Pathology of Infectious Disease*. Philadelphia: Elsevier/Saunders; 2015.)

be efficacious, but the results of clinical trials differ. Current recommendations state that nebulized hypertonic saline may be used in hospitalized patients with bronchiolitis, but should not be used in the emergency room setting.

There is often concern regarding the risk of developing a serious bacterial infection in patients hospitalized with an RSV infection and whether or not to treat with antibiotics. However, studies have shown that concurrent serious bacterial infections are rare (<1%) in hospitalized children. Therefore, the empiric use of antibiotics is unnecessary, and broad-spectrum antibiotic use actually increases the risk of bacterial superinfection.

Case Point 52.5

The result of the rapid testing sent from the ED is reported and confirms the suspicion of RSV infection.

Diagnosis: Respiratory syncytial virus bronchiolitis.

A variety of viruses can cause bronchiolitis, including influenza, parainfluenza, rhinovirus, adenovirus, bocavirus, human metapneumovirus, and RSV. RSV is the most common cause of bronchiolitis and is responsible for approximately 50% of cases.

RSV is an enveloped, medium-sized RNA virus with a nonsegmented, single-stranded, negative-sense genome. There are two major glycosylated surface proteins, F protein and G protein, that play a major role in the pathogenesis of RSV. The G protein is primarily involved in attachment of the virus to host cells. The F protein also plays a role in attachment but, once attached, undergoes structural changes that allow for viral penetration by fusing the viral and host cellular membranes. This promotes further fusion of infected cells to uninfected cells, which results in the characteristic RSV syncytia to form—hence, the name of this viral process (Fig. 52.6).

What is the pathogenesis of respiratory syncytial virus?
RSV is spread through close contact or direct inoculation. In a patient infected with RSV, the virus can aerosolize as large particles and spread via coughing or sneezing to others within

approximately a 3-foot radius. The long distance spread of aerosols is less likely. However, self-inoculation into the eyes or nose can also occur by touching objects contaminated with infectious secretions. Given these modes of infectivity, hospitalized patients suspected or diagnosed with RSV should be placed under droplet precautions. The average incubation period of RSV is 2 to 8 days, and shedding duration is typically 7 to 10 days.

RSV replicates in the respiratory epithelium and triggers a cascade of events that leads to the development of bronchiolitis. The first defense against RSV is the innate immune system, which is the respiratory epithelium. This initial step triggers alterations in gene expression that allow for the production of cell surface markers that initiate the release of cytokines and chemokines. These cytokines and chemokines recruit inflammatory cells to the respiratory tract. As noted, these inflammatory infiltrates accumulate at the bronchioles and cause edema, mucous plugs, and necrosis of the epithelium, resulting in obstruction of the bronchioles.

What are the possible complications of respiratory syncytial virus bronchiolitis?
Apnea is the most common complication associated with RSV infection and is a leading cause for the need for hospitalization. Certain conditions predispose children to have an increased risk of developing apnea and respiratory failure. Preterm gestation, with or without chronic lung disease, is a major risk factor. Infants with a gestational age of less than 36 weeks are three or more times more likely to become hospitalized when infected with RSV. Children with a gestational age less than 32 weeks are more likely to require intensive care. Congenital heart diseases, especially cyanotic heart conditions with pulmonary hypertension, are among the top reasons why infants require hospitalization with an RSV infection. Immunosuppressive conditions or other chronic diseases that affect the handling of respiratory secretions, such as neuromuscular disease, also put patients at higher risk.

Various social and environmental factors have been shown to increase the risk for a more severe RSV clinical infectious course. These include male gender, crowded living conditions, lower socioeconomic status, exposure to tobacco smoke, exposure to other young children in the home or daycare, and lack of breastfeeding.

Case Point 52.6

Over the course of the next 24 hours, the patient's oxygenation, work of breathing, and tachycardia improve. He is weaned from $HFNCO_2$ to oxygen via a nasal cannula. His breastfeeding and urine output return to baseline. He is eventually weaned to room air and is discharged on the 7th day from the start of his illness.

Can future respiratory syncytial virus infections be prevented?
Palivizumab, a neutralizing, humanized, murine monoclonal antibody, provides passive immunoprophylaxis against RSV and is strongly indicated for children at risk for severe RSV infections, including premature infants born at less than 29 weeks, preterm infants (<32 weeks) with bronchopulmonary dysplasia (BPD), and infants with hemodynamically significant congenital heart disease. Children who are immunocompromised or with neuromuscular or pulmonary disease, impairing the ability to clear airway secretions, may be considered for prophylactic treatment. Palivizumab is administered monthly for 5 months during RSV season (until March) during the first year of life. Immunoprophylaxis until the second year of life is recommended for BPD and immunocompromised patients.

Case Summary
Complaint/History: A 4-month-old male infant is brought to the ED for fever and difficulty breathing.

Findings: The patient has nasal secretions, coughing, tachypnea, tachycardia, hypoxia, fever, and signs of moderate dehydration.

Lab/Tests: Chest x-ray shows bilateral patchy infiltrates, hyperinflation, and signs of air trapping in the left lower lobe; a rapid RSV enzyme immunoassay (EIA) is positive.

Diagnosis: Respiratory syncytial virus (RSV) bronchiolitis.

Treatment: Conservative management includes IV fluid, nasal suctioning, supplemental oxygen, and humidified, high-flow, nasal cannula oxygen.

BEYOND THE PEARLS

- The American Thoracic Society (ATS) has recommended avoiding use of the term *rhonchi*. Wheezing (high-pitched) and rhonchi (low-pitched) both describe adventitious sounds during expiration. Both are caused by intrathoracic airway obstruction. There is no clinical utility in differentiating between the two sounds.
- Mechanisms of action of HFNCO$_2$ include filling airway dead space with oxygen-rich and carbon dioxide–depleted gas and generating positive end-expiratory pressure (PEEP) for distention of the collapsed airway.
- Palivizumab is a humanized monoclonal (IgG) that recognizes the A antigenic site of RSVs F protein. Phase II clinical trials have shown a decrease in 45% to 55% of hospitalization stays among palivizumab-treated children.
- At room temperature, secretions from patients infected with RSV may survive on nonporous surfaces for 3 to 30 hours, whereas on porous surfaces this usually lasts less than 1 hour.
- Transplacentally acquired anti-RSV maternal immunoglobulin G serum antibodies, if present in high concentration, appear to provide partial but incomplete protection, which accounts for the decreased severity of RSV infections in the first several months of life.

Bibliography

Crowe K. *Nelson's Textbook of Pediatrics*. 20th ed. Philadelphia: Elsevier; 2016.

Hall Caroline Breese, et al. Risk of secondary bacterial infection in infants hospitalized with respiratory syncytial viral infection. *J Pediatr*. 1988;113(2):266–271.

Kliegman R, Stanton B, St Geme J, et al. *Nelson's Textbook of Pediatrics*. 20th ed. Philadelphia: Elsevier; 2016.

Mc Gee S. *Evidence-Based Physical Diagnosis*. 4th ed. Philadelphia: Elsevier; 2018.

Piedimonte G, Perez MK. Respiratory syncytial virus infection and bronchiolitis. *Pediatr Rev*. 2014; 35(12):519–530.

Purcell K, Fergie J. Concurrent serious bacterial infections in 2396 infants and children hospitalized with respiratory syncytial virus lower respiratory tract infections. *Arch Pediatr Adolesc Med*. 2002;15(4):322.

Ralston SL, Lieberthal AS, Meissner HC, et al. Clinical Practice Guideline: The diagnosis, management, and prevention of bronchiolitis. *Pediatrics*. 2015;136(4):782.

Wagner T. Bronchiolitis. *Pediatr Rev*. 2009;30(10):386–395.

Walsh E, Hall C. *Mandell, Douglas, and Bennett's Principles and Practice of Infectious Disease*. 8th ed. Philadelphia: Elsevier; 2015.

7-Year-Old Female With Right-Sided Headache, Ear Pain, and Eye Deviation

Rebecca Graves ▪ Cynthia Stotts ▪ James Homans

A 7-year-old female presents to the emergency department with a 3-week history of right temporal headaches and right ear pain, as well as eye crossing since the day prior to presentation. Two weeks prior, she was seen by her primary care provider (PCP) and treated with a 5-day course of an unknown oral antibiotic and ear drops. These resulted in a brief period of improvement in her otalgia and headaches.

What condition had the patient's primary care provider diagnosed?
The PCP diagnosed the patient with acute otitis media (AOM), an infection of the middle ear with bacterial and viral causes (Table 53.1).

What is the recommended medical management of acute otitis media?
Antibiotic treatment is indicated when AOM causes severe symptoms, including a fever of 39°C or higher, severe otalgia for more than 2 days, toxic appearance, and/or inability to ensure a follow-up evaluation within 48 hours. In children ages 6 to 24 months with unilateral AOM and an absence of severe symptoms, the PCP may decide whether to treat with antibiotics or to treat symptomatically with analgesics and close monitoring for worsening of symptoms. Children older than 24 months, with either unilateral or bilateral nonsevere AOM, can also be treated with antibiotics or analgesia and watchful waiting. If there is no improvement in pain within 2 to 3 days, antibiotics should be started. Children younger than 6 months, younger than 24 months with bilateral AOM, or with severe disease symptoms should be started on antibiotic therapy immediately.

Amoxicillin (80–90 mg/kg per day bid) is the antibiotic of choice. For cases presenting after 30 days, amoxicillin plus clavulanate should be used. If there is no improvement in symptoms after 2 to 3 days of amoxicillin, treatment can be changed to amoxicillin with clavulanic acid. The recommended duration of antibiotic therapy is typically 10 days for children younger than 2 years, 7 days for children ages 2 to 5 years, and 5 to 7 days for children older than 6 years.

CLINICAL PEARL   **STEP 1**

The most common pathogens involved in otitis media are *Streptococcus pneumoniae*, nontypeable *Haemophilus influenzae*, and *Moraxella catarrhalis*. *S. pneumoniae* shows increasing resistance to penicillin due to changes in penicillin-binding proteins, whereas *H. influenzae* may produce β-lactamase–causing penicillin (or amoxicillin) resistance. Pneumococcal immunization of young children has led to a decrease in the relative frequency of pneumococcal otitis media.

TABLE 53.1 ▪ **Bacteria and Viruses in Acute Otitis Media (AOM)**

Bacteria	Viruses
Streptococcus pneumoniae	Respiratory syncytial virus
Haemophilus influenzae	Influenza
Moraxella catarrhalis	Parainfluenza
Staphylococcus aureus	Adenovirus
Group A *Streptococcus*	Rhinovirus
Alpha-hemolytic *Streptococcus*	
Pseudomonas aeruginosa	

CLINICAL PEARL   **STEP 2/3**

The peak incidence of otitis media is from 6 to 20 months of age. There is a subsequent decline in incidence, but a second peak occurs between the ages of 4 to 6 years, when children enter school. By 3 years of age, more than 80% of children will have had at least one episode of otitis media.

Case Point 53.1

On review of systems (ROS), the patient reports three episodes of nonbloody, nonbilious emesis, decreased appetite, and decreased energy. She denies fever, neck pain, stiffness, or known sick contacts. The remaining ROS is negative.

CLINICAL PEARL   **STEP 2/3**

Headache, vomiting, neck pain or stiffness, or altered mental status should alert the health care provider to the possibility of central nervous system infection, in particular meningitis. Fever, neck pain or stiffness, and altered mental status are all important signs and symptoms of meningitis.

Case Point 53.2

She was born full term, received all recommended vaccinations, and has a past medical history significant for a single episode of ear infection 4 months prior, reportedly treated with ear drops. Family history is negative for immunodeficiency. There are no smokers in the household. She has no allergies and is currently not taking any medications.

CLINICAL PEARL   **STEP 2/3**

Risk factors for otitis media include exposure to second-hand smoke, lack of pneumococcal vaccination, male gender, lower socioeconomic status, lack of breastfeeding, and exposure to other children.

Case Point 53.3

On physical examination, the patient is afebrile and well-appearing, with normal mental status. Her right tympanic membrane appears thickened, and fluid is visualized behind it. Her left tympanic membrane is only partially seen due to the presence of cerumen. There is no posterior auricular tenderness or displacement of the pinnae. Pupils are equal, round, and reactive to light. When asked to look to the right, her left eye moves freely to the right, but her right eye remains midline. When asked to look to the left, both eyes move freely to the left. On lateral gaze toward either side, as well as on downward gaze, she reports double vision. The remainder of the physical examination is normal.

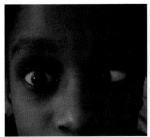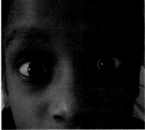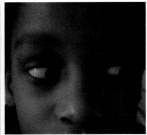

Fig. 53.1 Abducens palsy. The patient is unable to abduct her right eye, indicating right lateral rectus palsy. The lateral rectus muscle is innervated by the abducens nerve (cranial nerve VI). (From Vitale M, Amrit M, Arora R, Lata J. Gradenigo's syndrome: a common infection with uncommon consequences. *Am J Emerg Med.* 2017;35(9):138e1–1388e2.)

Which cranial nerve is affected, and how do you explain the examination findings?
The patient has abducens palsy (cranial nerve VI). The abducens nerve controls the lateral rectus muscle, which abducts the eye. When damaged, abduction is impaired. There is unopposed action of the medial rectus muscle, so the affected eye is pulled medially toward the nose (Fig. 53.1). Horizontal diplopia is also a common symptom of abducens nerve palsy. Although less common, slight vertical diplopia may also be seen.

What is the differential diagnosis?
In a patient with otitis media who is now experiencing otalgia and headaches, lack of response to therapy or progression of the disease process should be considered. In view of the cranial nerve involvement, mastoiditis with resulting inflammatory compression of adjacent neurovascular structures should be strongly considered. Focal neurologic deficits can also be caused by any process that leads to increased intracranial pressure, so tumor and intracranial abscess should be excluded.

CLINICAL PEARL   **STEP 2/3**

In a patient presenting with headache, focal neurologic deficits, in particular of the cranial nerves, should raise concern that the patient may have increased intracranial pressure. Head imaging is indicated. A computed tomography (CT) scan of the head is the imaging modality of choice in a situation in which information is needed quickly, such as when there is trauma or concern for an acute intracranial bleed. Because CT scanning delivers significant ionizing radiation exposure, MRI is safer for children and is often preferred in nonurgent situations. Additionally, because MRI depicts soft tissue anatomy in far greater detail, it is in general a more sensitive diagnostic tool.

Case Point 53.4

Laboratory testing shows a normal white blood cell count of 10.5×10^9/L, with 70% neutrophils and 21% lymphocytes, normocytic anemia with a hemoglobin level of 9.9 g/dL, and a platelet count of 601×10^9/L. Magnetic resonance imaging (MRI) of the brain reveals bilateral mastoid effusions, right greater than left, as well as a 14- × 4- × 7-mm fluid collection in the right petrous apex of the temporal bone with surrounding inflammatory changes extending to the right Meckel's cave, foramen ovale, Dorello canal, and right internal auditory canal. There is no venous sinus thrombosis, cerebral parenchymal, or orbital involvement identified.

Diagnosis: Complicated case of acute otitis media leading to mastoiditis and Gradenigo syndrome.

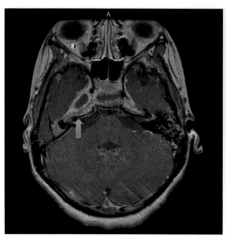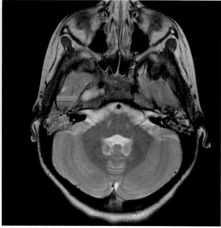

Fig. 53.2 Magnetic resonance imaging (MRI) of Gradenigo syndrome. The MRI scan shows fluid opacification of the right mastoid air cells, demonstrating otomastoiditis. Additionally, there is erosion of the right petrous apex with adjacent fluid collection, consistent with petrous apicitis and abscess formation. (From Vitale M, Amrit M, Arora R, Lata J. Gradenigo's syndrome: a common infection with uncommon consequences. *Am J Emerg Med.* 2017;35(9):138e1–1388e2.)

What is Gradenigo syndrome?

Gradenigo syndrome is a rare complication of otitis media or mastoiditis in which the intracranial spread of infection leads to abducens palsy and pain in the distribution of the ophthalmic branch of the trigeminal nerve. These findings are secondary to inflammatory changes in the region of the petrous apex (petrous apicitis) and cranial base, where the abducens and trigeminal nerves course is best seen on MRI (Fig. 53.2).

What physical examination findings not seen in this patient might you expect to encounter in a patient with mastoiditis?

Patients with mastoiditis are typically febrile. Additionally, postauricular tenderness, erythema, swelling, and fluctuance are commonly seen. Inflammation above the ear or a fluctuant mass overlying the mastoid bone may lead to displacement of the pinna. In children younger than 2 years, mastoiditis leads to downward and outward displacement of the pinna (Fig. 53.3), whereas children 2 years of age and older have an anterior and upward displacement (Fig. 53.4).

What is the pathophysiologic process whereby otitis media can lead to mastoiditis and subsequent intracranial involvement?

Because the mastoid bone is adjacent to the distal end of the middle ear and communicates with it through the aditus, otitis media is almost always accompanied by fluid in the mastoid causing inflammation in the air cells. Persistent inflammation leads to the accumulation of purulent exudates in the cells. Additionally, obstruction to middle ear drainage by eustachian tube dysfunction or a cholesteatoma can lead to increased pressure in the mastoid air cells and thus to mastoiditis. Infection can then spread to the periosteum, causing periosteitis. If untreated or inadequately treated, destruction and necrosis of the thin septae of the mastoid air cells occurs, called *coalescent mastoiditis*. Abscess cavities may then develop, followed by extension of purulent material into adjacent structures and leading to various complications, including meningitis, epidural abscess, lateral sinus thrombosis, subdural empyema, brain abscess, and petrous apicitis (Fig. 53.5).

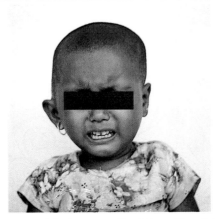

Fig. 53.3 Mastoiditis. Note the outward displacement of the right ear. (From Spicer WJ. *Clinical Microbiology and Infectious Diseases*. London: Elsevier; 2008.)

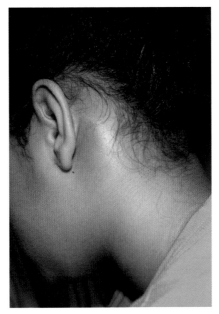

Fig. 53.4 Mild swelling with tenderness and erythema behind the left ear in mastoiditis. (From Nelson D, Jeanmonod R. Bezold abscess: a rare complication of mastoiditis. *Am J Emerg Med.* 2013;31(11):1626.e3–1626.e4.)

Case Point 53.5

Due to concern for possible resistant organisms and the intracranial spread of infection, treatment was initiated with intravenous (IV) vancomycin, cefepime, and metronidazole. On the second day of hospitalization, she underwent a right-sided mastoidectomy and bilateral tympanostomy tube placement. The abscess seen on the MRI scan was too deep to be accessible. There was no growth on bacterial culture of bone scrapings of the surgical site after 48 hours. The patient was discharged with a plan to receive a 6-week course of IV antibiotics as an outpatient. Repeat MRI at 3 weeks demonstrated a decrease in abscess size. Her abducens palsy and diplopia resolved after 2 weeks. She continues to do well, with no evidence of recurrence.

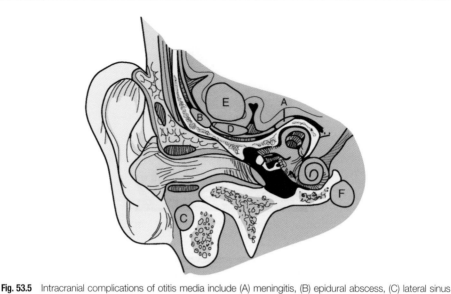

Fig. 53.5 Intracranial complications of otitis media include (A) meningitis, (B) epidural abscess, (C) lateral sinus thrombosis, (D) subdural empyema, (E) brain abscess, (F) and petrous apicitis. (Adapted from Vazquez E, Castellote A, Piqueras J, et al: Imaging of complications of acute mastoiditis in children. *RadioGraphics*. 2003;23:359–372.)

CLINICAL PEARL	STEP 1/2/3

The most common pathogens involved in mastoiditis are *Streptococcus pneumoniae, Streptococcus pyogenes, Staphylococcus aureus* (including methicillin-resistant *S. aureus*), and nontypeable *Haemophilus influenzae*. In cases of chronic mastoiditis, *Pseudomonas aeruginosa*, enteric gram-negative rods, and anaerobes should also be considered. In highly endemic areas, *Mycobacterium tuberculosis* complex is a common cause of chronic otitis media and mastoiditis.

What treatments options are indicated for a diagnosis of mastoiditis?

In the absence of periosteitis, mastoiditis typically resolves spontaneously or with outpatient antimicrobial therapy, which at this early stage would be the same as indicated for a child with AOM. Although cases of uncomplicated mastoiditis were much more common before the antibiotic era, today most children with mastoiditis develop periosteitis. If the child has a suppurative complication or history of failed antimicrobial treatment for AOM, drainage of the middle ear via tympanocentesis or myringotomy is usually indicated. In this situation, aerobic and anaerobic bacterial cultures and, in some cases, cultures for mycobacteria and fungi should be performed. Drainage of the middle ear is diagnostic and therapeutic. Middle ear fluid cultures are important for guiding and narrowing antimicrobial therapy. The procedure relieves pressure and otalgia. Tympanostomy tubes may be placed if longer-term drainage is deemed necessary.

Given the emergence of penicillin-resistant *Streptococcus pneumoniae* and methicillin-resistant *Staphylococcus aureus*, vancomycin is frequently included in empiric parenteral antimicrobial therapy. If there is a history of recurrent AOM, chronic perforation, recent antibiotic use, immunocompromise, or severe toxicity, an antipseudomonal agent such as cefepime should be added to the vancomycin. If there is evidence of intracranial spread of infection, metronidazole should also be added to treat anaerobes. The recommended duration of antibiotic treatment varies, depending on the clinical situation. A 4-week course with at least 7 days of IV antibiotics is usually indicated. A longer duration of IV antibiotics may be necessary for patients with intracranial complications.

If symptoms persist or progress despite drainage of middle ear fluid and appropriate antimicrobial treatment for 24 to 48 hours, mastoidectomy is usually indicated. It is also indicated for extracranial suppurative complications, such as cranial nerve palsy or labyrinthitis or intracranial complications, such as those shown in Fig. 53.5.

Case Summary

Complaint/History: A 7-year-old female is brought to the emergency department for right ear pain, headaches, and having "crossing of her eyes." She was given antibiotics by primary care physician 2 weeks prior.

Findings: The examination shows a thickened right tympanic membrane, with effusion. A cranial nerve examination shows inability for the right eye to perform a right lateral gaze.

Labs/Tests: Magnetic resonance imaging shows bilateral mastoid effusions, right greater than left, and a 14- × 4- × 7-mm fluid collection in the right petrous apex of the temporal bone, with surrounding inflammatory changes.

Diagnosis: Acute otitis media causing mastoiditis and Gradenigo syndrome.

Treatment: Intravenous antibiotics with vancomycin, cefepime, and metronidazole for 6 weeks; a right mastoidectomy and bilateral tympanostomy tube placement are performed.

BEYOND THE PEARLS

- The availability of the polymerase chain reaction (PCR) assay has identified viruses in effusions of children with acute otitis media (AOM). Viral pathogens impair eustachian tube function and local immune defenses and increase bacterial adherence. It is hypothesized that viruses are precursors to bacterial infection leading to AOM.
- Mastoiditis was common in the preantibiotic area and was a frequent cause of hospitalization in children. It was only treatable with surgical decompression and often led to severe complications, including death. It is slightly more common in areas where the watchful waiting approach for otitis media has become the standard of care.
- Middle ear fluid should always be collected prior to initiating antibiotic treatment for mastoiditis. The specimen should be sent for Gram staining and aerobic and anaerobic culture to ascertain the causative organism(s) and narrow antimicrobial therapy.
- Bacterial strains that produce biofilm result in antibiotic-resistant cases of AOM and mastoiditis. Biofilms are communities of interacting bacteria encased in a matrix of exopolysaccharides, which protects them from phagocytosis, immunoglobulins, complement factors, and antibiotics. These cases require mechanical debridement as part of the treatment.
- A major complication of mastoiditis is hearing loss. Hearing loss may be transient due to middle ear effusion or may be permanent due to damage to the ossicles or cochlea.

Bibliography

Anderson KJ. Mastoiditis. *Pediatr Rev.* 2009;30(6):233–234.

Bluestone C, Simmons J, Healy G. *Complications and Sequelae of Otitis Media. Bluestone and Stool's Pediatric Otolaryngology.* 5th ed. 2014.

Bunik M. Mastoiditis. *Pediatr Rev.* 2014;35(2):94–95.

Drew N, Jeanmonod R. Bezold abscess: a rare complication of mastoiditis. *Am J Emerg Med.* 2013;31(11):1626.

Elder C, Hainline C, Galetta SL, et al. Isolated abducens nerve palsy: update on evaluation and diagnosis. *Curr Neurol Neurosci Rep.* 2016;16(8):69.

Kerschner JE, Preciado D. *Otitis Media. Nelson's Textbook of Pediatrics.* 20th ed. Elsevier; 2016:3085–3100.

Lieberthal AS, et al. The diagnosis and management of acute otitis media. *Pediatrics.* 2013;131(3):964–991.

Rosa-Olivares J, Porro A, Rodriguez-Varela M, et al. Otitis media: to treat, to refer, to do nothing: a review for the practitioner. *Pediatr Rev.* 2015;36(2):480–488.

Wald ER, Conway JR. *Mastoiditis. Principles and Practice of Pediatric Infectious Diseases.* 4th ed. 2012.

Wood WA, Raz Y. Intracranial complications of otitis media. In: Myers E, ed. *Operative Otolaryngology: Head and Neck Surgery.* Philadelphia: Elsevier; 2008.

20-Day-Old Premature Male Infant Who Develops Feeding Intolerance

Rebecca Meyer ■ Jennifer Shepherd

A male infant born at 29{5/7} weeks with a birth weight of 1450 g is now 20 days old in the neonatal intensive care unit (NICU). Enteral feeds with breast milk via a nasogastric tube were initiated on the second day of life. The caloric density of his feeds was recently increased from 22 to 24 cal/oz. With his most recent feed, he has a gastric residual of 12 mL, more than his usual volume of 1 to 2 mL.

What are some causes of feeding intolerance in a premature infant?
Feeding intolerance is the inability to digest feedings associated with increased gastric residuals, abdominal distention, and/or emesis. In preterm infants, gastric emptying and intestinal motility are immature, which can result in gastrointestinal reflux, gastric residuals, distension, delayed passage of meconium, bowel distension, and benign feeding intolerance. Sepsis in a neonate can cause a functional ileus, which can present with increased gastric residuals. Necrotizing enterocolitis (NEC) can also present with gastric residuals as an early sign.

BASIC SCIENCE PEARL   **STEP 1**

Preterm infants have decreased gastric acid secretion, impairing the activity of enterokinases, enzymes secreted by the duodenum that are necessary for the activation of pancreatic enzymes, which aid in digestion. Enterokinases require an acidic environment for proper functioning.

Case Point 54.1

The patient has been having increased number of apneic episodes, tachypnea, tachycardia, and an increased oxygen requirement. His temperature is 97.7°F, blood pressure is 78/36 mm Hg, mean arterial pressure is 50 mm Hg, pulse rate is 183 beats/min, respiration rate is 66 breaths/min, and oxygen saturation is 96% on 1 L/min of oxygen via nasal cannula. Patient is minimally reactive, tachypneic with subcostal retractions, and tachycardic. His abdomen is full, soft, and nontender, with bowel sounds.

What studies are important for further evaluation of an infant with new-onset feeding intolerance and clinical deterioration?
When an infant presents with feeding intolerance in the context of clinical deterioration, it should not be attributed to physiologic feeding intolerance due to prematurity without further investigation to

rule out more serious causes. This investigation should include evaluation for infection with a complete blood count (CBC), C-reactive protein (CRP) level, blood culture, and abdominal x-ray (AXR).

Case Point 54.2

CBC, CRP level, coagulation studies, capillary blood gas values, blood culture, and chemistry panel are sent (Table 54.1). The AXR demonstrates dilated bowel loops, pneumatosis intestinalis (air in the bowel wall), and portal venous air (Fig. 54.1). The patient passes a large, grossly bloody stool.

TABLE 54.1 ■ Laboratory Studies

Study	Result	Reference Value
Leukocyte count	3.2 K/μL	9–30 K/μL
Neutrophils	36%	3%–68%
Bands	19%	0%–15%
Lymphocytes	36%	26%–36%
Hemoglobin	7.7 g/dL	14–20 g/dL
Hematocrit	22.5%	42%–60%
Platelet count	451 K/μL	150–450 K/μL
C-reactive protein (high sensitivity)	9.1 mg/L	0–10 mg/L
Prothrombin time	19.4 sec	11.5–5.3 sec
International normalized ratio	1.67	0.86–1.22
Partial thromboplastin time	65.9 sec	35.1–46.3 sec
Fibrinogen	407 mg/dL	82–383 mg/dL
Sodium	127 mEq/L	130–145 mEq/L
Potassium	6.2 mEq/L	3.7–5.9 mEq/L
Chloride	93 mEq/L	97–108 mEq/L
Bicarbonate	19 mEq/L	20–4 mEq/L
Blood urea nitrogen	29 mg/dL	5–8 mg/dL
Creatinine	0.6 mg/dL	0.2–0.4 mg/dL
Glucose	132 mg/dL	50–90 mg/dL
Calcium	6.8 mg/dL	9–11 mg/dL
Magnesium	1.6 mg/dL	1.3–2.1 mg/dL
Phosphorus	7.8 mg/dL	4–6.5 mg/dL
Lactate	3.6 mmol/L	1.1–3.5 mmol/L
Capillary Blood Gas		
pH capillary	7.27	7.3–7.4
pco_2 capillary	51 mm Hg	35–45 mm Hg
po_2 capillary	30 mm Hg	
HCO_3 capillary	23 mEq/L	22–26 mEq/L
Base excess	–3.7 mEq/L	–2 to +2 mEq/L

What is necrotizing enterocolitis?

NEC is an acute inflammation and ischemia of the intestinal mucosa, often resulting in intestinal necrosis, and is a medical emergency. The overall incidence is 0.5 to 5/1000 live births and approximately 7% in infants with a birth weight less than 1500 g. The vast majority of cases of NEC occur in premature infants, with incidence and associated fatality rates inversely related to gestational age and birth weight. Surgical intervention for NEC is needed in up to 50% of cases.

In spite of numerous advances in the care of neonates, the morbidity and mortality due to NEC have remained essentially unchanged. The mortality rate associated with NEC approaches 30%, with significantly higher mortality in those requiring surgical intervention (35%) compared to those requiring medical treatment alone (21%).

What physical examination, laboratory, and radiographic findings are suggestive of necrotizing enterocolitis?

The examination findings in infants with NEC range from subtle signs to fulminant illness, with significant compromise. Gastrointestinal signs include feeding intolerance, delayed gastric emptying, abdominal distention, abdominal tenderness, discoloration of the abdominal wall, and bloody stools. Systemic symptoms include apnea, lethargy, respiratory distress, temperature instability, and decreased perfusion.

Patients with NEC can have abnormalities in their white blood cell count, which most often is decreased, but it can be elevated. Thrombocytopenia, prolongation of the prothrombin time, and hypofibrinogenemia can also be seen. Infants can present with hypoglycemia or hyperglycemia, hyponatremia, and metabolic acidosis. The CRP level is often elevated.

CLINICAL PEARL   **STEP 2/3**

The decreased white blood cell count in patients with NEC is due to decreased production and increased utilization of leukocytes.

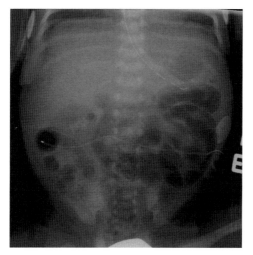

Fig. 54.1 This abdominal radiograph demonstrates loops of dilated bowel with the presence of pneumatosis in the right hemiabdomen and portal venous air. No free air is seen.

CLINICAL PEARL   **STEP 2/3**

Numerous biomarkers have been evaluated for their potential to diagnose NEC earlier and predict clinical course. However, to date, none are part of the standard evaluation of infants suspected of having NEC.

Findings on the AXR include pneumatosis intestinalis and portal venous gas. If bowel perforation is suspected, a two-view AXR should be obtained.

CLINICAL PEARL   **STEP 2/3**

Pneumatosis intestinalis is caused by hydrogen production by pathogenic bacteria. Pneumatosis intestinalis can also be seen in infants with Hirschsprung enterocolitis or severe gastroenteritis.

How is the severity of necrotizing enterocolitis classified?

Because of the wide spectrum of clinical presentations of NEC and lack of a uniform set of diagnostic criteria, Bell and colleagues, in 1978, proposed a system of classification. Table 54.2 lists the physical examination and radiographic signs associated with each stage of NEC.

TABLE 54.2 ■ **Staging of Necrotizing Enterocolitis (NEC)**

Stage	Classification of NEC	Systemic Signs	Abdominal Signs	Radiographic Signs
IA	Suspected	Temperature instability, apnea, bradycardia, lethargy	Gastric retention, abdominal distention, emesis, heme-positive stool	Normal or intestinal dilation, mild ileus
IB	Suspected	Same as above	Grossly bloody stool	Same as above
IIA	Definite, mildly ill	Same as above	Same as above, plus absent bowel sounds ± abdominal tenderness	Intestinal dilation, ileus, pneumatosis intestinalis
IIB	Definite, moderately ill	Same as above, plus mild metabolic acidosis, thrombocytopenia	Same as above, definite tenderness, ± abdominal cellulitis or RLQ mass	Same as IIA, plus ascites
IIIA	Advanced, severely ill, intact bowel	Same as above, plus hypotension, bradycardia, severe apnea, combined respiratory and metabolic acidosis, DIC, neutropenia	Same as above, plus signs of peritonitis, marked tenderness	Same as IIB
IIIB	Advanced, severely ill, perforated bowel	Same as IIIA	Same as IIIA	Same as IIIA, plus pneumoperitoneum

DIC, Disseminated intravascular coagulation; *RLQ,* right lower quadrant.
Adapted from Neu J. Necrotizing enterocolitis: the search for a unifying pathogenic theory leading to prevention. *Pediatr Clin North Am.* 1996;43:409–432.

What is the pathophysiology of necrotizing enterocolitis?
It has been suggested that a combination of numerous factors including genetics, immaturity of the intestinal tract and its functioning in preterm infants, alteration of the microbiome in premature infants, abnormal circulatory regulation, and an exaggerated inflammatory response to stimuli may all play a role in the development of NEC. The amount and diversity of bacteria in the neonate vary based on the mode of delivery, antibiotic exposure, diet, maternal flora, and even genetic background. Breastfeeding and vaginal birth contribute to more diversity, whereas antibiotic exposure decreases diversity. Very-low-birth-weight (VLBW) infants (those with birth weight <1500 g) are less likely than term infants to breast-feed after birth and are more likely to receive antibiotic therapy, resulting in less microbiome diversity. Additionally, preterm infants have more pathogenic organisms and fewer beneficial organisms.

What are the risk factors for developing necrotizing enterocolitis?
The most significant risk factors of developing NEC are prematurity, low birth weight, and enteral feeding. Risk is inversely related to birth weight and gestational age. The vast majority of NEC cases (>90%) present after the initiation of enteral feedings. Current neonatal practice uses a slow advancement of enteral feeding in an attempt to mediate the risk of enteral feeding.

CLINICAL PEARL   **STEP 2/3**

Up to 10% of cases of NEC occur in term infants, with clinical symptoms and pathologic findings similar to those found in preterm infants. Unlike in preterm infants, term infants usually have an underlying disorder or preexisting condition that predisposes them to developing NEC, such as perinatal asphyxia, congenital heart disease, myelomeningocele, polycythemia, exchange transfusion, intrauterine growth restriction, and gastroschisis.

Case Point 54.2

The infant is made NPO. Empiric antibiotic therapy is initiated with vancomycin, cefotaxime, and piperacillin-tazobactam. Over the course of the next 4 hours, the infant becomes increasingly lethargic, with worsening abdominal distention, abdominal tenderness, and erythema on the abdominal wall. Increasing apneic episodes necessitate intubation and mechanical ventilation.

How is necrotizing enterocolitis treated?
Basic NEC treatment consists of supportive care, antibiotic therapy, and frequent monitoring with clinical examination, laboratory studies, and radiologic evaluations. Supportive care includes bowel rest, decompression of the bowel, total parenteral nutrition, fluid and electrolyte management, correction of metabolic acidosis, support of the cardiovascular and respiratory systems, and correction of coagulopathies. The clinician should perform serial examinations and obtain regular radiographs to assess disease progression and for timely identification of pneumoperitoneum. Antibiotic therapy is a mainstay of NEC treatment. In general, therapy should include ampicillin and an aminoglycoside to cover both gram-positive and gram-negative organisms. However, due to the common use of ampicillin and gentamicin in premature infants in the NICU, pathogenic organisms can be resistant to these therapies. VLBW infants in the NICU are at risk for bacteremia from coagulase-negative *Staphylococcus*. Therefore, empiric treatment for NEC could consist of vancomycin, a third-generation cephalosporin, and an agent effective against anaerobic organisms.

For cases of suspected NEC (Bell's stage I), the duration of medical treatment is determined by the clinician based on clinical judgment. For definite cases of NEC (Bell's stage II or higher), medical treatment should continue for 7 to 14 days. If an infant has advanced disease, surgical intervention should be considered in addition to the other elements of treatment.

Case Point 54.3

> The patient is taken to the operating room for a laparotomy which reveals feculent material in the abdominal cavity and segments of necrotic bowel in the ileum, cecum, and right hemicolon requiring resection. A total of 50 cm of bowel is resected, including the ileocecal valve. A jejunostomy is created.

When does necrotizing enterocolitis require surgical intervention?
Surgical intervention for NEC is warranted when there is concern for bowel perforation or with worsening clinical status in spite of medical management. Perforation can be evident on an AXR with the presence of pneumoperitoneum (Fig. 54.2). In severe cases of pneumoperitoneum, a supine AXR can demonstrate the football sign, which occurs when the falciform ligament is outlined by intraperitoneal air (see Fig. 54.2). Pneumoperitoneum can also be suspected if the patient has significant abdominal distention, tenderness, or discoloration of the abdominal wall. Laboratory values including significant thrombocytopenia, metabolic acidosis, neutropenia, a left shift of segmented neutrophils, and hyponatremia are associated with more severe NEC and could warrant surgical exploration, even in the absence of obvious pneumoperitoneum. Bowel necrosis can be in a discrete segment of bowel—with the distal ileum being the most common site—in patchy areas on several portions of intestine, or may involve the entire gut, which is referred to as *necrotizing enterocolitis totalis* (NEC totalis).

Surgical intervention is usually done via a laparotomy with resection of the necrotic portions of bowel (see Fig. 54.2) and the creation of an intestinal stoma, although infrequently a primary anastomosis is performed. The other surgical intervention that can be considered is peritoneal drain placement.

CLINICAL PEARL   **STEP 2/3**

Even with appropriate medical management, 34% to 50% of patients with NEC require surgical intervention.

Case Point 54.4

> The infant's blood culture returns positive for *Streptococcus viridans*. He receives a total of 14 days of antibiotics after the first negative blood culture. Feeds are initiated with an elemental formula and advanced slowly. Once he reaches 100 mL/kg per day of enteral feeding, he develops loose watery output from his jejunostomy. Six weeks after his initial surgery, he has a reversal of his jejunostomy and reanastomosis of his intestines; however, he continues to have numerous watery stools daily and poor weight gain and is diagnosed with short bowel syndrome. He ultimately is discharged home with small-volume enteral feeds and long-term total parenteral nutrition.

What are the long-term sequelae of necrotizing enterocolitis?
Intestinal stricture is a common complication seen after an infant has developed NEC, with a rate of approximately 20%. Another common complication for infants after surgical intervention for NEC is the development of short bowel syndrome (SBS), defined as a reduction in gut function to a degree that prevents adequate growth, hydration, and/or electrolyte balance. The treatment of SBS focuses on ensuring appropriate nutrition, hydration, and electrolyte management

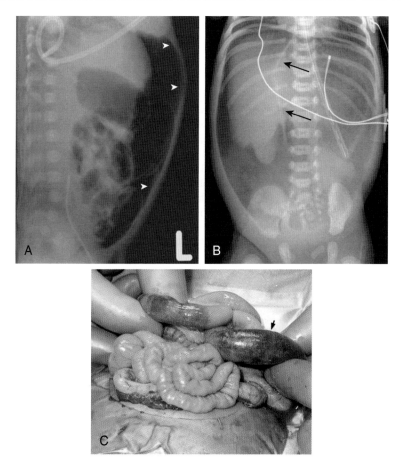

Fig. 54.2   (A) Free intraabdominal air on a lateral film *(arrowheads)*. (B) Free intraperitoneal air in an infant. The radiograph shows marked lucency and distention of the abdominal cavity. The falciform ligament *(arrows)* is seen outlined by air (football sign). (C) Clearly defined segments of bowel affected by NEC *(arrow)*. (A from Talmadge JC, Milla SS, Bixby SD. Imaging evaluation of common pediatric emergencies. In: Soto JA, Brian C, Lucey BC, eds. *Emergency Radiology: The Requisites*. 2nd ed. 2016:186–220; B from Donnelly LF. Gastrointestinal. In: Donnelly LF. *Pediatric Imaging: The Fundamentals*, Philadelphia: Saunders/Elsevier; 2009:86–124; C from Thakkar HS, Lakhoo K. The surgical management of necrotising enterocolitis (NEC). *Early Hum Dev.* 2016;97:25–28.)

while awaiting intestinal adaptation. Surgical lengthening techniques or intestinal transplantation may also be required. The most important factors in determining the outcome for patients with SBS are the length of bowel remaining after surgical resection and whether the ileocecal valve is present.

CLINICAL PEARL	STEP 2/3

For patients with short bowel syndrome, survival is increased if the length of the small intestine is at least 15 cm with a retained ileocecal valve, or if the length of the small intestine is at least 40 cm in the absence of the ileocecal valve.

Compared to other VLBW infants, infants with NEC are more prone to neurodevelopmental impairment later in life. Although the reason for this is unclear, damage to existing cerebral tissue by the acidosis, cytokine release, inflammation, fluctuations in glycemic regulation, and hypotension, all of which can accompany the acute phase of NEC, could play a role.

How can necrotizing enterocolitis be prevented?

The use of human milk—mother's own milk or donor breast milk—for feeding has been shown to decrease the risk of acquiring NEC compared to the use of formula. Fortification of breast milk is standard practice in the NICU to provide preterm infants with adequate calories and minerals. In an attempt to prevent NEC, enteral feeds for premature and VLBW infants are most often initiated at a very small volume and increased incrementally until the full volume is tolerated. One hypothesis that has been offered to support this incremental increase in feeds is that overdistention of the stomach with large volumes may impair splanchnic blood flow, leading to ischemia. Numerous studies have examined the effectiveness of probiotic supplementation for the prevention of NEC and, although a recent meta-analysis has suggested that probiotics may be effective for preventing NEC, lingering safety concerns and lack of consensus regarding which type of probiotic and in what dose has prevented universal acceptance of their use in the neonatal community.

BEYOND THE PEARLS

- The use of H2 blockers contributes to the development of NEC in VLBW infants. The proposed theory is that by creating a less acidic gastric environment, H2 blockers allow for bacterial overgrowth in the gastrointestinal tract, which can thereby lead to NEC.
- There is ongoing debate regarding the role of blood transfusion in the development of NEC. Although some studies have suggested that transfusion could be a risk factor for the development of NEC, others have suggested that significant anemia rather than the subsequent transfusion is the risk factor.
- Anal fissure and cow's milk protein allergy are also causes of hematochezia in a neonate. However, usually these infants are otherwise clinically well-appearing. Cow's milk protein allergy is uncommon in premature infants.
- Bowel perforation in a preterm infant during the first week of life or before the initiation of feeds is more likely to be spontaneous intestinal perforation (SIP) rather than NEC. Risk factors for SIP include birth weight less than 1500 g, prematurity, indomethacin exposure, and postnatal steroid exposure.
- Only approximately 17% of infants with NEC have a positive blood culture during the acute phase of NEC. Bloodstream infections in VLBW infants during the acute phase of NEC are much more likely to be due to gram-negative organisms than bloodstream infections that occur in VLBW infants that are not concurrent with NEC.

Case Summary

Complaint/History: A 20-day-old, 29-week gestational age premature infant develops increased residual feeds and apneic episodes.

Findings: Tachycardia, tachypnea, lethargy, prolonged capillary refill, erythema of the abdominal wall, bloody stool.

Labs/Tests: Laboratory studies show leukopenia, bandemia, and hyponatremia. Abdominal x-ray shows dilated loops of bowel, portal venous gas, and pneumatosis intestinalis; blood culture positive for *Streptococcus viridans*.

Diagnosis: Necrotizing enterocolitis.

Treatment: NPO, intravenous antibiotics, exploratory laparotomy with necrotic bowel resection, and jejunostomy.

Bibliography

Bell MJ, Ternberg JL, Feigin RD, et al. Neonatal necrotizing enterocolitis: therapeutic decisions based upon clinical staging. *Ann Surg.* 1978;187(1):1–7.

Bohnhorst B, Müller S, Dördelmann M, et al. Early feeding after necrotizing enterocolitis in preterm infants. *J Pediatr.* 2003;143(4):484–487.

Dimmitt RA, Moss RL. Clinical management of necrotizing enterocolitis. *Neoreviews.* 2001:1–10.

Frost BL, Modi BP, Jaksic T, et al. New medical and surgical insights into neonatal necrotizing enterocolitis. *JAMA Pediatr.* 2017;171(1):83–86.

Heida FH, Loos MHJ, Stolwijk L, et al. Risk factors associated with postnecrotizing enterocolitis strictures in infants. *J Pediatr Surg.* 2016;51(7):1126–1130.

Hull MA, Fisher JG, Gutierrez IM, et al. Mortality and management of surgical necrotizing enterocolitis in very low birth weight neonates: a prospective cohort study. *J Am Coll Surg.* 2014;218(6):1148–1155.

Lin PW, Stoll BJ. Necrotising enterocolitis. *The Lancet.* 2006;368(9543):1271–1283.

Maayan-Metzger A, Itzchak A, Mazkereth R, et al. Necrotizing enterocolitis in full-term infants: case–control study and review of the literature. *J Perinatol.* 2004;24(8):494–499.

Raval MV, Moss RL. Surgical necrotizing enterocolitis: a primer for the neonatologist. *Neoreviews.* 2013;14(8):e393–e401.

After Delivery, a Full-Term Newborn Is Lethargic, With Poor Respiratory Effort

Rebecca Meyer ■ Jennifer Shepherd

You are called to an emergency cesarean section for fetal distress at 39 3/7 weeks of gestation. A male infant is delivered through meconium-stained amniotic fluid. He is brought to the radiant warmer and is noted to be pale and floppy, with minimal respiratory effort and a heart rate more than 100 beats/min. You warm and stimulate him and provide bulb suctioning to clear his airway. He develops grunting, so you initiate continuous positive airway pressure (CPAP) at 5 cm H_2O with 21% oxygen. His work of breathing and color improve. He is transferred to the neonatal intensive care unit (NICU) for further management of respiratory distress.

What are common causes of respiratory distress in the neonate?

Respiratory distress in the neonate is common, affecting up to 7% of term infants. It can present with tachypnea, nasal flaring, retractions, or grunting and can be caused by pulmonary and nonpulmonary diseases. Transient tachypnea of the newborn (TTN) is caused by retained fetal lung fluid due to delayed clearance (Fig. 55.1A). It is a self-limited process and usually resolves within 48 hours. Respiratory distress syndrome (RDS) is caused by a deficiency of surfactant and is most common in preterm infants (Fig. 55.1B). Infants with RDS often require respiratory support, and some require administration of exogenous surfactant. Meconium aspiration syndrome (MAS) occurs when an infant passes meconium in utero and subsequently aspirates the meconium in utero or during delivery (Fig. 55.1C). It rarely occurs before 34 weeks of gestation. Meconium aspiration causes inflammation, surfactant deactivation, and obstruction of distal airways. For infants who have received positive pressure as part of the resuscitation at delivery and have respiratory distress, pneumothorax must also be considered (see Fig. 55.1D), although pneumothorax can also occur spontaneously. Infants with pneumothorax have diminished or absent breath sounds on the affected side and may have chest wall asymmetry on examination.

Numerous other disease states can present with respiratory distress (Box 55.1). Some common nonpulmonary causes of respiratory distress in a neonate include sepsis, hypoglycemia, congenital heart disease, and polycythemia.

BASIC SCIENCE PEARL   **STEPS 1/2/3**

The risk of respiratory disease among neonates decreases as gestational age increases. Among infants born at term, those born at 37 weeks have higher rates of RDS, TTN, pneumonia, RDS and use of high-frequency oscillatory ventilation compared to those born at 39 weeks.

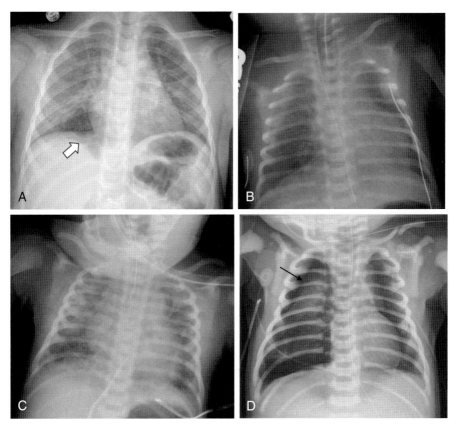

Fig. 55.1 (A) A 3-hour old, full-term boy born by cesarean section with transient tachypnea of the newborn (TTN). The frontal chest radiograph demonstrates bilateral pulmonary interstitial opacities and trace fluid *(arrow)* in the minor fissure. (B) Respiratory distress syndrome—diffusely hazy, with ground glass appearance and air bronchograms. (C) The chest x-ray (CXR) of this infant with meconium aspiration syndrome (MAS) demonstrates bilaterally patchy infiltrates and scattered asymmetric areas of both atelectasis and hyperinflation due to air trapping. (D) This infant has a right-sided pneumothorax. The CXR shows right-sided pleural air lacking peripheral lung markings. The *arrow* demonstrates the lung border. (A from Liszewski M, Stanescu AL, Phillips GS, Lee EY. Respiratory distress in neonates: underlying causes and current imaging assessment. *Radiol Clinics North Am.* 2017;55(4):629–644; B–D from Suprenant S, Coghlan MA. Respiratory distress in the newborn, an approach for the emergency care provider. *Clin Pediatr Emerg Med.* 2016;17(2):113–121.)

BASIC SCIENCE PEARL   **STEP 1**

Grunting occurs as an infant forces air against a partially closed glottis in an attempt to maintain adequate functional reserve capacity.

Case Point 55.1

On admission to the NICU, his vital signs are as follows: temperature is 97.7°F, blood pressure is 74/51 mm Hg, mean arterial pressure is 59 mm Hg, pulse rate is 167 beats/min, respiration rate is 76 breaths/min, and oxygen saturation is 94%, with nasal CPAP at 5 cm H_2O and Fio_2 of 30%. His birth weight is 3670 g. On physical examination, you see an appropriate for gestational age male, with decreased tone and reactivity to examination. His anterior fontanelle is soft and flat. He has a nasal cannula in place. He is tachypneic, with equal breath sounds, mild nasal flaring, intermittent grunting, and subcostal retractions. His cardiac examination is notable for absence of a murmur. His skin is pale.

BOX 55.1 ■ Differential Diagnosis of Respiratory Distress in the Newborn

Upper Airway:

Choanal atresia, nasal stenosis, Pierre-Robin anomaly, macroglossia, subglottic stenosis, external compression from mass, vascular rings, tracheoesophageal fistula

Pulmonary:

- *Congenital:* pulmonary hypoplasia, CDH, chylothorax, CPAM, BPS, surfactant deficiency
- *Acquired:* RDS, TTN, MAS, pneumonia, pneumothorax, PPHN, pleural effusion

Cardiovascular:

Cyanotic heart diseases, select acyanotic congenital heart defects, cardiomyopathy, pericardial effusion, tamponade

Neuromuscular:

Hypoxic-ischemic encephalopathy, hydrocephalus, narcotic withdrawal, medications (maternal sedation, antidepressants, magnesium), seizure, congenital myopathies

Hematologic:

Polycythemia, severe anemia

Metabolic:

Hypoglycemia, inborn errors of metabolism

Miscellaneous:

Sepsis, metabolic acidosis, hypothermia or hyperthermia

BPS, Bronchopulmonary sequestration; *CDH,* congenital diaphragmatic hernia; *CPAM,* congenital pulmonary airway malformation; *MAS,* meconium aspiration syndrome; *PPHN,* persistent pulmonary hypertension; *RDS,* respiratory distress syndrome; *TTN,* transient tachypnea of the newborn.

Adapted from Pramanik, AK, Rangaswamy, N, Gates, T. Neonatal respiratory distress: a practical approach to its diagnosis and management. *Pediatr Clin North Am.* 2015;62:453–469.

Case Point 55.2

A chest x-ray (CXR; Fig. 55.2) shows increased interstitial lung markings, without evidence of consolidation, effusion, or pneumothorax, and a normal cardiac silhouette. A complete blood count (CBC), capillary blood gas (CBG), blood glucose level, and blood culture were obtained at admission. Respiratory support is escalated to noninvasive positive-pressure ventilation. Because of his metabolic acidosis, you provide a normal saline bolus of 10 mL/kg and, to correct his hypoglycemia, you administer a bolus of dextrose 10% in water, 2 mL/kg, and start dextrose-containing intravenous fluids at 80 mL/kg per day. One hour later, his blood gas shows significant improvement in all parameters. His blood glucose level normalizes. You initiate antibiotic therapy with ampicillin, 50 mg/kg Q12H, and gentamicin, 4 mg/kg Q24H. At 12 hours of life, a C-reactive protein (CRP) level and repeat CBC are sent. The results of the laboratory studies are shown in Table 55.1.

What is neonatal sepsis?

Neonatal sepsis can be divided into two broad categories, each of which carries its own risk factors, pathophysiology, likely causative organisms, and treatment. Early-onset sepsis (EOS) is defined as signs or symptoms of sepsis with an associated positive culture within 72 hours of life; late-onset sepsis (LOS) is defined as signs or symptoms associated with sepsis at 72 hours after birth.

The diagnosis of sepsis is challenging due to the wide variety and severity of presenting features, many of which can mimic symptoms of other diseases. Although the gold standard of

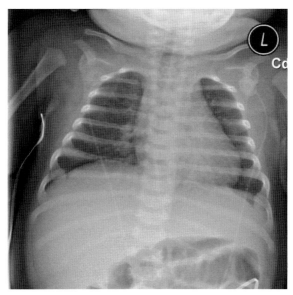

Fig. 55.2 This chest radiograph demonstrates appropriate lung volumes, with mildly increased interstitial lung marking bilaterally. There is no evidence of pneumothorax, pleural effusion, or focal consolidation. The cardiac silhouette is within normal limits.

TABLE 55.1 ■ **Laboratory Studies**

Study	Admission	12 Hours	Reference Value
Leukocyte count	8.3 K/μL	7.5 K/μL	9–30 K/μL
Neutrophils	37%	32%	38%–68%
Bands	26%	35%	0%–15%
Lymphocytes	27%	23%	26%–36%
Hemoglobin	13.5 g/dL	13 g/dL	14–20 g/dL
Hematocrit	40.5%	36.3%	42%–60%
Platelet count	195 × 10^9/L	154 × 10^9/L	150–450 × 10^9/L
C-reactive protein	—	7.8 mg/dL	0–0.5 mg/dL
Glucose	16 mg/dL		45–90 mg/dL
Capillary Blood Gas			
pH	7.03		7.3–7.4
pCO_2	74 mm Hg		35–45 mm Hg
pO_2	39 mm Hg		
HCO_3	14 mEq/L		22–26 mEq/L
Base excess	–12.6 mEq/L		–2 to +2 mEq/L

diagnosis for sepsis is a positive culture, a diagnosis of probable sepsis is often made based on the clinical presentation and evaluation of laboratory study results, even in the absence of a positive culture result.

The overall incidence of EOS is approximately 0.3 to 1/1000 live births, and the incidence increases with decreasing birth weight. For term infants, mortality due to EOS is approximately 3%; however, mortality reaches 30% to 54% in preterm infants. LOS occurs in approximately 36% of preterm infants with gestational age less than 28 weeks, and its incidence decreases with increasing birth weight and gestational age.

What is the clinical presentation of an infant with sepsis?

The symptoms of EOS generally present while the infant is still in the hospital after birth. LOS can present while an infant is still in the hospital or after discharge home. The clinical presentation of an infant with sepsis is nonspecific and can range from asymptomatic to shock. Some common symptoms include respiratory distress, hemodynamic instability, lethargy, poor feeding, metabolic acidosis, hypoglycemia, hyperglycemia, and jaundice. Neonates with meningitis may have a full fontanelle, seizures, irritability, and/or lethargy.

Case Point 55.3

You obtain additional history about the infant's mother. She is a 24-year-old G2P2 woman, with no significant medical history. Her only medication during the pregnancy was prenatal vitamins. She had appropriate prenatal care. The onset of labor was spontaneous, and the membranes ruptured 19 hours prior to the infant's delivery. Her prenatal laboratory results were unremarkable, including group B streptococci (GBS)–negative status.

What is the pathophysiology of sepsis?

EOS is thought to result from the vertical transmission of a causative organism, either through contaminated amniotic fluid or via exposure of the infant to flora from the mother's genitourinary tract. LOS can result from vertical transmission or horizontal transmission via contact with the environment or caregivers.

What risk factors are associated with sepsis?

The most significant risk factors for EOS are maternal colonization with group B streptococci (GBS), chorioamnionitis, maternal fever, prolonged rupture of membranes (>18 hours), and inadequate antibiotic prophylaxis during the intrapartum period. Additionally, premature infants and infants with lower birth weight are more susceptible to EOS.

Extreme prematurity is the greatest risk factor for LOS due to the impaired immune function of preterm infants, making them more vulnerable to invasive infection. Additional risk factors for LOS include mechanical ventilation, vascular catheters, hospitalization, surgery, and respiratory or cardiac disease.

Case Point 55.4

Approximately 17 hours after the infant's blood culture was sent to the laboratory, it is growing *Escherichia coli*, sensitive to gentamicin and cefotaxime. A repeat blood culture is sent and remains negative. Lumbar puncture is performed with a reassuring cell count glucose and protein from the cerebrospinal fluid (CSF). CSF culture is sent and remains negative. The antimicrobial therapy is changed to cefotaxime, 50 mg/kg bid.

Which infants should be evaluated for sepsis?

In EOS, evaluation should be performed if an infant has physical examination findings concerning for infection, if the infant is born in the setting of chorioamnionitis or maternal fever, even if asymptomatic, or if the mother is GBS-positive without adequate intrapartum antibiotic prophylaxis. The Centers for Disease Control and Prevention has released guidelines regarding the management of infants at risk for GBS sepsis and, based on the presence or absence of various perinatal risk factors, these guidelines recommend a full laboratory evaluation with empiric antibiotic therapy, laboratory evaluation alone, observation for 48 hours after birth, or routine care.

If the clinician is concerned about LOS in an infant, after obtaining laboratory studies and appropriate cultures, empiric antibiotic therapy should be initiated, particularly in the presence of risk factors such as the presence of an intravascular catheter or prolonged intubation.

What is the laboratory evaluation of infants suspected of having sepsis?

A CBC with differential should be sent to evaluate the white blood cell count and differential. Infants with EOS often demonstrate leukopenia and a high percentage of immature white blood cells. Infants with LOS may have a high or low white blood cell count, a high neutrophil count, and a high percentage of immature white blood cells.

Acute-phase reactants are often part of the evaluation of infants suspected of having EOS. The CRP level is a measure of the inflammatory response in a neonate; it begins to rise within 6 to 8 hours of exposure to infection and peaks at 24 hours following infection. The negative predictive value of two consecutive normal CRP levels has been reported as 99.7%; thus, if an infant has a consistently normal CRP level, the likelihood of bacterial sepsis is low. The CRP level is also useful for infants suspected of having LOS, and an elevated value is concerning for infection. Another serum biomarker used to evaluate infants suspected of having sepsis is procalcitonin. The procalcitonin concentration peaks at 2 to 12 hours after an infectious exposure and is more sensitive, but less specific than the CRP level for predicting bacterial sepsis.

CLINICAL PEARL   **STEPS 2/3**

The I/T ratio is the ratio of immature to total neutrophils. Immature neutrophils include bands, metamyelocytes, myelocytes, and promyelocytes. A value greater than 0.22 in infants younger than 32 weeks and greater than 0.27 in term infants is considered elevated and concerning for sepsis.

Cultures are required to identify a causative organism. A blood culture should be sent on any infant suspected of having EOS or LOS. A urine culture should not be sent routinely in infants suspected of having EOS, but should be sent on infants suspected of having LOS. The decision to perform lumbar puncture should be based on the infant's clinical presentation. However, if an infant has a positive blood culture, does not improve with antimicrobial therapy, or has laboratory findings that are strongly suggestive of bacterial sepsis, the infant should be evaluated for meningitis with a lumbar puncture. Lumbar puncture should also be performed in neonates with fever. If the infant is intubated, culture should also be sent on aspirate from the endotracheal tube.

CLINICAL PEARL   **STEPS 2/3**

In infants with bacteremia, as many as 23% have concurrent meningitis. In 38% of infants with meningitis, the blood culture is negative. It is uncommon for a neonate with meningitis to present with meningismus.

Which bacteria most commonly cause sepsis, and how is sepsis treated?

The two most common organisms that cause EOS are GBS and *E. coli*. Combined, they account for 62% of cases of EOS. Empiric therapy for EOS is usually ampicillin and gentamicin. For LOS, the most common pathogen is coagulase-negative staphylococci, which accounts for over

50% of LOS cases in the United States. Vancomycin and an aminoglycoside are commonly used as empiric therapy; however, a third-generation cephalosporin could be added if there is concern for gram-negative meningitis. Once a pathogen has been identified, antibiotic therapy should be tailored to the causative organism and susceptibilities for the duration of therapy.

For infants with uncomplicated bacteremia, treatment should be for 10 days. For cases of gram-negative bacteremia, treatment may extend to 14 days. For infants with uncomplicated GBS meningitis, treatment should continue for a minimum of 14 days, whereas those with gram-negative meningitis should be treated for 21 days or for 14 days after the first negative culture, whichever is longer. For infants whose clinical presentation, risk factors, and laboratory studies suggest sepsis, but whose culture does not grow an organism, the clinician must use his or her clinical judgment to determine the duration of therapy. In infants for whom empiric therapy has been initiated, but—based on laboratory results, clinical conditions, and negative culture results—the probability of sepsis has been determined to be low, antimicrobial therapy should be discontinued at 48 hours.

CLINICAL PEARL   **STEPS 2/3**

Antibiotic dosing for neonates is calculated based on an infant's weight, gestational age, and post-menstrual age. For infants suspected of having group B streptococci (GBS) meningitis, ampicillin is used at a dose of 200 to 300 mg/kg/day divided every 8 hours. Gentamicin has been associated with ototoxicity and nephrotoxicity. Close attention should be paid to an infant's renal function and hydration status while on gentamicin. Serum drug peak and trough levels should be monitored for infants undergoing prolonged therapy.

Case Point 55.5

The infant completes 14 days of antibiotic therapy. His laboratory studies normalize, and he is weaned off respiratory support to room air. He is discharged home after completion of antibiotic therapy.

How can bacterial sepsis be prevented?

The most significant intervention used to prevent EOS has been the routine use of intrapartum antibiotic prophylaxis for a mother colonized with GBS. Since the guidelines for intrapartum prophylaxis have been implemented, the incidence of EOS due to GBS has decreased by 80%. Neither the incidence of LOS due to GBS nor that of sepsis due to *E. coli* has changed with the routine use of intrapartum antibiotic prophylaxis.

Efforts to prevent LOS include careful hand hygiene and timely removal of unnecessary vascular catheters and endotracheal tubes.

What are the outcomes associated with neonatal sepsis?

Sepsis is one of the primary causes of neonatal mortality worldwide. Even with appropriate treatment, those who survive are at risk for long-term sequelae. Infants with sepsis have increased risk for delayed motor development, delayed cognitive development, and cerebral palsy. Those with meningitis have additional risks of hearing and vision impairment, seizures, neurodevelopmental impairment, and behavioral problems.

Case Summary

Complaint/History: A full-term newborn male has respiratory distress and pallor after delivery.
Findings: The infant is delivered with meconium-stained amniotic fluid. He is hypotonic, with minimal response to stimuli, tachycardic and tachypneic with nasal flaring and retractions.

Labs/Tests: Hypoglycemia, elevated C-reactive protein level, metabolic and respiratory acidosis; blood culture is positive for *E. coli;* chest x-ray shows bilateral interstitial markings.
Diagnosis: Early-onset neonatal sepsis.
Treatment: Intravenous antibiotics.

BEYOND THE PEARLS

- Although most bacteria that cause EOS arise from the mother's urogenital tract, some pathogenic bacteria can cross the placenta, such as *Treponema pallidum* and *Listeria monocytogenes.*
- By 24 hours after collection, 91% of pathogenic blood cultures will be positive, and 99% will be positive by 48 hours. A sample of at least 1 mL of blood should be collected for blood culture because infants often have a low colony count of bacteria. Therefore, a smaller sample volume could lead to a false-negative result.
- In neonates for whom a third-generation cephalosporin is indicated for therapy, ceftriaxone should be avoided because it has the potential to displace bilirubin from albumin, thereby increasing the potential for kernicterus. Cefotaxime could be used as an alternative.
- Fungemia, usually due to *Candida* spp., accounts for approximately 2.5% of bloodstream infections in very-low-birth-weight infants and should be considered in these infants when evaluating for LOS.
- Omphalitis, an infection of the umbilicus or surrounding tissue in neonates, can lead to systemic infection because bacteria can enter the bloodstream through the umbilical vessels.
- For infants being evaluated for sepsis in whom herpes simplex virus is on the differential diagnosis, acyclovir should be added to the empiric antimicrobial regimen until the infant's diagnostic study results are available.

Bibliography

Bentlin MR, de Souza Rugolo LMS. Late-onset sepsis: epidemiology, evaluation, and outcome. *Neoreviews.* 2010;11(8):e426–e435.

Dong Y, Speer CP. Late-onset neonatal sepsis: recent developments. *Arch Dis Child Fetal Neonatal Ed.* 2015;100(3):F257–F263.

Gerdes JS. Diagnosis and management of bacterial infections in the neonate. *Pediatr Clin North Am.* 2004;51(4):939–959.

Leonard EG, Dobbs K. Postnatal bacterial infections. *Fanaroff and Martin's Neonatal-Perinatal Medicine,* 10th ed. Richard J. Martin, Avroy A. Fanaroff, Michele C. Walsh, eds. Philadelphia: Elsevier; 2015: 734–750.

Mahoney AD, Jain L. Respiratory disorders in moderately preterm, late preterm, and early term infants. *Clinics in Perinatology.* 2013;40(4):665–678.

Mukhopadhyay S, Puopolo KM. Neonatal early-onset sepsis: epidemiology and risk assessment. *Neoreviews.* 2015;16(4):e221–e230.

Polin RA and the Committee on Fetus and Newborn. Management of neonates with suspected or proven early-onset bacterial sepsis. *Pediatrics.* 2012;129(5):1006–1015.

Reuter S, Moser C, Baack M. Respiratory distress in the newborn. *Pediatr Rev.* 2014;35(10):417–428.

Schrag SJ, Farley MM, Petit S, et al. Epidemiology of invasive early-onset neonatal sepsis, 2005 to 2014. *Pediatrics.* 2016;138(6):e20162013–e20162013.

Stoll BJ, Hansen NI, Sánchez PJ, et al. Early onset neonatal sepsis: the burden of group B Streptococcal and E. coli disease continues. *Pediatrics.* 2011;127(5):817–826.

4-Year-Old Male Has Right-Side Facial Weakness

Robyn Kuroki ▦ Cynthia H. Ho

A 4-year-old male presents with worsening right facial weakness for 5 days.

What is the differential diagnosis of facial weakness?
Facial weakness can be classified in the following ways: (1) unilateral or bilateral; (2) congenital or acquired; (3) central or peripheral nerve dysfunction. Most facial weakness is unilateral and has a peripheral nerve cause. Congenital facial weakness can be due to trauma during delivery or an inherited condition such as Moebius syndrome, which causes bilateral facial droop. Infections such as acute otitis media, Lyme disease (Fig. 56.1), varicella zoster virus (VZV), and human immunodeficiency virus (HIV) infection can cause facial nerve paralysis. Traumatic facial nerve palsy should be suspected in patients with a temporal bone fracture. Bell's palsy is an idiopathic facial palsy possibly associated with herpes simplex virus (HSV) infection (Fig. 56.2). It accounts for approximately 25% of cases of acute facial palsy in children.

CLINICAL PEARL   **STEP 1/2/3**

Normal mental status and involvement of both the upper and lower face suggest a peripheral nerve cause. Involvement of the lower motor neuron of a unilateral facial nerve (FN VII) causes the Bell's palsy, characterized by the inability to close the eyelid. The patient's affected eye gazes upward. Sparing of the upper portion of the face, mental status changes, and multiple cranial neuropathies suggest an upper motor neuron (UMN) lesion (see Fig. 56.2)

Case Point 56.1

The boy's mother reports that her son also has slurred speech, decreased energy, and a wide-based, unsteady gait. The child had a febrile illness 1 week ago.

CLINICAL PEARL   **STEP 2/3**

When evaluating a patient with facial weakness, it is important to perform a thorough review of symptoms with your differential diagnosis in mind. Parents and patients may focus on one symptom and may not mention other relevant symptoms unless asked.

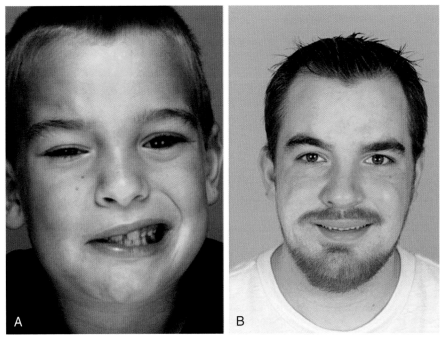

Fig. 56.1 Facial paralysis due to Lyme disease. (A) An 11-year-old boy with right facial paralysis due to Lyme disease diagnosed at 4 years of age. The patient underwent multimodality treatment, including intravenous antibiotics, cross-facial nerve grafting (CFNG), and botulinum toxin injections. (B) Patient at adulthood showing resolution of facial paralysis. (From Terzis J, Karypidis D. Therapeutic strategies in post-facial paralysis synkinesis in pediatric patients. *J Plast Reconstr Aesthet Surg.* 2012;65(8):1009–1018.)

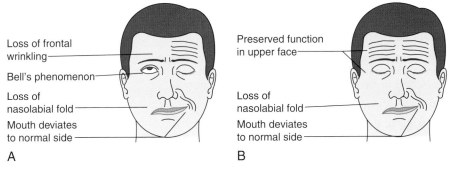

Fig. 56.2 Unilateral facial nerve VII paralysis. (A) Involvement of the lower motor neuron of the facial nerve results in an inability to close the affect eyelid. The patient's gaze points upward, with exposure of the conjunctiva below the cornea (Bell's palsy). (B) An upper motor neuron lesion showing sparing of the upper facial nerve function allows the patient to close the eyelid. (From Douglas G, Nicol F, Robertson C. *MacLeod's Clinical Examination.* 13th ed. London: Churchill Livingstone/Elsevier; 2013.)

CLINICAL PEARL	**STEP 2/3**

Decreased energy in a child may be a subtle sign suggesting a central nervous system (CNS) process.

TABLE 56.1 ▓ Pediatric Vital Signs

Age	Heart Rate (beats/ min)	Systolic Blood Pressure (mm Hg)	Diastolic Blood Pressure (mm Hg)	Respiratory Rate (breaths/min)
Premature	120–170	55–75	35–45	40–70
0–3 mo	100–150	65–85	45–55	35–55
3–6 mo	90–120	70–90	50–65	30–45
6–12 mo	80–120	80–100	55–65	25–40
1–3 yr	70–110	90–105	55–70	20–30
3–6 yr	65–110	95–110	60–75	20–25
6–12 yr	60–95	100–120	60–75	14–22
12+ yr	55–85	110–135	65–85	12–18

From Kliegman R, Stanton B, St. Geme J, eds. *Nelson Textbook of Pediatrics*. 20th ed. Philadelphia: Elsevier; 2016.

CLINICAL PEARL   **STEP 2/3**

Because many children have stranger anxiety, they may not respond to questions when asked by a clinician. Therefore, it is important to ask caregivers if the child's behavior is normal or whether she or he seems confused or irritable. Subtle changes in mental status are often detected only by family members or caregivers who know the child well.

Case Point 56.2

On review of systems, the boy's mother reports no seizure activity, mental status changes, vision changes, or abnormal eye movements.

CLINICAL PEARL   **STEP 2/3**

UMN conditions are associated with an alteration in mental status (encephalopathy). Facial nerve paralysis with encephalopathy raises suspicion for acute disseminated encephalomyelitis (ADEM), multiple sclerosis and, rarely, neurosarcoidosis.

Case Point 56.3

The lack of encephalopathy, other cranial neuropathies, and facial weakness involving the upper and lower face suggest a peripheral facial nerve palsy. The nurse hands you the following vital signs: temperature of 38.8°C, heart rate of 140 beats/min, respiratory rate of 24 breaths/min, blood pressure of 115/68 mm Hg, and oxygen saturation 98% on room air.

Which vital signs are abnormal?

You repeat the vital signs, ensure a properly sized blood pressure cuff, and obtain similar measurements (Table 56.1). The patient is febrile, tachycardic, and hypertensive for his age. These findings suggest autonomic dysfunction. Of pediatric patients with Guillain-Barré syndrome (GBS), also known as acute inflammatory demyelinating polyradiculopathy (AIDP), 50% present with signs of autonomic dysfunction, such as tachycardia, bradycardia, hypertension, ileus, bladder dysfunction, or abnormal sweating.

CLINICAL PEARL   STEP 2/3

Normal pediatric vital signs vary by age. The normal range of blood pressure measurements varies by gender, height, and age.

CLINICAL PEARL   STEP 2/3

You repeat the vital signs and they are often abnormal when a child is agitated while obtaining the heart rate, respiratory rate, and blood pressure. When you see vital signs that may be explained by agitation, repeat the vital signs when the child is in a position of comfort, usually in the parent's lap in a quiet room.

CLINICAL PEARL   STEP 2/3

An appropriate blood pressure cuff size has a bladder width measuring 40% of the arm circumference and cuff length of 80% of the arm. A large blood pressure cuff can give falsely low measurements, and a small blood pressure cuff can give falsely high blood pressure measurements.

Case Point 56.4

On examination, he is tired-appearing but playful and interactive. Right facial droop involves both the upper and lower face. His speech is dysarthric. Extraocular movements are intact, and the tongue is midline. He has normal tone, sensation, and muscle bulk. He is able to move against resistance in his upper extremities, but only antigravity movement is noted in the lower extremities. Upper extremity (biceps and triceps) deep tendon reflexes are slightly decreased, whereas lower extremity (patellar and Achilles) reflexes are absent. He is able to sit unsupported but unable to walk without assistance.

CLINICAL PEARL   STEP 2/3

In a young child, it is all right to perform the neurologic examination out of order and keep the child's comfort in mind because anxiety can affect his/her cooperation. Observe how the child interacts when you engage him/her with play. Watch how he/she reaches for an object or the child withdraws from you. Are movements symmetric? Much of the neurologic examination can be evaluated by observation alone. Get creative when performing a pediatric neurologic examination. For example, have the child walk toward the mother or father when you are trying to evaluate gait or have the child visually track a small toy to evaluate extraocular movements.

What is the difference between muscle tone and strength?
Tone is the length of the muscle at rest. Tone is evaluated by the amount of resistance during passive movement. Strength is the muscle's ability to contract in response to resistance. Patients with a lower motor neuron process or acute upper motor neuron injury or insult present with hypotonia. Hypertonia occurs as a result of dysfunction of inhibitory neurons and unopposed muscle contraction.

What is the significance of truncal (axial) versus appendicular (extremity) weakness?
Appendicular weakness (extremities only) suggests a peripheral nerve or muscle problem. In contrast, both truncal and appendicular weakness raises concern for a cerebellar or upper motor neuron lesion.

What are the causes of ataxia?

True ataxia is due to cerebellar pathology. With ataxia, gait is wide-based and unsteady. Ataxia due to cerebellar disease is associated with speech abnormalities, truncal instability, impaired coordination, decreased tone, tremor, and nystagmus. Ataxia should be distinguished from unsteady gait due to weakness or decreased sensation. In this patient, decreased strength and reflexes result in a wide-based gait. Lack of truncal instability, dyscoordination, change in tone, and nystagmus suggest a peripheral nerve lesion.

Case Point 56.5

> The patient's mother asks you what tests are going to be done to understand what is going on. You ensure her that you will need to consider all things in the history and physical examination before proceeding with a workup. You identify the following problems: right facial weakness for 5 days, bilateral lower extremity weakness, absent lower extremity reflexes, slurred speech, and fever.

What diagnoses are you considering in the differential diagnosis?

Bilateral lower extremity weakness and depressed reflexes, along with signs of autonomic dysfunction (fever, hypertension, and tachycardia), support the diagnosis of GBS. It is important to think of GBS because the weakness is ascending and can affect the respiratory muscles, leading to respiratory failure and posing a medical emergency. Tick paralysis is another diagnosis that can cause ascending weakness and should be considered in endemic areas or if travel history supports exposure. Spinal cord tumors and other spinal cord lesions, such as hematomas, hemorrhages, abscesses, and arteriovenous malformations, can all cause weakness secondary to the compression of nerve roots and are also medical emergencies. Fever is consistent with an epidural abscess and hematomas, hemorrhages, and arteriovenous malformations can potentially be superinfected, leading to fevers, although other findings of facial weakness and slurred speech are not consistent with these diagnoses. Transverse myelitis, acute postinfectious demyelinating encephalomyelitis (ADEM), and viral-related acute flaccid myelitis should also be considered, given the patient's recent infection 1 week ago, in addition to the neurologic symptoms. Additionally, toxins (e.g., lead, carbon monoxide, alcohol, inhalants), some medications (e.g., anticonvulsants, benzodiazepines), electrolyte abnormalities (e.g., hypokalemia, hypophosphatemia, hypocalcemia, hypoglycemia, hyponatremia, hypernatremia), and vitamin deficiencies (e.g., vitamin B_{12} deficiency) can lead to weakness. However, these present a more diffuse neuropathy and do not only affect lower extremities and unilateral facial weakness.

How would you proceed with your workup?

Initial laboratory tests that can give fast results can help provide information to support or refute diagnoses in your differential. Given that your patient has a fever, tachycardia, and hypertension, determination of a complete blood count (CBC) and inflammatory markers such as the C-reactive protein (CRP) level and erythrocyte sedimentation rate (ESR) can show signs of infection and inflammation. Although they are nonspecific, the differential is wide, and they may be important markers to trend over time if your patient is not responding to the appropriate treatment. Electrolyte levels are also important to check because abnormalities in sodium, potassium, glucose, calcium, and phosphorus levels can lead to weakness and abnormalities in the neurologic examination. With the signs and symptoms mentioned previously, it is necessary to carry out imaging of the brain and cerebellum to rule out masses.

In deciding between imaging modalities of the brain, several things need to be considered when weighing the risks and benefits of each. Head computed tomography (CT) is usually readily available and takes between 5 and 15 minutes. Children do not need to be sedated; however, CT is not the best test to visualize the cerebellum and exposes children to radiation. Magnetic resonance imaging (MRI), on the other hand, uses a magnetic field and radio waves to create images. It is a longer test, lasting approximately 45 to 60 minutes, but it is loud and tends to provoke stress and anxiety for patients with claustrophobia. Thus, it may require sedation to obtain usable images, especially in the pediatric population, for whom lying flat and still for an extended period is unlikely to occur. It is not always readily available and is contraindicated in patients with metallic foreign objects (e.g., pacemaker, implants, other devices). However, MRI does offer better visualization of the posterior fossa.

With fever and neurologic changes, lumbar puncture would help rule out infection with cerebrospinal fluid (CSF) culture. Given other considerations on the differential diagnosis, CSF studies are nonurgent, but could help support other diagnoses if infection is ruled out. A moderate CSF protein elevation can occur in ADEM, Guillain-Barré syndrome, and multiple sclerosis.

Case Point 56.6

Laboratory results reveal normal electrolytes. The complete blood count shows the white blood cell (WBC) count to be 13,500/µL, with 35% neutrophils, 55% lymphocytes, 9% monocytes, and 1% basophils; hemoglobin, 11.7 g/dL; platelets, $295 \times 10\ 3/\mu L$; ESR, 81 mm/h; and CRP, 5.9 mg/dL. Magnetic resonance imaging (MRI) scans are normal. The lumbar puncture is done, but the results are pending.

If there is any concern of increased intracranial pressure, head imaging should always be done prior to performing a lumbar puncture. Failure to do so could lead to herniation and subsequent morbidity.

After reviewing the results of the tests, you believe that GBS is the most likely diagnosis.

How can the diagnosis of Guillain-Barré syndrome be confirmed?
The diagnosis of GBS can be made on a clinical basis and further supported by CSF and electrophysiologic findings (Box 56.1). CSF analysis provides supportive evidence. It is normal early in the disease course, but an albuminocytologic dissociation with an elevated protein level without pleocytosis is evident 7 to 10 days after the onset of symptoms. Nerve conduction studies and electromyography are not necessary for diagnosis; these can also be normal if performed early in the disease course. Neuroimaging frequently shows gadolinium enhancement of the cranial and/or spinal nerve roots; however, these can also be normal if done very early on.

Case Point 56.7

Lumbar puncture reveals the following results: CSF analysis showed 1 WBC/mm³, 12 RBC/mm³, glucose level, 57 mg/dL, and protein level, 277 mg/dL.

BOX 56.1 ■ **Diagnostic Characteristics of Guillain-Barré Syndrome**

Hallmark Features of Diagnosis

> Progressive weakness of both legs and arms
> Areflexia

Clinical Features Supportive of Diagnosis

> Progression over days to 4 weeks
> Relative symmetry of symptoms and signs
> Mild sensory symptoms or signs
> Bifacial palsies
> Autonomic dysfunction
> Absence of fever at onset
> Recovery beginning 2 to 4 weeks after progression ceases

Laboratory Features Supportive of Diagnosis

> Elevated CSF protein levels, with <10 cells/µL
> Electrodiagnostic features of nerve conduction slowing or block

---

Adapted from Ashburry A, Cornblath D. Assessment of current diagnostic criteria for Guillain-Barré syndrome. *Ann Neurol.* 1990;27(Suppl): S21–S24.

What is the pathophysiology of Guillain-Barré syndrome?

Approximately two-thirds of GBS patients report a preceding event such as infection, surgery, or immunization 1 to 4 weeks prior to the onset of weakness. The inciting event causes an acute inflammatory response mediated by activated T helper cells and the formation of autoantibodies, which detect and facilitate destruction of axonal Schwann cell membranes by the complementary cascade (Fig. 56.3).

Case Point 56.8

Due to concerns for increasing weakness and signs of dysautonomia (e.g., bradycardia, hypertension), the patient is transferred to the pediatric intensive care unit (PICU) for closer monitoring.

How is Guillain-Barré syndrome treated?

The mainstay of treatment for GBS is supportive, although intravenous immunoglobulin (IVIG) and plasmapheresis, can be used in severe cases, such as when patients have progressive weakness, are unable to walk, or have significant respiratory compromise due to respiratory muscle involvement. These therapies, unfortunately, do not influence the ultimate outcome in terms of neurologic disability.

CLINICAL PEARL   **STEP 2/3**

IVIG is a blood product. Consent should be obtained, and it is important to inquire about immunoglobulin A (IgA) deficiency because giving IVIG to patients with an IgA deficiency can cause an anaphylactoid reaction.

CLINICAL PEARL   **STEP 2/3**

It is important to make sure that your patient is up to date with all vaccines prior to giving IVIG; otherwise, patients should wait 11 months after IVIG before giving a live vaccine.

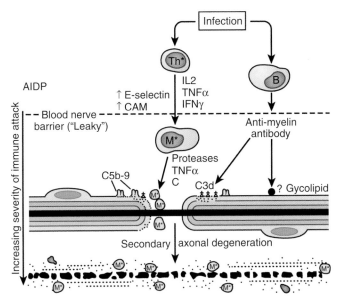

Fig. 56.3 Immune injury to nerve fibers in Guillain-Barré syndrome. A preceding infection incited the activation of T helper cells and production of antimyelin autoantibodies. Inflammatory cytokines and adhesion molecules facilitate the breakdown of the blood-nerve barrier to antibodies, T cells, and macrophages. Complement cascade activation (C3d, C5b-9 attack complex) leads to vesicular myelin changes, demyelination, and axonal degeneration. AIDP, Acute inflammatory demyelinating polyradiculopathy; CAM, intercellular adhesion molecule; IL2, interleukin-2; INFγ, interferon gamma; TNFα, tumor necrosis factor alpha. (From Bosch EP. Guillain-Barré syndrome: an update of acute immune-mediated polyradiculoneuropathies. *Neurologist.* 1998;4:211–226.)

Plasmapheresis is technically more difficult in the pediatric population, especially in young children; thus, IVIG is often preferred when treatment is necessary. If autonomic instability is involved, the patient needs to be monitored and given supportive care, as needed. Pain can also be present, and gabapentin (Neurontin) can be prescribed, although it is titrated up over 3 to 5 days, takes weeks to attain maximal effect and needs to be titrated up to effect.

Neurontin is used in GBS because the pain is neuropathic and secondary to nerve demyelination, not secondary to inflammation. It is thought to suppress the release of excitatory neurotransmitters that play a role in pain. Tylenol, a very common analgesic in pediatrics, does not work in treating GBS because it inhibits prostaglandin synthesis, which is not the mechanism of action of pain in GBS.

What are the complications of Guillain-Barré syndrome?
Usually, patients with GBS can display difficulty ambulating, paresthesias, gastrointestinal dysmotility, dysphagia, and bladder dysfunction. Nutrition needs to be maintained and, if bulbar and oromotor muscles are affected, the patient may benefit from a feeding tube to optimize nutritional status. Life-threatening complications include ascending paralysis affecting the respiratory muscles, leading to respiratory failure. Additionally, autonomic instability can lead to arrhythmias and hypotension. It is of paramount importance that the health care provider be aware of these potential sequelae and immediately transfer the patient to an intensive care setting for close monitoring and possible interventions.

Case Point 56.9

The patient is treated with IVIG, 400 mg/kg per dose, once daily for 5 days. His respiratory status is monitored by measuring forced vital capacity (FVC) every 6 hours while awake. He shows improvement in strength and autonomic stability within a few days of IVIG initiation. After 7 days of hospitalization, the patient's strength has improved markedly but is still less than baseline. He is discharged and will be followed by the pediatric neurologist as an outpatient.

BEYOND THE PEARLS

- Acute pandysautonomia, a variant of GBS, is rare and characterized by the rapid onset of sympathetic and parasympathetic failure (e.g., hypotension, heat intolerance, anhidrosis, xerostomia, fixed pupils, fixed heart rate, dysfunction of bladder and bowel function), without sensory and motor involvement.
- The most common cause of acute facial palsy is acute otitis media. In patients in an area where Lyme disease is endemic, it may be the most common cause of facial palsy.
- Unilateral facial nerve paralysis due to varicella zoster virus (VZV) infection is called Ramsay-Hunt syndrome.
- Postvaccine GBS has been the subject of much interest, although it must be emphasized that no definitive causal relationship has been established to date.
- Miller-Fisher syndrome is a variant of GBS; it is characterized by the triad of ophthalmoplegia, ataxia, and areflexia. The Miller-Fisher variant is considered to be a relatively benign condition, and IVIG therapy may not be necessary.
- The "20-30-40 rule" is used to identify GBS patients at risk for respiratory failure: FVC < 20 mL/kg or a 30% decline of baseline; maximal inspiratory pressure < 30 cm H_2O; maximal expiratory pressure < 40 cm H_2O.
- The mortality rate in GBS has dramatically decreased—from 33% to between 1% to 5%—after the introduction of positive-pressure ventilation in pediatric critical care medicine.

Case Summary:

Complaint/History: A 4-year-old male presents with 5 days of progressive right-sided facial weakness.

Findings: The examination reveals an alert, febrile child with right facial droop affecting the upper and lower parts of his face, dysarthric speech, decreased strength of lower extremities, and decreased and/or absent deep tendon reflexes of upper and lower extremities.

Labs/Tests: Cerebrospinal fluid shows elevated protein levels.

Diagnosis: Guillain-Barré syndrome.

Treatment: Intravenous immunoglobulin, 400 mg/kg daily × 5 days.

Bibliography

Ashburry A, Cornblath D. Assessment of current diagnostic criteria for Guillain-Barré Syndrome. *Ann Neurol.* 1990;27(suppl):S21–S24.

Katirji B. Disorder of peripheral nerves. *Bradley's Neurology in Clinical Practice.* 7th ed. Philadelphia: Elsevier; 2015.

Kliegman R, Stanton B, St. Geme J. *Nelson Textbook of Pediatrics.* 20th ed. Philadelphia: Elsevier; 2016.

Terzis J, Karypidis D. Therapeutic strategies in post-facial paralysis synkinesis in pediatric patients. *J Plast Reconstr Aesthet Surg.* 2012;65(8):1009–1018.

12-Year-Old Female With Rash and Joint Pain

Purva Chhibar ■ R. Michelle Koolaee

A 12-year-old female presents to urgent care with 6 weeks of a facial rash. Her mother mentions that she is avoiding playing soccer as her skin burns when she is out in the sun. The patient reports feeling tired and is unable to participate in sports like she used to before. She does not feel like going to school as she feels stiff, and her body has been hurting every morning for the past 2 months. The pain is worse in the morning and gets better with movement over a 2- to 3-hour period. She also reports hair thinning. She denies chest pain, shortness of breath, cough, fever, chills, nausea, and vomiting, and denies any recent illness. Her brother had the flu a few days ago. She has not traveled recently. She lives in Los Angeles with her parents, younger brother, and pet dog. She does not have any significant past medical history. She met all her milestones as a child. Menarche was 6 months ago. On physical examination, height is 59 inches, weight is 90 pounds, blood pressure is 122/75 mm Hg, pulse rate is 82 beats/min, respiration rate is 15 breaths/min, and oxygen saturation is 99% on room air. Her skin examination reveals an erythematous, macular rash on both cheeks, which spares the nasolabial folds bilaterally (Fig. 57.1). The musculoskeletal examination reveals mildly swollen elbows and knees bilaterally, slightly warm to the touch and tender to palpation. Her lungs are clear to auscultation. Breath sounds are equal bilaterally. A cardiovascular examination reveals normal heart sounds, with no murmurs, rubs, or gallops.

What are some causes of rash and joint pain in a 12-year-old?

There are various infectious and noninfectious causes of rash and arthritis in a 12-year-old. This includes, but is not limited to, the lists in Tables 57.1 and 57.2. It is important to pay attention to the clinical features of the disease and characteristics of the rash to help establish a differential diagnosis.

In general, when should you consider systemic lupus erythematosus as a diagnosis?

Systemic lupus erythematosus (SLE) is a multisystem autoimmune inflammatory disease. It is characterized by autoantibody- and immune-complex–mediated inflammation of the blood vessels and connective tissue. Of SLE cases, 15% to 20% are diagnosed in childhood and adolescence. There are classification criteria for adults with SLE, which were proposed by the American College of Rheumatology (ACR) in 1997, and later revised in 2012. These criteria are useful even for children and include both clinical and serologic criteria. The Systemic Lupus International Collaborating Clinics (SLICC) group classification criteria for SLE is a revised version of the ACR classification criteria and has been noted to have a higher sensitivity (97%) when used in children. Table 57.3 presents these classification criteria in more detail.

A detailed history and physical examination are essential in evaluating a patient with possible SLE. Also, be aware that the clinical manifestations of SLE can be mimicked by a number of other disorders (i.e., infections, malignancy, and other connective tissue diseases).

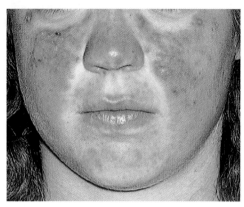

Fig. 57.1 Erythematous, macular rash on both cheeks that spares the nasolabial folds. (From Habif TP. Connective tissue diseases. In: Habif TP, ed. *Clinical Dermatology*. Philadelphia: Elsevier; 2016:673–712.)

TABLE 57.1 ■ Infectious Causes of Joint Pain and Rash in an Adolescent

Disease	Cause	Clinical Features
Fifth disease	Parvovirus B 19 virus	• Inflammatory arthritis for less than 6 weeks • Erythematous facial rash • Flu-like symptoms like fever, rhinorrhea, cough and arthralgias
Rubella virus		• Acute maculopapular rash, which begins on the face and spreads to involve the trunk, hands, and feet, while sparing the palms and soles • Lymphadenopathy • Arthritis, which is symmetrical, migratory, and additive, with resolution within 2 weeks • Arthralgias
Zika virus	Flavivirus	• Fever • Pruritic, erythematous maculopapular rash which may be present on the face, trunk, extremities, palms, and soles • Headache • Arthralgia • Arthritis • Myalgia • Conjunctivitis
Coxsackie virus and echovirus	Enterovirus	• Maculopapular rash • Arthritis/myalgias • Abrupt onset of fever • Headache • Constitutional signs and symptoms • Pharyngitis • Conjunctivitis • Nausea, vomiting, diarrhea • Abdominal pain • Myocarditis
Lyme disease	Spirochete *Borrelia burgdorferi* transmitted by hard-bodied Ixodes ticks	• Erythema migrans; target lesion on the skin around the area of the tick bite. • Arthritis/arthralgias • Neurologic symptoms in advanced disease like meningitis, cranial nerve palsy, and encephalomyelitis

TABLE 57.1 ■ **Infectious Causes of Joint Pain and Rash in an Adolescent—cont'd**

Disease	Cause	Clinical Features
Acute rheumatic fever (ARF)	Group A *Streptococcus* (GAS) pharyngitis	• Erythema marginatum–erythematous skin lesion presenting with rings on the torso, inner thighs, and arms • Migratory arthritis/arthralgias • Sydenham chorea • Subcutaneous nodules • Carditis • Fever • Elevated antistreptococcal antibody titers • Positive throat cultures supporting a recent GAS infection

TABLE 57.2 ■ **Noninfectious Causes of Rash and Joint Pain in an Adolescent**

Cause	Clinical Features
Familial Mediterranean fever (FMF), a hereditary autoinflammatory disorder	• Erysipelas-like rash • Inflammatory arthritis • Fever lasting 1–3 days occurring every 4–8 weeks • Serositis
Still disease, a seronegative inflammatory polyarticular arthritis	• Salmon-colored rash • Lymphadenopathy • Sore throat • Elevated inflammatory markers including erythrocyte sedimentation rate (ESR), C-reactive protein (CRP) and ferritin
Psoriatic arthritis	• Erythematous scaly plaques • Dystrophic nails • Inflammatory arthritis of peripheral joints, spine, and sacroiliac joints
Dermatomyositis	• Heliotrope rash • Erythematous, non-pruritic facial rash, which does not spare the nasolabial folds • Gottron's papules (erythematous, papulosquamous rash) on the dorsum of the MCP and PIP joints • Bilateral symmetric proximal muscle weakness • Arthritis • May be associated with interstitial lung disease • Elevated creatine kinase and aldolase
Systemic lupus erythematosus	• Erythematous, nonpruritic macular, malar rash, also called butterfly rash, which spares the nasolabial folds and is associated with photosensitivity • Nonerosive inflammatory arthritis • Serositis • Oral ulcers • Alopecia • Nephritis • Interstitial lung disease • Neurologic symptoms
Henoch-Schonlein purpura	• Palpable purpura in lower limbs • Inflammatory arthritis • Diffuse colicky abdominal pain • Nephritis

MCP, Metacarpophalangeal joint; *PIP*, proximal interphalangeal joint.

TABLE 57.3 ■ 2012 SLICC Classification Criteria[a]

Clinical Criteria

Acute cutaneous lupus	Malar rash sparing the nasolabial folds (see Fig. 57.1 for image of malar rash), bullous lupus, toxic epidermal necrolysis, maculopapular rash photosensitive rash
Chronic cutaneous lupus	Localized or generalized discoid rash (see Fig. 57.2 for image of discoid rash), hypertrophic rash, lupus panniculitis, mucosal lupus
Oral ulcers	Palate, buccal, tongue, or nasal *in the absence of other causes*
Nonscarring alopecia	Diffuse thinning or hair fragility
Arthritis	Synovitis involving two or more joints, characterized by swelling or effusion OR tenderness in two or more joints and 30 minutes or more of morning stiffness.
Serositis	Typical pleurisy for more than 1 day *or* Pleural rub or pleural effusion Typical pericardial pain (worse with recumbency and improved by sitting forward) for more than 1 day *or* Pericardial effusion or pericardial rub *or* Pericarditis by EKG *in the absence of other causes*
Renal	Urine protein/creatinine (or 24-hour urine protein) representing 500 mg of protein/24 hours OR Red blood cell casts
Neurologic	Seizures Psychosis Mononeuritis multiplex Myelitis Peripheral or cranial neuropathy Acute confusional state *in the absence of other causes*

Hemolytic anemia

Leukopenia
<4000/mm^3 at least once *in the absence of other causes*
OR
Lymphopenia
<1000/mm^3 at least once *in the absence of other causes*

Thrombocytopenia <100,000/mm^3 at least once *in the absence of other causes*

Immunological Criteria

ANA	Above laboratory reference range
1. Anti-dsDNA	Above laboratory reference range except ELISA: twice above laboratory reference range
2. Anti-Sm	
3. Antiphospholipid antibody	Any of the following: • Lupus anticoagulant • False positive RPR • Medium or high titer anticardiolipin (IgA, IgG, or IgM) • Anti-β2 glycoprotein I (IgA, IgG, or IgM)

TABLE 57.3 ■ 2012 SLICC Classification Criteria—cont'd

Clinical Criteria	
4. Low complement	Low C3 Low C4 Low CH50
5. Direct Coombs test	In the absence of hemolytic anemia

aLupus diagnosed based on fulfilling 4/17 criteria, including at least one clinical criterion and one immunologic criterion; OR biopsy-proven lupus nephritis.

ACR, American College of Rheumatology; *ANA,* antinuclear antibody; *Anti-dsDNA,* anti–double-stranded DNA; *Anti-Sm,* anti-Smith antibody; *CH,* hemolytic complement; *IgA,* immunoglobulin A; *IgG,* Immunoglobulin G; *IgM,* Immunoglobulin M; *RPR,* Rapid plasma regain; *SLICC,* Systemic Lupus International Collaborating Clinics.

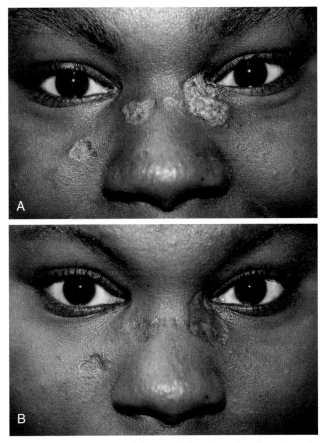

Fig. 57.2 Characteristic discoid lupus rash. (A) Characteristic indurated erythematous plaques with scaling on the face. (B) Healed discoid lupus lesions with atrophy and scarring. (From Hong J, Cordoro KM. Discoid lupus erythematosus in a teenager. *J Pediatr.* 2011;159[2]:350.)

CLINICAL PEARL	STEP 2/3

A mnemonic for SLE classification criteria is noted below:
"MAD MAN HAS Real Problems"
Malar rash
Alopecia
Discoid rash
Mucositis- Oropharyngeal ulcers
Antinuclear antibody, **A**nti–double-stranded DNA, **A**nti-Smith antibody, **A**ntiphospholipid antibody panel
Neurologic disorders
Hematologic disorders
Arthritis
Serositis
Renal disorder
Photosensitivity

CLINICAL PEARL	STEP 2/3

The classification criteria are extremely helpful while considering the diagnosis of SLE. However, these were designed for research purposes and are thus not validated diagnostic criteria. It is important to keep in mind that, for mild cases and for patients with early disease, the classification criteria may not be as sensitive, and the decision regarding whether to label someone with a diagnosis of SLE is based on clinical judgment.

What are some possible manifestations of systemic lupus erythematosus that were not included in the 2012 Systemic Lupus International Collaborating Clinics criteria?
Other possible manifestations of SLE may include (but are not limited to) the following:
- Constitutional symptoms—fevers, fatigue, weight loss, anorexia
- Other rashes (e.g., maculopapular rashes secondary to vasculitis or perivasculitis; these are usually present on sun-exposed areas, fingers, toes, and earlobes)
- Hypertension (particularly in patients with lupus nephritis)
- Lymphadenopathy
- Hepatomegaly/Splenomegaly
- Raynaud phenomenon
- Pancreatitis

What is the next best step to evaluate this patient's joint pain and rash?
In this particular case, the facial rash sparing the nasolabial folds and photosensitivity, as well as presence of an inflammatory arthritis, should warrant serologic evaluation, both for autoantibodies and the presence of possible target organ involvement.

Case Point 57.1

The results of laboratory testing are shown in Table 57.4.

How do you interpret these laboratory findings in the clinical context?
This is a 12-year-old girl with a malar rash sparing the nasolabial folds, photosensitivity, arthritis, leukopenia, thrombocytopenia, hemolytic anemia (as identified by low haptoglobin and elevated lactate dehydrogenase [LDH] levels), and acute kidney injury (AKI), with high suspicion for glomerulonephritis due to the presence of red blood cell casts in the urine sediment. The likelihood

TABLE 57.4 ■ **Laboratory Results**

Leukocyte count	2600/μL
Hemoglobin	8.4 g/dL
Mean corpuscular volume	87.4 fL
Platelet count	97,000/μL
Lactate dehydrogenase	500 U/L
Alkaline phosphatase	96 U/L
Aminotransferase, alanine (ALT)	20 U/L
Aminotransferase, aspartate	20 U/L
Blood urea nitrogen	25 mg/dL
Creatinine	1.71 mg/dL
Calcium	8.9 mg/dL
Haptoglobin	<20 mg/dL
Urinalysis	RBC >50 cells/mm^3
Spot urine protein/creatinine ratio	10 g/24 h

RBC, Red blood cell.

TABLE 57.5 ■ **Autoantibody Test Results**

Antinuclear antibodies	Positive (titer: 1:1280), speckled pattern
Anti–double-stranded DNA antibodies	Positive
Anti–Smith antibodies	Positive
C3 Complement	Low
C4 Complement	Low
Direct antiglobin (Coombs) test	Positive

is high for connective tissue disease, namely SLE, and autoantibody testing can help confirm this diagnosis.

Case Point 57.2

Autoantibody testing is performed; the results are shown in Table 57.5.

How is your assessment affected by these autoantibody results?

The high-titer antinuclear antibody (ANA) test, anti-Smith antibodies, hypocomplementemia, and elevated anti–double-stranded (ds) DNA antibodies, in conjunction with the clinical presentation thus far, help solidify a diagnosis of SLE. Hypocomplementemia and elevated anti-dsDNA antibodies are associated with increased disease activity. Furthermore, the presence of anti-dsDNA antibodies are associated with lupus nephritis.

Case Point 57.3

Diagnosis: Systemic lupus erythematosus.

CLINICAL PEARL   **STEP 2/3**

ANA is sensitive for the diagnosis of SLE but alone are not specific for disease. ANA titers do not correlate with disease activity and should not be monitored serially. ANA testing also has no known prognostic implications. Anti–double-stranded DNA antibodies may correlate with SLE disease activity (especially with the activity of lupus nephritis) and are monitored serially.

BASIC SCIENCE/CLINICAL PEARL   **STEP 1/2/3**

Erythrocyte sedimentation rate (ESR) and C-reactive protein (CRP) are not perfect markers of disease activity in SLE, and do not always correlate with active disease. It is important to always trend these laboratory tests for each individual patient. Sometimes, they do correlate with active disease, and this can help guide management, particularly when deciding whether to modify immunosuppression.

What is the significance of a positive Coombs test in this patient?
This patient has anemia, an elevated LDH level, and low haptoglobin, which points towards a hemolytic anemia. SLE patients can develop a secondary warm autoimmune hemolytic anemia. The pathophysiology involves the binding of immunoglobulin G (IgG) antibodies to the erythrocyte surface membrane molecules, which are then phagocytosed by macrophages. This causes erythrocytes to become progressively more spherocytic. They are then destroyed in the spleen. The direct antiglobulin (Coombs) test, tests for either IgG or C3 bound to erythrocytes and helps establish a diagnosis of an immune-mediated hemolytic anemia.

What are the indications for a renal biopsy and why would they be indicated in this case?
- Increasing serum creatinine level, without another identifiable cause.
- Proteinuria ≥ 1 g over a 24-hour period.
- Proteinuria ≥ 500 mg over a 24-hour period AND cellular casts or hematuria.

This patient has acute renal failure, with proteinuria and a high suspicion for glomerulonephritis. Obtaining a renal biopsy not only identifies the class of lupus nephritis (immunosuppression regimens may vary depending on the particular class of disease) but also provides information regarding activity and chronicity scores. In patients with high activity indices, there is more of a role for aggressive immunosuppression. In patients with biopsy findings more suggestive of chronic disease (e.g., scarring, sclerosis), there is less salvageable renal function, and thus there would be less of a role for aggressive immunosuppression.

Case Point 57.4

The patient undergoes a renal biopsy (Fig. 57.3). Results are as follows:
    Diffuse proliferative glomerulonephritis with immunofluorescence microscopy showing granular deposits in the subendothelial, mesangial, and subepithelial areas (IgG, IgM, IgA, C3, and C1q), which are confirmed by electron microscopy, and is classified as class IV lupus nephritis.

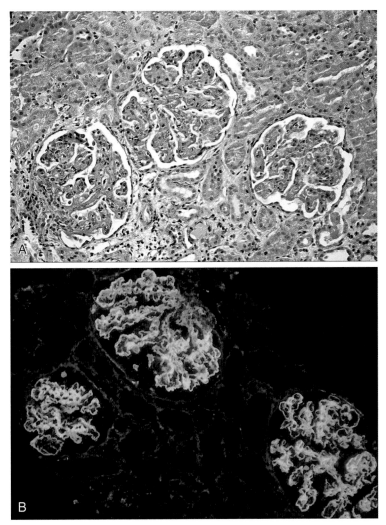

Fig. 57.3 Lupus nephritis class IV (diffuse lupus nephritis). (A) Low-power view showing the diffuse and global distribution of endocapillary proliferation, consistent with class IV disease (hematoxylin-eosin). (B) Diffuse and global deposition of IgG throughout the glomerular mesangium and outlining the peripheral capillary walls (immunofluorescence, anti-IgG). (From Salmon JE, Pricop L, D'Agati V. Immunopathology of systemic lupus erythematosus. In: Hochberg MC, et al, eds. *Rheumatology*. 7th ed. Philadelphia: Elsevier; 2019.)

What are the renal manifestations of systemic lupus erythematosus?

The International Society of Nephrology (ISN) and Renal Pathology Society (RPS) describe six classes of lupus nephritis as noted in Table 57.6 based on the severity of the disease.

CLINICAL PEARL   **STEP 2/3**

Childhood-onset SLE versus adult-onset SLE:
  Children present with more active disease compared to adults and also require treatment with more intensive drug therapy.

TABLE 57.6 ■ ISN/RPS 2004 Classification Criteria of Lupus Nephritis.

Class of lupus nephritis (ISN/RPS 2004)		Is treatment required?
Class I	Minimal mesangial lupus nephritis	No
Class II	Mesangial proliferative lupus nephritis	Rarely
Class III	Focal lupus nephritis	Yes
Class IV	Diffuse lupus nephritis or global lupus nephritis	Yes
Class V	Membranous lupus nephritis	Yes
Class VI	Advanced sclerosing lupus nephritis	May not benefit from treatment

ISN, International Society of Nephrology; *RPS,* Renal Pathology Society.

Case Point 57.5

The patient receives a pulse dose of methylprednisolone for 3 days, followed by prednisone 1 mg/kg daily, in combination with intravenous (IV) cyclophosphamide for 6 months.

How do you approach treatment for systemic lupus erythematosus?

The treatment of SLE is based on severity of disease, as well as specific organ involvement. High-dose glucocorticoid therapy is indicated for patients with organ-threatening or life-threatening manifestations, such as severe lupus nephritis, central nervous system (CNS) lupus, severe lupus-associated immune thrombocytopenic purpura (ITP), autoimmune hemolytic anemia (AIHA), acute pneumonitis, and diffuse alveolar hemorrhage (DAH). Cyclophosphamide is reserved for the most severe disease.

A variety of prednisone tapering schemes have been used, with the goal of taper within 6 to 9 months. In patients with mild disease (i.e., without organ-threatening disease), the choice of therapy depends on the systems involved. The goal is to use the minimum required immunosuppression to maintain clinical and laboratory remission. Some frequently used drugs in SLE include:

- **Glucocorticoids** are used in various doses, depending on the severity of disease.
- **Hydroxychloroquine** is an antimalarial drug, which is considered a standard therapy for SLE. All patients with any degree of SLE should be on hydroxychloroquine. It is effective for mild arthritis and skin disease but also helps in decreasing the frequency and severity of flares of SLE.
- **Belimumab** is a monoclonal antibody that inhibits the B lymphocyte stimulator (BLyS). It is most efficacious in patients with refractory skin manifestations and arthritis. Its use, however, is often limited by its cost.
- **Azathioprine** is used for the maintenance phase of lupus nephritis, hematologic manifestations of SLE, skin disease, and occasionally arthritis.
- **Methotrexate** is useful to treat arthritis in SLE.
- **Mycophenolate mofetil** has broad uses and may be considered for induction therapy and maintenance therapy for lupus nephritis. It is also used to treat hematologic, CNS, and skin manifestations of SLE.

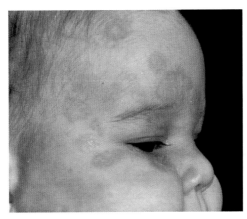

Fig. 57.4   Annular rash of neonatal lupus, which is an erythematous papulosquamous rash with fine scale and central clearing. (From Rajasingam D, Nelson-Piercy C Connective tissue diseases in pregnancy. In: Black M, et al, eds. *Obstetric and Gynecologic Dermatology.* 3rd ed. Philadelphia: Elsevier; 2008:99–106)

- **Cyclophosphamide** is used as induction therapy to treat CNS lupus, severe lupus nephritis, and diffuse alveolar hemorrhage. Infections, hemorrhagic cystitis, infertility, and future malignancy risk are adverse effects to be mindful of.
- **Rituximab** is an anti-CD 20 monoclonal antibody and is used to treat resistant cases of immune thrombocytopenia, hemolytic anemia, and sometimes lupus nephritis and CNS lupus.

What is the usual clinical course and outcome of systemic lupus erythematosus?
SLE has a relapsing and remitting course, with a 10-year survival of more than 90%. Most deaths are from infection, cardiac, renal, pulmonary, and CNS disease. The disease itself may lead to early-onset coronary artery disease due to inflammation causing accelerated atherosclerosis. SLE patients are often on long-term glucocorticoid therapy (tapering can often be a challenge), and so they can suffer from long-term side effects, including bone loss and avascular necrosis of bone (among many other steroidal side effects).

Case Point 57.6

The patient is tapered off prednisone by 6 months and is maintained on azathioprine 100 mg daily. Subsequently, her proteinuria improves to less than 500 mg in a 24-hour period. She is started on hydroxychloroquine and maintained on this indefinitely.

CLINICAL PEARL	**STEP 2/3**

Neonatal lupus is a disease of the developing fetus and newborn characterized by transplacental passage of maternal autoantibodies.
   The pathogenesis is linked to maternal anti-Ro (SS-A) and anti-La (SS-B) antibodies.
   Clinical features include complete congenital heart block, carditis, annular rash (an erythematous papulosquamous rash with fine scale and central clearing, as shown in Fig. 57.4), telangiectasias, thrombocytopenia, neutropenia, anemia, cholestatic hepatitis, hepatomegaly, macrocephaly, hydrocephalus, and spastic paresis.
   Any lupus patient with SS-A and/or SS-B antibodies undergoes frequent fetal echocardiograms during the second trimester to evaluate for congenital heart block. If identified early, there may be a role for glucocorticoids in first- or second-degree congenital heart block.

BEYOND THE PEARLS

- RNP antibody is specific for the diagnosis of mixed connective tissue disease, which may have features of SLE, scleroderma, and dermatomyositis.
- SS-A/Ro antibody and SS-B/La antibody are specific for Sjögren syndrome and neonatal lupus but may be positive in lupus patients with secondary Sjögren syndrome.
- Serum antiphospholipid antibodies, cerebrospinal fluid antineuronal antibodies, serum antiribosomal P antibodies, N-methyl-D-aspartate receptor (NMDAR) antibodies, and antiaquaporin 4/neuromyelitis optica (NMO) antibodies have been associated with CNS lupus.
- Common causes of death in SLE patients include infection (25%), active SLE (35%), cardiovascular disease (30%–40%), and malignancy (5%–10%).
- Exposure to acrolein, a urinary metabolite of cyclophosphamide, may result in hemorrhagic cystitis. To prevent this adverse effect, mesna (2-mercaptoethanesulfonic acid) is administered both before and after cyclophosphamide infusions. It interacts with acrolein to form an inactive product.
- Cyclophosphamide may lead to infertility from premature gonadal failure. To prevent premature gonadal failure in women, physicians may consider the use of leuprolide, a gonadotropin-releasing hormone, 10 days prior to each cyclophosphamide administration. In men, testosterone supplementation may be considered for the same reason.
- Immunizations are indicated in SLE patients preferably before starting immunosuppression. Human papilloma virus vaccine is recommended in patients who are younger than 26 years. Other vaccinations include hepatitis B vaccine, influenza vaccine, and pneumococcal vaccine. Do not administer live attenuated vaccines (measles, mumps, rubella, polio, BCG, herpes zoster, small pox, intranasal influenza vaccine, and yellow fever) in patients on immunosuppressive medications, and/or prednisone >20 mg/day, as they may not mount an immune response.
- Subacute bacterial endocarditis prophylaxis is indicated in patients with APLS antibodies and a heart murmur.
- Prophylaxis for *Pneumocystis carinii* should be considered in patients who are on cyclophosphamide and/or glucocorticoids (prednisone >15–20 mg/day).
- Drug induced lupus (DIL) can be caused by medications like hydralazine, isoniazid, and procainamide. Patients with DIL have antihistone antibodies.
- Tumor necrosis factor inhibitors may also cause DIL; these patients may have elevated anti-dsDNA antibodies.

Case Summary

Complaint/History: A 12-year-old female presents with facial rash, photosensitivity, fatigue, joint pain, and morning stiffness for 6 weeks.

Findings: Erythematous macular rash on her cheeks that spare the nasolabial folds; the elbows and knees are swollen and warm bilaterally.

Labs/Tests: Leukopenia, anemia, thrombocytopenia, positive direct Coombs test, elevated lactate dehydrogenase, low haptoglobin, and proteinuria of 10 g/24 h, a positive ANA, double-stranded DNA, and Smith antibody.

Diagnosis: Systemic lupus erythematosus with a positive ANA, double-stranded DNA, and Smith antibody, pancytopenia, autoimmune hemolytic anemia, malar rash, polyarticular arthritis, and class IV/diffuse proliferative lupus nephritis.

Treatment: Glucocorticoids, cyclophosphamide, azathioprine, and hydroxychloroquine.

Bibliography

Benseler SM, Silverman ED. Systemic lupus erythematosus. *Rheum Dis Clin North Am.* 2007;33(3):471–498.

Brunner HI, Gladman DD, Ibanez D, et al. Difference in disease features between childhood-onset and adult-onset systemic lupus erythematosus. *Arthitis Rheum.* 2008;58(2):556–562.

Hiraki LT, Benseler SM, Tyrrell PN, et al. Clinical and laboratory characteristics and long-term outcome of pediatric systemic lupus erythematosus: a longitudinal study. *J Pediatr*. 2008;152:550–556.

Petri M, Orbai A-M, Alarcón GS, et al. Derivation and validation of systemic lupus international collaborating clinics classification criteria for systemic lupus erythematosus. *Arthritis Rheum*. 2012;64(8):2677–2686.

Sag E, Tartaglione A, Batu ED, et al. Performance of the new SLICC classification criteria in childhood systemic lupus erythematosus: a multicentre study. *Clin Exp Rheumatol*. 2014;32(3):440–444.

11-Year-Old Female With New-Onset Difficulty in Swallowing and Speaking

Priya Shastry ■ Arthur Partikian

An 11-year-old female is brought to the emergency department by her parents for difficulty swallowing, an excessively nasal voice, and recent difficulty in comprehension of her speech. There is no history of trauma, ingestions, or fevers, and she is fully vaccinated.

What can cause difficulty swallowing and a change in the ability to speak normally?
Causes of dysphagia include esophageal foreign body, caustic substance ingestion, and infections; given the patient's history, these causes are less likely. Oropharyngeal infections and central nervous disorders, such as meningitis, encephalitis, or a cerebral abscess, can impair consciousness and the gag reflex, resulting in dysphagia. These infections generally present with fever, behavioral changes, and/or confusion.

Dysarthria may be caused by neuromuscular impairment secondary to a stroke, brain tumor, or disorder, such as cerebral palsy or myasthenia gravis (MG).

BASIC SCIENCE PEARL   **STEP 1**

Swallowing entails a complex set of actions involving the bulbar muscles, which include the muscles of the jaw and oropharynx. Oropharyngeal muscle weakness can cause impaired swallowing, which is referred to as *dysphagia,* as well as dysarthria, which is a change in speech quality, often due to palatal muscle dysfunction. The nasal speech quality—referred to as *dysphonia*—results from involvement of the laryngeal muscles. Dysarthria is often associated with dysphagia because both conditions frequently involve the same muscles and structures.

Case Point 58.1

Her difficulty swallowing solids and liquids is episodic and has evolved over 6 months, with an associated sensation of food being stuck in her chest. After eating, she has a cough, hoarse voice, throat pain, and chest pain. She is unable to speak in full sentences during these episodes. Her symptoms worsen in the evening.

Between these episodes, she feels well. Her mother notes that her daughter's upper eyelids started to droop about 5 years ago. She denies any recent travel and takes no medications.

What is the significance of her symptoms worsening in the evening?
Diurnal variation is a term to describe the change in symptoms during the day. It suggests increasing fatigability with continued use of her muscles during the day and with exertion, which is concerning for a neuromuscular disorder.

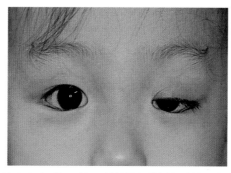

Fig. 58.1 Example of left-sided ptosis. (From Hayashi K, Katori N, Kasai K, et al. Comparison of nylon mono-filament suture and polytetrafluoroethylene sheet for frontalis suspension surgery in eyes with congenital ptosis. *Am J Ophthalmol.* 2013;155[4]:654–663.)

What is the significance of the upper eyelid drooping?

Drooping of the upper eyelid is referred to as ptosis (Fig. 58.1). The principal muscle involved in controlling the upper eyelid is the levator palpebrae. Ptosis can be congenital or acquired. Congenital ptosis is often unilateral and is due to the absence or hypoplasia of the levator palpebrae superioris muscle.

Acquired cases can be mechanical, neurologic, or myogenic in cause. Mechanical causes include inflammation, infections, and masses. Neurologic conditions affecting the muscle, neuromuscular junction (NMJ), cranial nerve (CN), or brainstem can also cause ptosis. Such conditions include an oculomotor (CN III) palsy, which can also cause diplopia, and ophthalmoplegia, as well as Horner syndrome. NMJ disorders include MG, Lambert-Eaton myasthenic syndrome, and botulinum toxin. Examples of myogenic causes are mitochondrial myopathy, oculopharyngeal muscular dystrophy, and myotonic dystrophy.

BASIC SCIENCE PEARL	STEP 1

Horner syndrome is the triad of ipsilateral ptosis, miosis, and anhidrosis due to disruption of the three-neuron oculosympathetic chain.

What is the differential diagnosis for muscle weakness?

The definition of weakness is a decreased ability to move muscles against resistance voluntarily and actively. The differential diagnosis of weakness includes upper and lower motor neuron disease and muscle disease (myopathy).

Upper motor neuron (UMN) weakness is present in lesions of the cerebral cortex and the corticospinal tracts above the anterior horn cell. Common acute findings in UMN lesions include decreased spinal cord reflexes and hypotonia, which evolve over weeks into chronic spasticity, hyperreflexia, and the Babinski sign. Cerebral cortex lesions include intracranial hemorrhage, stroke, brain tumors, Todd's paresis after a seizure, and hemiplegic migraines. Spinal cord lesions involving the descending corticospinal tracts include trauma, tumors, paraspinal infection/inflammation, and transverse myelitis.

Lesions involving the anterior horn cell, peripheral nerve, NMJ, or muscle cause lower motor neuron (LMN) weakness. LMN signs manifest as muscle weakness, hypotonia, and decreased spinal cord reflexes. Common causes of anterior horn lesions, which often cause fasciculations, include poliomyelitis and infections with other enteroviruses. Peripheral nerve causes include Guillain-Barré syndrome, peripheral nerve toxins such as heavy metals, and acute intermittent porphyria. Botulism, MG, organophosphate or carbamate poisoning, and tick paralysis are causes of NMJ disorders. Muscle causes for weakness include rhabdomyolysis and myositis.

Case Point 58.2

On physical examination, her extraocular muscles are intact and her pupils are round, and reactive to light and accommodation, with intact corneal reflexes. Her vision grossly is normal. She has bilateral ptosis. She is unable to close her eyes or raise her eyebrows against resistance and is unable to maintain a sustained upward gaze. She is coughing during the examination, and her speech is hoarse and dysphonic. She has a poor gag reflex. She is able to turn her head against resistance, with muscle strength of 4/5 in her bilateral upper extremities and 5/5 in her bilateral lower extremities. Her sensation is grossly intact to crude touch throughout. Reflexes are 2+, her gait is normal, and she has a negative Babinski.

How does her neurologic examination help narrow down the differential?

The absence of a Babinski sign, lack of spasticity (a velocity-dependent increase in passive muscle tone), normal deep tendon reflexes, and normal higher cortical function (e.g., normal ability to assemble sentences appropriately) make a UMN lesion unlikely. Instead, the patient's bilateral ptosis, poor gag, dysphonia, and dysphagia, as well as decreased upper extremity muscle strength, are suggestive of a LMN disorder.

It is important to distinguish between baseline and persistent weakness versus diurnal symptoms and fatigability, the latter of which are more specific for an NMJ disorder. The inability to close her eyes or raise her eyebrows against resistance indicates weakness with fatigability, which is confirmed by the inability to maintain a sustained upward gaze. Therefore, her examination findings and history of ptosis as a presenting symptom are consistent with a NMJ disorder, specifically MG. Other lower motor neuron processes, such as the Miller-Fisher variant of Guillain-Barré syndrome, which causes ophthalmoplegia and ataxia, other neuropathies, and myopathies do not usually have fluctuating or diurnal symptoms and fatigability on examination.

MG is categorized into pure ocular or generalized variants, depending on the affected areas. Ocular MG is more common in prepubertal children, and generalized weakness is more common in postpubertal adolescents and adults. Other symptoms of MG include dysphagia, dysarthria, extremity weakness, dysphonia, and respiratory failure in the absence of visible respiratory distress.

BASIC SCIENCE PEARL	**STEP 1**

The most common symptom seen in MG is ptosis.

BASIC SCIENCE/CLINICAL PEARL	**STEP 1/2/3**

Rapidly progressive NMJ symptoms suggest botulism and organophosphate poisoning.

Case Point 58.3

Diagnosis: Myasthenia gravis.
This is confirmed with testing (see later).

What is the pathophysiology of myasthenia gravis?

MG is an autoimmune condition wherein autoantibodies attack the postsynaptic membrane at the NMJ. The most common antibody seen in MG binds to the acetylcholine receptor (AChR; Fig. 58.2). The antibody binds to the α- and β-subunits of the AChR, leading to internalization

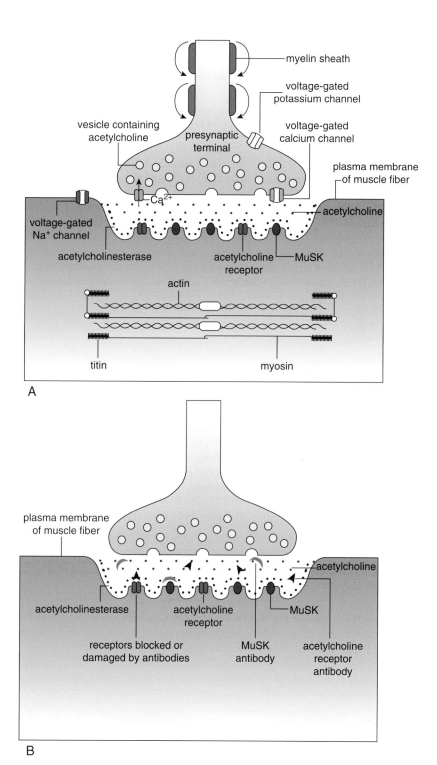

Fig. 58.2 Postsynaptic acetylcholine receptors and/or muscle-specific kinase affected by autoantibodies. Shown are (A) normal and (B) affected neuromuscular junctions. Most patients have antibodies to a single protein. *MuSK,* Muscle-specific kinase. (From Kang PB, Liew WKM, Oskoui M, Vincent A. Juvenile and neonatal myasthenia gravis. In: Darras BT, Jones R, Ryan MM, De Vivo DC, eds. *Neuromuscular Disorders of Infancy, Childhood, and Adolescence.* 2nd ed. London: Academic Press/Elsevier. 2014:482–496.)

and breakdown of the AChR. The antibodies can also directly impair the function of the AChR by simply binding to it.

BASIC SCIENCE PEARL	STEP 1

Acetylcholine is the primary neurotransmitter at the NMJ.

Another antibody implicated in MG, but less commonly found, is an immunoglobulin G (IgG) autoantibody to muscle-specific kinase (MuSK), which targets striated muscle protein (Fig. 58.2).

Ideally, which test should be performed clinically once the suspicion for myasthenia gravis is raised?
Serologic antibody tests should be sent (see later), and a bedside test using edrophonium—a short-acting ACh inhibitor that prolongs the presence of ACh in the neuromuscular synapse and thus allows for increased muscle contraction—is used to elicit a transient improvement in observable or measurable signs, such as ptosis, severe ophthalmoparesis, and dysphonia. A positive edrophonium test supports but does not confirm the diagnosis.

CLINICAL PEARL	STEP 2/3

Edrophonium enhances the muscarinic effects of ACh, producing bradycardia and bronchospasm. Cardiopulmonary monitoring should be used, and atropine should be immediately available at the bedside.

What other tests are used to diagnose myasthenia gravis?
Placing an ice bag on the eyelids of a patient with ptosis with resulting transient improvement—due to slowing the breakdown of ACh at the NMJ—is suggestive of MG. Electrophysiologic tests, including repetitive nerve stimulation and single-fiber electromyography, are less sensitive but more specific, allowing for diagnosis confirmation. The latter test is much more sensitive in both the ocular and generalized forms of MG. Finally, 85% of patients will have elevated anti-AChR antibody titers, which is predictive of a more severe clinical course.

Case Point 58.4

The patient's edrophonium test is positive. Serum tests show detectable anti-AChR antibody, confirming the diagnosis of myasthenia gravis.

What further workup is required now that she has been diagnosed with myasthenia gravis?
Patients with MG are often found to have thymic abnormalities, suggesting that the thymus may have a role in the pathogenesis of this disease—60% to 70% of patients have thymic hyperplasia and 10% to 12% have a thymoma. In patients who have a thymoma, there is a higher remission rate if the patient undergoes thymectomy (in adult studies). Even in most patients without a thymoma, a thymectomy is thought to improve the long-term prospects of remission or control of the disease.

Case Point 58.5

Further investigation into her past medical history reveals that she has been prescribed albuterol for presumed asthma due to a chronic cough, as well as having been given antibiotics for a pneumonia three times in the last 5 months. She was also admitted to the intensive care unit recently due to a pneumonia that required intubation for impending respiratory failure.

Are the diagnoses of asthma and pneumonia related to the patient's myasthenia gravis diagnosis?

The patient has oropharyngeal muscle weakness, likely leading to multiple episodes of microaspirations. Most of these episodes result in little more than a chronic cough, which in this case has led to a misdiagnosis of asthma. Some of the aspiration events were significant enough to result in pneumonia. One pneumonia was associated with respiratory failure requiring mechanical ventilation, which likely indicates an undiagnosed myasthenic crisis.

What is a myasthenic crisis?

Myasthenic crisis is a life-threatening condition in which a patient's respiratory muscles are so weak that the patient requires intubation and mechanical ventilation to ensure adequate oxygenation and ventilation. A crisis can be triggered by infection and by other stressors such as surgery, pregnancy, childbirth, and medications. Of patients with MG, 10% to 20% will experience a myasthenic crisis at some point during the course of disease.

BASIC SCIENCE/CLINICAL PEARL   **STEP 1/2/3**

Suspect myasthenic crisis in a patient with MG presenting with dyspnea, dysphagia, poor respiratory effort, paradoxical abdominal breathing, and low vital capacity.

The mainstays of treatment of a myasthenic crisis include plasma exchange and intravenous immunoglobulin (IVIG). Both therapies take effect within days, but the effects only last a few weeks, so patients are often started on glucocorticoids as well. Plasma exchange removes antibodies from the circulation but, without immunomodulatory treatment, the antibody levels will rise within a few weeks. The exact mechanism of action of IVIG in MG is unknown; however, possible mechanisms include neutralization of antibodies and effects on the complement system.

CLINICAL PEARL   **STEP 2/3**

Vital capacity measures the maximum amount of air that a person can expel from the lungs after a maximal inhalation; thus, it indicates the severity of respiratory muscle involvement in neuromuscular disease. In general, a vital capacity less than 20 mL/kg is an indication of impending respiratory failure in patients with myasthenia gravis.

What are the treatment options for myasthenia gravis?

Medications for the treatment of MG include anticholinesterases and immunosuppressive agents to manage symptoms and induce remission, respectively. The main cholinesterase inhibitor used currently for symptom management is pyridostigmine bromide, which blocks the action of acetylcholinesterase, allowing for higher levels of ACh in the NMJ that can bind to postsynaptic AChRs. Most patients will need immunosuppressive therapy eventually in their clinical course, typically starting with an oral glucocorticoid. Steroid-sparing immunosuppressive agents are not used as frequently in juvenile MG given their side effect profile but are generally used for poorly responsive or relapsed patients. A suggested treatment algorithm is shown in Fig. 58.3.

Case Point 58.6

The patient is started on pyridostigmine bromide, but significant symptoms of generalized weakness persist. Therefore, she is also treated with a 4-day inpatient course of IVIG and is started on an outpatient schedule of prednisone for chronic management of her autoimmune condition. She experiences slow but steady resolution of her fatigue over the next 10 days. She is discharged home with a plan to undergo magnetic resonance imaging to evaluate for a possible thymoma.

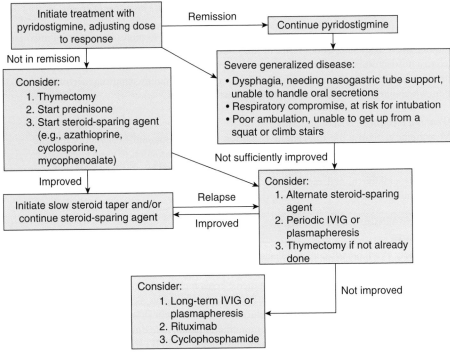

Fig. 58.3 Suggested approach to the treatment of myasthenia gravis. (From Silvestri NJ, et al. Acquired disorders of the neuromuscular junction. *IVIG,* Intravenous immunoglobulin. In: Swaiman KF, Ashwal S, Ferriero DM, et al, eds. *Swaiman's Pediatric Neurology.* 6th ed. Philadelphia: Elsevier; 2017:e2462–e2481.)

BEYOND THE PEARLS

- Anti-AChR antibodies are more likely to be detectable in patients with generalized disease (85% are positive) than in patients with only ocular symptoms (50% are positive).
- Although MG is an acquired autoimmune disorder, the presence of certain human leukocyte antigen group (HLA) antigens are overrepresented and thus suggest a hereditary disposition to developing MG.
- MG is commonly associated with other autoimmune diseases.
- There are congenital myasthenic syndromes that are due to genetic mutations that impair the function of the NMJ.
- Transient myasthenia of the newborn is seen in 10% to 20% of infants born to mothers with seropositive myasthenia gravis. It is due to maternal AChR antibodies that are transferred to the fetus. Symptoms include ptosis, hypotonia, poor feeding, a weak cry, and respiratory failure. Most symptoms abate within 4 weeks, but some manifestations may be permanent.

Case Summary

Complaint/History: An 11-year-old female presents with difficulty swallowing, an excessively nasal voice and difficulty in comprehension of her speech.

Findings: Bilateral ptosis, poor gag reflex, is unable to close her eyes or raise her eyebrows against resistance, unable to maintain a sustained upward gaze.

Labs/Tests: Anti–acetylcholine receptor-binding antibody positive.

Diagnosis: Myasthenia gravis.

Treatment: Pyridostigmine, intravenous immunoglobulin, oral glucocorticoids.

Bibliography

Chiang LM, Darras BT, Kang PB. Juvenile myasthenia gravis. *Muscle Nerve.* 2009;39(4):423–431.

Kang PB, Liew WKM, Oskoui M, Vincent A. Juvenile and neonatal myasthenia gravis. In: Darras BT, Jones R, Ryan MM, De Vivo DC, eds. *Neuromuscular Disorders of Infancy, Childhood, and Adolescence.* 2nd ed. San Diego: Elsevier Inc; 2014:482–496 [Chapter 27].

Liew WK, Kang PB. Update on juvenile myasthenia gravis. *Curr Opin Pediatr.* 2013;25(6):694–700.

Pershad J, Kriwanek KL. Peripheral neuromuscular disorders. In: Baren JM, Rothrock SG, Brennan JA, Brown L, eds. *Pediatric Emergency Medicine.* Philadelphia: Elsevier; 2008:391–396.

Vander Pluym J, Vajsar J, Jacob FD, et al. Clinical characteristics of pediatric myasthenia: a surveillance study. *Pediatrics.* 2013;132(4):e939–e944.

Newborn With Respiratory Distress

Loren Fox Yaeger ■ Priya Shastry ■ Smeeta Sardesai

You are called to evaluate a 10-minute-old term female infant with grunting and tachypnea born to a 29-year-old mother who had little prenatal care.

What is your initial differential in a newborn with respiratory distress?
Respiratory symptoms in a newborn may include apnea, tachypnea, grunting, nasal flaring, and intercostal retractions. The most common causes for respiratory distress in a newborn are transient tachypnea of the newborn (TTN), respiratory distress syndrome (RDS), meconium aspiration syndrome (MAS), infection, and persistent pulmonary hypertension of the newborn (PPHN). Certain congenital malformations, such as pulmonary hypoplasia, congenital emphysema, esophageal atresia, and congenital diaphragmatic hernia (CDH), can also lead to respiratory distress in the newborn.

TTN is secondary to retained lung fluid after delivery. It often resolves within 24 hours but may persist to 72 hours. RDS, most commonly seen in preterm infants, is due to surfactant deficiency. MAS is the result of aspiration of amniotic fluid stained with meconium, which can occur before, during, or immediately after birth. Respiratory symptoms are common in pneumonia, which is often the presenting infection in a neonate. PPHN occurs when pulmonary vascular resistance fails to decrease soon after birth. PPHN can be idiopathic, or secondary to other causes of respiratory distress.

BASIC SCIENCE/CLINICAL PEARL	STEP 1/2/3

Meconium is a viscous, dark-green substance composed of intestinal epithelial cells, lanugo, mucus, and intestinal secretions. In utero, fetal hypoxia can lead to the passage of meconium due to neural stimulation of the gastrointestinal tract. Respiratory distress in MAS immediately after delivery can be due to airway obstruction, surfactant dysfunction, chemical pneumonitis, and pulmonary hypertension.

Case Point 59.1

On arrival to the delivery room, you note that baby is cyanotic with a barrel-shaped chest. She is grunting, retracting, and tachypneic. Auscultation of her chest reveals poor air entry on the left side, with a shift of cardiac sounds over the right side. Her abdomen is scaphoid (Fig. 59.1). You do not notice any other physical anomalies.

What is the most likely diagnosis based on your examination?
The presence of a scaphoid abdomen, barrel-shaped chest and respiratory distress in any infant is suspicious for CDH. The clinical presentation of infants with CDH can vary from asymptomatic to severe respiratory failure at the time of delivery.

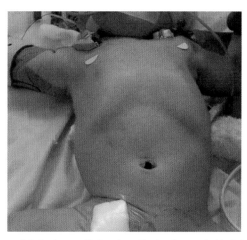

Fig. 59.1 Infant with congenital diaphragmatic hernia, with classic scaphoid abdomen with barrel shaped chest. (From Stone P. *High-Risk Pregnancy.* Philadelphia: Elsevier; 2011.)

Case Point 59.2

The baby is intubated in the delivery room and placed on mechanical ventilation with low peak pressures. An orogastric tube and an umbilical line are placed. The infant is placed in a warmer and immediately taken to the neonatal intensive care unit (NICU) for further evaluation and treatment. A consult is immediately placed for pediatric surgery evaluation.

Given your concern for congenital diaphragmatic hernia, what is important in managing this patient in the delivery room?

Optimal perinatal management requires a well-coordinated, multidisciplinary team with the immediate availability of neonatologists and pediatric surgeons. It is imperative that bag-mask ventilation be avoided to minimize gaseous gastric and intestinal distention. Instead, the infant should be intubated immediately following delivery for mechanical ventilation. Intestinal distention can worsen lung compression and the mediastinal shift, further worsening the respiratory distress. The infant should be ventilated with low peak pressures to minimize lung injury. A nasogastric or orogastric tube should be placed soon after delivery to facilitate intestinal decompression and promote the expansion of available lung tissue. Preductal saturations >70% for the first 1 to 2 hours are acceptable if the pH and arterial carbon dioxide levels are within normal limits.

Case Point 59.3

A chest and abdominal radiograph demonstrates the endotracheal tube in the correct position and bowel loops in the left thorax, with the tip of the orogastric tube in the chest cavity, heart shifted to the right, and liver in the abdominal cavity (Fig. 59.2).

What tests and imaging would help you make a definitive diagnosis?

A chest radiograph (CXR) is indicated in any infant with respiratory distress, especially when CDH is suspected. In left-sided CDH, a CXR reveals the presence of bowel loops in the left chest cavity with the heart shifted to the right side, as seen in Fig. 59.2. If the stomach is also a part of the hernia, the orogastric/nasogastric tube would be visualized within the thorax. If the liver is within the chest, the umbilical venous line may also take up an aberrant position. A right-sided CDH may be confused with diaphragmatic eventration or lobar consolidation.

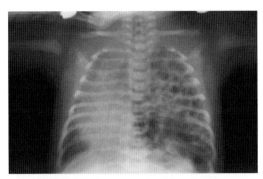

Fig. 59.2 X-ray of left-sided diaphragmatic hernia in a 1-day-old term infant. (From Crowley M. Neonatal Respiratory Disorders. In: Martin R, Fanaroff A, Walsh M, eds. *Fanaroff and Martin's Neonatal-Perinatal Medicine.* Philadelphia: Elsevier; 2015;1113–1136.)

BASIC SCIENCE/CLINICAL PEARL　　　　　　　　　　　　　　　**STEP 1/2/3**

In an infant with CDH, an echocardiogram should be performed within the first 24 hours to assess for pulmonary hypertension, right heart function, and congenital heart defects.

Case Point 59.4

Diagnosis: Bochdalek type of congenital diaphragmatic hernia.

What is congenital diaphragmatic hernia?

A CDH is a developmental defect secondary to failure of normal closure of the pleuroperitoneal folds between the fourth to tenth weeks of gestation. This allows the abdominal contents to enter the thoracic cavity. The incidence of CDH is 1 in 2000 to 3000 newborns. There are three CDH subtypes based upon the location of the defect (Fig. 59.3). The most common defect involves the posterolateral diaphragm resulting in a left-sided hernia (Bochdalek hernia). The retrosternal anterior defect results in a right-sided Morgagni hernia and the central defect results in a pars sternalis type. Herniation is most common on the left side (85% of cases), 13% are right-sided, and bilateral defects are rare and typically fatal. Both right- and left-sided hernias involve the bowel. The liver is often involved with right-sided herniation. In left-sided hernias, the stomach is often involved, although the liver may herniate as well.

BASIC SCIENCE/CLINICAL PEARL　　　　　　　　　　　　　　　**STEP 1/2/3**

A helpful mnemonic for remembering the features of a Bochdalek hernia is BBBBB: Bochdalek, big, back and medial (usually on the left side), baby, and bad (associated with pulmonary hypoplasia and prolonged hospital course).

What is the cause of respiratory distress in this patient with congenital diaphragmatic hernia?

The displacement of abdominal contents into the thorax during this critical time of lung development results in impaired pulmonary parenchymal and vascular structures, resulting in pulmonary hypoplasia. Pulmonary hypoplasia is most severe on the ipsilateral side to the hernia, although it may develop on the contralateral side if the mediastinum shifts and compresses the other lung. Arterial branching is reduced, resulting in muscular hyperplasia of the pulmonary arterial tree, which contributes to the increased risk of PPHN.

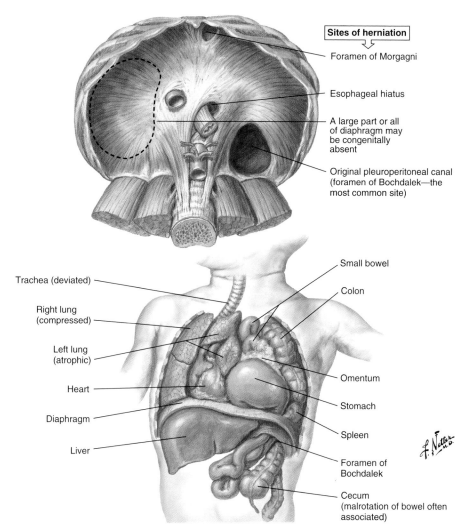

Sites of herniation

Foramen of Morgagni

Esophageal hiatus

A large part or all of diaphragm may be congenitally absent

Original pleuroperitoneal canal (foramen of Bochdalek—the most common site)

Trachea (deviated)

Right lung (compressed)

Left lung (atrophic)

Heart

Diaphragm

Liver

Small bowel

Colon

Omentum

Stomach

Spleen

Foramen of Bochdalek

Cecum (malrotation of bowel often associated)

Fig. 59.3 The type of congenital diaphragmatic hernia is determined by the site of the defect. (From Cochard LR. The respiratory system. In: Cochard LR. *Netter's Atlas of Human Embryology, Updated Edition.* Philadelphia: Elsevier/Saunders; 2012:113–129.)

BASIC SCIENCE PEARL	STEP 1

The time at which the CDH occurs, between the 4th and 10th weeks of gestation, is also a critical time of bronchial and pulmonary arterial development.

BASIC SCIENCE/CLINICAL PEARL	STEP 1/2/3

The clinical manifestations of CDH result from pulmonary hypoplasia. The severity of symptoms in CDH correlates with the degree of lung hypoplasia and the development of PPHN.

Can congenital diaphragmatic hernia be diagnosed prior to birth?

Most cases of CDH are diagnosed prenatally by antenatal ultrasound, typically between 16 to 24 weeks of gestation. Definitive diagnosis relies on the visualization of abdominal organs in the fetal chest. The hallmark for a left-sided CDH is a fluid-filled stomach just behind the left atrium and ventricle in the lower thorax, with a right mediastinal shift. Given that the liver is similar in echogenicity to the lung, and because the liver is the primary organ that herniates in a right-sided CDH, it is more common for right-sided CDHs to be missed or misdiagnosed. If a CDH is diagnosed prenatally, the baby should be delivered in a center with a level 3 NICU and experienced pediatric surgeons.

BASIC SCIENCE/CLINICAL PEARL   **STEP 1/2/3**

Peristalsis and fluid in the bowel within the thoracic cavity helps to distinguish CDH from other thoracic lesions, such as congenital cystic adenomatoid malformation, bronchopulmonary sequestration, bronchopulmonary foregut malformation, bronchogenic cysts, bronchial atresia, enteric cysts, and teratomas.

Case Point 59.5

The baby remains on conventional mechanical ventilation in the NICU, with preductal saturations between 85% and 90%. Her systemic blood pressures remain stable and she does not develop concurrent PPHN. The decision is made with a pediatric surgeon that she does not meet the criteria for extracorporeal membrane oxygenation (ECMO) at this time.

How are congenital diaphragmatic hernia patients managed?

Following immediate intubation and stabilization in the delivery room, the infant should be transferred to the NICU for further care and treatment. Venous access should be obtained for administering fluids and medications. Umbilical arterial catheter placement allows for blood pressure and blood gas monitoring. Both preductal and postductal arterial oxygen tension (Pao_2) saturations should be monitored, with preductal saturation goals between 85% and 95%. Monitoring only postductal Pao_2 can lead to an increased fraction of inspired oxygen (Fio_2). Systemic blood pressures should be managed based on the infant's gestational age. Conventional mechanical ventilation is the optimal initial ventilation strategy following delivery.

The paucity of pulmonary vasculature and remodeling of the vessels results in the fixed/irreversible component of PPHN in CDH. In infants older than 34 weeks gestational age, inhaled nitric oxide (iNO) is the first agent of choice for the treatment of PPHN. If medical management fails, ECMO is often used as a rescue therapy preoperatively and postoperatively for infants with CDH. To be a candidate for ECMO, the infant needs to be at least 34 weeks of gestation, weigh at least 2 kg, and have no associated major lethal anomalies.

Case Point 59.6

On day 2 of life, the baby is taken to the operating room and has her small muscular CDH closed. Her stomach and intestines are placed back within the abdominal cavity, resulting in some abdominal distention. However, the pediatric surgeon can close her abdominal sutures, and she does not require placement of a patch in either her diaphragm or abdomen. She returns to the NICU intubated.

BASIC SCIENCE/CLINICAL PEARL STEP 1/2/3

CDH repair depends on the size of the opening in the diaphragm and the amount of bowel/stomach/liver within the thorax. Small openings can undergo a primary repair, stitching together the existing muscle. Large defects may require additional native or synthetic tissue to cover the opening. A muscle flap repair uses the patient's own internal oblique or latissimus dorsi muscles. A patch repair uses a synthetic biocompatible material.

When can the patient undergo surgical repair?
Optimal timing of CDH repair can be difficult to determine, particularly in patients who require ECMO. Hernia reduction/repair is usually not offered until the patient is medically stable. Surgical repair is usually performed between 48 and 72 hours in medically stable neonates and can be deferred up to 5 to 10 days in neonates with more severe forms of pulmonary hypoplasia and PPHN.

Case Point 59.7

After the patient's successful surgery, her mother asks you about the long-term consequences of her daughter's condition.

What are the long-term consequences of congenital diaphragmatic hernia?
Outcomes in infants with CDH are dependent on the presence of associated anomalies (such as congenital heart disease), the extent of lung hypoplasia, and the position of the liver. CDH with liver herniation into the thoracic cavity is associated with a worse prognosis. Chronic lung disease, rebound pulmonary hypertension, obstructive pulmonary disease, and infection are common medical issues in CDH survivors. Recurrent hernia/patch problems, pectus and scoliosis postrepair, gastroesophageal reflux, aversion to oral feeds, gastrostomy tube feeding, and failure to thrive are also common. In addition to physical disabilities, neurologic sequelae commonly seen in this population include neurocognitive and functional delays, as well as hearing loss. Long-term outcomes also depend on the characteristics of the diaphragmatic defect. Recurrence rates and complications are negligible in patients with a small muscular defect that is easily approximated.

BEYOND THE PEARLS

- Surfactant replacement therapy should be considered for immature lungs with surfactant deficiency. However, the beneficial effect of surfactant replacement therapy in term infants with CDH is not well known.
- Maternal use of selective serotonin reuptake inhibitors (SSRIs) in the third trimester is associated with an increased incidence of infants with PPHN.
- ECMO is a cardiopulmonary bypass circuit that serves as an artificial lung and heart to provide oxygenation in patients whose intrinsic cardiopulmonary circuit is no longer functioning adequately for gas exchange and systemic perfusion.
- Approximately 40% of patients with CDH have other congenital anomalies. Trisomies are the most common chromosomal abnormalities associated with CDH. CDH may also be seen in many syndromes, such as Cornelia De Lange, Beckwith-Wiedemann, CHARGE, Goldenhar sequence, Simpson-Golabi-Behmel, Stickler, pentalogy of Cantrell, Pierre Robin sequence, and VACTERL anomalies.
- Given their complex medical and surgical histories, survivors of CDH require long-term follow-up with a multidisciplinary team for appropriate monitoring and screening of the sequelae of this complex disease.

Case Summary

Complaint/History: A 10-minute-old female is born with grunting and tachypnea.

Findings: The physical examination is notable for a barrel-shaped chest and a scaphoid abdomen. On auscultation, cardiac sounds are shifted to the right side of the chest, and there is poor air entry on the left side of the chest.

Labs/Tests: A chest radiograph shows bowel loops in the left thorax, with the heart shifted to the right side.

Diagnosis: Bochdalek type of congenital diaphragmatic hernia.

Treatment: Intubation in the delivery room without bag-mask ventilation, mechanical ventilation until stable for surgical repair.

Bibliography

Avery GB, MacDonald MG, Seshia MM, et al. Chapter 47: Respiratory failure in the term newborn. In: MacDonald MG, Mullett MD, Seshia MMK, eds. *Avery's Neonatology: Pathophysiology and Management of the Newborn*. Philadelphia, PA: Lippincott Williams & Wilkins; 2016:647–657.

Bojanić K, Pritišanac E, Luetić T, et al. Malformations associated with congenital diaphragmatic hernia: impact on survival. *J Pediatr Surg*. 2015;50(11):1817–1822.

Hedrick HL. Management of prenatally diagnosed congenital diaphragmatic hernia. *Semin Pediatr Surg*. 2013;22(1):37–43.

Lally KP, Engle W. Postdischarge follow-up of infants with congenital diaphragmatic hernia. *Pediatrics*. 2008;121(3):627–632.

Puligandla PS, Grabowski J, Austin M, et al. Management of congenital diaphragmatic hernia: a systematic review from the APSA outcomes and evidence based practice committee. *J Pediatr Surg*. 2015;50(11):1958–1970.

Snoek KG, Reiss IK, Greenough A, et al. Standardized postnatal management of infants with congenital diaphragmatic hernia in Europe: The CDH EURO Consortium Consensus-2015 Update. *Neonatology*. 2016;110(1):66–74.

3-Hour-Old, 31-Week Premature Infant Male With Tachypnea

Priya Shastry ▓ Anne Zepeda-Tiscareno ▓ Smeeta Sardesai

You are called to the neonatal intensive care unit (NICU) to evaluate a 3-hour-old infant male born at 31 weeks and 2 days via cesarean section to a mother with gestational diabetes. The nurse reports that she is concerned that the infant has been breathing fast for the last 20 minutes.

Case Point 60.1

On examination, you note that the infant is tachypneic and grunting, with subcostal retractions and nasal flaring. His heart rate is 140 beats/min, respiratory rate is 74 breaths/min, blood pressure is within normal parameters, and O_2 saturation is 88% on room air. On auscultation you hear coarse breath sounds bilaterally.

What is the significance of tachypnea, grunting, and retractions?

Tachypnea, retractions, and nasal flaring represent increased work-of-breathing and respiratory distress. Tachypnea in a newborn is defined as a respiratory rate greater than 60 breaths/min. It is a compensatory mechanism whereby the body responds to poor ventilation or oxygenation, making it a common but nonspecific finding in respiratory, cardiovascular, metabolic, or systemic diseases. Thoracic wall retractions during respiration are due to the forceful use of accessory muscles in the neck, rib cage, sternum, or abdomen when pulmonary compliance is low and airway resistance is high. Grunting is an expiratory sound generated when the infant is breathing with the glottis in a closed position to prevent alveolar atelectasis. Nasal flaring is a compensatory symptom in which the upper airway diameter is increased, and resistance to airflow is decreased.

CLINICAL PEARL   **STEP 2/3**

The volume of gas contained in the lung after a normal expiration, known as the *functional residual capacity* (FRC), is predominantly determined by the interaction between the elastic recoil of the chest and lungs. In the newborn, both the thorax and lung are very compliant, such that the FRC is very small. Newborns increase their FRC by grunting and by postinspiratory stimulation of inspiratory muscles during expiration, evident by retractions.

BASIC SCIENCE PEARL   **STEP 1**

Chest wall compliance of an infant is very high and decreases as the infant grows. In contrast, lung compliance is very low at birth and steadily increases throughout puberty.

What are the most common causes of respiratory distress?

The most common causes of respiratory distress in the newborn are respiratory distress syndrome (RDS) or hyaline membrane disease (HMD), transient tachypnea of the newborn (TTN), pneumonia, air leaks, meconium aspiration syndrome, pulmonary hemorrhage, and pulmonary hypertension.

The primary cause of RDS is inadequate pulmonary surfactant. Extremely preterm infants are at the greatest risk for RDS because surfactant production is developmentally regulated. Structurally immature and surfactant-deficient lungs have decreased compliance and a tendency to collapse between breaths. Microscopically, an eosinophilic membrane (hyaline membrane), composed of fibrinous matrix and cellular debris from injured epithelial cells, lines the air spaces—hence, this syndrome was named *hyaline membrane disease.* The most common signs and symptoms associated with RDS include tachypnea, grunting, nasal flaring, and use of accessory muscles.

Mild cases of RDS may be managed by continuous positive airway pressure (CPAP), but more severe cases require endotracheal intubation and the administration of exogenous surfactant into the lungs.

TTN is caused by the impaired clearance of fetal lung fluid. Late in gestation, or when the mother begins labor, there is reversal of chloride and fluid-secreting channels in the lung epithelium, which enhances fluid absorption from the alveoli. Infants delivered by cesarean section, especially without a trial of labor, have an increased risk for developing TTN. TTN presents with tachypnea, nasal flaring, mild retractions, and expiratory grunting. It often resolves within 24 to 72 hours of life. These infants may require supplemental oxygen and CPAP.

Pneumonia is another common cause of respiratory distress in the newborn. Neonatal pneumonia can be classified by the infant's age. Early-onset pneumonia (before 3 days of age) is generally acquired from the mother during labor or delivery. Late-onset pneumonia (after 3 days of age) is due to nosocomial organisms from previous colonization of the infant or transmission from care providers or contaminated equipment. Bacterial, viral, and fungal pathogens can cause neonatal pneumonia. Group B *Streptococcus* (GBS) is the most common cause of early-onset bacterial pneumonia. These infants require a sepsis evaluation, including a chest radiograph (CXR), complete blood count (CBC), blood culture, and empiric antibiotic therapy, which provides broad coverage for the most likely pathogens.

CLINICAL PEARL	STEP 2/3

Toxoplasma gondii, rubella, cytomegalovirus, herpes simplex virus (TORCH), *Mycobacterium tuberculosis, Treponema pallidum,* and *Listeria monocytogenes* are commonly transmitted via the transplacental route. GBS, *Escherichia coli, Staphylococcus aureus, Klebsiella* spp., *Haemophilus influenzae* (nontypeable), *Candida* spp., *Chlamydia trachomatis,* and *Ureaplasma urealyticum* are acquired at delivery.

The presence of maternal fever, prolonged rupture of membranes for more than 18 hours, chorioamnionitis, preterm delivery, and fetal tachycardia are risk factors for perinatal pneumonia. It is always important to review the maternal history to recognize at-risk infants.

Maternal colonization is the single most important risk factor for early-onset GBS infection. Hence, screening pregnant women for GBS colonization at 35 to 37 weeks of gestation and using intrapartum antibiotic prophylaxis (IAP) during labor for those colonized and those with specific risk factors for early-onset GBS infection is important.

What is the composition of a surfactant?

The active components of a surfactant are phospholipids and proteins. The most abundant surface-active phospholipid in the mature lung is dipalmitoylphosphatidylcholine (DPPC), which decreases surface tension in the individual alveoli. The four major proteins in surfactant are SP-A, SP-B, SP-C, and SP-D. SP-B and SP-C optimize the rapid adsorption and spreading of phospholipids on a surface. SP-A facilitates phagocytosis and the clearance of pathogens from the air space by macrophages, and SP-D functions as an innate host defense molecule.

Antenatal steroid administration at least 24 to 48 hours prior to delivery in pregnant women between 23 and 34 weeks of gestation, who are at increased risk of preterm delivery, decreases the risk of RDS by accelerating lung maturation, as well as the production and secretion of surfactant.

BASIC SCIENCE/CLINICAL PEARL	STEP 1/2/3

The five stages of lung development during gestation are the embryonic, pseudoglandular, canalicular, saccular, and alveolar stages. Surfactant is synthesized in the type II alveolar cells.

Case Point 60.2

After doing a chart review, you find that the mother has had prenatal care, with normal prenatal ultrasounds and laboratory findings. She arrived to the hospital after her contractions began and was given glucocorticoids on admission. However, her labor continued to progress, and the infant was delivered by cesarean section due to breech presentation 2 hours after arriving at the hospital.

What risk factors in this infant predispose him to respiratory distress syndrome?
The two most important risk factors for this infant are preterm delivery at 31 weeks of gestation and delivery within 2 hours of the administration of antenatal steroids. Antenatal steroids are most efficacious if delivery is 24 hours after or within 7 days of glucocorticoid administration. Meconium and blood in the alveoli, proteinaceous edema, and inflammatory products due to pneumonia can inactivat e surfactant and reduce the effective surfactant pool size.

CLINICAL PEARL	STEP 2/3

Prematurity is defined as any infant born before 37 weeks and 0 days. It is further divided into extremely preterm (<28 weeks), very preterm (28–<32 weeks), moderate to late preterm (32–<37 weeks).

What tests or imaging are indicated?
Determining blood gas levels to evaluate ventilation and oxygenation can be helpful, as well as a CBC, C-reactive protein (CRP) level, and blood culture to evaluate for infection. A CXR is helpful in diagnosing RDS and other causes of respiratory distress, such a pneumothorax, pneumonia, masses, and other congenital anomalies. In RDS, the CXR demonstrates a diffuse, bilateral, reticular granular or ground glass appearance (Fig. 60.1) and air-filled bronchi superimposed on the relatively airless alveoli presenting as air bronchograms. GBS pneumonia may have a similar appearance on CXR as RDS, so it is appropriate to initiate antibiotic therapy in the newborn with RDS.

What are the strategies used in the treatment of respiratory distress syndrome?
When approaching management of RDS, it is helpful to differentiate treatment into risk- reducing and supportive care. Risk-reducing treatment includes preventing premature birth and completion of an antenatal steroid course between 24 hours and 7 days prior to delivery. After birth, the mainstay of treatment remains supportive care, with supplemental oxygen and/or assisted ventilation, as well as exogenous surfactant administration. Exogenous surfactant is usually administered via the INSURE technique—*in*tubate-*sur*factant-*e*xtubate. The neonate is intubated, surfactant

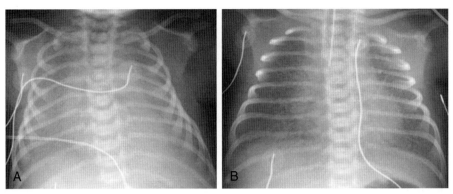

Fig. 60.1 Infant respiratory distress syndrome. (A) Initial chest radiograph in a premature newborn infant with respiratory distress shows hypoinflated lungs, with diffuse hazy granular opacities. (B) After intubation and surfactant administration, there is improved aeration of the lungs, but diffuse granular opacities persist. (Adapted from Chang PT, Sena L. Chest imaging. In: Walters M, Robertson R, eds. *Pediatric Radiology: The Requisites*. Philadelphia: Elsevier; 2017:6–61.)

is administered directly into the lungs via the endotracheal tube, and then the infant is extubated. Surfactant reduces the surface tension, thereby preventing alveolar collapse. Assisted ventilation provides positive pressure to maintain the airway and alveolar expansion through invasive or non-invasive support.

Case Point 60.3

His oxygen saturation increases to 95%, with an Fio_2 of 35% on a nasal cannula. After discussing with his mother, you perform an endotracheal intubation to deliver one dose of surfactant and promptly extubate to nasal CPAP with 21% Fio_2. He appears more comfortable and less tachypneic, and his O_2 saturation is 98%.

What types of ventilation strategies are useful in respiratory distress syndrome?
The goals of respiratory support are to prevent and reduce atelectasis. Nasal CPAP (nCPAP) is the preferred method to provide positive end-expiratory pressure (PEEP). The benefits of nCPAP include the reduction of laryngeal obstruction, improvement of oxygenation, establishment and maintenance of functional residual capacity (FRC), and release of surfactant stores. With nCPAP, there is also a reduction in barotrauma (trauma caused by pressure) and volutrauma (trauma caused by the amount of tidal volumes administered) and reduced risk of a secondary infection when compared to invasive ventilation. Nasal intermittent positive-pressure ventilation (NIPPV) may be a reasonable alternative to nCPAP. Preterm infants who fail CPAP may require invasive mechanical ventilation via an endotracheal tube.

Case Point 60.4

You update the mother with the progress of her son, and she asks you about complications associated with RDS.

What comorbid conditions and complications are seen with respiratory distress syndrome?
Most common acute complications of RDS are air leak syndromes. Air leaks are due to the rupture of an overdistended alveolus and may occur spontaneously or may be due to positive-pressure

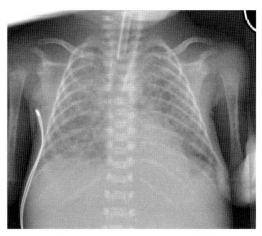

Fig. 60.2 Chest x-ray of newborn with bronchopulmonary dysplasia (BPD). Note the diffuse, coarse, interstitial opacities bilaterally. (Adapted from Rennie J, ed. *Rennie and Robertson's Textbook of Neonatology.* 5th ed. London: Churchill Livingstone/Elsevier; 2012:556.)

ventilation. The air from the ruptured alveoli dissects along the perivascular connective tissue sheath and in preterm infants, due to a loose perivascular space, may get trapped, resulting in pulmonary interstitial emphysema (PIE). A major chronic complication of RDS is bronchopulmonary dysplasia (BPD), defined clinically as the need for supplemental oxygen at 36 weeks' gestational age (Fig. 60.2). Many factors play a role in the cause of BPD—infection, inflammation, and oxygen toxicity, compounded by the structure of the premature lung, surfactant deficiency, and inadequate fluid clearance have all been implicated.

Case Summary

Complaint/History: A 3-hour-old, 31-week premature infant with tachypnea and respiratory distress.

Findings: The examination reveals hypoxia, increased work-of-breathing (subcostal retractions, nasal flaring, tachypnea), and tachycardia.

Labs/Tests: A CXR shows bilateral hypoinflated lungs, with diffuse granular opacities.

Diagnosis: Infant respiratory distress syndrome.

Treatment: Judicious oxygen supplementation, tracheal intubation, mechanical ventilation, and surfactant; after improvement with surfactant administration, the patient was extubated and placed on nasal CPAP with 21% Fio_2.

BEYOND THE PEARLS

- Systemic disorders causing respiratory distress, such as hypothermia, hypoglycemia, anemia, polycythemia, or metabolic acidosis, may be differentiated from RDS based on the history, physical findings, and appropriate laboratory evaluation.
- Other causes of respiratory distress include choanal atresia, tracheoesophageal fistulas, vocal cord paralysis, laryngeal or tracheal atresias, neck masses causing tracheal compression, and congenital diaphragmatic hernia. Congenital pulmonary adenomatous malformations (CPAMs) can cause pulmonary hypoplasia and lead to respiratory distress.
- Other organ systems can contribute to respiratory distress as well, including the musculoskeletal system (particularly chest wall abnormalities), cardiac system (acyanotic and cyanotic congenital heart defects), and neurologic system (birth trauma with spinal cord injury).

Bibliography

Carlo WA, Ambalavanan N. Respiratory distress syndrome (Hyaline Membrane Disease). In: Kliegman RM, Stanton BF, St Geme JW, Schor NF, eds. *Nelson Textbook of Pediatrics*. Philadelphia, PA: Elsevier; 2016:848–867.

Chang PT, Sena L. Chest imaging. In: Walters M, Robertson R, eds. *Pediatric Radiology: The Requisites*. Philadelphia: Elsevier; 2017:6–61.

Jobe A. Surfactant for respiratory distress syndrome. *NeoReviews*. 2014;15(6):e236–e245.

Reuter S, Moser C, Baack M. Respiratory distress in the newborn. *Pediatr Rev*. 2014;35(10):417–429.

Wambach JA, Hamvas A. Respiratory distress syndrome in the neonate. In: Martin R, Fanaroff A, Walsh M, eds. *Fanaroff and Martin's Neonatal-Perinatal Medicine*. Philadelphia: Elsevier; 2015:1074–1086.

Warren JB, Anderson JM. Core concepts: respiratory distress syndrome. *NeoReviews*. 2009;10(7):e351–e361.

INDEX

Note: Page numbers followed by "f" indicate figures and "t" indicate tables "b" indicate boxes.